INTERFERON THERAPY of MULTIPLE SCLEROSIS

INTERFERON THERAPY of MULTIPLE SCLEROSIS

edited by

ANTHONY T. REDER
University of Chicago
Chicago, Illinois

Library of Congress Cataloging-in-Publication Data

Interferon therapy of multiple sclerosis / edited by Anthony T. Reder.
    p.   cm.
    Includes index.
    ISBN 0-8247-9764-7 (hardcover : alk. paper)
    1. Multiple sclerosis—Immunotherapy. 2. Interferon—Therapeutic
use.   I. Reder, Anthony T.
    [DNLM: 1. Multiple Sclerosis—therapy. 2. Interferons–
–therapeutic use. 3. Interferons—pharmacology.   WL 360 I596 1997]
RC377.I553 1997
616.8′3406—dc21
DNLM/DLC
for Library of Congress
                           96-39953
                           CIP

The publisher offers discounts on this book when ordered in bulk quantities. For more information, write to Special Sales/Professional Marketing at the address below.

This book is printed on acid-free paper.

MARCEL DEKKER
270 Madison Avenue, New York, New York 10016

Current printing (last digit):
10 9 8 7 6 5 4 3

PRINTED IN THE UNITED STATES OF AMERICA

Preface

Multiple sclerosis (MS) affects 300,000 people in the United States and 1 million worldwide. It typically strikes an intelligent, educated woman just as her career and family life begin to flower.

Interferon-β (IFN-β) is the first and only FDA-approved therapy to change the course of MS. Its mechanism of action in MS is unknown. IFN-β has been approved for treatment of relapsing/remitting and relapsing/progressive MS, but this is only one part of a spectrum of demyelinating diseases. Arguably, "MS" includes monosymptomatic demyelination, optic neuritis, transverse myelitis, primary progressive MS, Devic's disease, postinfectious encephalomyelitis, and possibly Leber's optic atrophy, and adrenoleukodystrophy. Would interferons treat any or all of these?

Drug trials in MS are particularly difficult. Large numbers of patients must be studied over years—the time between exacerbations averages two years, and progression is typically slow (at least from the examiner's viewpoint). The Kurtzke disability rating scale is certainly nonlinear—the change from a Kurtzke rating of 4 to 5 is four times as fast as the change from 6 to 7. Experienced neurologists are required—disease symptoms encompass every function of the central nervous system, and attacks range from inconsequential to devastating. The natural history also changes over time—attack frequency declines, and relapsing disease becomes progressive. Finally, medical care and patient motivation and outlook affect the results; study patients taking a placebo drug do better than untreated patients.

The rationale for using IFNs to treat MS has evolved side by side with the most popular views of the cause of the disorder. In the early 1980s, IFN-α, IFN-β, and IFN-γ were all advanced as therapies for MS because of their antiviral effects, since many investigators hypothesized that MS was caused by a virus. Unfortunately, IFN-γ caused exacerbations, and the "virus" remains elusive. On the basis of relatively thin evidence, MS is now widely assumed to be caused by an immune reaction to brain antigens. All forms of IFN could alter this immune response, but do so in different directions. Regardless of their effects on immunity, the benefit from type I IFN therapy in MS does suggest that IFNs are somehow involved in the etiology of MS.

The type I IFN family contains four gene families (IFN-α, β, ω, and τ). In addition, there are multiple natural preparations and recombinant subtypes. IFNα-n3, IFNα-2a, and IFNα-2b are approved in the United States for various indications; IFNβ-1a and IFNβ-1b are approved for MS. The spectrum of indications for use of IFNs is even broader in Europe. Understanding IFN-receptor interactions, signaling, pharmacokinetics, and clinical effects should optimize treatment of MS and other diseases.

MS is the first inflammatory/autoimmune disease to be successfully treated with IFNs. Therapy with recombinant cytokines is in its infancy, yet much has been learned from our experience with IFNs. Although type I IFNs are not a cure for MS, they offer a building block. Interferons will potentially synergize with other treatments under study in MS, such as cytotoxic drugs/chemotherapy, glucocorticoids, cyclosporine, cAMP agonists, specific immunomodulators, anti-macrophage agents, copolymer-I, T-cell receptor/HLA/adhesion/costimulatory molecule blockade or elimination, oral tolerance to central nervous system antigens, and other cytokines or cytokine antagonists.

This book covers the role of interferons in the treatment of MS. It begins with the molecular biology of IFN binding to its receptors, the signal cascade within the cell, gene regulation, and the induction of IFN-stimulated genes. This is followed by a description of IFN pharmacokinetics. Next, response to IFNs is discussed at the cellular level in neurons, glia, and immune cells. Experimental allergic encephalomyelitis (EAE) is used as a model of MS for reviews of therapy with oral and systemic IFN-α, IFN-β, and IFN-γ, and the newly discovered IFN-τ. Finally, there are clinically oriented descriptions of the benefits and also the side effects of IFN-α, IFN β-1a, and IFN β-1b in MS, and the role of current and future magnetic resonance techniques for imaging MS lesions.

The target audience for this book is wide—basic scientists in biotechnology and academia, neurologists, other clinicians, and health care professionals who treat MS patients, and also pharmaceutical sales representatives, MS clinic personnel, and patient groups, such as MS Society chapters. Efforts were made to ensure clarity; each chapter was written in depth and should serve as reference source for its area.

Authors were selected because they are doing cutting-edge basic or clinical work in relevant areas. This was done to infuse each chapter with ideas from people actively investigating IFNs and MS rather than simply review the existing literature. The authors have analyzed the literature and have expanded on their own published and unpublished research. They have also addressed several common threads within their general topic. These include (1) comparisons of all forms of IFN, (2) the implications for treatment of MS, (3) synergy or interference with other agents, based on clinical experience or on basic/theoretical mechanisms, and (4) hypotheses on how IFNs prevent disease activity in MS. These ideas will suggest new and better ways to treat MS, and possibly lead us to the cause of the disease.

Anthony T. Reder

Contents

Contributors

Alfons Billiau, M.D., Ph.D. Professor of Microbiology and Immunology, Rega Institute, University of Leuven, Leuven, Belgium

Elana Brief, M.Sc. Department of Physics, The University of British Columbia, Vancouver, British Columbia, Canada

Staley A. Brod, M.D. Assistant Professor of Neurology, University of Texas Medical School at Houston, Houston Health Science Center, Houston, Texas

Richard Cirelli, M.D. Department of Microbiology and Immunology, University of Texas Medical Branch, Galveston, Texas

Stefan N. Constantinescu, M.D., Ph.D. Research Associate, Whitehead Institute for Biomedical Research, Cambridge, Massachusetts

Nachum Dafny, Ph.D. Professor of Neurobiology and Anatomy, University of Texas Medical School at Houston, Houston Health Science Center, Houston, Texas

Thomas Decker, Ph.D. Professor of Microbiology and Immunology, Vienna Biocenter, Institute of Microbiology and Genetics, Vienna, Austria

Luca Durelli, M.D. Associate Professor, Department of Neurosciences, Neurologic Clinic, University of Turin Medical School, Turin, Italy

James G. Files, Ph.D. Berlex Biosciences, Richmond, California

Diane S. Goldstein, Ph.D. Department of Psychiatry, The University of Chicago, Chicago, Illinois

Luigi M. E. Grimaldi, M.D. Head, Neuroimmunology Unit, DIBIT, Department of Neurology, San Raffaele Scientific Institute, Milan, Italy

Hubertine Heremans, Ph.D. Professor of Microbiology and Immunobiology, Rega Institute, University of Leuven, Leuven, Belgium

Robert M. Herndon, M.D. Department of Neurology, Jackson Veterans Administration Medical Center, Jackson, Mississippi

Kathleen B. Herne, M.D. Postdoctoral Fellow in Microbiology, University of Texas Medical Branch, Galveston, Texas

Jeremy C. Hobart, M.R.C.P. Welcome Fellow, Institute of Neurology, London, England

Howard M. Johnson, Ph.D. Graduate Research Professor, Microbiology and Cell Science, University of Florida, Gainesville, Florida

Lorne F. Kastrukoff, M.D. Associate Professor, Department of Medicine, The University of British Columbia, Vancouver, British Columbia, Canada

Robert L. Knobler, M.D., Ph.D. Professor, Department of Neurology, Jefferson Medical College, Philadelphia, Pennsylvania

Robert A. Koopmans, M.D., F.R.C.P.C. Department of Radiology, The University of British Columbia, Vancouver, British Columbia, Canada

David K. B. Li, M.D., F.R.C.P.C. Professor of Radiology, The University of British Columbia, Vancouver, British Columbia, Canada

Alex MacKay, Ph.D. Department of Physics, The University of British Columbia, Vancouver, British Columbia, Canada

Gianvito Martino, M.D. Research Assistant, Neuroimmunology Unit, DIBIT, Department of Neurology, San Raffaele Scientific Institute, Milan, Italy

Monica L. McCrary, M.D. Postdoctoral Research Fellow, Department of Microbiology, University of Texas Medical Branch, Galveston, Texas

Rachel M. McKenna, Ph.D. Director, Transplant Immunology Laboratory, and Associate Professor, Health Sciences Centre, Department of Medicine and Immunology, University of Manitoba, Winnipeg, Manitoba, Canada

Jeffrey W. Nelson, Ph.D. Berlex Biosciences, Richmond, California

Eirik Nestaas, Ph.D.   Berlex Biosciences, Richmond, California

Kjell Öberg, M.D., Ph.D.   Professor, Endocrine Oncology Unit, Department of Internal Medicine, University Hospital, Uppsala, Sweden

Joel J.-F. Oger, M.D., O.N.M., F.R.C.P.C.   Associate Professor, Division of Neurology, The University of British Columbia, Vancouver, British Columbia, Canada

Donald W. Paty, M.D.   Head, Division of Neurology, The University of British Columbia, Vancouver, British Columbia, Canada

Lawrence M. Pfeffer, Ph.D.   Professor and Director of Graduate Studies, Department of Pathology, University of Tennessee Health Science Center, Memphis, Tennessee

Neil H. Pliskin, Ph.D.   Director of Neuropsychology, Department of Psychiatry, The Brain Research Institute, The University of Chicago, Chicago, Illinois

Carol H. Pontzer, Ph.D.   Assistant Professor of Microbiology, University of Maryland, College Park, Maryland

Bertha Prieto-Gomez, Ph.D.   Professor of Physiology, Universidad Nacional Autónoma de México, Del Cayoacan, Mexico

Erno Pungor, Jr., M.D.   Berlex Biosciences, Richmond, California

Anthony T. Reder, M.D.   Associate Professor, Departments of Psychiatry and Neurology, The Brain Research Institute, The University of Chicago, Chicago, Illinois

Cruz Reyes-Vazquez, M.D., Ph.D.   Professor of Physiology, Universidad Nacional Autónoma de México, Del Cayoacan, Mexico

Peter Rieckmann, M.D.   Department of Neurology, University of Würzburg, Würzburg, Germany

Joel Schiffenbauer, M.D.   Associate Professor, College of Medicine, University of Florida, Gainesville, Florida

Jeanne M. Soos, Ph.D.   Center for Neurologic Diseases, Brigham and Women's Hospital, Boston, Massachusetts

Alan J. Thompson, M.D.   Senior Lecturer, Institute of Neurology, London, England

Stephen K. Tyring, M.D., Ph.D.   Professor of Microbiology/Immunology, Dermatology and Internal Medicine, University of Texas Medical Branch, Galveston, Texas

Timothy Vartanian, M.D., Ph.D.   Assistant Professor of Neurology, Harvard Medical School, Boston, Massachusetts

Irene Vavasour, M.Sc.   Department of Physics, The University of British Columbia, Vancouver, British Columbia, Canada

Ken Whittall, Ph.D.   Department of Physics, The University of British Columbia, Vancouver, British Columbia, Canada

Patricia L. Witt, Ph.D.   Associate Professor of Preventive Medicine, Medical College of Wisconsin, Milwaukee, Wisconsin

Guo Jun Zhao, M.D., Ph.D.   Department of Radiology, The University of British Columbia, Vancouver, British Columbia, Canada

The Molecular Biology of Interferon-β from Receptor Binding to Transmembrane Signaling

Lawrence M. Pfeffer

University of Tennessee Health Science Center, Memphis, Tennessee

Stefan N. Constantinescu

Whitehead Institute for Biomedical Research, Cambridge, Massachusetts

I. INTRODUCTION

Interferons (IFNs), which were independently discovered by two groups in the 1950s (1,2), are proteins capable of interfering with the viral infection of cells. Their discovery culminated many years of study on the basis for viral interference. Besides antiviral activity, the diverse biological actions of these cytokines also include inhibition of the proliferation of normal and transformed cells, regulation of differentiation, host responses to various pathogens, and modulation of the immune system (including activation of natural killer cells and macrophages). The human type I IFNs include 15 IFN-α subtypes, one IFN-β subtype, and two IFN-ω subtypes. Type I IFNs are acid stable, have similar protein structure and biological activities, bind and transduce signals through a common multiprotein cell surface receptor, are induced in response to viral and other inducers, and share a common gene locus on human chromosome 9. In contrast, type II IFN (or IFN-γ) is acid-labile and differs from type I IFNs in many of the above respects except that it shares similar biological actions. However, there are differences in biological potency of type I and type II IFNs. For example, type II IFN is considered more active in immunomodulation than type I IFN. In addition, the biological specific activities for the different type I IFN subtypes can vary by as much as three orders of magnitude on a $\log_{10}$ scale.

Several lines of evidence suggest that some of IFN's biological activities, such as the augmentation of natural killer cell activity, antiproliferative, and antiviral activities, can be elicited through different molecular pathways. IFNs elicit their effects by first binding to specific multiprotein receptors on the surface of target cells and then transducing a signal to the nucleus that results in selective gene expression (3–6). A family of early genes, the IFN-stimulated genes (ISGs), is transcriptionally activated within minutes by type I IFN. ISG transcriptional activation is mediated by the protein tyrosine kinase (PTK)–dependent phosphorylation of latent cytoplasmic transcriptional activators, termed the STAT proteins (for Signal Transducers and Activators of Transcription) (7,8). Type I IFNs activate STAT113 (M_r 113,000) and STAT91 (M_r 91,000), which then bind to the p48-DNA binding protein, forming the ISGF3 complex. This complex then moves into the nucleus and recognizes the highly conserved IFN stimulus–response element (ISRE) promoter element in ISGs directly to activate these genes (9,10). Immunologically related STAT proteins apparently function in the gene-activation pathway induced by other cytokines (11,12). Central to the IFN-α–activated PTK pathway are two Janus (JAK) PTKs, JAK1 and TYK2 (13,14), which apparently mediate the tyrosine phosphorylation of STATs, as well as other type I IFN receptor subunits (13–15).

Recent studies reveal that many cytokine receptors (including those for IFNs, erythropoietin [EPO], growth hormone [GH], colony-stimulating factors [CSFs], interleukins [ILs]) can associate with and activate members of the JAK family of cytoplasmic PTKs (13–15). These kinases are rapidly phosphorylated after receptor activation and share the unusual feature of having two kinase domains. EPO, GH, and IL-3 activate only JAK2. The ciliary neurotrophic factor (CNTF)/oncostatin M (OSM)/leukemia inhibitory factor (LIF)/IL-6 family of cytokines can activate JAK1, JAK2, and TYK2 in a cell type–dependent manner. IFN-γ responses involve JAK1 and JAK2, whereas IFN-α requires JAK1 and TYK2. Thus, both type I and type II IFNs activate JAK1 and the tyrosine phosphorylation of STAT91, whereas type I IFNs selectively activate TYK2 and the phosphorylation of STAT113. Furthermore, although both STAT proteins are involved in ISG activation, STAT113 and STAT91 are phosphorylated independently of one another (16). These data suggest that JAK1 is responsible for the phosphorylation of STAT91, whereas TYK2 is responsible for STAT113 phosphorylation. The JAK kinases appear to be the most proximal kinases activated in response to ligand, playing a critical and common role in mediating responses to all of these disparate but distantly related cytokines. A major question that arises from these findings is where is the specificity of cytokine signaling maintained if different cytokines with divergent biological effects all work through the JAK kinases. One possibility is that each member of the JAK family may have discrete substrate specificity. However, it is more plausible that specificity is dictated by the specific association of substrates with receptor subunits.

The role of the JAK/STAT pathway in ISG activation is described in detail in Chapter 2. The type I IFN–activated JAK/STAT pathway serves as a paradigm for cytokine signal transduction in general. IFNs are highly effective molecules; the occupancy of only a few receptors per cell triggers a biological response in IFN-responsive cells. Besides the activation of JAK PTKs, the type I IFNs also rapidly activate Ca^{2+}-independent protein kinase C (PKC) subspecies through the production of the lipid second-messenger DAG (17). Both PTK and serine/threonine kinases are involved in the regulation of IFN-α/β–induced ISG mRNA levels and in the establishment of antiviral activity in various human cells (17–20). It is unknown how these varied biological signals are integrated at the level of the type I IFN receptor (IFN$_I$R).

This chapter describes the molecular basis of IFN-β action with a focus on the roles of IFN$_I$R subunits at the levels of receptor structure and the components of the signaling pathway rapidly activated on ligand-receptor interaction. Since human IFNs (huIFNs) are clinically useful in the treatment of various human diseases (multiple sclerosis, hairy cell leukemia, laryngeal and genital papillomas, acquired immunodeficiency syndrome (AIDS), Kaposi's sarcoma, and chronic viral hepatitis), it is essential to understand how IFNs interact with cells. Knowledge of these interactions should expedite the therapeutic use of huIFN-β and provide a basis for developing new strategies in the treatment of multiple sclerosis (MS) with IFN-β alone or in combination with other agents.

II. DIFFERENCES IN BIOLOGICAL EFFECTS BETWEEN IFN-α AND IFN-β

Type I IFNs share a common ligand binding site and induce common biological effects. However, the intrinsic properties of all type I IFNs are not identical. For the purpose of this chapter we assume that all type I IFNs act on the IFN$_I$R in a similar manner, but we will emphasize any IFN-β–specific events that have been identified. For example, we and others have recently identified the tyrosine phosphorylation of a IFN$_I$R-associated protein that is induced by IFN-β but not by IFN-α2 or IFN-α8 (21–23). In addition, IFN-β may exert type I IFN actions at specific sites after autocrine secretion, and thus these effects may also be considered as IFN-β specific.

IFN-α and IFN-β differ markedly in their cell type–specific antiproliferative actions. IFN-β exerts greater antiproliferative activity on many cell types, such as embryonal carcinomas, melanomas, and melanocytes (24,25). IFN-β has been reported to bind with higher affinity to the common IFN-α/β binding sites and to stimulate peripheral blood stem cells of patients with hairy cell leukemia to differentiate into erythroid burst-forming cells (26). IFN-β, but not IFN-α, inhibits the growth of vascular smooth muscle cells (27). Autocrine secretion of IFN-β seems to be the physiological mechanism by which proliferative signals induced by prostaglandin F (PDGF), IL-1, or TNF-α are muted in vascular smooth muscle cells (27). IFN-β can block human immunodeficiency virus (HIV) infection at a step prior to the reverse transcription of viral RNA (28). This is important, since HIV develops a tat-dependent mechanism to overcome the type I IFN–induced restriction of HIV replication (29). IFN-β increases steroid receptor expression in breast cancer cells (30), and it has promising antiproliferative effects on prostate cancer cell lines (31). Taken together, these data show that IFN-β may be active in the treatment of cancers which are resistant to the antiproliferative effects of natural IFN-α. Furthermore, IFN-β induces IFN-α production in mice after systemic administration or in transgenic mice carrying an IFN-β gene under control of a metallothionen–enhancer/promoter, whereas IFN-α does not induce IFN-β (32).

Recently, in several large clinical trials, IFN-β was found to lower the frequency of relapses and improve the symptoms of relapsing-remitting multiple sclerosis (MS) (33–37). In contrast, IFN-γ exacerbated MS symptoms, and in some studies IFN-α was detrimental (38) (see Chapters 11–14). MS is an inflammatory demyelinating disease of the central nervous system which is clinically characterized by relapses and remissions and leads to chronic disability. The pathology of the disease has an autoimmune element, with a proposed defect in the suppressor T-cell subset. Importantly, mice that had an inactivated gene for IRF-1 (an ISG) showed abnormalities in the development of CD8 (T suppressor cells), which are implicated in the pathology of MS (39). Interestingly, early studies indicate a selective inhibition by IFN-β of the generation in vitro of T suppressor cells (40). The molecular basis for any differential effects of IFN-α versus β in MS is unknown.

Furthermore, IFN-α–resistant cell mutants remain partially sensitive to IFN-β activation of the JAK/STAT pathway and gene induction (14,41). Although both IFN-α and IFN-β induce the rapid tyrosine phosphorylation of IFN₁R subunits, a unique 105-kDa band is tyrosine phosphorylated only in response to IFN-β but not to several IFN-α subtypes (21–23).

III. TYPE I IFN RECEPTOR

A. Characterization

The four major antigenic types of IFNs (α, β, γ, and ω) are defined by the cellular source of their production. Type I IFNs (IFN α, β, and ω) compete with each other for cellular binding to IFN$_I$R and thus share at least some components of a common multisubunit cell surface IFN$_I$R, whereas the receptor for type II IFN (IFN-γ) is a distinct entity (42). Nearly all human cell lines and human tissues display the IFN$_I$R, varying in number from 500 to 20,000 high-affinity ($k_d \simeq 50$ pM) and 2000 to 100,000 low-affinity ($K_d \approx 1-10$ nM) receptors/cell. Chemical cross linking of iodinated IFN-α to human tumor cells has demonstrated that the IFN$_I$R apparently is composed of 100-, 110-, and 135-kDa glycoprotein subunits (21,43–45). The interaction of IFN with its cognate receptor is species specific, so that human cells respond preferentially to human type I IFNs over mouse IFNs. This suggests that a subunit (or subunits) of the hu-IFN$_I$R is responsible for the species-specific interaction. Studies with monoclonal antibodies (MoAbs) directed against huIFN$_I$R components suggest the existence of accessory proteins that may modulate the specificity of binding and signal transduction by the IFN$_I$R (46,47). Furthermore, structure-function analysis of type I IFN subtypes identifies regions required for IFN binding, as well as those involved solely in signal transduction (48), providing further evidence for the complexity of the IFN$_I$R structure.

Somatic cell genetics have established that both binding and transducing chains of IFN$_I$R map to human chromosome 21 (Ch21). Antisera generated to Ch21-encoded proteins block the biological activity of type I IFNs but not of type II IFN (49,50). Furthermore, the biological effect induced by type I IFNs in cells and the number of receptor subunits directly correlates with the copy number of Ch21 (51,52). In addition, MoAbs generated to IFN$_I$R components react with Ch21-encoded proteins (53,54). Furthermore, a gene on Ch21 in the region from q22.2 to q22.3 encodes a novel subunit of the IFN$_I$R required for type I IFN signaling (55). Although the binding subunit of the type II IFN receptor maps to human chromosome 6, accessory factors involved in type II IFN signal transduction also map to Ch21 (56,57).

The nomenclature used for the components of the type I IFN receptor (IFN$_I$R) is inconsistent and confusing, as shown in Table 1. The cDNAs coding for two IFN$_I$R chains have recently been cloned and named the IFNAR and IFNABR subunits by the groups that isolated the cDNAs (58,59). In addition, MoAbs have been generated against cells expressing

Table 1 Terms Used to Describe IFN$_I$R Subunits (Defined by Migration of Proteins from the Daudi Lymphoblastoid Cell Line)

New name	M_r (kDa)	Cross-linked complex (kDa)	cDNA Designation	Subunit by MoAb
IFN$_I$R-1	135[a]	150	IFNAR	α?
IFN$_I$R-2	100[b]	120	IFNABR	β
IFN$_I$R-3	110	130	Not cloned	α?

[a] Migration depends markedly on cell line examined, generally between 115 and 135 kDa.
[b] Present in U937 cell line as a 50-kDa protein. Thus it may exist as homodimers or heterodimers of $\approx$50-kDa subunits.

IFN$_I$R and identified by the ability either to precipitate IFN-α (or IFN-β) cross linked to cell surface IFN$_I$R, or block ligand binding to IFN$_I$R. The components of IFN$_I$R recognized by these MoAbs were termed the α and β subunits, respectively. In this chapter we have designated IFNAR as IFN$_I$R-1, and IFNABR as IFN$_I$R-2 on the basis of the order in which they were identified. It thus follows that the subunits of the type II IFN receptor should be called IFN$_{II}$R-1, 2, and so forth in the order of their discovery. In the following sections, we attempt to relate these subunits to findings made on the α and β subunits. We consider this as the appropriate nomenclature, because at the present time, the biological role of each individual huIFN$_I$R subunit in ligand binding and signal transduction has not been completely elucidated. Furthermore, our data suggest that a third component of the IFN$_I$R also exists, but the roles of these subunits alone or in concert have not been elucidated.

Partial purification and characterization of a ligand binding subunit of the IFN$_I$R from lymphoblastoid cell membranes has been achieved using a combination of wheat germ lectin and IFN-affinity techniques (60–62). The ligand binding subunit appears to be a highly asymmetrical membrane protein with a Stokes radius of $\approx$74 Å and a M_r of $\approx$110 kDa. These studies also provided evidence that the protein contains a sialic acid oligosaccharide moiety, a finding confirmed in affinity cross-linking studies (43). Using IFN-affinity chromatography, we have partially purified a ligand binding protein (IFN$_I$R-3) of similar M_r, which apparently is distinct from the two cloned chains of the IFN$_I$R (45).

B. Multisubunit Structure of IFN$_I$R

1. Affinity Cross Linking

Several lines of evidence indicate that the huIFN$_I$R binds the multiple type I IFNs (IFN-α subtypes, IFN-β, and IFN-ω) and consists of several subunits (43). Affinity cross linking of ^{125}I–IFN-α2 to cells with the homobifunctional reagents such as disuccinimidyl suberate DSS result in formation of a broad IFN receptor complex of 120–150 kDa on a variety of human cells (60,63). The specificity of complex formation has been confirmed by its precipitation with anti-IFN sera and by competition with excess unlabeled IFN-α2. The glycoprotein nature of the IFN$_I$R was demonstrated by the sensitivity of complex formation to the pretreatment of cells with trypsin and neuraminidase. In recent studies on the structure of the IFN$_I$R in various human tumor cell lines, the broad 120–150-kDa IFN-α receptor complex has been resolved into 100-, 110-, and 130-kDa glycoproteins (120-, 130-, and 150-kDa affinity cross-linked complexes, respectively), as illustrated in Figure 1 (43). Treatment of affinity cross-linked material with glycosidases demonstrates the glycoprotein nature of all IFN$_I$R subunits detected (43). In addition, numerous affinity cross-linking studies also identify high molecular weight IFN-α receptor complexes that reflect an association of receptor subunits, as illustrated by the ≈240-kDa complex in Figure 1. Affinity cross-linking studies with ^{125}I–IFN-β reveal IFN receptor complexes with similar electrophoretic mobility to those formed with IFN-α (62,64).

Partial solubilization of IFN-α receptor complexes with the nonionic detergents, digitonin or CHAPS, resolves a complex on high-performance chromatography with a relative size of ≈600 kDa. In addition, solubilization of cells or cell membranes with CHAPS yields a similar sized complex that is capable of binding type I IFN, with an IFN binding site–containing component of ≈95 kDa (65). However, we have found that CHAPS solubilizes only a low-affinity binding component of the IFN$_I$R. Use of the heterobifunctional Denny-Jaffe reagent to identify direct IFN receptor interaction reveals that a 110-kDa protein is selectively cross linked to IFN (66). The summary of results obtained by affinity cross-linking and gel chromatography shows that the IFN$_I$R is a multisubunit complex.

2. Anti-IFN$_I$R MoAbs Define Receptor Structure

Recent studies to define the exact structure of the IFN$_I$R have been aided by the generation of MoAbs against various receptor components. Two different strategies have been used successfully: (1) mice were injected with human cells that express high levels of IFN-α binding sites, and

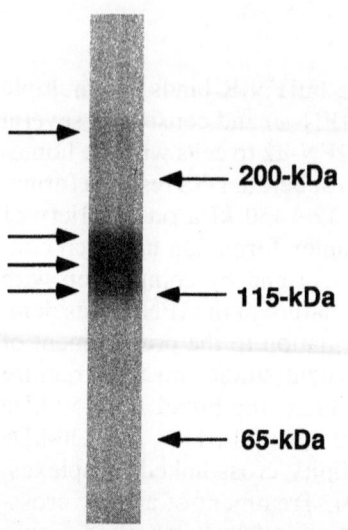

→ ← **200-kDa**

→
→
→ ← **115-kDa**

← **65-kDa**

Figure 1   Affinity cross linking of type I IFN receptors on Daudi lymphoblastoid cells. After incubation of cells with iodinated IFNCon1, IFN was cross linked to the cell surface with disuccinimidyl suberate. Proteins were analyzed by SDS-PAGE and autoradiographed. Molecular weight markers are indicated on the right of the figure and the arrows point to cross-linked complexes. The M_r of the receptor chains is calculated by subtracting the M_r of IFNCon1 (20 kDa) from that of the cross-linked complex.

hybridomas generated from the responding B cells were screened for the ability to block IFN-α binding or to immunoprecipitate affinity cross-linked material (53,54); or (2) mice were injected with baculovirus-expressed ectodomain of IFN$_I$R-1, and hybridomas were screened for the ability to detect IFN$_I$R-1 cell surface expression by flow cytometry (21,67,68). Using the first strategy, MoAbs that detect the so-called α and β subunits of the IFN$_I$R-1 were generated (53,54). Anti-α subunit MoAbs precipitate a 110-kDa protein from surface iodinated material, and a broad 130- to 150-kDa complex and $\approx$240-kDa complex from affinity cross-linked material. These MoAbs fail to precipitate the $\approx$100-kDa IFN$_I$R subunit detected as the 120-kDa affinity cross-linked complex shown in Figure 1. The high molecular weight complex ($\approx$240 kDa) presumably consists of the α subunit in association with another receptor subunit. Interestingly, the three individual anti-α subunit MoAbs were directed to one epitope, suggesting that this epitope is highly immunogenic. These results suggested that the α subunit was a 110-kDa protein, and distinct from the IFN$_I$R-1. Anti-β subunit MoAb blocks the binding and biological effects of several type I IFNs, including IFN-α2, IFN-α8, IFN-β, and IFN-ω. The β subunit detected by immunological techniques appears to correspond to a 100-kDa protein that is distinct from IFN$_I$R-1. In human U937 cells, another receptor form is expressed, consisting of a 55-kDa subunit, and the 100-kDa band is subsequently lost (69). The 55-kDa subunit may result from truncation or incomplete processing of the 100-kDa subunit.

We next studied the expression and signaling of huIFN$_I$R-1 with MoAbs generated to the baculovirus-expressed ectodomain of IFN$_I$R-1 (21). Immunoprecipitation and immunoblotting with MoAb of lysates from a variety of human cell lines showed that IFN$_I$R-1 has an apparent M_r which varies from 115 to 135 kDa depending on the cell line examined (see Table 1). Binding analysis with ^{125}I-labeled anti–IFN$_I$R-1 MoAb demonstrated high levels of cell surface expression of huIFN$_I$R-1 in human cells and in mouse cells transfected with IFN$_I$R-1 cDNA, whereas no cross reactivity was observed in control mouse L929 cells expressing only the endogenous mouse receptor. The subunit was rapidly downregulated by IFN-α (80% decrease within 2 hr) and degraded on internalization. The IFN$_I$R-1 chain appeared to be constitutively associated with a 110-kDa subunit of the IFN-α/β receptor, since the MoAbs coprecipitated this protein from surface-iodinated material. In a recent report using the anti-α subunit MoAb, it was suggested that IFN$_I$R-1 and the α-subunit may represent the same protein (70). However, since the α-subunit MoAb does not work in Western blots and has been reported not to detect baculovirus-expressed IFN$_I$R-1, the identification of the α-subunit as IFN$_I$R-1 must be viewed with caution.

To further characterize the huIFN$_I$R, in collaboration with Dr. Robert Schreiber of Washington University (St. Louis, MO) we generated polyclonal antibodies to subunits of the IFN$_I$R by injecting irradiated WA17 cells into syngeneic mice. WA17 cells are a mouse L-cell subline that contain three copies of human Ch21, which codes for the binding and signaling subunits of the IFN receptor. WA17 cells express ≈2500 binding sites for huIFN-α ($k_d \approx$ 50 pM), whereas the parental L-cell line expresses ≈75 binding sites for huIFN-α. The screening procedure for these MoAbs involved testing for the ability to (1) inhibit antiviral activity of IFN-α, immunoprecipitate IFN-α–cross-linked material; and (2) inhibit type I IFN binding. We generated a polyclonal serum (denoted IFNBaR) that not only completely blocks IFN-α binding to human cells but also precipitates a 110-kDa surface protein (possibly IFN$_I$R-3) that can be downregulated by type I IFN. The 110-kDa surface protein corresponds to the

130-kDa band detected by chemically cross linking IFN to cell surface receptors, and it is presumably the α subunit. This serum also coprecipitates the 95-kDa protein coded by the *vav*–proto-oncogene in lymphoblastoid cells. Vav is rapidly (within 2 min) tyrosine phosphorylated after IFN-α addition, and it becomes associated with the IFN_IR only after IFN-α treatment of cells. Its phosphorylation is blocked by the PTK inhibitor genistein. In addition, anti–α subunit MoAb also coprecipitates tyrosine-phosphorylated vav, suggesting that vav and the α subunit are closely linked (71).

Recently, a soluble 40-kDa huIFN-α/β binding protein (p40), which blocks the binding and the induction of antiviral activity of several type I IFNs, was purified from urine (59). Polyclonal sera raised to p40 immunoprecipitates a 100-kDa subunit detected in affinity cross-linking studies as a 120-kDa complex, which is sensitive to high concentrations of reductants. This serum also coprecipitates the IFN-activated JAK1 kinase. The cDNA of this second chain of the $huIFN_IR$ (IFN_IR-2) has been cloned and found to encode an $\approx$45-kDa conceptual translation product. Preliminary studies indicate that IFN_IR-2 binds IFN-α/β when expressed as a soluble ectodomain protein (p40), but the binding characteristics of the full-length transmembrane protein have not been clearly elucidated. Thus, whether the IFN_IR-2 chain alone binds IFN-α with high affinity or is a component of the high-affinity $huIFN_IR$ complex remains unexplored. In addition, the 100-kDa IFN_IR-2 subunit (denoted the β subunit in some studies) undergoes ligand-dependent tyrosine phosphorylation (22). In summary, of the three $huIFN_IR$ subunits detected by affinity cross linking, only the putative 110-kDa subunit (IFN_IR-3) has not yet been purified or its cDNA cloned.

C. IFN_IR Subunits as Members of the Cytokine Receptor Superfamily

Cytokine receptors have been classified into two groups on the basis of their structural similarity in their extracellular domains (72,73). The class I cytokine family includes receptors for growth hormone, prolactin, EPO, IL-2, IL-3, IL-4, IL-6, IL-7, granulocyte CSF, and granulocyte-macrophage CSF (GM-CSF). Members of this family are typified by a conserved tryptophan, N- and C-terminal cysteine pairs, and a membrane-proximal WS $\times$ WS box. The IFN_IR-1 and IFN_IR-2 chains, the receptor subunits responsible for binding and/or transducing the effects of IFN-γ, and the IL-10 receptor, constitute the class II cytokine receptor family, based on a characteristic 200–amino acid (AA) extracellular domain, termed D200 (72,73). Cytokine receptors form either homo- or heterodimeric structures

(74). Members of this family in general have a ligand binding α chain with either low or high affinity and at least one β chain involved in signal transduction, which has either relatively low binding affinity for the cytokine or no detectable binding activity at all. The IL-2 receptor is composed of at least three distinct polypeptides, whereas the receptors for IL-3, IL-5, and GM-CSF are heterodimeric, sharing a common β chain and having distinct α chains. Receptor activation by this family of cytokines requires interaction between receptor subunits. For example, activation of the family of receptors for IL-6/CNTF/OSM/LIF apparently requires the homodimerization of the gp130 signal transducing subunit or gp130 heterodimerization with the β subunit of the LIF receptor (75). Thus, one possibility is that huIFN$_I$R chains also homodimerize or form heterodimers. Studies in mouse or hamster cells expressing either the huIFN$_I$R-1 chain, a segment of Ch21 containing the IFN$_I$R-1 gene, or in cells in which the IFN$_I$R-1 chain is inactivated by genetic means have established that the IFN$_I$R-1 is not primarily responsible for IFN-α/β binding (21,68,76–78). Our working hypothesis is that the IFN$_I$R-1 chain functions as a β signal-transducing chain of the IFN$_I$R, whereas the IFN$_I$R-2 chain represents an α ligand binding chain.

An important general characteristic of these cytokine receptors is that they have no inherent enzyme activity but bind and generate cytoplasmic signals in combination with an additional molecular component(s). As illustrated in Figure 2, the extracellular region of the IFN$_I$R-1 chain consists of two repeated D200 domains. Each D200 has two conserved cysteines separated by seven AAs in the amino-terminal (SD100A) and two conserved cysteines separated by 20–22 AAs in the carboxyl-terminal (SD100B). In addition, two important conserved motifs, shown in Figure 3, are present within the intracellular domain of the IFN$_I$R-1 signal-transducing chain: (1) a membrane-proximal 50-AA block, which is also present in the IFN$_{II}$R-2 chain and the CRF2-4 orphan cytokine receptor chain (79); and (2) a tyrosine-activation motif of two tyrosines separated by 10 AAs (21), which is also present in signaling subunits of the T-cell and B-cell receptors (80,81).

D. IFN Downregulates IFN$_I$R Ligand Binding Sites

Several human tumor cell-lines have been compared for sensitivity to the antiproliferative action of type I IFN and the downregulation of huIFN$_I$R binding sites (82). IFN-sensitive and IFN-resistant cell lines have similar numbers (1000 to 4000 receptors per cell) of high-affinity (k_d ~20–75 pM) IFN$_I$R. In variant IFN-resistant Daudi cells and an IFN-resistant renal cancer (RC) cell line there is a one-to-one relationship between occupancy

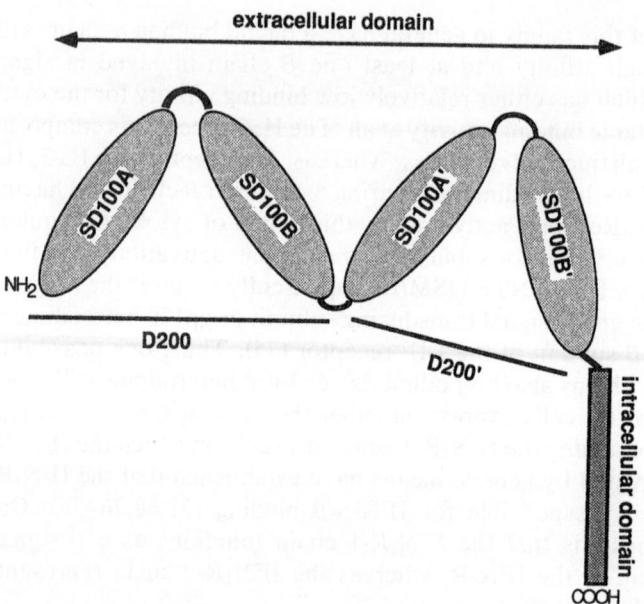

Figure 2 Schematic representation of the domain and subdomain structure of the IFN$_I$R-1 chain.

and IFN$_I$R downregulation. On removal from the cell surface, IFN binding sites are degraded inside the cell and do not recycle to the cell surface. In contrast, in IFN-sensitive Daudi cells and a highly IFN-sensitive RC cell line, at low IFN$_I$R occupancy (5%) there is high IFN$_I$R downregulation (60–80%). The results suggest that when type I IFN binds to fully functional receptors, it triggers cooperative interactions between IFN$_I$Rs leading to enhanced IFN$_I$R downregulation in sensitive cells; these interactions apparently do not occur in IFN-resistant cells. Furthermore, the association of the type I IFN-IFN$_I$R complex with cytoskeletal components prior to their internalization appears to be closely linked to cellular

KVFL<u>RCINYVFFPSLKPSSSIDEYFSEQPLKNLLLSTSEEQIEKCFIIENISTI</u> 54
ATVEETNQTDDHKKK<u><u>YSSQTSQDSGNYSNE</u></u>DESESKTSEELQQDFV 100

Figure 3 The 100–amino acid intracellular domain of the human IFN$_I$R chain. Tyrosine residues within conserved blocks are shown in boldface. The 50–amino acid membrane proximal conserved block is single underlined, and the 16–amino acid conserved serine-rich tyrosine activation motif is double underlined.

sensitivity to IFN action (83). For example, in IFN-resistant Daudi cells, the IFN-IFN$_I$R complex fails to associate with the cytoskeleton, and there is diminished internalization and receptor downregulation. These results are of special significance, since clinical responsiveness to IFN appears to correlate with the degree of IFN$_I$R downregulation (84). In addition, we found that downregulation of IFN-α binding sites is triggered by IFN-α covalently coupled to beads, which suggests that downregulation is independent of IFN internalization. The IFN$_I$R does not recycle to an appreciable extent, and thus after downregulation, the return of the IFN$_I$R to the cell surface requires both RNA and protein synthesis (85).

IV. CHARACTERIZATION OF BIOLOGICAL ACTIVITIES OF THE IFN$_I$R-1 AND IFN$_I$R-2 CHAINS

A. Transfection of the huIFN$_I$R-1 Chain into IFN-Nonresponsive Human or Mouse Cells Confers Sensitivity to the Antiviral Action to huIFN

The cDNA for the huIFN$_I$R-1 chain was originally isolated by detecting its ability to confer antiviral sensitivity to huIFN-α8 on mouse hepatoma cells (58). However, IFN$_I$R-1 was first described as the subunit responsible for binding and transducing the antiviral signal for IFN-α8 but not for IFN-α2 or IFN-β. This finding led to investigations on whether IFN$_I$R-1 chain bound several type I IFNs but only transduced the signal for IFN-α8, or whether IFN$_I$R-1 selectively bound and transduced the signal for only IFN-α8. However, the "ligand binding" conferred by huIFN$_I$R-1 chain was measured at 37°C by total cell-associated radioactivity. Steady-state binding measurements represent an equilibrium between ligand binding, dissociation, and internalization. Receptor-mediated internalization represents a large fraction of cell-associated radioactivity at 37°C (83). To minimize the contribution of ligand internalization to cell-associated radioactivity, ligand binding is routinely measured at 4 or 14°C. Using these conditions, we and others have shown that the huIFN$_I$R-1 chain does not confer high-affinity IFN binding when expressed in mouse, hamster, or monkey cells (21,68,76,77). The failure to bind IFN is not due to low levels of IFN$_I$R-1 expression, since these transfectants express abnormally high levels of the huIFN$_I$R-1 chain (21).

cDNAs encoding the human, mouse, and bovine homologues for the IFN$_I$R-1 chain have been cloned (58,86,87). Transfection of the huIFN$_I$R-1 chain into IFN-α–nonresponsive mouse or human cells produces antiviral sensitivity to several IFN-α subspecies (IFN-α2, IFN-α8, and IFN-Con1) without increasing cellular binding of any of these IFN-α subspecies in these cells (76). However, when we expressed the huIFN$_I$R-1 chain in huIFN-α–nonresponsive mouse NIH3T3 cells, it conferred low-affinity huIFN-α binding (68). Using MoAbs directed against the extracellular domain of the huIFN$_I$R-1 chain, we found that it represents a 115- to 135-kDa subunit of the IFN$_I$R, which undergoes rapid ligand-dependent tyrosine phosphorylation and acts as a species-specific transducer for gene induction by huIFN-α (21,76). These results clearly demonstrate that the IFN$_I$R-1 chain plays a crucial role in signal transduction through the IFN$_I$R.

To further characterize the function of this subunit, the full-length cDNA was transfected into the IFN-resistant human K-562 cell line (76). The acute myelocytic leukemia K-562 cell line has a complete homozygous deletion of IFN-α/β genes (88), so it does not secrete type I IFNs on induction by various stimuli. Although K-562 cells bind all huIFN-α subtypes, they are unresponsive to the antiviral and antiproliferative actions of IFN-α. Expression of the IFN$_I$R-1 chain in K-562 cells confers sensitivity to the antiviral action of several huIFN-α subtypes (IFN-$\alpha2$, IFN-$\alpha8$, and IFNCon1), but it did not increase cellular binding of any of these huIFN-α subtypes (76). Human IFN-$\alpha2$ resulted in a 4 log reduction in vesicular stomatitis virus (VSV) titer in two independent K-562 cell clones expressing the IFN$_I$R-1 chain as compared with no effect on VSV titer in empty vector transfectants. Surprisingly, transfected K-562 cells were not sensitive to the antiproliferative action of IFN-α.

Heterologous mouse L929 cells are highly responsive to the antiproliferative and antiviral actions of mouse type I IFN. Untransfected mouse cells bind low levels of huIFN-α (≈75 sites/cell) but do not respond to huIFN-α by either antiviral protection or the inhibition of cell proliferation. Expression of huIFN$_I$R-1 in L929 cells results in high sensitivity to antiviral protection by type I human IFN without affecting sensitivity to mouse IFN-α/β (76). Human IFNCon1 induced a 6500-fold reduction in VSV titer in two independent mouse L929 cells transfectants expressing the IFN$_I$R-1 chain as compared with a 50-fold reduction in viral titer in cells transfected with empty vector. Furthermore, 3000-fold less IFN-$\alpha8$ and 250-fold less IFNCon1 (and IFN-$\alpha2$) was required to result in 50% protection from the cytopathic effect of VSV in cells expressing the IFN$_I$R-1 chain when compared with empty vector transfectants. As originally reported (58), mouse IFN$_I$R-1 transfectants respond somewhat selectively to huIFN-$\alpha8$. Thus, a biological effect (reconstitution of antiviral sensitivity to type I IFNs) was obtained by transfecting the IFN$_I$R-1 chain into human and mouse cells, and its expression could be detected with anti–IFN$_I$R-1 MoAb (21).

B. huIFN$_I$R-1 Subunit of the huIFN$_I$R Undergoes Ligand-Dependent Phosphorylation

We also studied the signaling of huIFN$_I$R-1 with MoAbs generated to the baculovirus-expressed ectodomain of IFN$_I$R-1 (21). IFN-α/β treatment induced tyrosine phosphorylation of IFN$_I$R-1 within 1 min, with kinetics paralleling that of the IFN-activated protein tyrosine kinases JAK1 and TYK2. Ligand-induced tyrosine phosphorylation of IFN$_I$R-1 was blocked by the kinase inhibitors genistein or staurosporine. Having established the general characteristics of IFN-α/β–induced IFN$_I$R-1 chain tyrosine phosphorylation, it will be important to define which intracellular tyrosine residues are targets for tyrosine phosphorylation and define the role of the phosphorylation of these residues in type I signal transduction. Although IFN$_I$R-1 cDNA-transfected mouse cells express high levels of this subunit ($>$12,000 sites/cell) when compared with empty vector-transfected cells ($<$50 sites/cell), the number of high-affinity huIFN-α binding sites (50–75 sites/cell) was not increased in these cells. Human IFN-α induces the expression of a mouse IFN-α/β–responsive gene (the 204 gene) in mouse L929 cells transfected with the IFN$_I$R-1 cDNA but not in mock transfected cells (21). This suggests that the IFN$_I$R-1 subunit acts as a species-specific signal transduction component of the type I IFN receptor complex. The IFN$_I$R-1 chain has central importance in huIFN$_I$R structure and function based on findings that the huIFN$_I$R-1 chain undergoes rapid ligand-dependent tyrosine phosphorylation, acts as a species-specific transducer for gene induction and antiviral sensitivity to huIFN-α, is constitutively associated with a 110-kDa receptor subunit, and represents a 115–135-kDa subunit of the IFN$_I$R (21,76).

Signaling through the huIFN$_I$R-1 chain displays high IFN specificity, since (1) only type I IFN induces tyrosine phosphorylation of the IFN$_I$R-1 chain in cells sensitive to both type I and type II IFNs; and (2) only IFN-β induces the phosphorylation of a 105-kDa IFN$_I$R-1–associated protein in Daudi cells and U266 cells, whereas IFN-α and IFN-β induce IFN$_I$R-1 tyrosine phosphorylation, suggesting the phosphorylation of cell type–specific substrates. These rapid ligand-dependent phosphorylation events are inhibited by the PTK inhibitors staurosporine and genistein. Although the apparent M_r of the IFN$_I$R-1 chain is lower in U266 cells as compared with Daudi cells (115 and 135-kDa, respectively), the mobility of the 105-kDa phosphoprotein is similar in these cells. In any case, we propose that the loci of ligand-induced IFN$_I$R-1 tyrosine phosphorylation serve as docking sites for signaling proteins. Interestingly, although IFN$_I$R-1, the 105-kDa IFN$_I$R-1–associated protein, JAK1, and TYK2 are all tyrosine phosphorylated with a peak at 5 min, STAT113 and STAT91 are tyrosine phosphorylated with a maximum at 60 min. This might be due to sequential tyrosine phosphorylation by PTKs other than JAK1 or TYK2 of the IFN$_I$R-1 chain at different residues and of the STAT proteins (i.e., the TAM motif of IFN$_I$R-1, the Tyr 690 of STAT113, and Tyr 791 of STAT91 are all preceded by a lysine residue) or to sequestration of STAT proteins into a phosphatase-inaccessible compartment (i.e., accumulation in the nucleus). Nevertheless, these data show that IFN-induced tyrosine phosphorylation is temporally regulated. In addition, we found that tyrosine-phosphorylated IFN$_I$R-1 did not bind glutathione-S-transferase fusion proteins containing the SH2 domains of GAP, crk, or abl, suggesting that these SH2-containing proteins do not associate with tyrosine-phosphorylated IFN$_I$R-1.

By chemical cross linking ^{125}I–IFN-α to a variety of human cell lines, we showed that the huIFN$_I$R consists of multiple glycoproteins of 100, 110, and 135 kDa (43). Thus, our results indicate that the 135-kDa protein observed as the 150-kDa ^{125}I–IFN-α–cross-linked complex represents the IFN$_I$R-1 chain of the huIFN$_I$R. Furthermore, a 110-kDa (IFN$_I$R-3) and not a 135-kDa protein is precipitated by huIFN-α–coupled beads, providing more evidence that the IFN$_I$R-1 chain is not a high-affinity IFN-α binding site. Using the convention applied to other cytokine receptors in the class II cytokine family, we consider the IFN$_I$R-1 chain as a β subunit of the IFN$_I$R, since it is not primarily involved in high-affinity ligand binding but functions as a transducer in type I IFN signaling.

To determine if the antiviral effects of huIFN can be completely explained by expression of the IFN$_I$R-1 chain, we assayed the antiviral activity of several IFN subtypes in WA17 mouse cells, which contain three copies of human Ch21. When WA17 cells are compared with parental L929 cells and mouse IFN$_I$R-1 transfectants, WA17 cells are much more sensitive to all huIFN-α/β subtypes. In contrast, mouse transfectants respond somewhat selectively to IFN-α8 and IFNCon1. These data indicate that other components of the huIFN$_I$R encoded on Ch21 are involved in the induction of antiviral activity by type I IFN. Furthermore, whereas mouse transfectants are not sensitive to the antiproliferative action of type I IFN, WA17 cells are.

C. Structural Analysis of IFN$_I$R-1 Identifies Common Intracellular Motifs Common to Other Cytokine Receptor Signal Transducing Chains

Receptor-chains responsible for binding and/or transducing the effect of IFNs have previously been defined as members of the type II cytokine receptor family (i.e., IFN$_I$R-1 and -2, IFN$_{II}$R-1 and -2, CRF2 orphan receptor chain [CRF2-4], the IL-10R, and tissue factor) based on the characteristic D200 extracellular domain (73). The IFN$_I$R chain contains two intracellular motifs present in the signal transducing chains of other cytokine receptors: (1) a membrane-proximal 50-AA region (79); and (2) a 16-AA tyrosine-activation motif (TAM) (21). The continuous 50-AA membrane-proximal motif encompasses three conserved blocks (A, B, and C) in IFN$_I$R-1, IFN$_{II}$R-2, and CRF2-4, indicating it may interact with signaling molecules, such as the JAK PTKs and STAT proteins (79). Therefore, this domain may act in the same way as the juxtamembrane "box 1" and "box 2" motifs of certain type I cytokine receptor chains, which are critical to the binding of JAK PTKs.

Since IFN$_I$R-1 and IFN$_{II}$R-2 are involved in IFN signal transduction, it is not surprising that they have similar intracellular domains. In addition, the homology in the corresponding CRF2-4 region suggests that CRF2-4 chain also functions in signal transduction by a cytokine receptor. The COOH-terminal sequences beyond this intracellular domain in IFN$_I$R-1 and CRF2-4 are unique to each protein and may provide further specificity to signaling by their respective receptor complexes. The TAM motif was first identified in signaling subunits of the T-cell and B-cell receptor and is believed to couple to SH2 domain-containing proteins involved in downstream signal transduction (80,81). This motif is fully conserved in the human, mouse, and bovine interspecies IFN$_I$R-1 homologues, and has Tyr, Ser, and Thr residues that may serve as targets for phosphorylation by PKC and PTK. Multiple phosphorylation events are important, since the specificity of PTKs can be determined by previous phosphorylation events at serine/threonine residues (89). We propose that the interactions of tyrosine-phosphorylated subunits of the IFN$_I$R with SH2 and SH3 domain-containing proteins couple the IFN$_I$R-1 to multiple downstream signaling pathways (90).

V.   ROLE OF IFN$_I$R SUBUNITS IN IFN-β BINDING

Transfection of the IFN$_I$R-1 into mouse cells or human cells does not increase the high-affinity binding of type I IFNs. However, the human or bovine IFN$_I$R-1 proteins expressed in frog oocytes can bind and form cross-linked complexes with iodinated IFN-α2 and IFN-α8 (91), confirming that IFN$_I$R-1 has a low intrinsic affinity for IFN. Recently, we and others found that high levels of expression of the IFN$_I$R-1 chain in NIH3T3 cells results in low-affinity binding for type I IFN (68,92). Anti–IFN$_I$R-1 MoAb blocks low-affinity type I IFN binding in transfected NIH3T3 cells but does not inhibit IFN binding in a variety of human cell lines. These results point to NIH3T3 cells as a cellular system in which the intrinsic low-affinity ligand binding properties of IFN_IR-1 chain can be studied. We assume that in many cells the IFN_IR-1 chain participates in a low-affinity recognition event which cannot be measured by the usual solution binding methods.

Several lines of evidence show that the human IFN_IR-1 chain is capable of interacting with mouse IFN_IR components in order to trigger human IFN-specific effects on mouse cells. Particularly, mouse cells transfected with human IFN_IR-1 do not become more sensitive to the effects of mouse IFNs but do induce a strong antiviral effect in response to human IFN-α8. In contrast, the human IFN_IR-1 chain in mouse cells is efficiently downregulated by mouse IFN but not by human IFN (68), suggesting that downregulation may be triggered by non–species-specific interactions between high-affinity binding sites for mouse IFN-α and the human IFN_IR-1 chain, resulting in the formation of interspecies IFN_IR complexes.

The role of the IFN_IR-1 chain in ligand binding has also been investigated by using CHO cells expressing a yeast artificial chromosome (YAC) which apparently encodes all known human IFN_IR subunits (77,78). In this system, knocking out the human IFN_IR-1 chain does not abolish high-affinity type I IFN binding (77). Transfection of the human IFN_IR-1 chain back into the knockout cells resulted in high expression of IFN_IR-1 and in a 2- to 2.5-fold increase in high-affinity IFN binding, suggesting a role of IFN_IR-1 in modulating ligand binding by other IFN_IR subunits. We demonstrated the expression of IFN_IR-1 and showed by Western analysis that it migrates as a 130- to 135-kDa protein in these cells. Furthermore, an alternatively spliced product of IFN_IR-1 mRNA coding for a shorter protein has been identified (77). It will be important to assay if this chain can modulate binding or function in the signal transduction of type I IFNs.

Studies with IFN_IR-1 knockout mice show that the IFN_IR-1 chain is required for the signaling of all type I IFNs, since these mice are completely unresponsive to all type I IFNs (93). However, cells from the knockout animals display high-affinity binding sites for type I IFNs. Thus, the IFN_IR-1 chain is clearly not the high-affinity ligand binding component. In addition, these experiments demonstrated the critical role of type I IFNs in controlling viral infections and that type I and type II IFNs are involved in antiviral activity against different viruses in vivo. Transfection of the IFN_IR-1 chain into cells from these knockout mice restores antiviral sensitivity to type I IFN (94).

As a summary of the data on the components of the IFN_IR, the IFN_IR-1 chain is the 115 to 135-kDa component of IFN_IR, which functions predominantly in signal transduction but may bind type I IFN with only low affinity. The IFN_IR-2 chain (previously called β subunit) is 100-kDa receptor subunit, which seems to function in ligand binding and has not been shown to act in signal transduction. Transfection of the IFN_IR-2 chain into heterologous cells does not confer type I IFN sensitivity, showing that it is not a transducing chain. Our data point to a novel 110-kDa protein as a high-affinity binding chain (IFN_IR-3). This protein has similar mobility to IFN_IR-1 in certain cell lines (U266 or mouse transfectants expressing huIFN_IR-1) but can be resolved from IFN_IR-1 in Daudi cells.

The so-called α subunit was initially proposed to function in high-affinity binding (53,95), but it has been recently reported to be IFN_IR-1 (70). However, there are some discrepancies between the reported characteristics of IFN_IR-1 and the α subunit. For example, the α subunit is not downregulated by IFN-α treatment in U937 cells (69,95), whereas the IFN_IR-1 chain is efficiently downregulated (by 90%). The α subunit does not become tyrosine phosphorylated in U937 cells (69), whereas IFN_IR-1 becomes tyrosine phosphorylated in U937 cells within minutes of type I IFN addition. Furthermore, since the IFN_IR-1 chain functions as a classic β transducing chain, it is particularly confusing to designate the IFN_IR-1 chain as the α subunit and the IFN_IR-2 (a ligand binding chain) as the β subunit. Taken together, the cloned IFN_IR proteins are of 100–135 kDa, and a high-affinity binding chain remains unidentified.

An interesting issue is the possible contribution of the TYK2 PTK to the correct assembly of the IFN_IR receptor complex. Mutant cell lines that lack TYK2 do not respond to the gene-inducing activity of IFN-α and bind IFN-α poorly as compared with the parental cell line. However, these mutant cells remain partially sensitive to IFN-β (13,14). Transfection of TYK2 restores the IFN-α response and "normal" IFN-α binding in these mutant cells (96). Moreover, the N-terminus kinase-like domain (KL) of TYK2, but not the classic kinase (KD) domain at the C-terminus, appears to be responsible for restoring ligand binding. Both kinase domains of TYK2 are required to restore the gene-inducing activity of type I IFNs in TYK2-deficient cells. These results suggest that KL domain of TYK2 may play a role in the IFN_IR structure. However, since the increased cell-associated radioactivity was measured at 37°C in TYK2-complemented mutants, it is unclear if the results reflect ligand binding or internalization, and if the increase in binding is for low- or high-affinity binding. We have previously shown that IFN-sensitive cells (i.e., Daudi cells) rapidly internalize high levels of surface bound IFN at 37°C in a cooperative manner (82). In contrast, internalization is slower in resistant cells and is triggered by a one-to-one relationship between receptor occupancy and downregulation. These data are potentially important, since some cytokine receptor subunits are basally associated with JAK kinases.

For example, the EPO receptor is basally associated with JAK2 (97). Thus, preassociation of TYK2 might contribute to correct assembly of the IFN_IR complex.

VI. CONFORMATION OF THE IFN-IFN$_I$R COMPLEX

A. Three-Dimensional Structure of Murine and Human IFN-β

The availability of large amounts of recombinant DNA–derived IFN proteins has facilitated the elucidation of their three-dimensional structure by use of x-ray crystallography. The structure of hexagonal crystals of murine recombinant IFN-β (MuIFN-β) has recently been solved using the multiple isomorphous replacement method to a resolution of 2.6 Å (98). The structure of MuIFN-β is a bundle of five α helices, and it apparently represents a basic structural framework of all type I IFNs. The spatial arrangement described for MuIFN-β is similar to the arrangement of α helices of other helical cytokines such as IFN-γ, IL-2, or GH. IFNs-α and IFN-β show 26% homology at the amino acid level, and the homology is present over the entire sequence, indicating a common ancestry of type I IFNs (99). Structure-activity relationships of type I IFNs by site-directed mutagenesis previously identified three functionally important segments that are closely located in the spatial structure (100–102).

A major challenge will now be to locate the important regions of IFN-β involved in receptor binding, as well as in its interaction with signal-transducing chains. IFN-β shares common signaling events with IFN-α as well as having distinct signaling events. Thus, future studies will have to relate amino acid sequence differences in a particular helix or loop to the activation of distinct signaling events by IFN-β versus IFN-α (i.e., tyrosine phosphorylation of a 105-kDa IFN_IR-1–associated phosphoprotein by IFN-β but not by IFN-α).

We first discuss the three-dimensional crystal structure of MuIFN-β (98,102) in relation to receptor binding and subsequent transmembrane signaling. As depicted in Figure 4, the five helices of MuIFN-β are helix A (residues 6–23), helix B (49–65), helix C (77–91), helix D (112–131), and helix E (138–158). Likewise, the loops are AB, BC, CD, and DE. Since loop AB is relatively long (27 AAs), helices A and B are parallel, whereas the other helices are sequentially antiparallel to each other. A spatially continuous binding site for the IFN_IR is formed by regions of loop AB, helix D, and loop DE (98). The core of the structure can be considered a bundle of four tightly interacting helices with A, E, B, and C arranged clockwise (103). Interestingly, the remaining α helix D interacts with the helix bundle by making contacts with the parallel helix B

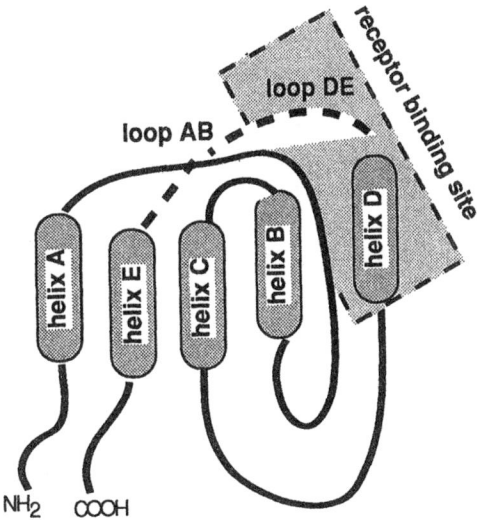

Figure 4 Representation of the packing scheme for murine IFN-β.

and with antiparallel helix E. The hydrophobic interaction of Tyr 120 and Tyr 121 in helix D with Trp 138 of helix E attaches helix D to the bundle. This framework is also compatible with the pattern of disulfide bonds observed in IFN-α but absent in IFN-β. For example, introducing a disulfide bond (analogous with the Cys 29–Cys 136 of IFN-α) into the sequence of MuIFN-β by a double mutation to Cys results in an 15-fold increase in the antiviral activity (104). Furthermore, the residues comprising the type I IFN binding site as defined by x-ray crystallography are also the biologically important residues elucidated by hybrid scanning and site-directed mutagenesis of type I IFNs (102). These residues are highly conserved in type I IFNs and form the interdomain interface in the three-dimensional crystal structure of IFN-β. The importance of loop AB (in particular residues 32–46) in receptor binding has been demonstrated by epitope mapping studies with anti–IFN-β–neutralizing antibodies (105). In addition, several studies (102,106–109) also show the biological significance of residues 36–41 (loop AB) and residues 112–148 (helix D and loop DE).

The multisegment nature of the binding site for the type I receptor (loop AB, helix D, and loop DE) explains why peptide fragments of IFN-α (generated by cyanogen bromide cleavage or by chemical synthesis) lack biological activity (99). The target cell specificities of hybrids of IFN-α subtypes show that IFNs have two distinct binding regions—one located in the COOH-terminal half and another in the NH-terminal half (110). Moreover, biological activity is preserved in naturally occurring IFN-α species that either lack 10–11 AA at the COOH-terminus, the 4 AAs at the NH-terminus, or the Cys 1–Cys 99 bridge of IFN-αA. However, the second bridge of Cys 29 (N-terminal region of loop AB) and Cys 139 (middle of loop CD) must be important to maintain proximity of loops AB and DE. Furthermore, an antibody binding to the 150- to 166-AA region of human IFN-α1 belonging to helix E can bind IFN even when it is bound to cells (102). Thus, although helix E is exposed, it is not directly involved in receptor interaction. Thus, all available evidence shows that the receptor binding epitope is three dimensional rather than simply a linear epitope.

The three-dimensional structures of cytokines, such as IFN-β and GH, which contain four α helix bundles, can be considered closely related. Thus, the recently solved crystal structure of the GH receptor (GHR):GH complex also provides some important structural hints for the interaction of type I IFN with its cognate receptor. The structure of the GHR:GH complex is a dimeric arrangement of receptor subunits which cradles the GH helix bundle (111). Each GHR subunit interacts with a unique helix of the ligand. GHR subunit 1 interacts with COOH-terminal helix 4 of GH, whereas subunit 2 interacts with NH-terminal helix 1. The two distinct sites of GH also appear as a continuous functionally important area. These results suggest that in IFN receptor interaction, distinct chains of the IFN$_1$R may be required for high-affinity binding and others for transmembrane signaling. The spatially continuous area of loop AB, helix D, and loop DE may be binding to two receptor subunits involved in high-affinity binding. The binding area of IFN-β is relatively large, with the horizontal distance between interacting regions in helix D and loop A being 25 Å, whereas the vertical distance between interacting regions of loop AB is 15 Å, which is also very long. Thus, a receptor would be required to have a very large contact area (15 × 25 Å) with a deep V-shaped cleft, which indicates that one IFN molecule may interact with two distinct receptor subunits (102).

The evolutionary behavior of IFN-α and IFN-β sequences provides some hints about the evolution of their receptors. First, the rules that govern the evolution of IFN molecules seem to be different from those of other proteins. Helices B and E of IFN-β are buried (hydrophobic), whereas helices A, C, and E are amphipathic (102). However, the exposed residues in IFN-β are not any more variable than the hydrophobic ones, as the general rule for protein evolution is conservation of exposed residues (102). Although there is only 50% homology between human and MuIFN-β, the interspecies homology for other cytokines is also relatively low when compared with the values for other proteins: only 28% for CSF,

50% for GM-CSF and IL-6, and 75% for M-CSF, G-CSF, and IL-5 (102). Furthermore, when considering specific AA residues, the Cys 29–Cys 139 disulfide bond present in all human IFN-α and IFN-β examined so far are converted in MuIFN-β into Asn and Tyr, respectively (102). Thus, the requirement for conservation is less stringent in cytokines than in structural proteins and enzymes, and this suggests that the low-sequence conservation of cytokines reflects the unique manner in which these proteins act. Although, part of the molecule provides a binding site for the receptor or accessory factor, the rest of the cytokine molecule only seems to provide a helical framework (102).

B. Model of IFN Binding to Receptor

Based on the x-ray crystallography, site-directed mutagenesis, and hybrid scanning studies of type I IFNs, a model for interaction between IFN-α/β and the two subunits of IFN_IR has been recently proposed (94). The functionally important area of IFN-β structure (loop AB, helix D, and possibly loop DE) seems to mediate the initial interaction of IFN with the ligand binding component of the receptor. Since IFN_IR-1 acts a species-specific transducer, the regions involved in the recognition event between IFN_IR-1 and the IFN–ligand binding site complex can be identified using data on bioassays with hybrid IFNs when IFN_IR-1 is expressed in heterologous cells. For example, transfecting bovine IFN_IR-1 into human cells increases sensitivity to human IFN-α1, to which bovine cells are not normally very sensitive. Residues 16–29 of IFN-α1 are responsible for its species-specific activity, and encompass the last two turns of helix A and the proximal part of loop AB. In addition, we found that transfection of huIFN_IR-1 into mouse cells impairs the high cross reactivity of human IFN-α1 on mouse cells, suggesting that human IFN-α1 interacts in a nonproductive manner with human IFN_IR-1. Furthermore, the IFN-α8 (1–62): IFN-α1 (63–92): IFN-α8 (93–166) hybrid is active on mouse cells, whereas IFN-α8 is inactive (112). The double mutation, changing individual residues to those of IFN-α8 (K84 to E84 and Y90 to D90), abolished the activity of the hybrid on mouse cells, but it did not abolish its activity on mouse cells transfected with human IFN_IR-1 (which are highly sensitive to human IFN-α8) (94). The hybrid differs from parental IFN-α8 by four positions which are surface exposed on helix C (112). The three-dimensional structure of murine IFN-β shows that residues in helices A and C are surface exposed on one side of the molecule, and that residues in the AB and D domains are surface exposed on the other side. Since helices A and C of type I IFNs are apparently critical for species-specific signaling through the IFN_IR-1 chain, they probably mediate a low-affinity interaction between IFN$_I$R-1 and IFN (94). Transfection of huIFN$_I$R-1 into mouse NIH3T3 cells confers low-affinity IFN binding ($k_d \approx 5$ nM), which can be blocked by anti–IFN$_I$R-1 MoAb. This MoAb does not block high-affinity ligand binding ($k_d \approx 50$ pM) or signal transduction.

An important assumption in this model is that there are only two chains in the IFN$_I$R complex. However, our studies indicate that a third chain (110-kDa protein) may play a role in high-affinity ligand binding. In this case, the rather large functionally important area of IFN-β, which includes loop AB, helix D, and loop DE (25 × 15Å, horizontal × vertical), might interact with two ligand binding chains as originally proposed (102), whereas IFN$_I$R-1 may instead interact with helices A and C. This provides the opportunity to explore IFN-β–specific signaling through the IFN$_I$R-1 chain. We and others (21–23) have observed with different reagents that IFN-β, but not IFN-α, induces the tyrosine phosphorylation of a 100- to 105-kDa band which becomes associated with the IFN$_I$R-1 chain on IFN binding. This band is not IFN$_I$R-1 (21,23), although originally believed to be based on its association with the α subunit (22). We also showed that this protein is not the IFN$_I$R-2 chain or the 110-kDa putative IFN-α binding site. Surface biotinylation demonstrated that this protein is a cell surface chain (23), whereas our preliminary data show that it is N-glycosylated (68).

Therefore, IFN-β must interact differently with components of the IFN$_I$R when compared with other type I IFNs. Using two-dimensional gel electrophoresis, we have detected several IFN-β–specific tyrosine phosphoproteins that become associated with IFN$_I$R-1. Therefore, we propose that the IFN-β–specific tyrosine phosphorylation events reflect a means whereby IFN-β interacts differently with IFN$_I$R-1 than other type I IFNs. IFN-α/β hybrids and IFN-β mutants have been produced, and their antiviral and antiproliferative activities assayed (113). Their use may yield important new information on the precise residues which mediate the IFN-β–specific interaction with IFN$_I$R-1. These data suggest that IFN-β interacts with both the binding and transducing chains of IFN$_I$R.

C. Topology of the Ligand Binding Domain of the IFN$_I$R

The ligand binding domain of the IFN$_I$R-1 may be approximated based on the three-dimensional crystal structure of the GH-GHR complex (111). All members of the cytokine receptor superfamily have an extracellular domain (D200) composed of two 100-AA subdomains (SD100A and SD100B). Each SD100 domain is folded into a β barrel consisting of two β sheets: one sheet contains three β strands, and the second sheet contains four β strands. The β strands are antiparallel. Since the β strand length is conserved, it is possible to predict the position of interstrand loops. In the GH-GHR structure, the ligand binding site forms in the groove between the two SD100 domains (A and B) consisting of inter-β strand loops. Since each subdomain folds into a barrel, the loops close to the hinge region and the proximal parts of the β strands present a surface for ligand binding (see Fig. 2). However, since IFN_IR-1 has a duplication of the D200 domain and therefore has four barrels of domains A, B, A', B', hinges between A and B, A' and B', and B and A' are possible binding regions. The last region is unlikely to contribute to the ligand binding domain, since a MoAb recognizing this region does not block binding, and the loop between B and A' is short and has multiple glycosylation sites. In a preliminary results, helix A of IFN seems to interact with the A,B hinge region (94). The duplication of D200 domains in IFN_IR-1 makes it difficult to speculate on the interacting sites based on GH-GHR structure. The IFN_IR-2 chain is also a member of the class II cytokine family and has a single D200 domain. However, since the IFN_IR-2 chain reportedly forms dimers (either with itself or with another chain of similar size), the IFN_IR-2 subunit also may provide two other D200 domains for ligand interaction. As an additional complication to any model of IFN-receptor interaction, there is the possible involvement of glycosphingolipids in ligand binding (114).

VII. TRANSMEMBRANE SIGNALING BY THE IFN_IR

A. Signal Transduction Involving Protein Tyrosine Kinases

The involvement of protein phosphorylation in ISG activation was first suggested by our finding that the protein kinase inhibitor staurosporine completely blocks the transcriptional activation of ISGs (17,18) by blocking STAT activation (18). Transfection of the cDNAs encoding the nonreceptor TYK2 and JAK1 PTKs reverse the signaling defects in genetically selected IFN-α–nonresponsive mutant cell lines (13,14). These findings revealed that each of these PTKs is necessary for signal transduction by type I IFN. One likely possibility is that the IFN_IR-1 signal transducing chain, on the activation of JAK kinases, serves to recruit distinct sets of potential substrates. As illustrated in Figure 5, PTKs mediate the IFN-α–induced rapid tyrosine phosphorylation of STAT91 and STAT113 and the activation of ISG transcription (7,8). The STAT proteins contain SH2 and SH3 regions (8), modular noncatalytic domains of about 100 AA that are found in nonreceptor PTKs, structural proteins, and other cytoplasmic signaling proteins (115). SH2 domains mediate high-affinity interactions

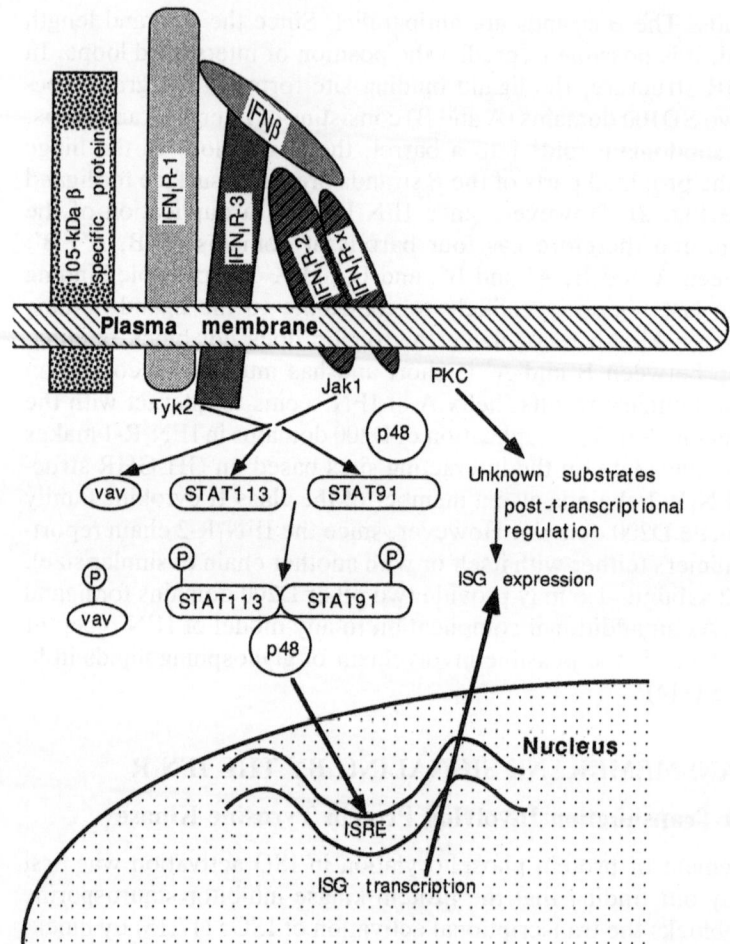

Figure 5 Schematic representation of the type I IFN system.

of cytoplasmic effectors with unique phosphotyrosine residues in activated cell surface receptors (115,116). By this mechanism, the activated receptors acquire the ability to recruit to the membrane a number of cytoplasmic signal-transducing proteins via SH2 domains.

The SH2 domains of cytoplasmic effectors (i.e., phosphatidylinositol 3-kinase, phospholipase Cγ, Ras GTPase-activating protein, vav, shc, GRB-2, and src-like PTKs) recognize phosphotyrosine motifs with specificity dictated by the primary sequence immediately COOH-terminal from the phospho-Tyr. These motifs, identified by using degenerate phospho-peptide libraries, are also present in the cytoplasmic domains of various cell surface receptors (117). The separate docking sites for the binding domains of SH2 from different signaling molecules have been mapped on many receptors. Ligand binding to the IFN$_I$R results in the rapid tyrosine phosphorylation of receptor subunits and intracellular proteins, including IFN$_I$R-1 and IFN$_I$R-2, STATs, and the vav guanine nucleotide exchange factor (7,8,21,58,71,118). We have found that the STAT91 and STAT113 proteins are detected in anti–IFN$_I$R-1 immunoprecipitates of IFN-α–treated Daudi cells. An attractive hypothesis is that JAK1 and PTKs mediate the phosphorylation of the highly conserved TAM motif in IFN$_I$R-1 subunit, creating a multifunctional docking site for SH2 domain-containing cytoplasmic effectors (13,75,97).

Several groups reported that TYK2 is associated with the IFN$_I$R-1 chain (23,70) and JAK1 is associated with the IFN$_I$R-2 chain (59). Complementation experiments have shown that JAK1 also is required for type I IFN signaling, whereas type II IFN requires JAK1 and JAK2 (13,14,41). In cell lines sensitive to both type I and II IFNs, we found that only type I IFNs are able to induce tyrosine phosphorylation of IFN$_I$R-1, although all IFNs activate JAK1. IL-3 and EPO receptors transduce overlapping signals through JAK2 activation, but only EPO will phosphorylate the EPO receptor (15,97). The present model of cytokine signaling predicts that receptors are associated with JAK kinases, and these kinases remain localized in the activated receptor complex. This provides the basis for the specificity of substrate protein phosphorylation, since proteins will only become phosphorylated if they attach to the cytokine receptor complex. In Daudi cells, we have observed that IFN-β activates JAK1 more than IFN-α does, as assayed by its tyrosine phosphorylation. This leads us to speculate that JAK1, which is basally associated with the IFN$_I$R-2 chain, may function somewhat selectively in signaling by IFN-β compared with IFN-α. Consistent with this, cells defective in TYK2 retain partial sensitivity to IFN-β (these cells still express JAK1) while being insensitive to IFN-α (14). IFN-β appears to be evolutionarily closer to ancestral IFN than IFN-α, and JAK1 is probably closer to the initial signaling pathway used by ancestral IFN (94). In this respect, the recruitment of TYK2 in the IFN signal transduction pathway would represent an evolutionary diversification of biological function.

B. Signal Transduction Involving Protein Kinase C

In early studies, we showed that type I IFN effects a rapid and transient increase in the plasma membrane rigidity of target cells (119) and also stimulates lipid turnover and synthesis (120). Recent evidence in several IFN-sensitive human cell lines has established that IFN rapidly induces transient increases of the lipid-derived second-messenger diacylglycerol (DAG), a physiological activator of PKC (17,121). PKC comprises a family of related serine/threonine kinases with pivotal roles in cell signaling, as well as in a variety of cellular responses (122). PKC subspecies belong to three major groups: conventional (α, β, and γ), nonconventional (δ, ϵ, η, and θ), and atypical (ζ and λ). Individual PKC subspecies exhibit distinct requirements for cofactors (Ca^{2+}, phospholipids) and activators (phorbol esters), tissue-specific distributions, and enzymological properties, including substrate specificity (123–127).

The lipid source for the increase in DAG has not been definitely identified and could have several origins (128). In human cells, the involvement of IFN-α–induced inositol phospholipid turnover has been ruled out as a source for the increase in cellular DAG mass (17,121). In HeLa cells, IFN-α rapidly increases phosphatidylcholine (PC) hydrolysis, as well as inducing the appearance of phosphorylcholine, DAG, and phosphatidic acid (121). In Daudi cells, a phospholipase D (PLD) pathway seems to be involved, since the IFN-α–induced DAG increase can be inhibited by propranolol, a phosphatidic acid phosphohydrolase inhibitor. However, a ceramide-dependent pathway is also involved in IFN-α signaling, since the DAG transient is accompanied by an increase in ceramide content. Ceramide metabolism has been shown to play an important role in the signaling pathway induced by other cytokines (129).

Direct evidence for a role of PKC activation in IFN-α action has been provided by our discovery that IFN-α activates selective PKC subspecies (17,121). The cellular distribution of PKC subspecies was identified in various human cells by antipeptide antisera to specific PKC subspecies. In HeLa cells, IFN-α rapidly (within 5 min) induced the selective translocation of PKC-β, but not PKC-α, from the cytosol to the particulate fraction of cells as determined by immunoblot analysis (121). IFN-α treatment of IFN-sensitive Daudi cells results in a time-dependent increase in PKC-ϵ immunoreactivity, apparently through its phosphorylation, without any PKC-ϵ translocation (17). PKCs α, β, ζ, and θ are present in Daudi cells, but are unaffected by IFN-α. In contrast, IFN-α treatment of the IFN-resistant Daudi subclone did not result in PKC-ϵ activation. Furthermore, we found that IFN-α only transiently activates ISG gene expression in IFN-resistant Daudi cells, whereas IFN treatment of sensitive Daudi lymphoblastoid cells induces prolonged and high levels of ISG expression (19). These results suggest a role of PKC-ϵ in a process following the initiation of ISG transcription, perhaps on mRNA stability. Activation of selective PKC subspecies in different cell lines is similar to the activation of several JAK kinases by IL-6 in different cell lines (15).

C. Protein Phosphorylation Through PTK and PKC Pathways Is Required for Type I IFN-induced ISG Expression and Antiviral Activity

Our studies establish that transcriptional and posttranscriptional regulation of ISGs by type I IFN is triggered by protein phosphorylation. We showed that staurosporine, a potent protein kinase inhibitor, blocked induction and accumulation of ISGs (17,18). It was demonstrated subsequently that JAK PTKs are involved in ISG transcriptional activation, and we found that Ca^{2+}-insensitive PKC subspecies are involved in the accumulation of ISGs in IFN-α–sensitive cells. Pretreatment of IFN-responsive cells with staurosporine largely blocks the steady-state accumulation of ISG mRNAs and impairs the transcriptional activation of ISGs. Staurosporine blocks STAT activation in both HeLa and Daudi cells by blocking a phosphorylation event necessary for activation (18); namely, STAT tyrosine phosphorylation (7,8). In contrast, H8, an inhibitor of cAMP- and cGMP-dependent protein kinases, and HA1004, a weak protein kinase inhibitor, have no effect on the transcriptional activation of ISGs and ISG mRNA accumulation.

The selective PKC inhibitor, H7, inhibits late ISG transcription ($\geq$4 hr after IFN addition) and mRNA accumulation in IFN-sensitive Daudi cells but does not affect STAT activation or initial ISG transcriptional activation. These results demonstrate that the action of PKC in type I IFN signaling occurs temporally after the initiation of ISG transcription (18). However, although the STAT activation is unaffected by H7, induction of ISGF2 (IRF-1) is completely blocked. ISGF2 is an IFN-inducible gene whose induction pathway is distinct from that of ISGs. The ISGF2 gene does not contain an ISRE within its promoter (130), but it does contain several NF-κB binding sites, sites that can be regulated through a PKC-dependent pathway. Furthermore, expression of the adenovirus E1A oncoprotein blocks the IFN-α–induced transcription of ISGs (131,132) but does not affect ISGF2 transcription (133). Our initial studies suggest that IFN-α–induced ISGF2 gene expression occurs through a PKC-dependent pathway. Interestingly, although the kinetics of tyrosine phosphorylation of $IFN_I R$-1, TYK2, and JAK1 are similar with a maximum at 5 min, tyrosine phosphorylation of STAT113 and STAT91 is maximal at 1 hr. The high intrinsic sensitivity of several human lymphoblastoid cell lines (Daudi, MOLT4) to IFN-α seems related to the marked activation of a serine/threonine kinase–dependent pathway (possibly involving MAP kinase and/or PKC), which amplifies signaling through IFN-activated PTKs.

D. Defective ISG Expression in IFN-resistant Cells May Involve a Defect in the PKC Pathway that Modifies Posttranscriptional Regulation

We have compared the type I IFN response pathway in IFN-sensitive and IFN-resistant cell lines. The IFN resistance of these cells is not due to a failure to bind type I IFN, as all cells studied display high-affinity IFN binding sites (500–3000 receptors/cell, $k_d \sim 50$ pM). IFN treatment of sensitive cells results in rapid STAT activation and enhanced ISG transcription. In some resistant cell lines, IFN does not induce STAT activation, and thus fails to activate ISG transcription (132). Surprisingly, we found that the level of ISG mRNA induction at 30 min after IFN addition in IFN-sensitive and IFN-resistant Daudi cells is comparable. Only at later times (>2 hr) after type I IFN addition, are marked differences in ISG expression apparent between sensitive and resistant Daudi cells. The time course of the IFN-induced tyrosine phosphorylation of the STAT113 is also similar in both resistant and sensitive Daudi cells. However, in sensitive cells, the steady-state levels of ISG mRNA increase nearly linearly for 12 hr after IFN addition, whereas in resistant cells, the mRNA levels peak within 2 hr and decrease to near basal levels by 12 hr. ISG transcription in sensitive Daudi cells remains high for extended periods (≥20 hr). An inability to maintain high ISG expression in IFN-resistant cells appears to reflect a selective inability to activate a PKC pathway, for they do activate a PTK pathway (95).

We also established that ISG induction in some cells is protein synthesis dependent. In human monocytic U937 cells, whereas type I IFN induces only slight antiviral protection, IFN-γ pretreatment markedly potentiates the antiviral activity of type I IFN (134). The protein synthesis inhibitor cycloheximide blocks type I IFN–induced ISG transcription and mRNA accumulation in U937 cells. Although IFN-γ alone does not induce ISG transcription, IFN-γ pretreatment markedly hastens and increases ISG expression. Our recent studies show that the early IFN-signaling pathway is intact in U937 cells (i.e., tyrosine phosphorylation of STAT proteins and IFN$_I$R-1). STAT activation rapidly appears at low levels in nuclear extracts of U937 cells on type I IFN treatment in gel shift assays. A late increase in STAT activity ultimately correlates with the type I IFN–induced synthesis of the p48 ISG-specific DNA-binding protein. IFN-γ induces p48 synthesis at much greater levels, which accounts for the dramatic effect of IFN-γ pretreatment on ISG induction by type I IFN.

REFERENCES

1. Issacs A, Lindenmann J. Virus interference I: the interferon. Proc Roy Soc Lond 1957; 147:258–267.
2. Nagano Y, Kojima Y. Inhibition de l'infection vaccinale par un facteur liquide dans le tissu infect par le virus homologue. C R Soc Biol 1958; 152: 1627–1629.
3. Aguet M. High affinity binding of ^{125}I-labeled mouse interferon to a specific cell surface receptor. Nature 1980; 284:459–461.
4. Langer J, Pestka S. Interferon receptors. Immunology 1988; 9:875–878.
5. Pfeffer LM. Mechanisms of Interferon Action. Boca Raton, FL: CRC Press, 1987.
6. Rubinstein M, Orchansky P. The interferon receptors. CRC Crit Rev Biochem 1986; 21:249–275.
7. Schindler C, Shuai K, Prezioso VR, Darnell JE. Interferon-dependent tyrosine phosphorylation of a latent cytoplasmic transcription factor. Science 1992; 257:809–813.
8. Fu X-Y. A transcription factor with SH2 and SH3 domains is directly activated by an interferon α–induced cytoplasmic protein tyrosine kinase(s). Cell 1992; 70:323–335.
9. Friedman RL, Stark GR. α-Interferon–induced transcription of HLA and metallothionein genes containing homologous upstream sequences. Nature 1985; 314:637–639.
10. Reich NC, Evans B, Levy DE, Fahey D, Knight E, Darnell JE. Interferon-transcription of a gene encoding a 15-KD protein depends on an upstream enhancer element. Proc Natl Acad Sci USA 1987; 84:6394–6398.
11. Sadowski HB, Shuai K, Darnell JE Jr, Gilman MZ. A common nuclear signal transduction pathway activated by growth factor and cytokine receptors. Science 1993; 261:1739–1743.
12. Larner AC, David M, Feldman GM, et al. Tyrosine phosphorylation of DNA binding proteins by multiple cytokines. Science 1993; 261:1730–1736.
13. Muller M, Briscoe J, Laxton C, et al. The protein tyrosine kinase JAK1 complements defects in the interferon-α/β and -γ signal transduction. Nature 1993; 366:129–135.
14. Velazquez L, Fellous M, Stark GR, Pelligrini S. A protein tyrosine kinase in the interferon α/β signaling pathway. Cell 1992; 70:313–322.
15. Ihle JN, Witthuhn BA, Quelle FW, et al. Signaling by the cytokine receptor superfamily: JAKs and STATs. TIBS 1994; 19:222–229.
16. Improta T, Schindler C, Horvath CM, Kerr I, Stark GR, Darnell JE. Transcription factor ISGF-3 formation requires phosphorylated Stat91, but Stat113 protein is phosphorylated independently of Stat91. Proc Natl Acad Sci USA 1994; 91:4776–4780.
17. Pfeffer LM, Eisenkraft BL, Reich NC, et al. Transmembrane signaling by interferon α involves diacylglycerol production and activation of the ε isoform of protein kinase C in Daudi cells. Proc Natl Acad Sci USA 1991; 88: 7988–7992.

18. Reich NC, Pfeffer LM. Evidence for involvement of protein kinase C in the cellular response to interferon α. Proc Natl Acad Sci USA 1990; 87: 8761–8765.

19. Wang C, Constaninescu SN, MacEwan DJ, et al. Interferonα induces protein kinase C-ε (PKC-ε) gene expression and a 4.7-kb PKC-ε–related transcript. Proc Natl Acad Sci USA 1993; 90:6944–6948.

20. Pfeffer LM, Wang C, Fu X-Y, Reich NC, MacEwan DJ, Constantinescu SN. Interferonα-induced gene expression and antiviral activity require distinct protein tyrosine kinase- and protein kinase C-dependent pathways. 1996.

21. Constantinescu SN, Croze E, Wang C, et al. The role of the interferon α/β receptor chain 1 in the structure and transmembrane signaling of the interferon α/β receptor complex. Proc Natl Acad Sci USA 1994; 91: 9602–9606.

22. Platanias LC, Uddin S, Colamonici OR. Tyrosine phosphorylation of the α and β subunits of the type I interferon receptor: interferon-β selectively induces tyrosine phosphorylation of an α subunit-associated protein. J Biol Chem 1994; 269:17761–17764.

23. Abramovich C, Shulman LM, Ratovitski E, et al. Differential tyrosine phosphorylation in response to interferon-α and interferon-β of a surface protein associated with the IFNAR chain of the type-I interferon receptor. EMBO J 1994; 13:5871–5877.

24. Belhumeur P, Lanoix J, Blais Y, Forget D, Steyaert A, Skup D. Action of spontaneously produced beta interferon in differentiation of embryonal carcinoma cells through an autoinduction mechanism. Mol Cell Biol 1993; 13:2846–2857.

25. Garbe C, Krasagakis K. Effects of interferons and cytokines on melanoma cells. J Invest Dermatol 1993; 100:239S–244S.

26. Liberati AM, Schippa M, Portuesi MG, et al. IFN-beta induced biochemical and immunological modifications in hairy leukemia patients. Hematology 1991; 76:375–382.

27. Palmer H, Libby P. Interferon beta. A potential autocrine regulator of human vascular smooth muscle cell growth. Lab Invest 1992; 66:715–721.

28. Vieillard V, Lauret E, Rousseau V, De Maeyer E. Blocking of retroviral infection at a step prior to reverse transcription in cells transformed to constitutively express interferon beta. Proc Natl Acad Sci USA 1994; 91: 2689–2693.

29. Popik W, Pitha PM. Transcriptional activation of the tat-defective human immunodeficiency type 1 provirus. Virology 1992; 189:435–437.

30. Sica G, Iacopino F, Amadori D, et al. Steroid receptor enhancement by natural interferon-beta in advanced breast cancer. Eur J Cancer 1993; 29: 329–333.

31. Nakajima Y, Konno S, Perruccio L, et al. Effects of IFN beta on growth of human prostatic JCA-1 cells. Biochem Biophys Res Commun 1994; 200: 467–474.

32. Asano M, Hayashi M, Yoshida E, Kawade Y, Iwakura Y. Induction of interferon-α by interferon-β, but not of interferon-β by interferon-α in the mouse. Virology 1990; 176:30–38.
33. Connelly JF. Interferon beta for multiple sclerosis. Ann Pharm 1994; 28: 610.
34. Clanet M, Blancher A, Calvas P, Rascol O. Interferons and multiple sclerosis. Biomed Pharm 1989; 43:355.
35. Traugott U, Lebon P. Multiple sclerosis: involvement of interferons in lesion pathogenesis. Ann Neurol 1988; 24:243.
36. Panitch HS. Interferons in multiple sclerosis—a review of the evidence. Drugs 1992; 44:946–962.
37. IFNB Multiple Sclerosis Study Group. Interferon beta-1b is effective in relapsing-remitting multiple sclerosis. Neurology 1993; 43:655–661.
38. Kinnunen E, Timonen T, Pirttila T, et al. Effects of recombinant α-2b-interferon therapy in patients with progressive MS. Acta Neurol Scand 1993; 87:457–460.
39. Reis LFL, Ruggner H, Aguet M, Weissman C. The interferon system lacking IRF-1. J Interferon Res 1994; 14:S45.
40. Knop J, Taborski B, De Maeyer-Guignard J. Selective inhibition of the generation of T suppressor cells of contact sensitivity in vitro by interferon. J Immunol 1987; 138:3684–3687.
41. Pelligrini S, John J, Shearer M, Kerr IM, Stark GR. Use of a selectible marker regulated by alpha interferon to obtain mutants in the signaling pathway. Mol Cell Biol 1989; 9:4605–4612.
42. Branca AA, Faltynek CR, D'Alessandro SB, Baglioni C. Interaction of interferon with cellular receptors: internalization and degradation of cell-bound interferon. J Biol Chem 1982; 257:13291–13296.
43. Vanden Broecke D, Pfeffer LM. Characterization of interferon-α binding sites on human cell lines. J Interferon Res 1988; 8:803–811.
44. Platanias LC, Pfeffer LM, Cruciani R, Colamonici OR. Characterization of the α subunit of the IFN-α receptor: evidence of N- and O-linked glycosylation and association with other surface proteins. J Immunol 1993; 150: 3382–3388.
45. Constantinescu SN, Blatt LM, Pfeffer LM. The 110-kDa subunit of the interferon-alpha (IFNα) receptor corresponds to an IFNα binding site. 1996.
46. Benoit P, Maguire D, Plavec I, Kocher H, Tovey M, Meyer F. A monoclonal antibody to recombinant IFN-α receptor inhibits the biological activity of several species of human IFN-α, IFN-β, and IFN-ω. J Immunol 1993; 150:707–716.
47. Platanias LC, Pfeffer LM, Barton KP, Vardiman JW, Golomb HM, Colamonici OR. Expression of the IFNα receptor in hairy cell leukemia. Br J Hematol 1993; 82:541–546.
48. Wang L, Hertzog PJ, Galanis M, Overall M, Waine GJ, Linnane AW. Structure-function analysis of human IFN-α: mapping of a conformational epitope by homologue scanning. J Immunol 1994; 152:705–715.

49. Revel M, Bash D, Ruddle FH. Antibodies to a cell surface component coded by human chromosome 21 inhibit action of interferon. Nature 1976; 260: 139–141.

50. Razziuddin A, Sarkar FH, Dutkowski R, Shulman L, Ruddle FH, Gupta SL. Receptors for human α and β interferon but for for γ interferon are specified by human chromosome 21. Proc Natl Acad Sci USA 1984; 81: 5504–5508.

51. Yap WH, Teo TS, McCoy E, Tan YH. Rapid and transient rise in diacylglycerol concentration in Daudi cells exposed to interferon. Proc Natl Acad Sci USA 1986; 83:7765–7769.

52. Tan YH, Schneider EL, Tischfield J, Epstein CJ, Ruddle FH. Human chromosome 21 dosage: effect on the expression of the interferon induced antiviral state. Science 1974; 186:61–63.

53. Colamonici OR, D'Alessandro F, Diaz MO, Gregory SA, Neckers LM, Nordan R. Characterization of three monoclonal antibodies that recognize the interferon α2 receptor. Proc Natl Acad Sci USA 1990; 87:7230–7234.

54. Colamonici OR, Domanski P. Identification of a novel subunit of the type I interferon receptor localized to human chromosome 21. J Biol Chem 1993; 268:10895–10899.

55. Hertzog PJ, Hwang SY, Holland KA, Tymms MJ, Iannello R, Kola I. A gene on human chromosome 21 located in the region of 21q22.2 to 21q22.3 encodes a factor necessary for signal transduction and antiviral response to type I interferons. J Biol Chem 1994; 269:14088–14093.

56. Soh J, Donnelly RJ, Kotenko S, et al. Identification and sequence of an accessory factor required for activation of the human interferon γ receptor. Cell 1994; 76:793–802.

57. Hemmi S, Bohni R, Stark G, Di Marco F, Aguet M. A novel member of the interferon receptor complements functionality of the murine interferon γ receptor in human cells. Cell 1994; 76:803–810.

58. Uzé G, Lutfalla G, Gresser I. Genetic transfer of a functional human interferon α receptor into mouse cells: cloning and expression of its cDNA. Cell 1990; 60:225–234.

59. Novick D, Cohen B, Rubinstein M. The human interferon α/β receptor: characterization and molecular cloning. Cell 1994; 77:391–400.

60. Faltynek CR, Branca AA, McCandless S, Baglioni C. Characterization of an interferon receptor on human lymphoblastoid cells. Proc Natl Acad Sci USA 1983; 80:3269–3273.

61. Traub A, Feinstein S, Gec M, Lazar A, Mizrahi A. Purification and characterization of the alpha-interferon receptor of human lymphoblastoid (Namalva) cells. J Biol Chem 1984; 259:13872–13877.

62. Zhang ZQ, Fournier A, Tan YH. The isolation of human interferon-beta receptor by wheat germ lectin affinity and immunoabsorbent column chromatographies. J Biol Chem 1986; 261:8017–8021.

63. Joshi AR, Sarkar FH, Gupta SL. Interferon receptors. Crosslinking of human leukocyte interferon alpha-2 to its receptor on human cells. J Biol Chem 1982; 257:13884–13887.

64. Thompson MR, Zhang ZQ, Fournier A, Tan YH. Characterization of human beta-interferon-binding sites on human cells. J Biol Chem 1985; 260: 563–567.

65. Eid P, Mogenson K. Detergent extraction of the human interferon-alpha/beta receptor: a soluble form capable of binding interferon. Biochem Biophys Acta 1990; 1034:114–121.

66. Langer J. Radiolabeling of the interferon-α receptor. Biochem Biophys Res Commun 1988; 157:1264–1270.

67. Croze E, Constantinescu SN, Pfeffer LM, et al. Characterization of the type I IFN receptor using monoclonal antibodies. 1996.

68. Pfeffer LM, Basu L, Croze E, Constantinescu SN. The IFNaR1 chain binds human IFNα when expressed in specific cellular contexts. 1996.

69. Colamonici OR, Domanski P, Krolewski JJ, et al. IFNα signalling in cells expressing the variant form of the type I IFN receptor. J Biol Chem 1994; 269:5660–5665.

70. Colamonici O, Yan H, Domanski P, et al. Direct binding to and tyrosine phosphorylation of the α subunit of the type I IFN receptor by p135^{tyk2} tyrosine kinase. Mol Cell Biol 1994; 14:8133–8142.

71. Platanias LC, Sweet ME. Interferon α induces rapid tyrosine phosphorylation of the *vav* proto-oncogene product in hematopietic cells. J Biol Chem 1994; 269:3143–3146.

72. Bazan JF. Structure design and molecular evolution of a cytokine receptor superfamily. Proc Natl Acad Sci USA 1990; 87:6934–6938.

73. Bazan JF. Shared architecture of hormone binding domains in type I and II interferon receptors. Cell 1990; 61:753–754.

74. Taga T, Kishimoto T. Cytokine receptors and signal transduction. FASEB J 1992; 6:3387–3396.

75. Stahl N, Yancopoulos GD. The alphas, betas, and kinases of cytokine receptor complexes. Cell 1993; 74:587–590.

76. Colamonici OR, Porterfield B, Domanski P, Constantinescu SN, Pfeffer LM. Complementation of the IFNα response in resistant cells by expression of the cloned subunit of the IFNα receptor: central role of this subunit in IFNα signalling. J Biol Chem 1994; 269:9598–9602.

77. Cleary CM, Donnelly RJ, Soh J, Mariano TM, Pestka S. Knockout and reconstitution of a functional human type I interferon receptor complex. J Biol Chem 1994; 269:18747–18749.

78. Soh J, Mariano TM, Lim J-K, et al. Expression of a functional type I interferon receptor in hamster cells: application of functional yeast artifical chromosome (YAC) screening. J Biol Chem 1994; 269:18102–18110.

79. Mullersman JE, Pfeffer LM. A novel cytoplasmic homology domain in interferon receptors. TIBS 1995; 20:55–56.

80. Wange RL, Malek SN, Desiderio S, Samelson LE. Tandem SH2 domains of ZAP-70 bind to the T cell antigen receptor ζ and CD3ε from activated Jurkat T cells. J Biol Chem 1993; 268:19797–19801.

81. Weiss A. T cell antigen receptor signal transduction: a tale of tails and cytoplasmic protein-tyrosine kinases. Cell 1993; 73:209–212.

82. Pfeffer LM, Donner DB. The down-regulation of interferonα receptors in human lymphoblastoid cells: Relation to cellular responsiveness to the antiproliferative action of α-interferon. Cancer Res 1990; 50:2654–2657.

83. Pfeffer LM, Stebbing N, Donner DB. Cytoskeletal association of human α-interferon–receptor complexes in interferon-sensitive and -resistant lymphoblastoid cells. Proc Natl Acad Sci USA 1987; 84:3249–3253.

84. Bartsch HH, Pfizenmaier K, Hanusch A, Scheurich P, Ucer U, Nagel GA. Sequential therapy with recombinant interferons gamma and alpha in patients with unfavorable prognosis of chronic myelocytic leukemia: clinical responsiveness to recombinant IFN-α correlates with degree of receptor downregulation. Int J Cancer 1989; 43:235–240.

85. Branca AA, D'Alessandro SB, Baglioni C. Internalization and degradation of human interferon alpha-A bound to bovine MDBK cells: regulation of the decay and resynthesis of receptors. J Interferon Res 1983; 3:465–471.

86. Uzé G, Lutfalla G, Bandu M-T, Proudhon D, Mogensen K. Behavior of a cloned murine α/β receptor expressed in homospecific or heterospecific background. Proc Natl Acad Sci USA 1992; 89:4774–4778.

87. Mouchel-Viehl E, Lutfalla G, Mogensen KE, Uzé G. Specific antiviral activities of the human alpha interferons are determined at the level of receptor (IFNAR) structure. FEBS Lett 1992; 313:255–259.

88. Diaz MO, Ziemin S, Le Beau MM, et al. Homozygous deletion of the alpha and beta1-interferon genes in human leukemia and derived cell lines. Proc Natl Acad Sci USA 1988; 85:5259–5263.

89. Donella-Deana A, Marin O, Brunati AM, Cesaro L, Piutti C, Pinna LA. Phosphorylated residues as specificity determinants for an acidophilic protein tyrosine kinase. A study with src and cdc2 derived phosphopeptides. FEBS Lett 1993; 330:141–145.

90. Pearson RB, Kemp BE. Protein kinase phosphorylation site sequences and consensus specificity motifs: tabulations. Methods Enzymol 1991; 200: 62–81.

91. Lim J-K, Xiong J, Carrasco N, Langer JA. Intrinsic ligand binding properties of the human and bovine alpha interferon receptors. FEBS Lett 1994; 350:281–286.

92. Hertzog PJ. 1995: unpublished observations.

93. Muller U, Steinhoff U, Reis LFL, et al. Functional role of type I and type II interferons in antiviral defense. Science 1994; 264:1918–1921.

94. Uzé G, Lutfalla G, Mogenson KE. The α/β interferons and their receptor and their friends and relatives. J Interferon Res 1995;15:3–26.

95. Colamonici OR, Pfeffer LM, D'Alessandro F, et al. Multichain structure of the IFN-α receptor on hematopoietic cells. J Immunol 1992; 148:2126–2132.

96. Velazquez L, Barbieri G, Mogenson KE, Uzé G, Fellous M, Pellegrini S. How does interferon tickle Tyk? J Cell Biochem 1994; S18B:203.

97. Witthuhn BA, Quelle FW, Silvonnoinen O, et al. JAK2 associates with the erythropoietin receptor and is tyrosine phosphorylated and activated following stimulation with erythropoietin. Cell 1993; 74:227–236.

98. Senda T, Shimazu T, Matsuda S, et al. Three-dimensional crystal structure of recombinant murine interferon-β. EMBO J 1992; 11:3193–3201.

99. Pestka S, Langer JA, Zoon KC, Samuel CE. Interferons and their actions. A Rev Biochem 1987; 56:727–777.

100. Staehlin T, Hobbs DS, Kung H-F, Lai C-Y, Pestka S. Purification and characterization of recombinant human leukocyte interferon (IFLrA) with monoclonal antibodies. J Biol Chem 1981; 256:9750–9754.

101. Ortaldo JR, Mason A, Rehberg E, et al. Effect of recombinant human leukocyte interferons on cytotoxic activity on Natural Killer cells. J Biol Chem 1983; 258:15011–15015.

102. Mitsui Y, Senda T, Shimuza T, Matsuda S, Utsumi J. Structural, functional and evolutionary implications of the three dimensional crystal structure of murine interferon-β. Pharm Ther 1993; 58:93–132.

103. Presnell SR, Cohen FE. Topological distribution of α-helix bundles. Proc Natl Acad Sci USA 1989; 86:6592–6596.

104. Day C, Schwartz B, Li B-L, Pestka S. Engineering disulfide bond greatly increases specific activity of recombinant murine interferon-β. J Interferon Res 1992; 12:139–143.

105. Redlich PN, Hoeprich PD, Colby CB, Grossberg SE. Antibodies that neutralize human β interferon biologic activity recognize a linear epitope: analysis by synthetic peptide mapping. Proc Natl Acad Sci USA 1991; 88: 4040–4044.

106. Arnheiter H, Thomas RM, Leist T, Fountoulakis M, Gutte B. Physiochemical and antigenic properties of synthetic fragments of human leucocyte interferon. Nature 1981; 294:278–280.

107. Ackerman SN, Nedden DZ, Heintzelman M, Hunkapiller M, Zoon K. Biological activity in a fragment of human interferon α. Proc Natl Acad Sci USA 1984; 81:1045–1047.

108. Eichman F, Majarov UA, Kozhlich AT, Noll F, Zav'yalov VP. Biologic activity of synthetic peptides of the sequence of human interferon-alpha. Immunol Lett 1990; 24:233–236.

109. Cheethman BF, McInnes B, Mantamadiotis T, et al. Structure-function studies of human interferon-α enhanced activity on human and murine cells. Antiviral Res 1991; 15:27–40.

110. Streuli M, Hall A, Boll W, Stewart II WE, Nagata S, Weismann C. Target cell specificity of two species of human interferon alpha produced in *E. coli* and of hybrid molecules derived from them. Proc Natl Acad Sci USA 1981; 78:2848–2852.

111. De Vos AM, Ultsch M, Kossiakoff AA. Human growth hormone and extracellular domain of its receptor. Crystal structure of the complex. Science 1992; 255:306–311.

112. Meister A, Uzé G, Mogenson KE, et al. Biological activities and receptor binding of two human recombinant interferons and their hybrids. J Gen Virol 1986; 67:1633–1643.

113. Stewart AG, Adair JR, Catlin G, et al. Chemical mutagenesis of human

interferon-β. Construction, expression in *E. coli*, and biological activity of sodium bisulfite-induced mutations. DNA 1987; 6:119–128.

114. Ghislan J, Lingwood CA, Fish EN. Evidence for glycosphingolipid modification of the type 1 interferon receptor. J Immunol 1994; 153:3655–3663.

115. Koch CA, Anderson D, Moran MF, Ellis C, Pawson T. SH2 and SH3 domains: elements that control interactions of cytoplasmic signaling proteins. Science 1991; 252:668–674.

116. Pawson T, Schlessinger J. SH2 and SH3 domains. Curr Biol 1993; 3: 434–442.

117. Songyang Z, Shoelson SE, McGlade J, et al. Specific motifs recognized by the SH2 domains of Csk, 3BP2, fps/fes, GRB-2, HCP, SHC, Syk, and Vav. Mol Cell Biol 1994; 14:2777–2785.

118. Platanias LC, Colamonici OR. Interferon α induces rapid tyrosine phosphorylation of the α subunit of its receptor. J Biol Chem 1992; 267: 24053–24057.

119. Pfeffer LM, Landsberger FR, Tamm I. Beta-interferon-induced time-dependent changes in the plasma membrane lipid bilayer of cultured cells. J Interferon Res 1981; 1:613–620.

120. Pfeffer LM, Kwok BCP, Landsberger FR, Tamm I. Interferon stimulates cholesterol and phosphatidylcholine synthesis but inhibits cholesterol ester synthesis in HeLa-S3 cells. Proc Natl Acad Sci USA 1985; 82:2417–2421.

121. Pfeffer LM, Strulovici B, Saltiel AR. Interferon-α selectively activates the β isoform of protein kinase C through phosphatidylcholine hydrolysis. Proc Natl Acad Sci USA 1990; 87:6537–6541.

122. Nishizuka Y. Intracellular signaling by hydrolysis of phospholipids and activation of protein kinase C. Science 1992; 258:607–614.

123. Sekiguchi K, Tsukuda M, Ase K, Kikkawa U, Nishizuka Y. Model of activation and kinetic properties of three distinct forms of protein kinase C from rat brain. J Biochem (Tokyo) 1988; 103:759–765.

124. Bacher N, Zisman Y, Berent E, Livneh E. Isolation and characterization of PKC-L, a new member of the protein kinase C-related gene family specifically expressed in lung, skin and heart. Mol Cell Biol 1991; 11:126–133.

125. Osada S, Mizuno K, Saido TC, et al. A phorbol ester receptor/protein kinase, nPKC-eta, a new member of the protein kinase C family predominantly expressed in lung and skin. J Biol Chem 1990; 265:22434–22440.

126. Schaap D, Parker PJ, Bristol A, Kriz R, Knopf J. Unique substrate specificity and regulatory properties of PKC-ϵ: a rationale for diversity. FEBS Lett 1989; 243:351–357.

127. Parker PJ, Kour G, Marais RM, et al. Protein kinase C—a family affair. Mol Cell Endocrinol 1992; 65:1–11.

128. Exton JH. Signalling through phosphatidylcholine breakdown. J Biol Chem 1990; 265:1–4.

129. Schutze S, Potthoff K, Machleidt T, Berkovic D, Weigmann K, Kronke M. TNF activates NF-κB by phosphatidylcholine-specific phospholipase C-induced "acidic" sphingomyelin breakdown. Cell 1992; 71:765–776.

130. Sims SH, Cha Y, Romine MF, Gao P-Q, Gottlieb K, Deisseroth AB. A novel interferon-inducible domain: structural and functional analysis of the human interferon regulatory factor 1 gene promoter. Mol Cell Biol 1993; 13:690–702.

131. Gutch MJ, Reich NC. Repression of the interferon signal transduction pathway by the adenovirus E1A oncogene. Proc Natl Acad Sci USA 1992; 88: 7914–7918.

132. Kessler DS, Pine R, Pfeffer LM, Levy DE, Darnell JE. Cells resistant to interferon are defective in activation of a promoter-binding factor. EMBO J 1988; 7:3779–3783.

133. Haque SJ, Williams BR. Evidence for two distinct interferon-α-signalling pathways. J Interferon Res 1992; 12:S105.

134. Improta T, Pine R, Pfeffer LM. Interferon-γ potentiates the antiviral activity and the expression of interferon-stimulated genes induced by interferon-α in U-937 cells. J Interferon Res 1992; 12:87–94.

2

The Molecular Biology of Type I Interferons (Interferon-α/β) (Gene Activation, Promoters, Proteins Induced)

Thomas Decker

Vienna Biocenter, Institute of Microbiology and Genetics, Vienna, Austria

I. INTRODUCTION

To understand how interferon-β (IFN-β) acts to influence the course of multiple sclerosis, one has to consider several biological levels of its activity. In this Chapter, I focus on a level at the very basis of any complex phenotype: how genes are turned on or off to express or repress their products, ultimately causing an altered behavior of cells and an entire organism. Although we do not precisely know the mechanism by which IFN-β influences the course of multiple sclerosis, it is next to certain that regulating gene expression is a major component. This assumption is based on what we have learned in two decades of molecular IFN research, the finding that none of the changes in cells IFNs are known to elicit, be it the antiviral response, the altered growth or differentiation behavior, or the modulated functions of cells within the immune system, are possible without changing the levels of gene products by directly regulating their transcription. Additional ways of regulating gene expression through the control of mRNA processing or translation exist but will not be considered here, because their relevance to the IFN biology is not yet well understood.

IFNs are subdivided into distinct types (type I IFNs, IFN-α/β; type II IFN, IFN-γ) that are defined by structural relationship and by interaction with cell surface receptors. There are several distinct members of the

41

IFN-α family of cytokines, whereas IFN-β and IFN-γ each comprise a single species only. The receptors for individual IFN-α species and for IFN-β are composed of several distinct components. These subunits are shared between IFN-α and IFN-β receptors, and the two IFN species compete for cell surface binding. However, recent findings indicate that receptor events in response to IFN-α and IFN-β may not be identical (see Chapter 1). In contrast, there are very limited data comparing postreceptor events leading to transcription factor activation and transcriptional regulation between the subtypes IFN-α and IFN-β. In fact, the current paradigm in this field assumes a general validity of studies with either IFN-α or IFN-β for type I IFNs in general. I follow this paradigm, because the major molecular events in transcriptional regulation have been shown to occur in response to both IFN species. However, there is a caveat to the generalization of all findings with IFN-α for IFN-β and vice versa. Differences observed in clinical applications between the subtypes of IFN-α and IFN-β, not only in the treatment of multiple sclerosis but also in cancer therapy, may originate from not so obvious or even subtle differences in the transcriptional response of cells to these cytokines (Section V.A).

Transcriptional control usually occurs at a gene's promoter region, the DNA that is upstream (5') of the mRNA initiation site. It requires the interaction between DNA and transcription factors, proteins that specifically recognize a short sequence of promoter nucleotides. Transcription factor association with these DNA binding sites (DNA elements) is thought to affect the structure of the promoter in a way that interactions with other proteins, the basal transcription factors required for the association of RNA polymerase with the gene, are either promoted or repressed. A transcriptional activator will increase binding of basal factors and thus the association and activity of RNA polymerase, whereas a transcriptional repressor will interfere with these processes. The major questions to be dealt with in this chapter thus address the DNA elements in promoters of IFN-α/β–regulated genes and the transcription factors recognizing these elements. We will see that the current understanding of these topics is fairly complete. However, IFN-α/β is only one of many players within the so-called cytokine network affecting the course of multiple sclerosis. Therefore, one would like to understand crosstalk between the molecular components required for transcriptional control by IFN-α/β and those utilized by other cytokines. In this latter area, we are only beginning to understand how things might happen.

II. THE SYNTHESIS OF IFN-α/β–INDUCED mRNAs

Studies addressing transcriptional regulation by IFN-β began when several laboratories succeeded in the molecular cloning of cDNAs corresponding to IFN-inducible mRNAs during the 1980s (reviewed in ref. 1). Most of these cDNAs were obtained by differential screening methods, and the functions of their encoded products were at the time unknown. It became possible, however, to use these cDNAs as probes to investigate general patterns of transcriptional induction in response to type I IFN in nuclear run-on assays. These assays measure transcription rates in the absence of further mRNA processing and therefore allow accurate statements about promoter activity. It became clear that IFN-α/β did indeed stimulate the transcription rate of specific genes (2–4). In a seminal paper, Larner et al. (4) established the rules of transcriptional regulation in response to IFN-α/β: (1) mRNA induction occurs within minutes; (2) it does not require the synthesis of new proteins, because it resists protein synthesis inhibition by cycloheximide (CHX); (3) transcriptional activity is transient. Peak mRNA synthesis occurs about 1 hr after IFN treatment, and within the next 5–8 hr, transcription rates are repressed back to basal values; (4) repression is an active process, because it will not occur if the synthesis of new proteins is inhibited by CHX during the period of transcriptional activity; (5) genes that have gone through one cycle of induction and repression are refractory for several days to a further induction by IFN. This state of insensitivity to transcriptional gene induction is not due to a downregulation of type I IFN receptors.

These rules have been confirmed by a large number of studies on many IFN-α/β–inducible genes in a variety of cell types. They provided researchers with a useful paradigm for the transcriptional induction of type I–responsive genes despite some cell type–specific variations, especially in the kinetics of the repressive phase. It was clear from there on that understanding an IFN response required a close look at transcriptional regulation.

III. IFN-α/β–REGULATED PROMOTERS

In a first step toward understanding IFN regulation of genes at the level of protein-DNA interactions, phage or cosmid clones were obtained from genomic DNA libraries that contained promoters of IFN-inducible genes. The promoters were analyzed by fusing the DNA to a reporter gene and assaying IFN-regulated activity during transient transfection of IFN-treated cell lines. Systematic introduction of progressive deletions into promoters confined the IFN-responsive region to small stretches of DNA. Sequence comparisons between response regions of different promoters finally allowed definition of a minimal element required for inducibility by type I IFNs. Using this approach, a Friedman-Stark consensus sequence for IFN inducibility was proposed in 1985 for the metallothionein and HLA-A genes (3). Further work, mostly on the promoters of the

Table 1 Examples of IFN-α/β-Inducible Genes

Gene[a]	ISRE[b]: AGTTTCNNTTTCNY[c]	GAS[d]: TTA/CNNNT/GAA[c]	Function of product	References
huISG15	AGTTTCGGTTTCCC		Ubiquitin homologue	6, 143
huISG54	AGTTTCACTTTCCC		Unknown	9
huISG56	AGTTTCACTTTCCC		Unknown	9
hu6-16	AGTTTCATTTTCCC		Unknown	8
hu9/27 (Leu-13)	AGTTTCTATTTCCT		Antiproliferative	11, 105
huHLA-A	AGTTTCTTTTCTCC		MHC class I protein	3, 144
huOASe	GGTTTCGTTTCCTC		RNAaseL Activation	7, 86
huIRF-2	AATTTCATTTTCGC		Transcriptional repressor	32, 145
mu202	AGTTTCTCATTTAC		Antiproliferative (RB-binding)	5, 103
muH-2D	AGTTTCACTTTGC		MHC class I protein	1, 9, 144
muMx	AGTTTCGTTTCTGA		Antiviral (GTPase)	85, 106, 146
muGBP	AGTTTCACTTTCAC	TTTCCCAGCA	Unknown (GTPase)	51, 112, 113, 146
huGBP	ACTTTCAGTTTCAT	TTACTCTAAA	Unknown (GTPase)	12, 111, 112, 113
huICSBP		TTCTCGGAAA	Transcriptional repressor	39, 40, 41
huIRF-1		TTCCCCGAAA	Transcriptional (co)activator	37, 129, 148
muIRF-1		TTCCCCGAAA	Transcriptional (co)activator	31, 145
huIFP53		TTCTCAGAAA	Tryptophanyl-tRNA synthetase	28, 149, 150, 151
muLy6A/E		TTCCTGTAAG	T-cell activation	152
huPKR	NOT CHARACTERIZED		Translational control	86, 93
huRNAaseL	NOT CHARACTERIZED		dsRNA degradation	90, 92

[a] Abbreviated designations; ISG, interferon-stimulated gene; OASe, 2'-5' oligoadenylate synthetase; IRF, interferon regulatory factor; GBP, guanylate-binding protein; ICSBP, interferon consensus sequence–binding protein; IFP, interferon-induced protein; PKR, protein kinase R (= eIF-2α kinase).
[b] Interferon-stimulated response element; N, any nucleotide; Y, pyrimidine nucleotides.
[c] Consensus DNA sequence; N, any nucleotide; Y, pyrimidine nucleotides.
[d] IFN-γ activation sequence (also a type I IFN–responsive element, see text for further explanations).

murine 202 gene (5), the 2′,5′-oligoadenylate A synthetase (2′,5′-oligoade-nylate synthetase [2′,5′-OAS]) (6), and the 6–16 (7), ISG 15 (8), and ISG 54 genes (9) resulted in delineating what has been accepted as a minimal element for type I IFN inducibility: a 14-bp sequence designated inter-feron-stimulated response element (ISRE); (7,9) (Table 1). The ISRE was able to confer type I IFN inducibility on a heterologous minimal promoter containing only the elements required for basal factor association (10,11). A saturating mutagenesis confirmed its crucial role in the response of transfected promoters to type I IFN (10). Thus, the ISRE is both necessary and sufficient for a transcriptional response to IFN-α/β.

Most promoters known to respond to type I IFN contain an ISRE (see Table 1). However, it is now clear that a second, distinct response element also fulfills the purpose of interferon stimulation. This element was origi-nally detected in the promoter of the human gene encoding a guanylate-binding protein (GBP) that responds to both IFN types (see Section VI.D). The promoter contains an ISRE and a second, overlapping *cis* element designated interferon-γ activation site (GAS) (12) (see Table 1). The origi-nal notion was that the ISRE was needed to respond to IFN-α/β, whereas IFN-γ inducibility required both the GAS and the ISRE. Subsequent anal-yses showed that the response of the GBP promoter to type I IFN also required both response elements (13). Moreover, a GBP-GAS oligonucleo-tide was able to confer IFN-α/β inducibility on a heterologous minimal promoter (13). During the last 2 years, several genes have been cloned that entirely rely on a single GAS element in their promoters for type I IFN inducibility (see Table 1). Thus, like the ISRE, the GAS can be both necessary and sufficient for a response to type I IFN. The human GBP gene has remained the only clear example where a cooperation of GAS and ISRE is required for a full-blown transcriptional induction by both IFN types.

IV. TRANSCRIPTION FACTORS INTERACTING WITH IFN RESPONSE ELEMENTS

A. ISGF3 and STATs

The first IFN response element to be thoroughly studied with respect to protein association was the ISRE. Short fragments of promoter DNA or synthetic ISRE oligonucleotides were used in electrophoretic mobility shift assays (EMSAs) to detect constitutively present or IFN-regulated proteins in nuclear extracts that specifically bind to the ISRE (Table 2). Several laboratories reported protein/ISRE complexes, and it took years of research to sort out the identity of the complexes binding to different

Table 2 IFN-α/β–Responsive Transcription Factors

Designation	Subunits	Synonyms	DNA specificity	Function
ISGF3		E	ISRE	Primary transcriptional activator
	STAT1α	α-Component, p91		Receives activating signal
	STAT1β	α-Component, p84		Functional equivalent to STAT1α
	STAT2	α-Component, p113		Receives activating signal
	P48	γ-Component		DNA binding
AAF		—	GAS	Primary transcriptional activator
	STAT1α DIMER			Receives activating signal; DNA binding
	p48 (GBP-GAS)			DNA binding?[a]
AAF2			GAS	Primary transcriptional activator?[b]
	STAT3 DIMER?[c]	—		Receives activating signal; DNA binding
IRF-1	—	ISGF2	CORE-ISRE[d]	Coactivator (maintainance factor?)[e]
IRF-2	—	ISGF1	CORE-ISRE	Transcriptional repressor
ICSBP	—	—	CORE-ISRE	Transcriptional repressor

[a] p48 has exclusively been detected in AAF/GBP-GAS complexes (28). Its function in these complexes is unclear.
[b] An assumption based on kinetic experiments. There are no hard data to support this assumption yet.
[c] An assumption based on experiments from independent studies (refs. 28–30). Formally, the identity of AAF2 with STAT3 dimer has not been shown.
[d] The central nine base pairs of the ISRE (TTTCNNTTT).
[e] See section IV B.

ISREs found and named in individual laboratories (9,14,15). I will not follow the history of each of the ISRE-associated proteins, but I will focus on what we know now and use the nomenclature that prevails in current literature.

The main interest after the identification of the ISRE was to find the major activating protein for interferon-induced genes. One protein/ISRE complex, designated E (14) or ISGF3 (9), fulfilled the criteria of a bona fide primary transcriptional activator: its DNA binding activity appeared rapidly after IFN-α/β treatment but not after IFN-γ treatment, with kinetics resembling those of transcription rates of IFN-α/β–stimulated genes. Activation of the factor took place in the cytoplasm and was rapidly followed by nuclear translocation (14,16). Several cell lines selected for resistance to the biological effects of type I IFNs were shown to be defective in ISGF3 activation (17). Purified ISGF3 had the ability to stimulate ISRE-dependent transcription in vitro (18). Moreover, a mutagenesis approach taken by Ian Kerr, George Stark, and their collegues (described below) confirmed the crucial role of ISGF3 in IFN-α/β–stimulated transcription. These studies provided ample evidence that ISGF3 was indeed the activating transcription factor for IFN-α/β–stimulated genes.

ISGF3 was purified and biochemically characterized in the laboratory of James Darnell, Jr. at the Rockefeller University. It turned out to be a protein complex containing species of 113, 91, 84 and 48 kDa (18,19). Using oligonucleotides complementary to peptide sequences from the purified proteins, all components were molecularly cloned from cDNA libraries. The 91- and 84-kDa proteins were shown to be alternatively spliced products from the same gene with the 84-kDa protein lacking 38 amino acids at the carboxy-terminus (20). The 113-kDa protein is highly homologous to the 91-kDa component with an amino acid identity of 42% in an overlapping 715–amino acid region (21). More strikingly, the 113-kDa and 91/84-kDa proteins both contain SH2 and SH3 domains in the carboxy-terminal half, and heptad leucine repeats with the potential to form an amphipathic helix toward the amino-terminus. These unique structural features together with the mode of activation by cytoplasmic tyrosine kinases (see below) made the 91- and 113-kDa proteins the first cloned members of a family of cytokine-responsive transcription factors termed the signal transducer and activator of transcription (STAT) family (Fig. 1). They were renamed STAT1 and STAT2, respectively (see Table 2). The 91- and 84-kDa proteins are distinguished as STAT1α and STAT1β. Several regions within STAT1 have been shown to be necessary for the formation of the ISGF3 complex. These include the heptad leucine repeat, the SH2 domain, and tyrosine 701 which receives the activating phosphate group (22). The 48-kDa ISGF3 protein (p48), also designated γ component for reasons outlined in Section VII.B, was similarly purified and cloned (23). Earlier experiments had suggested that the protein might be the DNA binding subunit of the ISGF3 complex owing to its ability to bind to the ISRE with low affinity in the absence of STAT1 and STAT2 (19). This was confirmed both with the purified and with the recombinant in vitro translated protein (23). The amino-terminus containing the DNA binding domain of p48 had structural similarity both to the functionally analogous domains of the IRF family proteins, which also bind to the ISRE sequence (see below), and to the DNA binding domain of the c-Myb oncoprotein (23,24). The region of p48 required for the interaction with STAT1 and/or STAT2 for the formation of ISGF3 was mapped to amino acids 217–377. Intact ISGF3 differed somewhat in its DNA se-

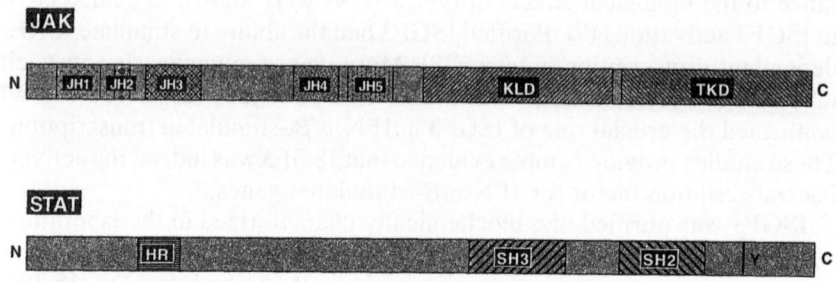

Figure 1 Prototype structure of JAKs and STATs. JH, JAK-homology region; KLD, kinase-like domain; TKD, tyrosine kinase domain; HR, heptad repeat; SH, SRC-homology domain; Y, tyrosine residue receiving the activating phosphorylation.

quence specificity with respect to uncomplexed p48, indicating that the STAT proteins contribute to DNA binding of the complex (24).

Owing to its original role in the transcriptional IFN-γ response, the other IFN response element, the IFN-γ activation site (GAS), was first instrumental in the detection of IFN-γ–regulated transcription factors. An IFN-γ activation factor (GAF) was identified (25). Like ISGF3 after IFN-α/β stimulation, GAF was rapidly activated in the cytoplasm of IFN-γ–treated cells. With the help of antibodies against the recombinant ISGF3 proteins, GAF was shown to be a dimer of tyrosine-phosphorylated STAT1 (26,27). The same STAT family transcription factor thus has the ability to form complexes of different DNA binding specificities depending on whether it forms homodimeric or heterooligomeric complexes. In IFN-α–treated cells, a factor with indistinguishable properties from GAF was rapidly and transiently activated to bind to the GAS and designated IFN-α activation factor (AAF) (13). It was shown to contain either STAT1 only or to contain the 48-kDa protein in addition (28). The composition of AAF apparently depends on the details of the GAS sequences found in different promoters. At the present time, the GAS found in the promoter of the IFN-inducible guanylate-binding protein (see Section VI.D) is the only example of a GAS sequence that forms complexes involving STAT1 and p48.

STAT1 thus plays a dual role in IFN-α/β–stimulated transcriptional induction, because it acts on the ISRE as part of the ISGF3 complex and on the GAS, presumably either as a dimer or in a complex of unknown stoichiometry with p48. A second, IFN-α–stimulated transcription factor which binds to a subset of GAS elements was also identified (28). This factor, designated AAF2, did not contain the STAT1 protein. Recent data suggest it might be identical with another member of the growing STAT family, STAT3, which has been shown in some cell types to be activated by IFN-α/β (29,30) and which possesses the ability of heterodimerizing with STAT1 (30). Different STAT family members thus may contribute to transcriptional induction via GAS sequences, and some of these may be activated in a cell type–dependent manner.

B. IRF Family Proteins

Transcription factors belonging to the interferon regulatory factor (IRF) family were cloned and characterized as proteins binding to the virus-responsive region in the promoter of the IFN-β gene (31,32). A "southwestern" screening of a cDNA expression library resulted in the detection of two cDNAs coding for proteins (IRF-1 and IRF-2) that bind to the positive regulatory domain I (PRDI) element within the IFN-β promoter. This DNA element resembles the core ISRE sequence (see Table 1). In transfection experiments, IRF-1 had a stimulatory effect on a cotransfected IFN-β promoter, whereas IRF-2 had a repressive effect (32). A model in which IRF-1 induction by viral infection leads to displacement of IRF-2 from the DNA was proposed. As a result, IRF-1 exerts a stimulatory effect. With levels of IRF-1 declining, IRF-2 takes over its repressive role again and silences the promoter. Although transcriptional induction of the IFN-β promoter is by far more complex and involves a number of proteins in addition to IRFs (33), a number of experimental systems suggest that the IRFs do indeed antagonize each other (32,34).

Early studies on proteins binding to ISREs from different IFN-inducible genes showed that besides ISGF3 at least two other complexes bound specifically to the response element in an EMSA. Constitutive complexes were designated either C1/C2 or ISGF1 (9,35). Complexes induced by either IFN-α/β or IFN-γ were designated M, G, or ISGF2 (9,36). The appearance of the inducible M, G, or ISGF2 complexes in IFN-treated cells was delayed and sensitive to the simultaneous presence of CHX (9,36). Therefore, none of them qualified as containing primary transcriptional activators of IFN-stimulated genes. Purification and cloning of ISGF2 demonstrated that this factor is identical to IRF-1 (37). Reagents to recombinant IRF-2 proved that the protein is a constituent of ISGF-1 or C1/C2, whereas complexes M and G were shown at least for some ISREs to contain both IRF-1 and IRF-2 (38).

A distinct IRF family member was obtained in an expression cloning approach using the ISRE from a murine major histocompatibility (MHC) class I gene (39). This protein is about 50% identical to mouse IRF-1 and IRF-2 in the amino-terminal DNA binding domain. It was designated interferon consensus sequence-binding protein (ICSBP). In contrast to both IRF-1 and IRF-2, its expression is restricted to cells from hematopoietic lineages. Like IRF-2, the ICSBP is constitutively expressed and further inducible by IFN-γ owing to a GAS sequence in its promoter (40). Moreover, it appears that ICSBP and IRF-2 are functionally equivalent. Both ICSBP and IRF-2 efficiently repress IFN-α/β– or IFN-γ–stimulated transcription in transfection experiments (41,42). ICSBP associates with both IRF-1 and IRF-2 in vivo, and the resulting complexes have higher affinity for the ISRE than ICSBP alone. Moreover, ICSBP inhibits binding of the 48-kDa ISGF3 subunit to the ISRE (43). Thus, the inhibitory activity of ICSBP might not only result from a constitutive occupation of the ISRE but also from formation of transcriptionally inactive complexes with other IRF family members.

With the exception of the 48-kDa ISGF3 protein, the role of the IRF family proteins in inducing IFN-α/β–stimulated genes is still not entirely clear. Particularly a repressive effect of IRF-2 or ICSBP in vivo awaits further confirmation. Mice containing a targeted disruption of the IRF-2 gene (IRF-2 k/o) showed no obvious derepression or altered induction kinetics of IFN-α/β–stimulated genes (44). On the other hand, overexpression of IRF-2 in cell lines increases their potential for anchorage-independent growth and tumor formation in nude mice. This was proposed to result from a constitutive repression of IRF-1–stimulated genes which control growth or may be required for apoptosis (45,46). The stimulatory role for IRF-1 on type I IFN-inducible genes has been suggested by cotransfection experiments with ISRE-dependent reporter plasmids or by IRF-1 transgenic cell lines (47–49). Fibroblasts from mice with a disrupted IRF-1 gene showed normal induction for some type I IFN-stimulated genes (1–8; 2′,5′-OAS, pKR [44,50]), but in a different study, the IFN-α inducibility of the murine GBP gene was reduced in ES cells from IRF-1 k/o mice compared with wild-type controls (51). A more drastic effect of the IRF-1 null allele is seen in the IFN-γ inducibility of some genes containing the ISRE in their promoters. mRNAs corresponding to the genes encoding iNOS or the mouse GBP the mouse GBP were barely detectable under these conditions (50,52).

How ISGF3 and IRF-1 might interact to stimulate transcription from ISRE-containing promoters has not been clarified. Since ISGF3 appears in the nucleus early after IFN treatment, its role might be to induce an open promoter conformation which then allows other proteins like IRF-1 to participate in maintaining an elevated transcription rate. This model is especially appealing in the case of the IFN-γ response of the GBP gene where interactions between GAS and ISRE most likely involve GAF and IRF-1. In vivo footprinting experiments showed that the human GBP gene GAS is occupied for less than 2 hrs after IFN-γ treatment, whereas transcription rates stay up for more than 48 hr (53). This indicates a likely role for maintainance factors of transcription in the IFN response, and IRF-1 might be one example of such a factor.

C. Differences Between Individual Genes in the Transcriptional Response to IFN-α/β

The sections above have introduced transcription factors and response elements required for responsiveness to IFN-α/β. These factors represent a common denominator for transcriptional induction, but the contribution of individual proteins to the induction of a given gene may vary. Affinities of ISRE or GAS sequences for STAT or IRF proteins differ due to variations in the consensus sequence (38). For the ISRE, the sequences found in the GBP and 9/27 genes represent extreme examples: the GBP ISRE has low affinity for ISGF3 but high affinity for IRFs, whereas the exact opposite is true for the 9/27 ISRE (36,54). Factors M and G have been shown to differ for the 9/27 and 6–16 ISREs, representing either the 48-kDa ISGF3 protein not complexed to STAT1 and STAT2 (9/27) or complexes containing IRF-1 and IRF-2 (6-16, [38]). The exact implications of these variations are unknown. In the GBP gene, the low affinity for ISGF3 might explain the requirement for the GAS in IFN-α–stimulated transcriptional induction. Sequences outside the consensus ISRE may also contribute to the induction of gene expression. Transcription of the 2′,5′-OAS gene in response to IFN-α is less reduced in IFN-resistant cell lines defective in ISGF3 activation than for example transcription of the 6-16 gene. The DNA sequence required for OASe gene transcription in these cells might lic upstream of the ISRE (55).

With exception of a three-base-pair palindrome (TT A/C . . . T/G AA), the GAS sequence varies considerably between different promoters. However, all known GAS bind AAF, the STAT1 dimer (with or without p48). Differences are found in the affinity for AAF2 (STAT3?); some GAS do not bind this protein at all (e.g., GBP), whereas others bind it with high affinity (e.g., IFP53 [28]). Owing to this difference, the response of individual promoters with GAS elements to IFN-α can also be expected to vary. This has not been thoroughly tested.

STATs and IRF family transcription factors thus provide a potential for variation in transcriptional induction by type I IFNs which is exploited differently by individual genes owing to the detailed sequence of their response elements. Additionally, the response of genes to either type of IFN can be controlled by the maturation or differentiation state of a cell. Particularly cells of the monocyte/macrophage lineage show increased activation of STAT transcription factors or gene transcription mediated by GAS- or ISRE sequences as they progress to the more mature stages of differentiation (55a,55b).

V.   ACTIVATION OF TRANSCRIPTION FACTORS IN CELLS TREATED WITH TYPE I IFNs

Research conducted during the past 3 years to reveal the events occurring between ligand binding of type I IFN receptors and the activation of the transcription factors that mediate rapid induction of IFN-responsive genes has entirely focused on the STAT family proteins. This is justified by the overwhelming evidence for the role of these proteins as primary transcriptional activators. IRF-1 activity in IFN-treated cells appears to be regulated by de novo synthesis of the protein, although a posttranslational event that influences its ability to stimulate gene expression can not be ruled out. At any rate, the IRF-1 effect in the context of an IFN response is delayed and sensitive to protein synthesis inhibition; there is no indication that IRF-1 might contribute to the rapid onset of transcription occurring minutes after signals from the receptor have been generated.

Two independent strategies have been developed to identify the molecules involved in ISGF3 activation. A biochemical approach identified signaling proteins with the help of reagents produced against recombinant proteins. A second approach to the problem used a combination of mutagenesis and genetic complementation to reconstitute IFN-α/β signaling in cultured fibrosarcoma cells. It may not be surprising that the rapid progress in the field was achieved by combining the two strategies and through productive interactions among the contributing scientists (reviewed in refs. 56, and 57). For the genetic complementation approach, the HT1080 fibrosarcoma cell line was manipulated to express the *gpt* gene under the control of the ISRE from the 6-16 gene promoter. The cells were then mutagenized and subsequently selected in IFN-α + 6-thioguanine for the inability to induce *gpt* expression (58). With this, or a similar procedure based on the inability to induce a cell surface marker under the control of an IFN-γ–responsive promoter (59,60), a number of mutations were selected over the years with defects in type I IFN signaling, type II IFN signaling, or both (Table 3). Using cell fusion techniques, the individual mutant cell lines were subdivided into different complementation groups. The success of the approach was apparent from the fact that mutagenized lines were derived with defects in any one of all three ISGF3 proteins (57,61,62).

Table 3 Mutant Cell Lines with Known Signaling Defects in the Response to IFN-α/β

Complementation group	Phenotype	Complementing protein
U1	IFN-α^-, IFN-$\beta^{+/-}$, IFN-γ^+	TYK2
U2	IFN-$\alpha^{+/-}$, IFN-$\beta^{+/-}$, IFN-$\gamma^{+/-}$	p48
U3	IFN-α^-, IFN-β^-, IFN-γ^-	STAT1
U4	IFN-α^-, IFN-β^-, IFN-γ^-	JAK1
U5	IFN-α^-, IFN-β^-, IFN-γ^+	IFNAR2[a]
U6	IFN-α^-, IFN-β^-, IFN-γ^+	STAT2
γ1	IFN-α^+, IFN-β^+, IFN-γ^-	JAK2
γ2	IFN-α^+, IFN-β^+, IFN-γ^-	?

[a] Lutfalla G, et al. EMBO J 1995;14:5100–5108.
Source: Adapted from refs. 57 and 137.

A major breakthrough and the first experimental evidence concerning the kinases responsible for STAT activation came from the complementation of the U1 (1,11) cell line. U1 cells are unusual, because gene activation occurs normally in response to IFN-γ, partially in response to IFN-β, and not at all after IFN-α treatment. This phenotype could be corrected by complementation with genomic DNA containing a protein tyrosine kinase (PTK) gene designated *tyk2* (63). A *tyk2* cDNA had been isolated earlier using a polymerase chain reaction (PCR)–based strategy with primers to tyrosine kinase domain consensus sequences (64). However, a function for the kinase in cellular signaling had remained elusive. It is still a matter of investigation why U1 cells retain some responsiveness to IFN-β. The answer may lie in the structural role the TYK2 protein plays in the type I IFN receptor (see Chapter 1). U1 cells show strongly reduced cell surface binding of IFN-α which can be restored with a TYK2 protein lacking the tyrosine kinase domain (S. Pellegrini, personal communication). A possible explanation for the remaining activity of IFN-β might thus be that receptor association of this cytokine is less affected by the absence of TYK2.

The cloning of TYK2 precipitated numerous experiments to investigate the PTKs' role in cytokine signaling. Further movement in the field was caused by the fact that two TYK2 homologues were found in sequence data bases. Both had been cloned in screenings for pTK-homologous proteins by PCR. Like TYK2, these two kinases, designated JAK1 and JAK2 (JAK, just another kinase or Janus kinase [65]), had the distinctive feature of two domains with homology to catalytic PTK domains (see Fig. 1). Therefore, PTKs of the JAK family turned into promising candidates for cytokine-induced signaling paths (66). Within a short period, several labo-

ratories reported data to support the idea of a "JAK-pot" in signaling
paths toward STAT transcription factors (depicted for type I IFNs in Fig.
2).

IFN-α/β stimulates tyrosine phosphorylation and activation of the
TYK2 and JAK1 kinases. As a direct consequence, STAT1 and STAT2
are phosphorylated on a single and corresponding tyrosine residue (Y_{701}
in STAT1 and Y_{690} in STAT2, [22,67–69]). Tyrosine phosphorylation leads
to dimerization of STAT1 to form AAF or to oligomerization of STAT1,
STAT2, and p48 to form ISGF3. The STAT1 SH2 domain is required for
dimerization because this process can be competed with phosphopeptides
containing Y_{701} (27). As mentioned above, the formation of ISGF3 requires both the STAT1 heptad repeat sequence and the SH2 domain. IFN-
γ treatment of cells also leads to activation of JAK1, but the second activated PTK in this case is JAK2 (59,70–72). As a consequence, only STAT1
is phosphorylated on Y_{701}. This leads to formation of GAF, which like
AAF contains or consists of dimerized STAT1.

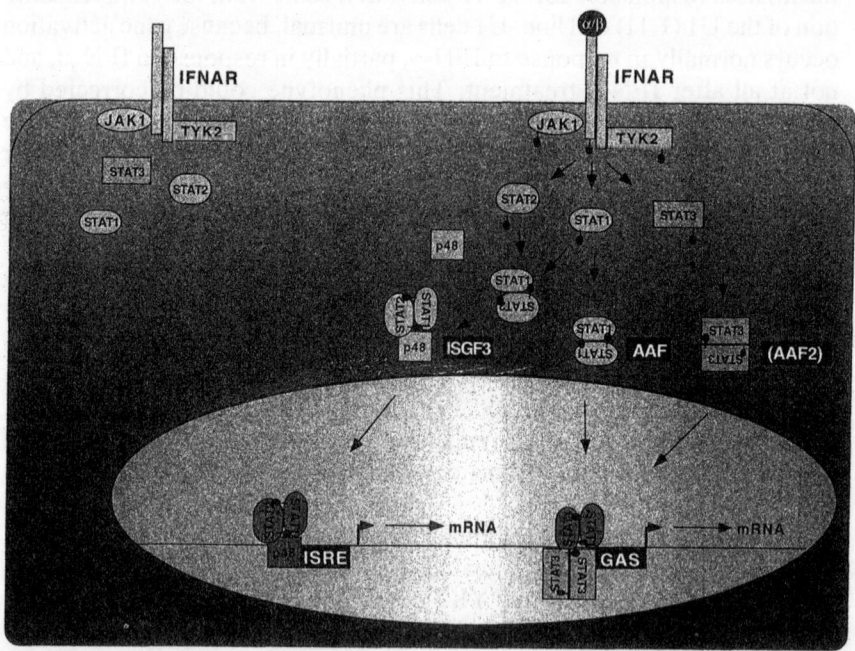

Figure 2 The IFN-α/β responsive JAK-STAT pathway. Black, closed circles
indicate IFN-induced tyrosine phosphorylation events. The identity of AAF2 with
the STAT3 homodimer is unclear and STAT1-STAT3 heterodimers, which are
formed in vivo, have not been depicted. Further explanation is provided in the
text. IFNAR, type I IFN receptor.

This model of JAK-STAT signaling leaves a number of questions unanswered, but the involvement of its major players rests on firm ground. Biochemical data showed tyrosine phosphorylation and activation of the JAK family kinases in response to both IFN types, with TYK2 and JAK1 activated in response to IFN-α/β and JAK1 and JAK2 activated in response to IFN-γ(59,70–72). Overexpression of either JAK1 or JAK2 leads to transcriptional activation of a GAS-dependent reporter gene (72). Several lines of evidence suggest a direct association of JAK family kinases with IFN receptors (see Chapter 1). In an in vitro system, activation of STAT1 and STAT2 required only a cellular membrane fraction, whereas formation of ISGF3 required both IFN-treated membranes and cytoplasm (73,74). This suggests that all components required for STAT activation may be more or less strongly associated with the plasma membrane, but in addition ISGF3 formation requires cytoplasmic p48.

The strongest support for the JAK-STAT path came from further complementation of the cell lines selected for defective IFN signaling. One complementation group (U4), defective in IFN-α/β and IFN-γ signaling, could be restored with a JAK1 cDNA, and another one (γ1), selected for unresponsiveness to IFN-γ but normal in its response to IFN-α, could be restored with a JAK2 cDNA (59,71). Therefore, JAK kinases must be essential components in the path between IFN receptors and the STAT proteins. The data further prove the involvement of TYK2 and JAK1 in IFN-α/β–mediated ISGF3 activation and the role of JAK1 and JAK2 in IFN-γ–mediated GAF activation.

Despite the overwhelming progress that has recently been made, there are still numerous open questions in the scenario of events leading to STAT activation and transcription factor formation. The known components may not be all that is needed to activate JAK kinases or STAT factors. A (tyrosine) dephosphorylation step has been suggested in ISGF3 activation on the basis of order of inhibitor addition experiments in the IFN-α–dependent in vitro activation system of STATs (74). Interestingly, no vanadate-sensitivity (sensitivity to the inhibition of tyrosine phosphatases) was found in the activation of TYK2 (75). Crosstalk between the JAK kinases and kinases in other IFN-responsive signaling paths (e.g., PKC [76,77]) may also be possible. Serine kinases have been shown to modulate the DNA-binding activity of the STAT1 dimer in differentiating macrophages (78). STAT3, which is tyrosine phosphorylated in response to a variety of cytokines, including type I IFNs, undergoes a modification that is sensitive to the serine/threonine kinase inhibitor H7 in addition to tyrosine phosphorylation when activated by interleukin-6 (IL-6) (78a). Serine residue 727 of both STAT1 and STAT3 was recently shown to be phosphorylated in a regulated fashion, thus increasing the transactivating potential of both transciption factors (78b). Moreover, the mitogen-activated protein serine kinase (MAPK) ERK2 was found associated with the type I IFN receptor and to bind and phosphorylate STAT1 (78c). These results suggest that multiple signaling paths, originating from the same or from different cell surface receptors, converge on STATs to activate and modulate their activity.

Within the JAK-STAT path, the order of activation of the individual proteins has not been established. Assuming a direct enzyme-substrate relationship between JAKs and STATs (which has not been formally shown in IFN signaling), JAK activation should precede STAT activation. However, it is absolutely unclear whether stimulation of JAK1 and TYK2 occurs simultaneously, or one after the other, or whether one JAK family kinase is substrate for the other. Experiments aimed at clarifying this relationship have unambiguously shown a stringent interdependence of the activation of both kinases in type I IFN signaling. U1 cells (TYK2 deficient) cannot activate JAK1 in response to IFN-α/β. Vice versa, U4 cells (JAK1 deficient) cannot activate TYK2 (71). JAK1 overexpression leads to (auto?)activation of both JAK1 and JAK2 and vice versa (TYK2 has not been examined in this study, [72]). One explanation for this interdependence might lie in the role of JAK kinases in assembling the multisubunit receptor complex needed for signaling. Consistent with this, the interdependence of JAK family kinase activation is not seen after stimulation of cells with IL-6. Signals leading to JAK activation after IL-6 treatment are transmitted by a single protein, gp130 (79). A structural role for JAK kinases in assembling intact IFN receptor complexes is also suggested by the somewhat puzzling finding that U4 cells can be complemented with a kinase-negative JAK1 (79a). It appears that although both kinase *proteins* are needed for signaling, the same may not be true for their enzymatic activity.

In the process of ISGF3 formation, STAT1 tyrosine phosphorylation depends on the presence of (tyrosine phosphorylated?) STAT2. This is indicated by the inability of IFN-α/β to phosphorylate STAT1 on tyrosine in cells of the U6 complementation group (STAT2 defective [57]). In contrast, STAT2 tyrosine phosphorylation occurs in the U3 complementation group, although its nuclear translocation is less efficient compared with normal control cells (22). Despite these findings, there cannot be a general dependence of STAT1 phosphorylation on STAT2, because a variety of cytokines, including IFN-γ, activate STAT1 but not STAT2. In fact, STAT2 is one of few (the only?) examples of a STAT family transcription factor whose activation has only been observed in response to a single cytokine. Transcriptionally active ISGF3 can either contain STAT1α or STAT1β, because the U3 complementation group can be functionally reconstituted with either cDNA (62). A strikingly different result was obtained for the STAT1 dimer (AAF, GAF). U3 cells reconstituted with a STAT1α cDNA produced transcriptionally active STAT1 dimer, whereas reconstitution with STAT1β cDNA produced an IFN-responsive dimer with the ability to bind to the GAS but unable to stimulate transcription from a GAS-dependent reporter gene (69). STAT1β might thus be a naturally occurring antagonist to STAT1α activity on GAS-dependent transcription.

A. Differences Between IFN-α and IFN-β in STAT Factor Activation

As pointed out in the introduction to this chapter, there is no published evidence that STAT factor activation in response to either IFN-α subspecies or IFN-β involves different molecular events. However, recent findings in Schindler's (personal communication) laboratory indicate that significant differences may exist in the balance of IFN-α- or IFN-β–activated ISRE- and GAS-binding transcription factors. At concentrations of IFN-α and IFN-β that produce equal amounts of activated ISGF3, IFN-β induces much higher levels of the GAS-binding factors, STAT1 dimer (AAF), STAT3 dimer, and STAT1-STAT3 heterodimer. The higher amount of AAF is probably due to a more efficient tyrosine phosphorylation of STAT1 in response to IFN-β. It will be an important future task to investigate the cause of these phenomena in the STAT activation paths and to unravel the effect of a stronger activation of GAS-dependent transcription on cellular functions.

B. Downregulation of IFN-α/β–Induced Transcription

There are two ways to repress or downregulate promoters of inducible genes (excluding changes of chromatin structure). The first is to inactivate the activating transcription factor by either degrading it, removing the activating modification, or by the association of an inhibitory factor. The second is to produce or activate repressors that compete with activators for binding to the response element. Both mechanisms have been suggested to play a role in gene regulation by IFNs, but their relative contributions are unclear. In many cells, the activation/deactivation cycle of ISGF3 corresponds quite well with transcription rates of IFN-induced genes (9). How deactivation of ISGF3 occurs and whether the STAT proteins cycle between active and inactive forms remains to be elucidated. A nuclear tyrosine phosphatase involved in the dephosphorylation of STAT1 has been suggested based on cell fractionation and vanadate inhibition studies (80). Whether nuclear dephosphorylation will target the STAT proteins for degradation or allow them to leave the nucleus for another round of activation is an interesting question still to be answered. Inactivating ISGF3 might not be enough to silence IFN-stimulated genes if IRF-1 is able to maintain transcription. The antagonistic action of repressors like IRF-2 or ICSBP is conceptually appealing but is rendered unlikely by the lack of derepression in IRF-2 k/o animals (see above). Redundant proteins might take over the role of IRF2, but such proteins have so far only been found in hematopoietic cells that express ICSBP.

A new and interesting aspect in the negative regulation of IFN-α/β–induced genes has emerged from a recent study by Larner's laboratory (81). A number of cervical cancer cell lines produced only low levels of ISGF3 EMSA activity following stimulation with IFN-α/β, but they were shown to contain normal levels of activated STATs. The cells expressed a "transcriptional knockout" (TKO) activity, inhibiting STAT association with the 48-kDa ISGF3 subunit. In addition, TKO inhibited binding of IRF-1 and IRF-2 to the ISRE, indicating that it might keep all IRF family proteins from binding to their DNA recognition sites. Whether TKO can be part of a physiological IFN response, or whether tumor cells are selected to express a protein which is not normally expressed to function within the IFN system in order to acquire resistence to the growth inhibitory activity of IFN-α/β, remains to be established.

VI. FUNCTIONS OF IFN-α/β–INDUCED PROTEINS

There have been fairly extensive reviews on some of the proteins induced by IFNs (82–86), and their pharmacokinetics are discussed in Chapter 3. In this section, I will not attempt to review all that is known about these proteins, but rather give a brief overview concerning their role in the cellular IFN response and indicate recent developments as to their functions and regulation.

A. 2′,5′-Oligoadenylate Synthetase and 2′,5′-Oligoadenylate–Dependent RNAase

In human cells, IFN-α/β induces the synthesis of several isoforms of a synthetase that oligomerizes adenylates via a 2′,5′-phosphodiester bond (2′,5′-oligoadenylate synthetase, [2′,5′-OASe], reviewed in ref. 86). The enzyme contains a binding domain for double-stranded (ds) RNA (87), and binding of certain species of cellular or viral dsRNAs is required for enzymatic activity. 2′,5′-OAS might play a role in physiological processes like RNA splicing (88); however, in the context of the IFN response, its best studied function is to promote the resistance to certain viruses (89). This occurs through activation of an RNAase by the OAS product 2′,5′A.

Following 2',5'A binding, the oligoadenylate-dependent RNAase (RNAase L) degrades mRNAs transcribed from both viral genomes and from cellular genes thought to be involved in growth control. RNAase L protein is significantly increased in IFN-α/β-treated cells. A cDNA encoding the 83.5-kDa RNAase L enzyme has been obtained, and the corresponding mRNA is induced by type I IFN (90). Stable overexpression of an RNAase L cDNA, coding for a truncated enzyme lacking the carboxy-terminal catalytic domain, inhibited the function of the endogenous ribonuclease L. This dominant-negative mutant inhibited not only the IFN-induced response to encephalomyocarditis virus but also the antiproliferative effect in murine SVT2 cells (91). These experiments thus confirmed an earlier notion that the importance of RNAase L activity in the IFN response goes beyond a role in producing the antiviral state (reviewed in ref. 92).

B.   dsRNA-Dependent eIF-2α Protein Kinase

A well-studied biological effect of type I IFN is to downregulate cellular translation—an effect thought to disturb predominantly the synthesis of viral proteins. A target for translational inhibition is the initiation factor eIF-2α. IFN-α/β-treated cells contain elevated levels of a protein kinase with the ability of selectively phosphorylating eIF-2α on a single serine residue (reviewed in refs. 84 and 86), thereby keeping it from recycling to an active form in translational initiation. Protein kinase activity depends on the presence of dsRNA species. The enzyme, now designated pKR, has been purified as a 68-kDa protein and cloned (93). It contains a binding domain for dsRNA which is unrelated to that of OASe (87,94). DsRNA binding leads to autophosphorylation and activation of enzymatic activity. Several viral RNAs have been shown to activate pKR (84 and refs. therein). However, some viruses produce RNAs that inhibit the kinase like the Epstein-Barr virus EBER1 RNA or the adenoviral VAI RNA. Moreover, some viruses can either synthesize inhibitory proteins or induce the synthesis of cellular proteins which inhibit pKR and thus abolish its antiviral effect (84 and refs. therein).

   A function for pKR not only in the antiviral response but also in cellular growth control is again suggested by overexpression of a mutant kinase. The mammalian enzyme can act as a growth suppressor in yeast by functionally replacing the yeast homologue GCN2 in eIF-2α phosphorylation (95). In two studies, a dominant negative mutation abolishing enzymatic activity caused a transformed phenotype in murine NIH3T3 cells (96,97). In further support of a possible function of pKR in growth control, the same dominant-negative pKR has been shown to abolish the growth-inhibitory effect of IRF-1 (98). However, mice with a targeted disruption of the pKR locus show no apparent abnormalities, which would indicate a redundant function of the enzyme in the control of cellular proliferation (99).

A recently reported role of pKR might be to enhance the induction of cytokine genes containing binding sites for the transcription factor NF-κB in their promoters, like for example the IFN-β gene (100) or the tumor necrosis factor-α (TNF-α) gene. One of many NF-κB inducers are dsRNAs like synthetic poly rI–poly rC. Several lines of evidence now suggest a role of pKR in inactivating the NF-κB inhibitor IκB (101). Support for this idea also comes from studies with cells from pKR k/o mice in which NF-κB activation does not occur in response to dsRNA. Interestingly, it can be restored by pretreating cells with IFN-α (99), indicating that IFN may induce a functional substitute for pKR.

C. Other Proteins with a Potential Role in the Growth Inhibitory Effect of IFN-α/β—202 and 9/27 (Leu-13) Gene Products

A potential link to the inhibition of cellular proliferation has recently been suggested for two other IFN-induced genes. The mouse 202 gene belongs to a cluster of type I IFN-inducible genes on mouse chromosome 1 (102). It encodes a protein of 50 kDa which accumulates in the cell nucleus. Data presented at a recent meeting showed that the 202-encoded p50 contains a LXCXE consensus motif found in proteins that bind to the Rb tumor suppressor gene product. The 50 kDa protein binds to the hypophosphorylated form of Rb in vitro (103). It may thus be a candidate protein for the inhibition of Rb phosphorylation that was reported to occur in response to IFN-α/β (104). Underphosphorylated Rb cannot function in the G_1/S transition during the cell cycle.

The second protein suggested as an effector of the antiproliferative response to IFN-α/β is the 9/27 gene product. It encodes a 17-kDa membrane protein shown to be identical to the Leu-13 surface antigen present on B and T cells and endothelial cells. Antibodies to this 17-kDa protein reduce the cellular growth rate and potentiate the antiproliferative effect of IFN-α/β (105).

D. Mx and GBP Proteins

Mx and GBP proteins fall into one group by virtue of their common ability to bind and hydrolyze GTP. There is no structural relationship between Mx and GBP. Moreover, although Mx has a well-documented role in antiviral responses, an antiviral role of GBP is still unclear and mostly suggested by biochemical analogy to Mx.

Most species contain several distinct Mx proteins which are induced almost exclusively by type I IFN (reviewed in refs. 88 and 106). Mouse Mx was the first to be discovered as being decisive in determining susceptibility or resistance to influenza virus. Further studies showed that Mx proteins confer resistance also to other groups of viruses including Rhabdoviridae like vesicular stomatitis virus (reviewed in refs. 106 and 107). Their antiviral activity requires an intact GTP binding site (88). Mx proteins reside either in the cytoplasm or the cell nucleus and, depending on their subcellular localization, block different steps in influenza virus replication (108). In the nucleus, primary influenza transcription is inhibited, and a direct interaction with the viral polymerase has been proposed. It is noteworthy that not all Mx proteins display an identical spectrum of antiviral activities. For example, the human MxA confers resistence to both influenza and VSV, whereas the murine Mx2 only affects the VSV life cycle. Other Mx proteins, like the rat Mx, inhibit neither influenza nor VSV replication (107). The molecular basis for this is currently not known but appears to reside in subtle changes of the primary amino acid sequence. Functions of Mx proteins besides their contribution to the antiviral state are unclear. A more general role in protein trafficking has been proposed, mainly based on a homology between Mx proteins and the yeast VPS1 protein, which is involved in vacuolar protein sorting (109).

In contrast to the Mx proteins, GBPs are induced by both IFN types (110,111). They have been identified through their specific binding to affinity matrices containing guanine nucleotides. GBPs do not contain a canonical tripartite GTP binding site; they lack one consensus motif (112). A very unusual feature is their mode of hydrolyzing GTP—GMP is produced instead of GDP (113). Another interesting finding is a CAAX motif at the C-terminal end which can be modified by farnesylation (113). GBPs may thus be constitutively membrane associated or have regulated subcellular localization.

VII. INTERACTIONS OF TYPE I IFN WITH OTHER CYTOKINES

Complex inflammatory pathogenesis like that leading to multiple sclerosis (MS) involves the activity of numerous cytokines. The effect of IFN-β on the course of this disease can only be understood if one knows how it influences the biological activity of other cytokines. Interactions of particular interest are those leading to an influence of IFN-β on the proinflammatory cytokines, IFN-γ and TFN-α, which are thought to make a major contribution to MS progression. These interactions may occur at the level of synthesis, or through suppression or enhancement of a biological effect. (Also see chapter 7.)

A.   Influence of IFN-β on Its Own Synthesis

IFN-β induces very little transcription of its own gene. However, it was noted that type I IFNs can "prime" cells for higher IFN-β production during viral infection (114). The molecular basis of the priming phenomenon has been studied and found to reside within the same region of the IFN-β promoter that is required for virus inducibility. Particularly, the PRDI element, an IRF-1 binding site, is able to mediate a priming effect (115). Increasing the levels of IRF-1 might thus be how IFN-β stimulates its own synthesis on viral infection. Signals elicited by the virus activate transcription factors like NF-κB which interact with IRF-1 in promoter stimulation (37,48). In cells with a constitutively expressed IRF-1 transgene, the protein induces little, but detectable, synthesis of IFN-β message and biologically active protein (49). Several cytokines, including TNF-α, can induce higher levels of IRF-1 and thus exert either a priming or an activating effect on the transcription of the IFN-β gene (116).

B.   Interactions with IFN-γ

There are multiple levels of influence of IFN-β on the pleiotropic activity of IFN-γ. Through yet unknown mechanisms, IFN-β can influence IFN-γ synthesis. With respect to biological activity, IFN-β and IFN-γ may act both in a synergistic or antagonistic fashion. For example, the antiviral or antiproliferative effects can be strongly enhanced if cells are treated simultaneously with both IFN types. In the activation of macrophages, IFN-β either promotes or suppresses the activating effect of IFN-γ depending on the concentration at which the two cytokines are present (117). Moreover, primed macrophages may produce type I IFNs and thus be capable of autocrine stimulation.

   The antagonistic activity of IFN-α/β and IFN-γ in the induction of MHC class II (MHC II) genes might be of extreme importance for the course of MS. A role for microglial MHC II proteins in autoimmune demyelination was recently confirmed in mice. Twitcher mice are a murine model of globoid cell leukodystrophy and develop severe demyelinating lesions. MHC II–negative twitcher mice, generated by mating to I-A$_\beta^{0/0}$ animals, showed a strong reduction in the severity of demyelinating lesions (118). A mechanistic explanation is beginning to emerge. It has been known for some time that IFN-α/β can counteract IFN-γ–induced MHC II synthesis in macrophages (119). Antagonism of IFN-α/β to IFN-γ–induced MHC II upregulation was more recently also demonstrated for both IFN-β and TGF-β in human astrocytoma cells (120,121). These studies also indicated that suppression occurs at the level of transcription (120,122). Thus, IFN-β is likely to influence activities of factors that regulate MHC II transcription. Proteins with a decisive role in directing both expression and repression of MHC II genes, designated CIITA and YB-1, respectively, have been identified and cloned (123–126). An influence of IFN-β on their activity can now be tested.

MHC II gene transcription in response to IFN-γ occurs by a mechanism that does not seem to involve ISRE or GAS sequences (reviewed in ref. 127). In contrast to the antagonism of the two IFN types on transcription of MHC II genes, IFN-α/β and IFN-γ enhance each other's activity on promoters with ISRE and/or GAS sequences, especially when suboptimal concentrations are used for stimulation (111). The molecules mediating the additive or even synergistic effect of the two IFN types are, at least in part, known. In some cell types, IFN-γ induces the synthesis of the 48-kDa ISGF3 protein, which was therefore also designated the ISGF3 γ component (128). IFN-γ also increases transcription of the STAT1 gene but not of the STAT2 gene (129). For these reasons, a "superinduction" of type I IFN–responsive genes can be observed in cells that have been pretreated with IFN-γ. It is much more pronounced in the case of genes regulated by the ISRE sequence, indicating that the 48-kDa protein is rate limiting for the assembly of ISGF3 in some cell types. Interestingly, IFN-γ also influences the repression of genes following stimulation with IFN-α/β, and this antirepressive effect on transcription is directly correlated with an antideactivating effect on ISGF3 (111). It is possible that IFN-γ represses a phosphatase activity leading to a reversible deactivation of ISGF3.

C. Interactions with Other Cytokines

Until now there is very limited knowledge about an influence of type I IFN on molecular mechanisms involved in the synthesis or biological effects of cytokines with a strong proinflammatory activity. One exception is the gene encoding IL-8. Transcription of the IL-8 gene is induced by various agents, including TNF-α or IL-1. If added simultaneously with these cytokines, IFN-β suppresses transcriptional induction through a mechanism involving the IL-8 promoter NF-κB binding site (130,131). This suppressive effect is of transient nature and, it is not observed if IFN-β is added long before TNF-α. In fact, the synthesis of IL-8 mRNA in response to certain bacterial lipopolysaccharides is increased in IFN-β–preincubated ("primed") cells (132). Many biological activities of the inflammatory cytokines TNF-α and IL-1 require the activation of transcription factor NF-κB (reviewed in ref. 133). This protein complex is therefore an attractive target for antiinflammatory cytokines. However, a repressive effect of IFN-α/β on the synthesis or activation of NF-κB has, to my knowledge, not been reported. In contrast, NF-κB and IFN-induced transcription factors (IRF-1) cooperatively activate some promoters, like those of MHC I genes, and of the IFN-β gene itself (100,134,135).

Available experimental evidence suggests that TNF, IL-1, or IL-8 form a class of polypeptide ligands that do not activate JAKs and STATs. Therefore, crosstalk with those cytokines that act via JAKs and STATs may occur by fundamentally different mechanisms compared with crosstalk between cytokines that activate JAK-STAT signaling paths. Consistent with the assumption that JAK-STAT paths form an interactive network, multiple cytokines and growth factors are able to activate JAK kinases and STAT factors (136; reviewed in refs. 57 and 137). Among these is ciliary neurotrophic factor (CNTF), which activates STAT1 in neuroblastoma cells (138). Most STATs differ somewhat in their binding specificity, so GAS elements can be subdivided into distinct types depending on which STATs they bind besides the STAT1 dimer (139). Since most, or even all, GAS elements bind several STATs, and most STATs can be activated by several cytokines, a GAS element will make a gene subject to regulation by multiple cell surface stimuli. A good example for this is provided by the GAS element in the gene encoding the FcγRI receptor. This sequence binds several distinct STATs activated by many different stimuli (136). Among these are IFN-γ and IL-10, which stimulate FcγRI transcription, and granulocyte-macrophage colony-stimulating factor (GM-CSF), IL-3, and IL-4, which exert a repressive effect (136,140).

The implications of the JAK-STAT network for type I IFNs are that, in principle, many cytokines are able to impinge on the cellular response to type I IFNs either through their own activation of STATs or through an effect on the activation of STATs by IFN-α/β. Vice versa, IFN-α/β is likely to affect responses to other cytokines using the same JAKs or STATs (see Fig. 2). Mutual influences may be costimulatory, repressive, or modulatory, and it is therefore hard to predict the behavior of a GAS-regulated gene in a cell that is stimulated with several cytokines either simultaneously or sequentially. Experimental support for these assumptions is provided by several studies showing that type I IFN–inducible genes are transcribed in response to other cell surface ligands (141,142). However, besides the IFN-α and IFN-γ interactions described in Section VII.B, there have not been many studies investigating transcription in a situation of combined treatment with type I IFNs and other cytokines. One rare example of such a study reports a repressive effect of IL-4 on IFN-α/β–induced transcription of the ISRE-containing ISG54 gene and links this effect to the inability of IFN-α/β to activate ISGF3 after pretreatment of monocytes with IL-4 (141).

VIII. CONCLUSIONS

The scientific work I have tried to integrate in this chapter has generated a wealth of knowledge about the molecular biology of type I IFNs. We now know many of the genes regulated by IFNs and have delineated the DNA sequences required for their transcriptional regulation. The transcription factors binding to these sequences have been cloned and crucial signals and signaling molecules required for their activation have been established. Progress has also been made concerning the biological activities of the IFN-induced proteins even though we still have no function for several of them. The challenging task for the future will be to put all the parts and modules of the IFN system together and place them into the proper cellular context and biological activity. This will include interactive effects with the cytokines determining the onset and the course of MS. The JAK-STAT signaling path leading to gene activation will provide a valuable basis for rapid progress towards this goal.

ACKNOWLEDGMENTS

I thank Manuela Baccarini (Vienna Biocenter) and Mathias Müller (Veterinary Medical University, Vienna) for helpful comments to the manuscript and Alexander von Gabain (Vienna Biocenter) for support. Because of space limitations, I have frequently cited reviews. I apologize to many colleagues whose original work does not appear in the reference list.

REFERENCES

1. Revel M, Chebath J. Interferon-activated genes. Trends Biochem Sci 1986; 11:166–170.
2. Friedman RL, Manley SP, McMahon M, Kerr IM, Stark GR. Transcriptional and posttranscriptional regulation of interferon-induced gene expression in human cells. Cell 1984; 38:745–755.
3. Friedman RM, Stark GR. α-Interferon–induced transcriptional of HLA and metallothionein genes containing homologous upstream sequences. Nature 1985; 314:637–639.
4. Larner AC, Chaudhuri A, Darnell JE. Transcriptional induction by interferon. J Biol Chem 1986; 261:453–459.
5. Gribaudo G, Toniato E, Engel DA, Lengyel P. Interferons as gene activators. Characteristics of an interferon-activatable enhancer. J Biol Chem 1987; 262:11878–11883.
6. Reich NC, Evans B, Levy DE, Fahey DE, Knight E, Darnell JE. Interferon-induced transcription of a gene encoding a 15 KDa protein depends on an upstream enhancer element. Proc Natl Acad Sci USA 1987; 84:6394–6398.

7. Cohen B, Peretz D, Vaiman D, Benech P, Chebath J. Enhancer-like interferon responsive sequences of the human and murine (2'-5') oligoadenylate synthetase gene promoters. EMBO J 1988; 7:1411-1419.

8. Porter ACG, Chernajovski Y, Dale TC, Gilbert CS, Stark GR, Kerr IM. Interferon response element of the human gene 6-16. EMBO J 1988; 7: 85-92.

9. Levy DE, Kessler DS, Pine R, Reich N, Darnell JE Jr. Interferon-induced nuclear factors that bind a shared promoter element correlate with positive and negative transcriptional control. Genes Dev 1988; 2:383-393.

10. Kessler DS, Levy DE, Darnell JE Jr. Two interferon-induced nuclear factors bind a single promoter element in interferon-stimulated genes. Proc Natl Acad 1988; 85:8521-8525.

11. Reid LE, Brasnett AH, Gilbert CS, Porter ACG, Gewert DR, Stark GR, Kerr IM. A single DNA response element can confer inducibility by both α- and γ-interferons. Proc Natl Acad Sci USA 1989; 86:840-844.

12. Lew DJ, Decker T, Strehlow I, Darnell JE Jr. Overlapping elements in the guanylate-binding protein gene promoter mediate transcriptional induction by alpha- and gamma interferons. Mol Cell Biol 1991; 11:182-191.

13. Decker T, Lew DJ, Darnell JE Jr. Two distinct IFN-α-dependent signal transduction pathways may contribute to activation of transcription of the GBP gene. Mol Cell Biol 1991; 11:5147-5153.

14. Dale TC, Imam AM, Kerr IM, Stark GR. Rapid activation by interferon α of a latent DNA-binding protein present in the cytoplasm of untreated cells. Proc Natl Acad Sci USA 1989; 86:1203-1207.

15. Rutherford MN, Hannigan GE, Williams BRG. Interferon-induced binding of nuclear factors to promoter elements of the 2-5A synthetase gene. EMBO J 1988; 7:751-759.

16. Levy DE, Kessler DS, Pine R, Darnell JE Jr. Cytoplasmic activation of ISGF-3, the positive regulator of interferon-α- stimulated transcription, reconstituted in vitro. Genes Dev 1989; 3:1362-1371.

17. Kessler DS, Pine R, Pfeffer LM, Levy DE, Darnell JE Jr. Cells resistant to interferon are defective in activation of a promoter-binding factor. EMBO J 1988; 7:3779-3783.

18. Fu X-Y, Kessler DS, Veals SA, Levy DE, Darnell JE Jr. ISGF-3, the transcriptional activator induced by interferon-α consists of multiple interacting polypeptide chains. Proc Natl Acad Sci USA 1990; 87:8555-8559.

19. Kessler DS, Veals SA, Fu X-Y, Levy DE. Interferon-α regulates nuclear translocation and DNA-binding affinity of ISGF-3, a multimeric transcriptional activator. Genes Dev 1990; 4:1753-1765.

20. Schindler C, Fu X-Y, Improta T, Aebersold RH, Darnell JE Jr. The proteins of ISGF-3: one gene encodes 91 and 84 kDa ISGF-3α proteins. Proc Natl Acad Sci 1992; 89:7836-7839.

21. Fu X-Y, Schindler C, Improta T, Aebersold RH, and Darnell JE Jr. The proteins of ISGF-3, the IFN-α induced activator define a new gene family of signal transducers. Proc Natl Acad Sci USA 1990; 89:7840-7843.

22. Improta T, Schindler C, Horvath CM, Kerr IM, Stark GR, Darnell JE Jr.

Transcription factor ISGF-3 formation requires phosphorylated Stat 91 protein, but Stat 113 protein is phosphorylated independently of Stat 91 protein. Proc Natl Acad Sci 1994; 91:4776–4780.

23. Veals SA, Santa Maria T, Levy DE. Two domains of ISGF3γ that mediate protein-DNA and protein-protein interactions during transcription factor assembly contribute to DNA-binding specificity. Mol Cell Biol 1993; 13: 196–206.

24. Veals SA, Schindler C, Leonard D, Fu X-Y, Aebersold R, Levy DE. Subunit of an IFN-α-responsive transcription factor is related to IRF and Myb families of DNA-binding proteins. Mol Cell Biol 1992; 12:3315–3324.

25. Decker T, Lew DJ, Mirkovitch J, Darnell JE Jr. Cytoplasmic activation of GAF, an IFN-γ-regulated DNA-binding factor. EMBO J 1991; 10:927–932.

26. Shuai K, Schindler C, Prezioso V, Darnell JE Jr. Activation of transcription by IFN-γ: Tyrosine phosphorylation of a 91-kD DNA-binding protein. Science 1992; 258:1808–1812.

27. Shuai K, Horvath C, Tsai-Huang LH, Qureshi SA, Cowburn D, Darnell JE Jr. Interferon activation of the transcription factor Stat91 involves dimerization through SH2-phosphotyrosyl peptide interactions. Cell 1994; 76: 821–828.

28. Seegert DS, Strehlow I, Klose B, Levy DE, Schindler C, Decker T. A novel, IFN-α-regulated, DNA-binding protein participates in the regulation of the IFP53/tryptophanyl-tRNA synthetase gene. J Biol Chem 1994; 269: 8590–8595.

29. Harroch S, Revel M, Chebath J. Interleukin-6 signaling via transcription factors binding palindromic enhancers of different genes. J Biol Chem 1994; 269:26191–26195.

30. Raz R, Durbin JE, Levy DE. Acute phase response factor and additional members of the interferon-stimulated gene factor 3 family integrate diverse signals from cytokines, interferons, and growth factors. J Biol Chem 1994; 269:24391–24395.

31. Miyamoto M, Fujita T, Kimura Y, Maruyama M, Harada H, Sudo Y, Miyata T, Taniguchi T. Regulated expression of a gene encoding a nuclear factor, IRF-1, that specifically binds to IFN-β gene regulatory elements. Cell 1988; 54:903–913.

32. Harada H, Fujita T, Miyamoto M, Kimura Y, Maruyama M, Furia A, Miyata T, Taniguchi T. Structurally similar but functionally distinct factors, IRF-1 and IRF-2 bind to the same regulatory elements of IFN and IFN-inducible genes. Cell 1989; 58:729–739.

33. Du W, Thanos D, Maniatis T. Mechanism of transcriptional synergism between distinct virus-inducible enhancer elements. Cell 1993; 74:887–898.

34. Harada H, Kitagawa M, Tanaka N, Yamamoto H, Harada K, Ishihara M, Taniguchi T. Anti-oncogenic and oncogenic potentials of interferon-regulatory factors-1 and -2. Science 1993; 259:971–974.

35. Dale T, Rosen JM, Guille MJ, Lewin AR, Porter AGC, Kerr IM, Stark GR. Overlapping sites for constitutive and induced DNA binding factors involved in interferon-stimulated transcription. EMBO J 1989; 8:831–839.

36. Imam AMA, Ackrill A, Dale TC, Kerr I, Stark GR. Transcription factors induced by interferons α and γ. Nucleic Acids Res 1990; 18:6573–6580.

37. Pine R, Decker T, Kessler DS, Levy DE, Darnell JE Jr. Purification and cloning of interferon-simulated gene factor 2: ISGF2 (IRF-1) can bind to the promoters of both interferon-β and interferon-stimulated genes but is not a primary transcriptional activator of either. Mol Cell Biol 1990; 10: 2448–2457.

38. Parrington J, Rogers NC, Gewert DR, Pine R, Veals SA, Levy DE, Stark GR, Kerr IM. The interferon-stimulable response elements of two human genes detect overlapping sets of transcription factors. Eur J Biochem 1993; 214:617–626.

39. Driggers PH, Ennist DL, Gleason SL, Mak W, Marks MS, Levi B, Flanagan JR, Apella E, Ozato K. An interferon-gamma regulated protein that binds the interferon-inducible enhancer element of major histocompatibility complex class I genes. Proc Natl Acad Sci USA 1990; 87:3743–3747.

40. Kanno Y, Kozak CA, Schindler C, Driggers PH, Ennist DL, Gleason SL, Darnell JE, Ozato K. The genomic structure of the murine ICSBP gene reveals the presence of the gamma interferon-responsive element to which an ISGF3α subunit (or similar) protein binds. Mol Cell Biol 1993; 13: 3951–3963.

41. Nelson N, Marks MS, Driggers PH, Ozato K. Interferon consensus sequence-binding protein, a member of the interferon regulatory factor family, suppresses interferon-induced gene transcription. Mol Cell Biol 1993; 13: 588–599.

42. Weisz A, Marx P, Sharf R, Appella E, Driggers PH, Ozato K, Levi BZ. Human interferon consensus sequence binding protein is a negative regulator of enhancer elements common to interferon-inducible genes. J Biol Chem 1992; 267:25589–25596.

43. Bovolenta C, Driggers PH, Marks MS, Medin JA, Politis AD, Vogel SN, Levy DE, Sakaguchi K, Appella E, Coligan JE, Ozato K. Molecular interactions between interferon consensus sequence binding protein and members of the interferon regulatory factor family. Proc Natl Acad Sci USA 1994; 91:5046–5050.

44. Matsuyama T, Kimura T, Kitagawa M, Pfeffer K, Kawakami T, Watanabe N, Kündig TM, Amakawa R, Kishihara K, Wakeham A, Potter J, Furlonger CL, Narendran A, Suzuki H, Ohashi PS, Paige CJ, Taniguchi T, Mak TW. Targeted disruption of IRF-1 or IRF-2 results in abnormal type I IFN gene inducion and aberrant lymphocyte development. Cell 1993; 75:83–97.

45. Kirchhoff S, Schaper S, Hauser H. Interferon regulatory factor 1 (IRF-1) mediates cell growth inhibition by transactivation of downstream target genes. Nucleic Acids Res 1993; 21:2881–2889.

46. Tanaka N, Ishihara M, Kitagawa M, Harada H, Kimura T, Matsuyama T, Lamphier MS, Aizawa S, Mak TW, Taniguchi T. Cellular commitment to oncogene-induced transformation or apoptosis is dependent on the transcription factor IRF-1. Cell 1994; 77:829–839.

47. Harada H, Willison K, Sakakibara J, Miyamoto M, Fujita T, Taniguchi T.

Absence of the type I interferon system in EC cells: transcriptional activator (IRF-1) and repressor (IRF-2) genes are developmentally regulated. Cell 1990; 63:303–312.

48. Reis LFL, Harada H, Wolchok JD, Taniguchi T, Vilček J. Critical role of a common transcription factor, IRF-1, in the regulation of IFN-β and interferon-inducible genes. EMBO J 1992; 11:185–193.

49. Pine R. Constitutive expression of an ISGF-2/IRF-1 transgene leads to interferon-independent activation of interferon-inducible genes and resistance to virus infection. J Virol 1992; 66:4470–4478.

50. Reis LFL, Ruffner H, Stark G, Aguet M, Weissmann C. Mice devoid of interferon-regulatory factor 1 (IRF-1) show normal expression of type I interferon genes. EMBO J 1994; 13:4798–4806.

51. Briken V, Ruffner H, Schultz U, Schwarz A, Reis LFL, Strehlow I, Decker T, Staeheli P. Transcription factor IRF-1 is required for mouse GBP gene activation by interferon-gamma. Mol Cell Biol 1995;15:975–982.

52. Kimura T, Nakayama K, Penninger J, Kitagawa M, Harada H, Matsuyama T, Tanaka N, Kamijo R, Vilček J, Mak TW, Taniguchi T. Involvement of the IRF-1 transcription factor in antiviral responses to interferons. Science 1994; 264:1921–1924.

53. Mirkovitch J, Decker T, Darnell JE Jr. Interferon induction of gene transcription analyzed by in vivo footprinting. Mol Cell Biol 1992; 12:1–9.

54. Strehlow I, Decker T. Transcriptional induction of IFN-γ-responsive genes is modulated by DNA surrounding the interferon stimulation response element. Nucleic Acids Res 1992; 20:3865–3872.

55. Guille MJ, Laxton CD, Rutherford MN, Williams BRG, Kerr IM. Functional differences in the promoters of the interferon-inducible (2'-5')A oligoadenylate synthetase and 6-16 genes in interferon-resistant Daudi cells. Eur J Biochem 1994; 219:547–553.

55a. Eilers A, Seegert D, Schindler C, Baccarini M, Decker T. The response of the gamma interferon activation factor (GAF) is under developmental control in cells of the macrophage lineage. Mol Cell Biol 1993;13:3245–3254.

55b. McDowell MA, Lucas DM, Nicolet CM and Paulnock DM. Differential utilization of IFN-γ-responsive elements in two maturationally distinct macrophage cell lines. J Immunol 1995;155:4933–4938.

56. Pellegrini S, Schindler C. Early events in signalling by interferons. TIBS 1993; 18:338–342.

57. Darnell JE Jr, Kerr IM, Stark GR. Jak-STAT pathways and transcriptional activation in response to IFNs and other extracellular signaling proteins. Science 1994; 264:1415–1421.

58. Pellegrini S, John J, Shearer M, Kerr IM, Stark GR. Use of a selectable marker regulated by alpha interferon to obtain mutations in the signaling pathway. Mol Cell Biol 1989; 9:4605–4612.

59. Watling D, Guschin D, Müller M, Silvennoinen O, Witthuhn BA, Quelle FW, Rogers NC, Schindler C, Stark GR, Ihle JN, Kerr IM. Complementation by the protein tyrosine kinase jak2 of a mutant cell line defective in the interferon-γ signal transduction pathway. Nature 1993; 366:166–170.

60. Mao C, Davies D, Kerr IM, Stark GR. Mutant human cells defective in induction of major histocompatibility complex class II genes by interferon γ. Proc Natl Acad Sci USA 1993; 90:2880–2884.

61. John J, McKendry R, Pellegrini S, Flavell D, Kerr IM, Stark GR. Isolation and characterization of a new mutant human cell line unresponsive to alpha and beta interferons. Mol Cell Biol 1991; 11:4189–4195.

62. Müller M, Laxton C, Briscoe J, Schindler C, Improta T, Darnell JE, Stark GR, Kerr IM. Complementation of a mutant cell line: central role of the 91 kDa polypeptide of ISGF3 in the interferon-α and -γ signal transduction pathways. EMBO J 1993; 12:4221–4228.

63. Velazquez L, Fellous M, Stark GR, Pellegrini S. A protein tyrosine kinase in the interferon α/β signaling pathway. Cell 1992; 70:313–322.

64. Firmbach-Kraft I, Byers M, Shows T, Dalla Favera R, Krolewski JJ. Tyk2, prototype of a novel class of non-receptor tyrosine kinase genes. Oncogene 1990; 5:1329–1336.

65. Wilks AF, Harpur A, Kurban RR, Ralph SJ, Zurcher G, Ziemiecki A. Two novel protein-tyrosine kinases, each with a second phosphotransferase-related catalytic domain, define a new class of protein kinase. Mol Cell Biol 1991; 11:2057–2065.

66. Stahl N, Yancopoulos GD. The alphas, betas, and kinases of cytokine receptor complexes. Cell 1993; 74:587–590.

67. Schindler C, Shuai K, Prezioso VR, Darnell JE Jr. Interferon-dependent tyrosine phosphorylation of a latent cytoplasmic transcription factor. Science 1992; 257:809–813.

68. Fu X-Y. A transcription factor with SH2 and SH3 domains is directly activated by an interferon-α-induced cytoplasmic protein tyrosine kinase(s). Cell 1992; 70:323–335.

69. Shuai K, Stark GR, Kerr IM, Darnell JE Jr. A single phosphotyrosine residue of Stat91 required for gene activation by interferon-γ Science 1993; 261:1744–1746.

70. Shuai K, Zimiecki A, Wilks A, Harpur AG, Sadowski HB, Gilman MZ, Darnell JE Jr. Polypeptide signalling to the nucleus through tyrosine phosphorylation of Jak and Stat proteins. Nature 1993; 366:580–583.

71. Müller M, Briscoe J, Laxton C, Guschin D, Zimiecki A, Silvennoinen O, Harpur AG, Barbieri G, Witthuhn BA, Schindler C, Pellegrini S, Wilks A, Ihle JN, Stark GR, Kerr IM. The protein tyrosine kinase jak1 complements defects in interferon α/β and -γ signal transduction. Nature 1993; 366: 129–135.

72. Silvennoinen O, Ihle JN, Schlessinger J, and Levy DE. Interferon-induced nuclear signalling by Jak protein tyrosine kinases. Nature 1993; 366: 583–585.

73. David M, Larner A. Activation of transcription factors by interferon-alpha in a cell-free system. Science 1992; 257:813–815.

74. David M, Romer G, Zhang ZY, Dixon JE, Larner AC. In vitro activation of the transcription factor ISGF3 by interferon-α involves a membrane-

associated tyrosine phosphatase and tyrosine kinase. J Biol Chem 1993; 268:6593–6599.

75. Barbieri G, Velazquez L, Scrobogna M, Fellous M, Pellegrini S. Activation of the protein tyrosine kinase tyk2 by interferon α/β. Eur J Biochem 1994; 223:427–435.

76. Reich NC, Pfeffer LM. Evidence for involvement of protein kinase C in the cellular response to interferon α. Proc Natl Acad Sci USA 1990; 87: 8761–8765.

77. Pfeffer LM, Strulovici B, and Saltiel AR. Interferon-α selectively activates the β isoform of protein kinase C through phosphatidylcholine hydrolysis. Proc Natl Acad Sci 1990; 87:6537–6541.

78. Eilers A, Georgellis D, Klose B, Schindler C, Ziemiecki A, Harpur AG, Wilks AF, Decker T. Differentiation-regulated serine phosphoporylation of STAT 1 promotes GAF activation in macrophages. Mol Cell Biol 1995;15: 3579–3586.

78a. Lütticken C, Coffer P, Yuan J, Schwartz C, Schindler C, Kruijer W, Heinrich PC, Horn F. Interleukin-6-induced serine phosphorylation of transciption factor APRF: evidence for a role in interleukin-6 target gene induction. FEBS Lett 1995;360:137–143.

78b. Wen Z, Zhong Z, Darnell JE Jr. Maximal activation of transciption by Stat1 and Stat3 requires both tyrosine and serine phosphorylation. Cell 1995;82: 241–250.

78c. David M, Petricoin EF, III Benjamin C, Pine R, Weber MJ, Larner AC. Requirement for MAP Kinase (ERK2) activity in interferon α and interferon-β-stimulated gene expression through SAT proteins. Science 1995; 269:1721–1723.

79. Guschin D, Rogers N, Briscoe J, Witthuhn B, Watling D, Horn F, Pellegrini S, Yasukawa K, Heinrich P, Stark GR, Ihle JN, Kerr IM. A major role for the protein tyrosine kinase JAK1 in the JAK/STAT signal transduction pathway in response to interleukin-6. EMBOJ. 1995;14:1421–1429.

79a. Briscoe J, Rogers NC, Witthuhn BA, Watling D, Harpur AG, Wilks AF, Stark GR, Ihle JN, Kerr I. Kinase negative mutants of JAK1 can sustain interferon γ-inducible gene expression but not an antiviral state. EMBO J 1996;15:799–809.

80. David M, Grimley P, Finbloom DS, Larner AC. A nuclear tyrosine phosphatase downregulates interferon-induced gene expression. Mol Cell Biol 1994; 13:7515–7521.

81. Petricoin E III, David M, Fang H, Grimley P, Larner AC, Vande Pol S. Human cancer cell lines express a negative transcriptional regulator of the interferon regulatory factor family of DNA-binding proteins. Mol Cell Biol 1994; 14:1477–1486.

82. Lengyel P. Enzymology of interferon action-A short survey. Methods Enzymol. 1981; 79:135–148.

83. Pestka S, Langer JA, Zoon KC, and Samuel CE. Interferons and their actions. Ann Rev Biochem 1987; 56:727–777.

84. Katze M. The war against the interferon-induced, dsRNA-activated protein kinase: Can viruses win? J Interferon Res 1992; 12:241–248.
85. Staeheli P, Pitossi F, and Pavlovic J. Mx proteins: GTPases with antiviral activity. Trends Cell Biol 1993; 3:268–272.
86. Hovanessian AG. Interferon-induced and double-stranded kinase-activated enzymes: a specific protein kinase and 2',5'-oligoadenylate synthetases. J Interferon Res 1994; 11:199–205.
87. Patel RC, and Sen GC. Identification of the double-stranded RNA-binding domain of the human interferon-inducible protein kinase. J Biol Chem 1992; 11:7671–7676.
88. Sperling J, Chebath J, Arad-Dann H, Offen D, Spann P, Lehrer R, Goldblatt D, Jolles B, Sperling R. Possible involvement of (2'-5') oligoadenylate synthetase activity in pre mRNA splicing. Proc Natl Acad Sci USA 1991; 88: 10377–10381.
89. Chebath J, Benech P, Reve M, and Vigneron M. Constitutive expression of (2'-5') oligo A synthetase confers resistance to picornavirus infection. Nature 1987; 330:587–590.
90. Zhou A, Hassel BA, Silverman RH. Expression cloning of 2-5A–dependent RNAase: a uniquely regulated mediator of interferon action. Cell 1993; 72: 753–765.
91. Hassel BA, Zhou A, Sotomayor C, Maran A, and Silverman RH. A dominant-negative mutant of 2-5A-dependent RNase suppresses antiproliferative and antiviral effects of interferon. EMBO J 1993; 12:3297–3304.
92. Williams BRG, Silverman RH (eds.). The 2-5A System: Molecular and Clinical Aspects of the Interferon-Regulated Pathway. New York: Alan RL Riss, 1984.
93. Meurs E, Chong K, Galbru J, Thomas NS, Kerr IM, Williams BR, Hovanessian AG. Molecular cloning and characterization of the human double-stranded RNA-activated protein kinase induced by interferon. Cell 1990; 62:379–390.
94. Feng G-S, Chong K, Kumar A, Williams B. Identification of double-stranded RNA-binding domains in the interferon-induced double-stranded RNA-activated p68 kinase. Proc Natl Acad Sci USA 1992; 89:5447–5451.
95. Chong KL, Feng L, Schappert K, Meurs E, Donahue TF, Friesen JD, Hovanessian AG, Williams BR. Human p68 kinase exhibits growth suppression in yeast and homology to the translational regulator GCN2. EMBO J 1992; 11:1553–1562.
96. Koromilas AE, Roy S, Barber GN, Katze MG, Sonenberg N. Malignant transformation by a mutant of the IFN-inducible dsRNA-dependent protein kinase. Science 1992; 257:1685–1689.
97. Meurs E, Galbru J, Barber GN, Katze MG, Hovanessian AG. Tumor suppressor function of the interferon-induced double-stranded RNA-activated protein kinase. Proc Natl Acad Sci USA 1990; 90:232–236.
98. Kirchhoff S, Koromilas A, Köster M, Schaper F, Sonenberg M, Hauser H. The double-stranded RNA-dependent protein kinase PKR mediates the

antiproliferative action of the tumor suppressor IRF-1. J Interferon Res 1994; 14(suppl 1):161.

99. Yang Y-L, Reis LFL, Pavlovic J, Aguzzi A, Schäfer R, Kumar A, Williams BRG, Aguet M, Weissman C. Deficient signaling in mice devoid of double-stranded RNA-dependent protein kinase. EMBO J 1995; 14:6069–6106.

100. Visvanathan KV, Goodbourne S. Double-stranded RNA activates binding of NF-kB to an inducible element in the human β-interferon promoter. EMBO J 1989; 8:1129–1135.

101. Kumar A, Haque J, Lacoste J, Hiscott J, Williams BR. Double-stranded RNA-dependent protein kinase activates transcription factor NF-κ B by phosphorylating IκB. Proc Natl Acad Sci USA 1994; 91:6288–6292.

102. Choubey D, Snoddy J, Chaturvedi V, Toniato E, Opdenakker G, Thakur A, Samanta H, Engel DA, Lengyel P. Interferons as gene activators. Indications for repeated gene duplication during the evolution of a cluster of interferon-activatable genes on murine chromosome 1. J Biol Chem 1989; 264: 17182–17189.

103. Choubey D, Lengyel P. Binding of an interferon-inducible protein (p202) to the retinoblastoma protein. J Biol Chem 1995;270:6134–6140.

104. Resnitzky D, Tiefenbrun N, Berissi H, Kimchi A. Interferons and interleukin 6 suppress phosphorylation of the retinoblastoma protein in growth-sensitive hematopoietic cells. Proc Natl Acad Sci USA 1992; 89:402–406.

105. Deblandre G, Marinx O, Leo O, Caput D, Huez GA, Wathelet MG. Cloning of the cDNA coding for a 17kDa membrane protein implicated in the antiproliferative activity of interferons. J Interferon Res 1994; 14(suppl 1):160.

106. Pavlovic J, Staeheli P. The antiviral potential of Mx proteins. J Interferon Res 1991; 11:215–219.

107. Horisberger MA. Mx protein: function and mechanism of action. In: Baron S, Coppenhaver DH, Dianzani F, Fleischmann WR, Hughes TK, Klimpel GR, Niesel DW, Stanton GJ, Tyring SK, eds. Interferon Principles and Medical Application. Galveston: The University of Texas Medical Branch at Galveston, Department of Microbiology, 1992:215–224.

108. Zürcher T, Pavlovid J, Staeheli P. Mechanism of human MxA protein action: variants with changed antiviral properties. EMBO J 1992; 11: 1657–1661.

109. Rothman JH, Raymond CK, Gilbert T, O'Hara PJ, Stevens TH. A putative GTP binding protein homologous to interferon-inducible Mx proteins performs an essential function in yeast protein sorting. Cell 1990; 61:1063–1074.

110. Cheng Y-SE, Becker-Manley MF, Chow TP, Horan DC. Affinity purification of an interferon-induced human guanylate-binding protein and its characterization. J Biol Chem 1985; 260:15834–15839.

111. Decker T, Lew DJ, Cheng Y-SE, Levy D, Darnell JE Jr. Interactions of α- and γ-interferon in the transcriptional regulation of the gene encoding a guanylate-binding protein. EMBO J 1989; 8:2009–2014.

112. Cheng Y-SE, Patterson CE, Staeheli P. 1. Interferon-induced guanylate-binding proteins lack an N(T)KXD consensus motif and bind GMP in addition to GDP and GTP. Mol Cell Biol 1991; 11:4717–4725.

113. Schwemmle M, Staeheli P. The interferon-induced 67-kDa guanylate-binding protein (hGBP1) is a GTPase that converts GTP to GMP. J Biol Chem 1994; 269:11299–11305.
114. Stewart WE, Gosser BL, Lockart RZ Jr. Priming: a nonantiviral function of interferon. J Virol 1971; 7:792–801.
115. Dron M, Lacasa M, Tovey M. Priming affects the activity of a specific region of the promoter of the human beta interferon gene. Mol Cell Biol 1990; 10:854–858.
116. Fujita T, Reis LFL, Watanabe N, Kimura Y, Taniguchi T, Vilček J. Induction of the transcription factor IRF-1 and interferon-β mRNAs by cytokines and activators of second messenger pathways. Proc Natl Acad Sci 1989; 86:9936–9940.
117. Yoshida R, Murray HW, Nathan CF. Agonist and antagonist effects of interferon-α and β on activation of human macrophages. J Exp Med 167: 1171–1185.
118. Matsushima GK, Taniike M, Glimcher LH, Grusby MJ, Frelinger JA, Suzuki K, Ting JPY. Absence of MHC class II molecules reduces CNS demyelination, microglial/macrophage infiltration, and twitching in murine globoid cell leukodystrophy. Cell 1994; 78:645–658.
119. Ling PD, Warren MK, Vogel SN. Antagonistic effect of interferon-β on the interferon-γ-induced expression of Ia antigen in murine macrophages. J Immunol 1985; 135:1857–1863.
120. Devajyothi C, Kalvakolanu I, Babcock GT, Vasavada HA, Howe PH, Ransohoff RM. Inhibition of interferon-gamma–induced major histocompatibility complex class II gene transcription by interferon-beta and type beta 1 transforming growth factor in human astrocytoma cells. Definition of cis-element. J Biol Chem 1993; 268:18794–18800.
121. Ransohoff RM, Devajyothi C, Estes ML, Babcock GT, Rudick RA, Frohman EM, Barna BP. Interferon-beta specifically inhibits interferon-gamma-induced class II major histocompatibility complex gene transcription in a human astrocytoma cell line. J Neuroimmunol 1991; 33:103–112.
122. Fertsch-Ruggio D, Schoenberg DR, Vogel SN. Induction of Ia antigen expression by rIFN-gamma and down-regulation by IFN-alpha/beta and dexamethasone are regulated transcriptionally. J Immunol 1988; 141: 1582–1589.
123. Steimle V, Otten LA, Zufferey M, Mach B. Complementation cloning of an MHC class II transactivator mutated in hereditary MHC class II deficiency (or bare lymphocyte syndrome) Cell 1993; 75:135–146.
124. Silacci P, Mottet A, Steimle V, Reith W, Mach B. Developmental extinction of major histocompatibility complex class II gene expression in plasmocytes is mediated by silencing of the transactivator gene CIITA. J Exp Med 1994; 180:1329–1336.
125. Chang C-H, Fontes JD, Peterlin M, Flavell RA. Class II transactivator (CIITA) is sufficient for the inducible expression of major histocompatibility complex class II genes. J Exp Med 1994; 180:1367–1374.
126. Ting JP-Y, Painter A, Zeleznik-Le NJ, MacDonald G, Moore TM, Brown

A, Schwartz BD. YB-1 DNA-binding protein represses interferon γ activation of class II major histocompatibility complex genes. J Exp Med 1994; 179:1605–1611.

127. Kara CJ, Glimcher LH. Regulation of MHC class II gene transcription. Curr Opin Immunol 1991; 3:16–21.

128. Levy DE, Lew DJ, Decker T, Kessler DS, Darnell JE Jr. Synergistic interaction between interferon-α and interferon-γ through induced synthesis of one subunit of the transcription factor ISGF3. EMBO J 1990; 9:1105–1111.

129. Pine R, Canova A, Schindler C. Tyrosine phosphorylated p91 binds to a single element in the ISGF2/IRF-1 promoter to mediate induction by IFNα and IFNγ, and is likely to autoregulate the p91 gene. EMBO J 1994; 13: 158–167.

130. Oliviera IC, Sciavolino PJ, Lee TH, Vilček J. Downregulation of interleukin 8 gene expression in human fibroblasts: unique mechanism of transcriptional inhibition by interferon. Proc Natl Acad Sci USA 1992; 89:9049–9053.

131. Oliviera IC, Mukaida M, Matsushima K, Vilček J. Transcriptional inhibition of the interleukin-8 gene by interferon is mediated by the NF-kB site. Mol Cell Biol 1994; 14:5300–5308.

132. Tamura M, Tokuda M, Nagaoka S, Takada H. Lipopolysaccharides of Bacteroides intermedius (Prevotella intermedia) and Bacteroides (Porphyromonas) gingivalis induce interleukin-8 gene expression in human gingival fibroblast cultures. Infect Immun 1992; 60:4932–4937.

133. Bäerle PA. The inducible transcription activator NF-kB: regulation by distinct protein subunits. Biochem Biophys Acta 1991; 1072:63–80.

134. Girdlestone J, Isamat M, Gewert D, Milstein C. Transcriptional regulation of HLA-A and -B: differential binding of members of the Rel and IRF families of transcription factors. Proc Natl Acad Sci USA 1993; 90:11568–11572.

135. Johnson JR, and Pober JS. HLA class I heavy chain gene promoter elements mediating synergy between tumor necrosis factor and interferons. Mol Cell Biol 1994; 14:1322–1332.

136. Larner AC, David M, Feldman GM, Igarashi K-I, Hackett RH, Webb DSA, Sweitzer SM, Petricoin EF/III, Finbloom DS. Tyrosine phosphorylation of DNA-binding proteins by multiple cytokines. Science 1993; 261:1730–1733.

137. Müller M, Ibelgaufts H, Kerr IM. Interferon response pathways—a paradigm for cytokine signalling? J Viral Hepatitis 1994; 1:87–103.

138. Bonni A, Frank DA, Schindler C, Greenberg ME. Characterization of a pathway for ciliary neurotrophic factor signaling to the nucleus. Science 1993; 262:1575–1579.

139. Rothman P, Kreider B, Azam M, Levy D, Wegenka U, Eilers A, Decker T, Horn F, Kashleva H, Ihle J, Schindler C. Cytokines signal through tyrosine phophorylation of a family of related transcription factors. Immunity 1994; 1:457–468.

140. Lehmann J, Seegert D, Strehlow I, Schindler C, Lohmann-Matthes M-L, Decker T. Interleukin-10-induced factors belonging to the p91 family of proteins bind to interferon-gamma-responsive promoter elements. J Immunol 1994; 153:165–172.

141. Larner AC, Petricoin EF, Nakagawa Y, and Finbloom DS. IL-4 attenuates the transcriptional activation of both IFN-alpha and IFN-gamma–induced cellular gene expression in monocytes and monocytic cell lines. J Immunol 1993; 150:1944–1950.

142. Heuson F, Pohler U, Decker T, Just U, Ostertag W, and Baccarini M. Coordinate expression of the lineage-specific growth factor CSF-1 and its receptor selectively promotes macrophage maturation during GM-CSF mediated differentiation of multipotential progenitor cells. Cell Growth Diff 1994; 5:1119–1126.

143. Loeb KR, Haas KL. The interferon-inducible 15kDa ubiquitin homolog conjugates to intracellular proteins. J Biol Chem 1992; 267:7806–7813.

144. David-Watine B, Israel A, Kourilsky P. The regulation and expression of MHC class I genes. Immunol Today 1990; 11:286–292.

145. Harada H, Takahashi E-I, Itoh S, Harada K, Hori T-H, Taniguchi T. Structure and regulation of the human interferon regulatory factor-1 (IRF-1) and IRF-2 genes: implications for a gene network in the interferon system. Mol Cell Biol 1993; 14:1500–1509.

146. Hug H, Costas M, Staeheli P, Aebi M, and Weissmann C. Organization of the murine Mx gene and characterization of its interferon- and virus-inducible promoter. Mol Cell Biol 1988; 8:3065–3079.

147. Nicolet CM, Paulnock DM. Promoter analysis of an interferon-inducible gene associated with macrophage activation. J Immunol 1994; 152:153–162.

148. Sims SH, Cha J, Romine MF, Gao P-Q, Gottlieb K, Deisseroth AB. A novel interferon-inducible domain: structural and functional analysis of the human interferon regulatory factor 1 gene promoter. Mol Cell Biol 1993; 13:690–702.

149. Buwitt U, Flohr T, and Boettger EC. Molecular cloning and characterization of an interferon-induced human cDNA with sequence homology to a mammalian peptide chain release factor. EMBO J 1992; 11:489–496.

150. Kisselev L, Frolova L, Haenni AL. Interferon inducibility of mammalian tryptophanyl-tRNA synthetase: new perspectives. TIBS 1993; 18:263–267.

151. Strehlow I, Seegert D, Frick C, Bange F-C, Schindler C, Boettger EC, Decker T. The gene encoding IFP 53/tryptophanyl-tRNA synthetase is regulated by the gamma-interferon activation factor. J Biol Chem 1993; 268: 16590–16595.

152. Dad Khan K, Shuai K, Lindwall G, Maher SE, Darnell JE, Bothwell ALM. Induction of the Ly6A/E gene by interferon α/β and γ requires a DNA element to which a tyrosine-phosphorylated 91-kDa protein binds. Proc Natl Acad Sci USA 1993; 90:6806–6810.

3

Pharmacokinetics of Interferon-β and the Biological Markers It Induces

Patricia L. Witt

Medical College of Wisconsin, Milwaukee, Wisconsin

I. INTRODUCTION

Interferon-β (IFN-β) has shown therapeutic effectiveness in decreasing the exacerbation rate and magnetic resonance imaging (MRI) lesions of multiple sclerosis (MS). In one study, 8 million units (MU) IFN-β-1b was administered subcutaneously every other day to 372 patients (1,2), and in another study, 1 MU natural fibroblast IFN-β was administered intrathecally once a week to 69 patients (3). These doses and routes were selected on the basis of pharmacokinetic studies of IFN-β and IFN-induced proteins, which defined the dose dependence and duration of the effective biological response to IFN-β versus the side effects. These biological responses to IFN include increased 2′,5′-oligoadenylate synthetase (2,5-OAS) activity in peripheral blood mononuclear cells (PBMCs), β_2-microglobulin and neopterin in serum, and HLA class I and II surface antigens on monocytes. Further consideration of IFN-β pharmacokinetics and biological response may reveal more effective dose/schedule combinations of IFN-β for MS, as well as IFN's mechanism of action.

II. PHARMACOKINETICS OF IFN IN VIVO

A. Effects of Route of Administration

IFN-β has been systemically administered by intravenous (i.v.), intramuscular (i.m.), and subcutaneous (s.c.) routes. Generally, the measurable serum IFN concentration is higher and detected sooner after i.v. than s.c. or i.m. administration; however, it appears that all routes are biologically effective. After i.v. injection of IFN-β, serum concentrations can be measured within minutes and peak at approximately 5 mins. A typical example is shown in Fig. 1a (4) of nine healthy male volunteers who received an i.v. injection of 90 MU IFN β-1b*; the peak concentration (mean, 1490 U/ml) was found at the earliest sampling time, 5 min. The mean $t_{1/2}$ was 4.3 ($\pm$ SD 2.3) hr. In contrast, after an s.c. injection of the same 90 MU dose, the peak serum concentration was 40 U/ml with peak times from 1–3 hr (Fig. 1b). After eight consecutive daily s.c. doses, mean peak serum concentration was 44 U/ml, suggesting no bioaccumulation of IFN-β over multiple doses. IFN-α, like IFN-β, is detectable in serum within minutes after i.v. bolus injection and remains detectable for 12–48 hr.

Similar pharmacokinetics were observed in a crossover study of 16 cancer patients (5) who received 45 and 180 MU IFN β-1b (old units) administered i.v. and s.c. The mean peak serum IFN-β concentration after the 180 MU dose was 1800 U/m for i.v. and 25 U/ml for s.c. administration, and after the 45-MU dose was 350 U/ml for i.v. and undetectable for s.c. administration (Table 1). The peak time was 5 min, the earliest timepoint measured after i.v. administration. Despite dramatic differences in serum IFN concentration after i.v. versus s.c. routes, however, increases in IFN-induced proteins in this study were similar for the two routes of administration, as discussed below.

Pharmacokinetics of 1 MU IFN β-1b (old units) by i.v., i.m., and s.c. routes were compared in African green monkeys infected with simian varicella virus (6). The peak serum concentration was higher after a single i.v. administration, 2500 U/ml, compared with 250 U/ml after i.m. and 140 U/ml after s.c. However, 6 hr later, the serum concentrations were similar (about 100 U/ml). Total bioavailability, as measured by AUC (area under the curve), was less after i.m. and s.c. administration; mean $AUC_{s.c.}$ was 30% of mean $AUC_{i.v.}$ and mean $AUC_{i.m.}$ was 50% of mean $AUC_{i.v.}$. However, s.c. or i.m. administration were as effective as i.v. in diminishing viremia and virus-associated rash in these animal models.

After a 4-hr i.v. infusion of 30 MU IFN-β (Cetus rIFN-β-1b, Chiron

---

* Reevaluation in 1993 of the titer of the IFN β-1b preparation used, compared with the WHO standard, resulted in an approximately fivefold decrease in specific activity (i.e., 45 MU [old units] is now titered at 8 MU [new units]).

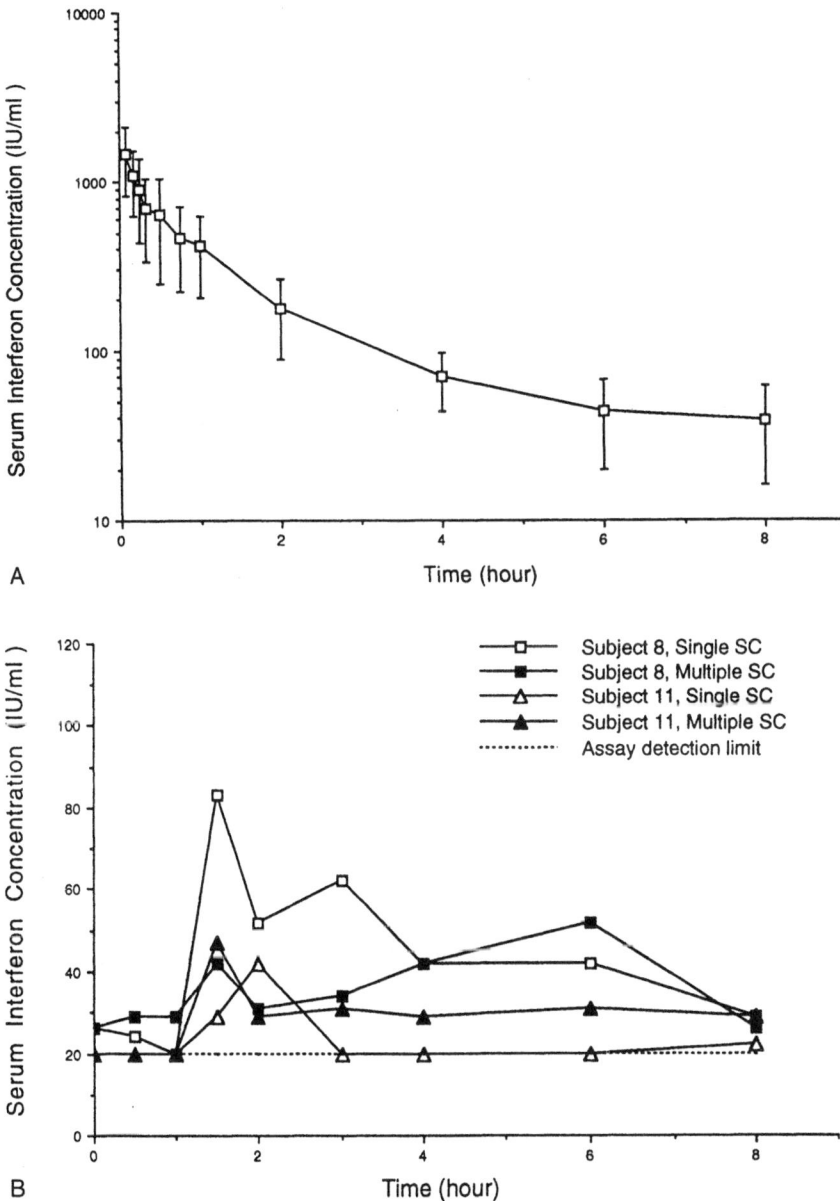

Figure 1 (A) Mean serum interferon concentration-time profile following a single i.v. administration of 90 MU (old units) IFN β-1b. Values are for nine subjects, with vertical bars indicating standard deviation. (B) Serum interferon concentration-time profiles following single and multiple s.c. doses of 90 MU (old units) IFN β-1b to two representative subjects. (From ref. 4.)

Table 1 Dose-Response in Serum IFN Concentrations After s.c.and i.v. Administration of IFN βser in Cancer Patients

Dose of IFN-β (IU/ml [old units])	Peak IFN (IU) (mean ± SE) s.c. (n = 8)	Peak IFN (IU) (mean ± SE) i.v. (n = 8)	IFN (IU) (range)
45 × 10^6	0	357 ± 69	208–667
180 × 10^6	25 ± [a]	1833 ± 386	1000–3333

Peak value occurred in the first sample, drawn 5 min after the IFN injection.
[a] Five of eight patients had no rise in antiviral activity above baseline. Three patients had increases to 21, 26, and 28 IU.
Source: From ref. 5.

Corp., Emeryville, CA) the mean peak serum IFN-β concentration of approximately 150 U/ml occurred at 4 hr after start of treatment (7). After low doses of IFN-β (4–10 MU purified fibroblast IFN) by i.v. infusion, serum IFN levels peaked at the end of the 30-min infusion and returned to preexisting levels by 120 min; after the highest doses (160–320 MU), serum IFN levels peaked again at the end of a 30 min infusion but remained elevated until 24–48 hr after treatment (8). Continuous infusions of IFN-αA, administered either i.v. or s.c. have achieved steady-state concentrations of 10^2–10^4 U/ml (9,10).

The pharmacokinetics of i.m. administration of IFN-β has not been well studied. However, when IFN-α is administered i.m., the peak of serum IFN is approximately 6 hr, much later than the i.v. route. The peak concentration is lower, with a mean peak serum of IFN-α concentration of 50 U after i.m. administration of 3 MU (11,12). Nonetheless, i.m. administration of Serono IFN β-1a induced similar biological responses to i.v., as described below (13).

In rabbits, human IFN-β (fibroblast) injected i.m. led to 10-fold lower serum titer than the same amount (10^6 U) of IFN-α (human lymphocyte, Cantell) (13a). This difference was attributed to greater retention of IFN-β than IFN-α in tissue rather than more rapid clearance, since the two IFNs injected i.v. into rabbits were cleared at similar rates.

B. Clinical Side Effects and Toxicity

The major dose-limiting side effects of type I IFNs are fatigue, malaise, and fever in most cancer patients. These are more pronounced early in treatment and diminish with repeated administration, which remains unexplained, since biological (biochemical) responses do not diminish (see Section III and Chapter 16). The maximum tolerated dose (MTD) of IFN β-1b, defined by clinical toxicity, was found by Kinney et al. (14) to be 2.5

mg (450 MU old units) when administered three times a week by 2 hr i.v. infusion; this dose was later decreased after cumulative toxicity. Other studies with cancer patients found the MTD of IFN β-1b was 180 MU (old units) as a single dose and 90 MU (old units) with repeated every other day administration (5).

III. BIOLOGICAL RESPONSE TO IFN-β

IFN induces the production of 15–20 new mRNAs, proteins, and metabolites, several of which have been measured in clinical trials to assess biological response to IFNs. These mediate IFN's antiviral, antiproliferative, and immunomodulatory activities elsewhere in this book. Increases in 2,5-OAS activity in PBMCs and serum after IFN-α, IFN-β, and to a lesser extent after IFN-γ are well documented in numerous studies. β_2-Microglobulin, part of the HLA class I molecule, is increased in serum after IFN-α, IFN-β, and IFN-γ; this increase represents increased turnover, increased surface concentration, or both. Neopterin, a product of the IFN-induced enzyme GTP cyclohydrolase, is secreted by activated macrophages after IFN-α, IFN-β, and IFN-γ treatment.

A. Duration of Biological Response to Single Dose

Measurements of 2,5-OAS, β_2-microglobulin, and neopterin as well as other IFN-induced proteins suggest that biological activity of IFN persists for several days after a single injection and does not accumulate to higher levels after repeated injections. In one study defining the kinetics of the biological response to IFN β-1b, groups of eight healthy volunteers received single s.c. injections of 0.09, 0.9, 9.0, and 45.0 MU IFN β-1b (old units) (15). Responses were measured at 24, 48, and 72 hr and 7 days after a single injection, and were compared with responses at 24 and 48 hr after 4 every other day injections. 2,5-OAS, neopterin, and β_2-microglobulin levels were significantly elevated over pretreatment values at 24, 48, and 72 hr, but they returned to baseline by 7 days, indicating the persistence of a biological response for at least 3 days (Fig. 2). When escalating doses (1–46 MU) of natural IFN-β (produced by a foreskin cell line) were given to 15 cancer patients (16), the β_2-microglobulin level peaked at 24 hr and remained significantly elevated at 72 hr ($p = .001$), whereas neopterin remained significantly elevated at 96 hr. These results suggest that an every other day or two times a week schedule would be sufficient to maintain IFN's biological activity.

After i.m. administration of 6 MU IFN β-1a (Bioferon, Laupheim, Germany, and Biogen USA, Cambridge, MA, CHO-derived), induction of

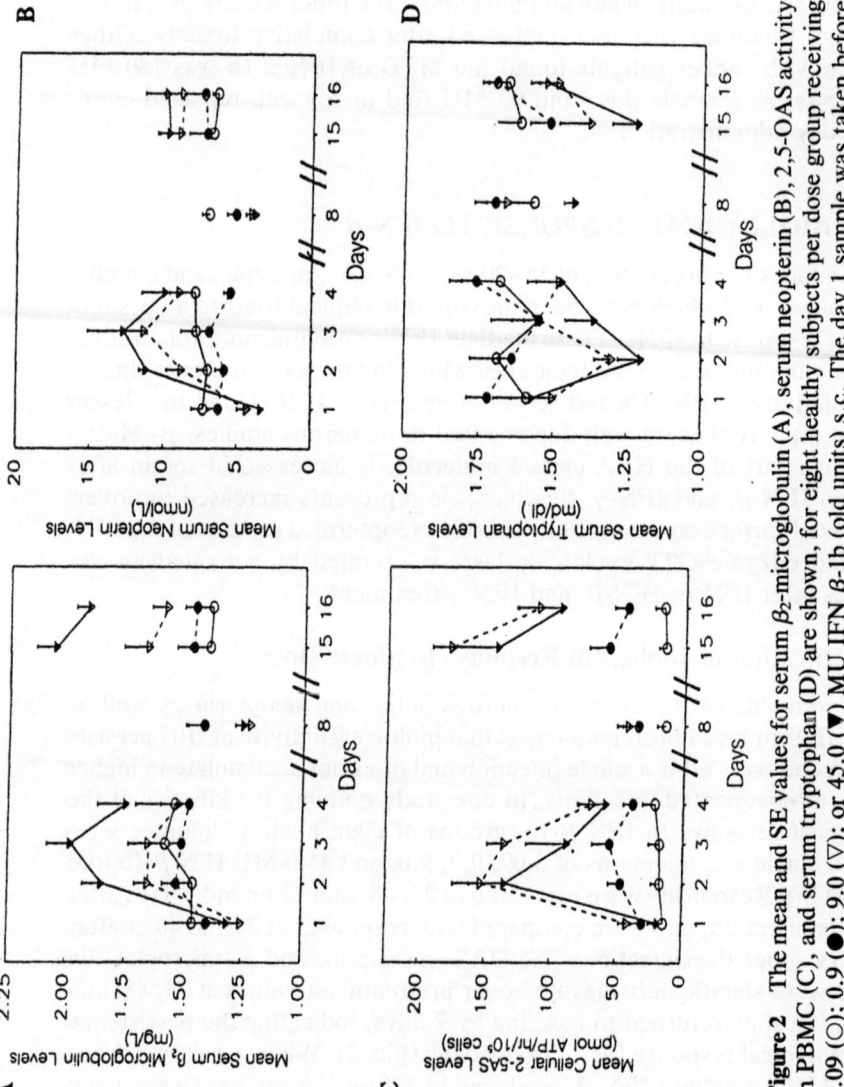

Figure 2 The mean and SE values for serum β_2-microglobulin (A), serum neopterin (B), 2,5-OAS activity in PBMC (C), and serum tryptophan (D) are shown, for eight healthy subjects per dose group receiving 0.09 (○); 0.9 (●); 9.0 (▽); or 45.0 (▼) MU IFN β-1b (old units) s.c. The day 1 sample was taken before the first injection; samples on days 2, 3, 4, and 8 follow that single injection. Subjects received further injections on days 8, 10, 12, and 14; samples were assayed on days 15 and 16 following these every other day injections. (From ref. 15.)

β_2-microglobulin remained significantly above baseline for 2 days (40% elevated, mean of five patients) and slightly elevated (15%) for 7 days (17). This increase in β_2-microglobulin was comparable in extent and duration to that induced by a comparable dose (45 old units or 8 MU new units) of IFN β-1b administered s.c. to healthy volunteers in the study described above (15). On this basis, weekly i.m. administration of Bioferon/Biogen IFN β-1a was chosen for a trial in 290 active relapsing, minimally disabled MS patients.

B. Effects of Repeated Administration on Biological Response

Increases in 2,5-OAS, β_2-microglobulin, and neopterin at 24 or 48 hr after a single injection of IFN β-1b were not statistically different from increases after 4 every other day s.c. injections of the same dose, suggesting that there is neither accumulated nor diminished biological effect (see Fig. 2: compare days 15 and 16 with days 2 and 3; [15]). Continuous daily administration of IFN β-1b maintained 2,5-OAS activity and β_2-microglobulin at approximately their 24-hr peak levels for up to 8 weeks (18). Over several weeks of administration of fibroblast IFN-β, cumulative increases in neopterin but not β_2-microglobulin were observed (19). However, surface expression of MHC class II decreased on monocytes after extended (2–3 weeks) administration of IFN β-1b (20). In 64 patients with metastatic renal carcinoma, 2,5-OAS, β_2-microglobulin, natural killer (NK) and killer (K) cell cytotoxicity, and HLA-DQ on monocytes, but not HLA-DR, remained at the 24- to 48-hr peak level over 10 days of daily treatment with IFN-β (21). HLA-DQ, but not HLA-DR, has been linked to activity of a suppressor T-cell population (22), which may be part of the therapeutic effect of IFN-β. These studies suggest that the biological response persists over long-term administration of IFN, whereas many clinical side effects diminish.

C. Effects of Dose on Biological Response

Some, but not all, studies have shown dose-dependent increases in the biological response; measured as IFN-induced proteins or activation of immune cell functions. When the biological response over the range of 0.09–45.0 MU IFN β-1b (old units) was studied (15), the lowest biologically effective dose was 0.9 MU s.c.; significant ($p < .02$) increases were observed at 24 hr in β_2-microglobulin and 2,5-OAS activity. At the two higher doses, 9 and 45 MU, changes were observed at 24 hr in neopterin as well ($p < .01$). A dose-dependent increase ($p < .01$) was observed in these biological responses over the range of 0.09–45.0 MU, and changes in neopterin, β_2-microglobulin, and cellular 2,5-OAS correlated significantly with each other. After i.m. administration of 6 MU IFN β-1a (Bioferon and Biogen), β_2-microglobulin was significantly elevated for 2 days and slightly elevated up to 7 days. 3 MU IFN β-1a was insufficient to maintain this extended biological effect (17).

Dose-dependent increases in the biological response have been observed in many, but not all, studies of IFN-β in cancer patients. A dose response in 2,5-OAS activity, but not NK cell cytotoxicity, was observed in renal cancer patients treated with 0.01–150 MU/m² IFN β-1b (old units) (18). A dose-dependent increase in β_2-microglobulin, but not in neopterin, was observed after i.v. administration of a purified fibroblast IFN-β in the range of 1–46 MU (16). 180 MU IFN β-1b (old units) induced greater increases in 2,5-OAS activity and neopterin, but not β_2-microglobulin, compared with 45 MU IFN β-1b (old units) (5). However, no dose-dependent increase was measured in patients with advanced malignancy after 3–30 MU i.v. IFN β-1b (old units) (23) or comparing 4.5 and 90.0 MU IFN β-1b (old units) (21).

These differences between trials probably reflect the impact of individual variability on the relatively small sample size. Individual variability in response can be dramatic; for example, 32 healthy volunteers had baseline 2,5-OAS activity levels of between 1 and 78 U and showed increases in 2,5-OAS activity of 4- to 25-fold over baseline after 45 MU IFN β-1b (old units) (15). Lack of a dose response may also reflect a plateau of the biological effect at higher doses. Many factors undoubtedly contribute to the potential for immunoactivation, including the presence of ongoing viral infection, which can increase the patients' baseline activity, or other chronic conditions diminishing health. Personalized dosing may be more effective, with higher doses for patients with initially smaller increases in the biological response. When biological mechanisms underlying IFN-β activity in MS are understood, we may define the threshholds of critical factors.

D. Effects of Route on Biological Response

IFN-β administered s.c. was as effective as i.v. administration in increasing a number of IFN-induced biological responses (5). In this study, comparable increases in HLA class II or β_2-microglobulin on monocytes, tryptophan degradation, non-MHC restricted killing (NK cells and antibody-dependent cell-mediated cytotoxicity [ADCC]), and serum β_2-microglobulin concentration were observed after 45 or 180 MU IFN-β (old units). The s.c. route resulted in greater increases in 2,5-OAS ($p = .02$), while the i.v. route resulted in greater increases in HLA-DR expression on monocytes and serum neopterin concentration ($p = .01$ and $p = .0002$). This study suggested that the s.c. route, which was easier for self-administration by patients, would have equivalent clinical effectiveness.

E. Comparisons of Biological Response to Natural and Recombinant IFN-β

Biological responses to a natural IFN-β and a mammalian-derived recombinant IFN β-1a administered i.m. (both from Serono, Geneva, Switzerland) were similar in crossover-design, double-blind studies. When 6 MU was administered i.m. to 12 healthy volunteers (13), neopterin and β_2-microglobulin in serum and 2,5-OAS and human Mx protein in PBMCs were increased between 24 and 72 hr by both subtypes of β IFN; the increases induced by the two IFNs were not statistically different. When administered i.v. in a separate study to 12 healthy volunteers (24), there were as well no statistical differences in induction of 2,5-OAS, β_2-microglobulin, or neopterin induced by the two types of β IFNs. Neither of the subtypes of IFN-β induced interleukin-1α (IL-1α) or IL-1β. One study found natural IFN-β more antigenic than recombinant IFN-β ([25]; see also Section IV).

F. Intrathecal Administration and the Blood-Brain Barrier

If antiviral or immunoregulatory activity in the central nervous system (CNS) is important in the treatment of MS, then it is important to establish whether IFN or IFN-activated cells reach this site. The clinical effectiveness of systemically administered IFN β-1b (1,2) as well as intrathecally (i.t.) administered IFN β-1a (3,26) suggests that IFN, or IFN-activated cells, do cross the blood-brain barrier. In a clinical study of IFN-αA (18 MU) administered i.v., IFN was readily detected in serum (peak 9000 pg/ml at 10 min) but not in ventricular cerebrospinal fluid (CSF) (<15 pg/ml; [27]). However, IFN administered i.v., s.c., or intraperitoneally (i.p.) to mice increased 2,5-OAS in the brain, a more sensitive measure of IFN activity, demonstrating that IFN can cross the blood-brain barrier (28). Conversely, IFN injected intracranially increased 2,5-OAS activity in the spleen as well (28); again suggesting that IFN crosses the blood-brain barrier. IFN-β (fibroblast, Roswell Park Memorial Institute, Buffalo, NY) administered i.t. (3–6 MU, once per week) resulted in pleocytosis and increases in CSF protein, although it could not be determined whether the cells were attracted from the periphery (3). Human IFN-β (fibroblast) injected i.t. in monkeys was found to diffuse rapidly through the CSF, including around the brain, although little IFN was detected in the superficial cortex and deeper parenchyma (29). IFN-β (3–23 IU) was detected in patients' CSF during the first month of i.t. administration of 1 MU IFN-β semiweekly by lumbar puncture (26). Since the precise etiology of MS is not yet defined, the site—whether peripheral and/or CNS—and mechanism of action of IFN-β remain unclear.

G. Oral Administration of IFN

Investigation of whether IFN administered orally is biologically effective has yielded conflicting results. Orally administered human IFN conferred a protective effect on neonatal mice and kittens subsequently exposed to viral challenge (30,31). However, studies in adult African green monkeys and beagle dogs have failed to demonstrate measurable serum levels of IFN-α after oral administration of 6 $\times$ 10^6 U/kg (32,33). In patients with acquired immune deficiency syndrome (AIDS), reports showed that a low dose of oral IFN-α decreased progression of the disease and increased weight (34,35). IFN-αA/D has suppressed peripheral white blood cell (WBC) counts when administered orally, and this is thought to reflect suppression in bone marrow (36). However, in six healthy human volunteers, oral administration of 2.5 or 7.5 mg recombinant IFN β-1b did not induce measurable levels of IFN in serum, nor did it significantly induce β_2-microglobulin and neopterin in serum, or 2,5-OAS in PBMCs, which are more sensitive measures of IFN than serum IFN concentration (37). Two sources of difference could be the use of extremely low doses, and holding the IFN in the mouth for an extended time for increased transmucosal penetration in the AIDS studies. Also, immune functions may be able to be increased to baseline from lower levels in immunocompromised subjects but are not able to be increased further above normal, for example, in healthy subjects. This effect has been reported for other immunomodulators, such as levamisole (38). Finally, oral IFN at low doses could act directly on oral or gastrointestinal immune cells (see Chapter 10).

H. Administration by Inhalation

IFN-β (3–100 MU) was administered by inhalation to eight patients with thoracic malignancy (39). No IFN was detectable in serum after inhalation, and no other biological effects except for a slight increase in body temperature and a decrease in peak expiratory flow rate in one patient.

IV. Effect of Antibodies to IFN on Biological and Clinical Activity

A. Antibodies to IFN-α

Some patients develop binding or neutralizing antibodies to IFN during treatment; neutralization is typically tested in antiviral assays. The effect of antibodies to IFN-α on clinical effectiveness has been evaluated in leukemia patients. In chronic myelogenous leukemia (CML) patients treated with 5 MU IFN-α2b, 8 of 27 developed neutralizing antibodies to IFN after 4–20 months of treatment (40); neutralizing antibodies were more prevalent in patients who became refractory to treatment (5 of 9). Resistance to rIFN-α2a in hairy cell leukemia patients was also associated with anti-IFN antibodies; resistance to IFN therapy was present in 6 of 16 patients with neutralizing antibodies but not in 20 patients without antibodies (41).

Hairy cell leukemia patients who became refractory to treatment with recombinant IFN-α2a and had developed neutralizing anti-IFN antibodies remained responsive to subsequent treatment with natural IFN-α (42), suggesting that changing IFN type is one approach to restoring clinical responsiveness. Another study suggested that over time, the presence of anti-IFN antibodies diminished without other intervention. Steiss et al. (43) observed loss of antibodies in all nine previously antibody-positive hairy cell leukemia patients after a median of 14.5 months of continuous treatment with IFN-α. The loss of antibodies is suggestive of loss of clinical side effects which also occurs over time. We can conclude from these studies that the presence of antibodies which neutralize antiviral activity may not always neutralize other clinical activity, and that tolerance to IFN may develop over time.

B. Antibodies to IFN-β

The influence of several factors on antigenicity of IFN-β have been investigated, including glycosylation (present on natural or recombinant mammalian-derived, but not on *Escherichia coli*–derived IFNs) and route of administration. One study suggested that antibody formation may be more common when IFN is administered i.m. than i.v. Two of 36 cancer patients developed antibody after i.v. administration of 3–30 MU IFN β-1b for 5 days every 2 weeks or 14 days every 4 weeks. In contrast, 20 of 25 patients developed binding antibody after i.m. administration of 10–100 MU daily (44). In a study of 34 melanoma patients treated with 2–3 MU natural IFN-β (Fiblaferon, Rentschler, Laupheim, Germany) i.v. or s.c. three times a week and 50 μg rIFN-γ (Polyferon, Bioferon) s.c. on 3 consecutive days every 4 weeks, 56% developed antibodies to IFN-β but none to IFN-γ (45). Neutralizing antibodies were found in 6 of 20 (30%) of patients receiving IFN-β i.v. compared with 13 of 14 (92%) of those receiving IFN-β s.c.

Some studies found that no patients made antibodies to IFN-β. For example, none of six patients with chronic-phase CML receiving 3–12 MU/day IFN-β-1a s.c. (Bioferon, recombinant, CHO-derived), developed antibodies up to 12 weeks (46). In the large study of 372 MS patients who received E. coli–derived IFN β-1b s.c. (2), 11% of the placebo sera, 47% of the 1.6 MU sera, and 45% of the 8-MU sera had neutralizing activity to IFN-β at some time during treatment. No relationship was found between neutralizing antibodies and exacerbation severity or timing during the first

2 years of the study, unlike the trials of IFN-α in cancer patients described above. However, 5-year data suggest that neutralizing activity is associated with a rebound in relapses to the rate in the placebo group (47). Longer term follow-up and a more reliable assay are pending. Another study compared natural IFN-β (Fiblaferon) with recombinant IFN-β-1a (Betaferon, Rentschler) both given 3 MU/week s.c. to patients with malignant melanoma (25). Neutralizing antibodies were found after 12 weeks in 62% of patients receiving nIFN-β and no patients receiving rIFN-β; after 24 weeks, the percentages were 95% in nIFN-β and 29% in rIFN-β patients, respectively, suggesting nIFN-β was more antigenic. The presence of antibodies also correlated with smaller elevations of 2,5-OAS, β_2-microglobulin, and neopterin, suggesting that antibodies decreased the biological response to IFN-β.

These studies suggest further work is needed regarding route of administration, natural versus recombinant molecules, and whether neutralization of antiviral activity is a good model for other clinical activities of IFN. Low titers of neutralizing antibody may be unimportant and will be better evaluated when a reliable assay is developed. The development of anti-IFN antibodies may be another factor in individual response to IFN, again suggesting that personalized dosing may be effective.

V.   DIFFERENCES IN BIOLOGICAL RESPONSE BETWEEN IFN-β and IFN-α

The therapeutic mechanism of IFN-β in MS remains an active area of discussion and experimentation. Ideas include stabilization of T-lymphocyte suppressor activity associated with MS, downregulation of IFN-γ effects, and/or clearing CNS viral infection which may influence exacerbation rate. Several differences in biological response between IFN-β and IFN-α may shed light on why IFN-β has shown clinical effectiveness, although IFN-α may also prove effective as well. Unlike IFN-α, IFN-β induces HLA class II on peripheral blood monocytes, astrocytes, and other cells, but to a lesser extent than IFN-γ ([20]; our unpublished results). In addition, IFN-β decreases the extent of induction of MHC class II by IFN-γ at the transcriptional level (48) and the level of surface MHC class II protein (49–52). The ability to upregulate MHC class II antigen on target cells and antigen-presenting cells, without fully activating macrophages as does IFN-γ, may be important. IFN-β was less effective than IFN α-2b in inducing IL-1 receptor antagonist protein (IL-1-Ra) in serum of CML patients but equally effective in inducing β_2-microglobulin and neopterin (46). Also, IFN-β had less clinical effectiveness than IFN α-2b in CML. Finally, IFN-β is a better inducer of 2,5-OAS than IFN-γ both in vivo and in vitro, and it is a better activator of antiviral pathways.

VI. SUMMARY

Route: Subcutaneous and i.m. dosing show similar biological effectiveness to i.v., although IFN is less detectable in the former. Intravenous dosing may lead to a lower incidence of antiviral-neutralizing antibodies, although the relevance of these antibodies to clinical activity is still unclear. Subcutaneous and i.m. dosing are simpler for patients to administer at home on a long-term basis. Induction of IFN-induced proteins in the brain (2,5-OAS [28]) and the clinical effectiveness of systemically administered IFN indicate that IFN or IFN-activated immune cells can reach CNS tissues.

Dose: In the large MS study (2), 8.0 MU IFN β-1b had greater clinical effectiveness than 1.6 MU, and both were better than placebo, especially in decreasing MRI-detected lesions. A small study also showed 16 MU was more effective than 8 MU IFN β (53). The MTD for IFN β-1b (defined primarily with cancer patients) is closer to 18 MU for long-term administration. Thus, it is possible that higher doses may yield greater decreases in the exacerbation rate and brain lesions in MS. However, there is difficulty in blinding a study at this dose.

Schedule: The biological response to both IFN β-1a and IFN β-1b, as measured by several IFN-induced proteins or metabolites, is increased significantly for 2–3 days and increased slightly for up to 1 week. More frequent (i.e., daily) IFN-β administration appears to be unhelpful in further inducing these proteins. Thus treatments once or twice a week were selected. Clinical studies utilizing high i.t. doses of IFN-β showed that 9 treatments in 6 months were about as effective as 13 treatments in 6 months (26), suggesting that even fewer treatments may be sufficient. There is no evidence on this point with systemic treatments. Other markers of biological response, especially changes in populations of specific effector cells, or induction of specific HLA, adhesion, or costimulatory molecules, may be more relevant to the mechanism of IFN-β in MS and remain to be defined in the future.

REFERENCES

1. Paty DW, Li DKB, UBC MS/MRI Study Group, IFNB Multiple Sclerosis Study Group. Interferon beta-1b is effective in relapsing-remitting multiple sclerosis II: MRI analysis results. Neurology 1993; 43:662–667.
2. IFNB Multiple Sclerosis Study Group. Interferon beta-1b is effective in relapsing-remitting multiple sclerosis I: Clinical results. Neurology 1993; 43: 655–661.
3. Jacobs L, Salazar AM, Herndon R, Reese P, Freeman A, Josefowics R, Cuetter A, Husain F, Smith WA, Ekes R, O'Malley JA. Multicentre double-

blind study of effect of intrathecally administered natural human fibroblast interferon on exacerbations of multiple sclerosis. Lancet 1986; 20:1411–1413.

4. Chiang J, Gloff CA, Yoshizawa CN, Williams GJ. Pharmacokinetics of recombinant human interferon-βser in healthy volunteers and its effects on serum neopterin. Pharm Res 1993; 10:567–572.

5. Goldstein D, Sielaff KM, Storer BE, Brown RR, Datta SP, Witt PL, Teitelbaum AP, Smalley RV, Borden EC. Human biologic response modification by interferon in the absence of measurable serum concentrations: a comparative trial of subcutaneous and intravenous interferon betaserine. J Natl Cancer Inst 1989; 81:1061–1068.

6. Chiang J, Gloff CA, Soike KF, Williams G. Pharmacokinetics and antiviral activity of recombinant human interferon-βser17 in African green monkeys. J Interferon Res 1993; 13:111–120.

7. Grunberg SM, Kempf RA, Venturi CL, Mitchell MS. Phase I study of recombinant beta-interferon given by four-hour infusion. Cancer Res 1987; 47: 1174–1178.

8. Abdi EA, Kamitomo VJ, McPherson TA, Konrad MW, Inoue M, Tan YH. Extended phase I study of human β-interferon in human cancer. Clin Invest Med 1986; 9:33–40.

9. Rohatiner AZS, Balkwill FR, Griffin DB, Malpas JS, Lister TA. A phase I study of human lymphoblastoid interferon administered by continuous intravenous infusion. Cancer Chemother Pharmacol 1982; 9:97–102.

10. Dhingra K, Duvic M, Hymes S, McLaughlin P, Rothberg J, Gutterman JU. A phase-I clinical study of low-dose oral interferon-α. J Immunother 1993; 14:51–55.

11. Maluish AE, Reid JW, Crisp EA, Overton WR, Levy H, Foon KA, Herberman RB. Immunomodulatory effects of poly(I,C)-LC in cancer patients. J Biol Response Mod 1985; 4:656–663.

12. Quesada JR, Gutterman JU. Clinical study of recombinant DNA-produced leukocyte interferon (Clone A) in an intermittent schedule in cancer patients. J Natl Cancer Inst 1983; 70:1041–1046.

13. Liberati AM, Horisberger MA, Palmisano L, Astolfi S, Nastari A, Mechati S, Villa A, Mancini S, Arzano S, Grignani F. Double-blind randomized phase I study on the clinical tolerance and biological effects of natural and recombinant interferon-β. J Interferon Res 1992; 12:329–336.

13a. Billiau A, DeSomer P, Edy VG, DeClercq E, Heremans H. Human fibroblast interferon for clinical trials: pharmacokinetics and tolerability in experimental animals and humans. Antimicrobial Agents Chemother 1979; 16:56–63.

14. Kinney P, Triozzi P, Young D, Drago J, Behrens B, Wise H, Rinehart JJ. Phase II trial of interferon-beta-serine in metastatic renal cell carcinoma. J Clin Oncol 1990; 8:881–885.

15. Witt PL, Storer BE, Bryan GT, Brown RR, Flashner M, Larocca AT, Colby CB, Borden EC. Pharmacodynamics of biological response in vivo after single and multiple doses of interferon-β. J Immunother 1993; 13:191–200.

16. Liberati AM, Fizzotti M, Proietti MG, DiMarzio R, Schippa M, Biscottini B, Senatore M, Berruto P, Canali S, Peretti G, Zanolo G. Biochemical host response to interferon-beta. J Interferon Res 1988; 8:765–777.

17. Jacobs L, Munschauer F. Treatment of multiple sclerosis with interferons. In: Rudick FA, Goodkin DE, eds. Treatment of Multiple Sclerosis: Trial Design, Results, and Future Perspectives. London: Springer-Verlag, 1992: 233–250.

18. Rinehart JJ, Young D, Laforge J, Colborn D, Neidhart JA. Phase I/II trial of interferon beta-serine in patients with renal cell carcinoma: immunological and biological effects. Cancer Res 1987; 47:2481–2487.

19. Talmadge JE, Tribble HR, Pennington RW, Phillips H, Wiltrout RH. Immunomodulatory and immunotherapeutic properties of recombinant gamma-interferon and recombinant tumor necrosis factor in mice. Cancer Res 1987; 47:2563–2570.

20. Spear GT, Paulnock DM, Jordan RL, Meltzer DM, Merritt JA, Borden EC. Enhancement of monocyte class I and II histocompatibility antigen expression in man by in vivo beta-interferon. Clin Exp Immunol 1987; 69:107–115.

21. Borden EC, Rinehart JJ, Storer BE, Trump DL, Paulnock DM, Teitelbaum AP. Biological and clinical effects of interferon betaser at two doses. J Interferon Res 1990; 10:559–570.

22. Hirayama K, Matsushita S, Kikuchi I, Iuchi M, Ohta N, Sasazuki T. HLA-DQ is epistatic to HLA-DR in controlling the immune response to schistosomal antigen in humans. Nature 1987; 327:426–430.

23. Borden EC, Hawkins MJ, Sielaff KM, Storer BM, Schiesel JD, Smalley RB. Clinical and biological effects of recombinant interferon beta administered intravenously daily in a phase I trial. J Interferon Res 1988; 8:357–366.

24. Liberati AM, Garofani P, DeAngelis V, DiClemente F, Horisberger M, Cecchini M, Betti AR, Palmisano L, Astofi S, Nastari A, Villa A, Arzano S. Double-blind randomized phase I study on the clinical tolerance and pharmacodynamics of natural and recombinantinterferon-beta given intravenously. J Interferon Res 1994; 14:61–69.

25. Fierlbeck G, Schreiner T. Incidence and clinical significance of therapy-induced neutralizing antibodies against interferon-β. J Interferon Res 1994; 14:205–206.

26. Jacobs L, O'Malley J, Freeman A, Ekes R. Intrathecal interferon reduces exacerbations of multiple sclerosis. Science 1981; 214:1026–1028.

27. Wills RJ, Smith RA. Pharmacokinetics of interferons. In: Smith RA, ed. Interferon Treatment of Neurologic Disorders. New York: Marcel Dekker, 1988:103–134.

28. Hovanessian AG, Marcovistz R, Riviere Y, Guillon J-C, Tsiang H. Production and action of interferon in rabies virus infection. In: Smith RA, ed. Interferon Treatment of Neurologic Disorders. New York: Marcel Dekker, 1988:157–208.

29. Billiau A. Interferon therapy: pharmacokinetic and pharmacological aspects. Arch Virol 1981; 67:121–133.

30. Schafer TW, Lieberman M, Cohen M, Came PE. Interferon administered orally: protection of neonatal mice from lethal virus challenge. Science 1972; 76:1326–1327.

31. Cummins JM, Tompkins MB, Olsen RG, Tompkins WA, Lewis MG. Oral use of human alpha interferon in cats. J Biol Response Mod 1988; 7:513–523.

32. Wills RJ, Spiegel HE, Soike KF. Pharmacokinetics of recombinant A interferon following IV infusion and bolus, IM and PO administration to African green monkeys. J Interferon Res 1984; 4:399–409.

33. Gibson DM, Cotler S, Spiegel HE, Colburn WA. Pharmacokinetics of recombinant leukocyte A interferon following various routes and modes of administration to the dog. J Interferon Res 1985; 5:403–408.

34. Koech DK, Obel AO, Minowada J, Hutchinson VA, Cummins JM. Low dose oral alpha-interferon therapy for patients seropositive for human immunodeficiency virus type-1 (HIV-1). Mol Biother 1990; 2:91–95.

35. Hutchinson V, Cummins JM. Low-dose oral interferon in patient with AIDS. Lancet 1987; 2:1530–1531.

36. Koren S, Fleischmann WRJ. Orally administered interferons suppress bone marrow function. Proc Soc Exp Biol Med 1993; 204:155–164.

37. Witt PL, Goldstein D, Storer BE, Grossberg SE, Flashner M, Colby CB, Borden EC. Absence of biologic effects of orally administered interferon-βser. J Interferon Res 1992; 12:411–413.

38. Schiller JH, Witt PL. Levamisole: clinical and biological effects. In: DeVita VT Jr, Hellman S, Rosenberg SA, eds. Biologic Therapy of Cancer Updates. vol. 2. Philadelphia, Lippincott, 1992:1–14.

39. Halme M, Maasilta P, Mattson K, Cantell K. Pharmacokinetics and toxicity of inhaled human natural interferon-beta in patients with lung cancer. Respiration 1994; 61:105–107.

40. Freund M, VonWussow P, Diedrich H, Eisert R, Link H, Wilke H, Buchholz F, LeBlanc S, Fonatsch C, Diecher H, Poliwoda H. Recombinant human interferon (IFN) alpha-2b in chronic myelogenous leukaemia: dose dependence of response and frequency of neutralizing anti-interferon antibodies. Br J Haematol 1989; 72:350–356.

41. Steis RG, Smith JWII, Urba WJ, Clark JW, Itri LM, Evans LM, Schoenberger C, Longo DL. Resistance to recombinant interferon alfa-2a in hairy-cell leukemia associated with neutralizing anti-interferon antibodies. N Engl J Med 1988; 318:1409–1413.

42. vonWussow P, Pralle H, Hochkeppel H-K, Jakschies D, Sonnen S, Schmidt H, Muller-Rosenau D, Franke M, Haferlach T, Zwingers T, Rapp U, Deicher H. Effective natural interferon-α therapy in recombinant interferon-α-resistant patients with hairy cell leukemia. Blood 1991; 78:38–43.

43. Steis RG, Smith JWII, Urba WJ, Venzon DJ, Longo DL, Barney R, Evans LM, Itri LM, Ewel CH. Loss of interferon antibodies during prolonged continuous interferon-α2a therapy in hairy cell leukemia. Blood 1991; 77: 792–798.

44. Konrad MW, Childs AL, Merigan TC, Borden EC. Assessment of the antigenic response in humans to a recombinant mutant interferon beta. J Clin Immunol 1987; 7:365–375.

45. Dummer R, Muller W, Nestle F, Wiede J, Dues J, Lechner W, Haubitz I, Wolf W, Vill E, Burg G. Formation of neutralizing antibodies against natural interferon-beta but not against recombinant interferon-gamma during adjuvant therapy for high-risk malignant melanoma patients. Cancer 1991; 67: 2300–2304.

46. Aulitzky WE, Peschel C, Despres D, Aman J, Trautman P, Tilg H, Rudolf G, Huttmann H, Obermeier J, Herold M, Huber C. Divergent in vivo and in vitro antileukemic activity of recombinant interferon beta in patients with chronic-phase chronic myelogenous leukemia. Ann Hematol 1993; 67: 205–211.

47. The IFNβ Multiple Sclerosis Study Group. Beta interferon 1b in the treatment of MS: Final outcome of the randomized controlled trial. Neurology 1995; 45:1277–1285.

48. Ransohoff RM, Devajyothi C, Estes ML, Babcock G, Rudick RA, Frohman EM, Barna BP. Interferon-beta specifically inhibits interferon-gamma-induced class II major histocompatibility complex gene transcription in a human astrocytoma cell line. J Neuroimmunol 1991; 33:103–112.

49. Ling PD, Warren MK, Vogel SN. Antagonistic effect of interferon-beta on the interferon-gamma-induced expression of Ia antigen in murine macrophages. J Immunol 1985; 135:1857–1861.

50. Naito Y, Baba T, Suzuki H, Ayeno K. The antagonistic effect of interferon-β on the interferon-γ-induced expression of HLA-DR antigen in a squamous cell carcinoma line. J Exp Pathol 1992; 6:75–87.

51. Inaba K, Kitaura M, Kato T, Watanabe Y, Kawade Y, Muramatsu S. Contrasting effect of alpha/beta and gamma interferons on expression of macrophage Ia antigens. J Exp Med 1986; 163:1030–1035.

52. Scotlandi K, Baldini N, Campanacci M, Lollini PL, Picci P, Serra M. Induction of HLA class II antigens in osteosarcoma cells by interferons and tumor necrosis factorα. Anticancer Res 1992; 12:767–772.

53. Knobler RL, Greenstein JI, Johnson KP, Lublin FD, Panitch HS, Conway K, Grant-Gorsen SV, Muldoon J, Marcus SG, Wallenberg JC. Systemic recombinant human interferon-β treatment of relapsing-remitting multiple sclerosis: pilot study analysis and six-year follow-up. J Interferon Res 1993; 13: 333–340.

4

Interferons and the Central Nervous System Glia

Timothy Vartanian

Harvard Medical School, Boston, Massachusetts

I. INTRODUCTION

This chapter focuses on the relationship between interferons (IFNs) and the glia of the central nervous system (CNS). We will discuss synthesis of IFNs by glia, the biological responses of glia to IFNs, and instances where type I and II IFNs generate opposing responses. We will begin with a brief review of the biology of glia.

In the CNS, astrocytes, oligodendrocytes, and ependyma comprise the macroglia. These cells are neuroectodermal in origin (1). Microglia, Cajal's third element, are resident phagocytes in the CNS and are mesenchymal in origin (2).

Astrocytes serve multiple roles in the developing and the adult CNS. During development, radial glia form a scaffolding which serves in neuronal guidance (1,3). Astrocytes are also a source of neurotrophic factors for developing neurons and oligodendrocytes (3). In addition, the blood-brain barrier, which consists of specialized endothelial cells joined by tight junctions, develops in part from the influence of one or more unknown factors derived from astrocytes. At synapses and nodes of Ranvier, astrocytes regulate homeostasis by maintaining pH and ion concentrations, as well as transporting and metabolizing excitatory amino acids (3). Most importantly, astrocytes are significant players in the cellular response to

CNS injury (4). In response to injury, astrocytes hypertrophy (to a lesser extent they may proliferate) and secrete numerous cytokines.

Myelin formed by the oligodendrocyte is crucial for high-efficiency saltatory conduction along axons (5). Loss of oligodendrocytes and the myelin they form results in slowed or blocked conduction of action potentials. Oligodendrocytes do not significantly proliferate in the normal adult, but they will proliferate at sites of injury such as the active margins of multiple sclerosis (MS) lesions. Remyelination occurs at the margins of some MS lesions, but for reasons which remain elusive, it is usually scant.

Microglia are bone marrow–derived cells in the monocyte-macrophage lineage which immigrate into the CNS during development to become resident phagocytes. There is little biochemically to distinguish microglia from blood-borne monocytes, although they are morphologically distinct. However, an important distinction exists between these cell types in their electrophysiology. Microglia possess an inward rectifying K^+ channel, distinct from the exclusively outward rectifying K^+ channel of monocytes (6,47). It is interesting to note that a subpopulation of monocyte precursors within the bone marrow can also be distinguished by this physiological difference, suggesting that some bone marrow cells within the monocyte lineage might be predetermined to become microglia.

II. EFFECTS OF INTERFERONS ON ASTROCYTES

Astrocytes have been the most intensely studied macroglial cell in terms of the production of, and the response to, cytokines. Astrocytes form the glial scar within chronic and chronic active MS lesions. In active MS lesions and at the margins of chronic active lesions, reactive astrocytes stain intensely for IFN-γ (7). In this section, we will review the relationship of IFNs and astrocytes as it applies to the biological response, the synthesis of IFNs and other cytokines, and the immune response.

A. Biological Responses of Astrocytes to Interferons

Astrocytes have receptors for both type I and type II IFNs (8). IFN-γ induces proliferation of human astrocytes in vitro, with maximal effects occurring at concentrations of 10 U/ml (9). Reactive astrogliosis, induced by corticectomy in adult mice and assessed by a marked increase in glial fibrillatory acidic protein (GFAP) immunoreactivity, was notably potentiated by IFN-γ (9,10). Other groups using similar methods have failed to observe a proliferative response of rodent astrocytes in vitro to IFN-γ (11). However, reactive gliosis, a poorly understood biological response, is marked by hypertrophy of existing astrocytes rather than their proliferation (5). Thus, in vivo, IFN-γ may contribute to gliosis by inducing hypertrophy of astrocytes.

A key role of the astrocyte is to control pH and the ionic microenvironment, particularly at synapses, nodes of Ranvier, and around neuronal somata. This process is carried out in part by one or more Na^+/H^+ exchange proteins. IFN-γ activates the type 1 Na^+/H^+ exchanger in astrocytes; this activation is followed by an efflux of glutamate (12). Glutamate is a well-described neurotoxin, and under certain conditions, it has been shown to kill oligodendrocytes (13). Yet, it is difficult to implicate glutamate as a sole mediator of oligodendrocyte injury in MS in light of the well-described neuronal sparing in MS.

IFN-γ, in combination with interleukin-1β (IL-1β) induces nitric oxide synthase (NOS) in cultured astrocytes (14, 15). NOS generates the free radical nitric oxide (NO·) from oxygen and the guanidino nitrogen of L-arginine. Nitric oxide, or reactive intermediates formed from nitric oxide, are cytotoxic to a number of neuronal cell types (16). Induction is dependent on protein kinase C (PKC) activity, as the PKC inhibitors H7 and genistein block NOS synthesis (15). Transcription of the gene encoding NOS in astrocytes is regulated in part by NOS activity itself. Inhibitors of NOS activity downregulate and exogenous NO· upregulates transcription of the NOS gene in astrocytes (17,18). Thus, IFN-γ could trigger in astrocytes the secretion of NO·, a second toxic agent potentially involved in damage to oligodendrocytes.

B. Synthesis of Interferons and Other Cytokines by Astrocytes

Traugott and Lebon have reported immunohistochemical staining of type I and type II IFNs in active chronic MS lesions (7). IFN-γ is localized to astrocytes in normal-appearing white matter adjacent to the active margin of MS lesions, but IFN-β is found in astrocytes within the boundaries of lesions. IFN-α is present within foamy macrophages at the active margins of lesions. However, Cannella and Raine have recently reported IFN-γ is also localized to microglia within MS lesions (19), which is consistent with findings from our laboratory (20).

Within both normal and transected optic nerve, Lewis rat astrocytes express IFN-γ (21). Other studies of the rodent CNS localize IFN-γ immunoreactivity only to a subset of circumventricular organ cells within the hypothalmus (22). It is well known that the Lewis rat, unlike many other rat species, is permissive for the formation of experimental autoimmune encephalopathy (EAE) (23) and the constitutive expression of IFN-γ may be related to the ease with which the Lewis rat develops EAE. Furthermore, in vitro, IFN-γ given in combination with IL-1β induces expression of tumor necrosis factor-α (TNF-α) in astrocytes derived from Lewis rats but not in astrocytes from Brown-Norway rats (24,25). Brown-Norway rats do not develop EAE, and thus Benveniste and colleagues suggest that astrocyte responsiveness to IFN-γ may relate to EAE susceptibility (25).

A number of other macromolecules, such as apolipoprotein E (26) and proenkephalin (27), are upregulated or downregulated in astrocytes in response to IFN-γ. The relationship of these macromolecules to diseases of myelin has not been an area of rigorous study.

C. Astrocytes, IFNs, and the Immune Response

There is an extensive body of work on major histocompatibility complex (MHC) antigen expression (see Chapter 7) by astrocytes and their involvement in the immune response, much of which is summarized in Table 1. The majority of this work is based on in vitro data. Robust MHC expression on normal astrocytes in vivo is not seen. One explanation for this dichotomy is that neurons interacting with astrocytes may suppress expression of MHC. It turns out that even in vitro, class I and class II MHC expression by astrocytes is significantly downregulated by coculture with neurons (28). Neurotransmitters, such as β-adrenergic agonists (29,30), and glutamate (31) inhibit the ability of astrocytes to express MHC antigens in vitro and in vivo. MHC antigens, however, appear on astrocytes in vivo after focal injury or cytokine injection. Injection of IFN-γ into mouse brain also induces H2 (MHC class I) expression on most astrocytes and Ia (MHC class II) expression on a subpopulation of astrocytes (33). In contrast, Uitdehaag and coworkers found that after injection of IFN-γ into the ventricles of Lewis rats, microglia, but not astrocytes, were the major population of cells expressing class II antigens (35). In MS, the major class II–expressing cell also appears to be the microglial cell rather than the astrocyte (36,37).

A substantial body of work in both humans and rodents has shown that astrocytes can present antigen to T lymphocytes in the context of class II (38, 39, and references therein). The ability of astrocytes to present antigen in vitro, however, depends on prior exposure to IFN-γ (40,41) or IL-2 (42). It is interesting in light of the dramatically opposite effects of type I and type II IFNs on the clinical course of MS, that IFN-β opposes the ability of IFN-γ to induce class II antigens on astrocytes in vitro (43). EAE and Theiler's virus–induced demyelination are two rodent models which share a few features with MS. Disease susceptibility among different strains of animals for both EAE and Theiler's virus correlates with the ability of IFN-γ to induce class II expression on astrocytes in vitro

(44,45). Although, as stated above, it is not clear that significant class II expression on astrocytes occurs in vivo.

A final note about astrocytes relates to their heterogeneity. There are several in vitro and in vivo studies which identify biological and molecular differences between astrocytes from different anatomical regions of the brain. For example, in response to transforming growth factor-β1 (TGF-β1), mouse brainstem astrocytes proliferate, whereas forebrain astrocytes do not (46). TGF-β1 blocks IFN-γ–induced class II antigen expression on brainstem astrocytes but not that of forebrain astrocytes (46). There are also regional differences between astrocytes in the expression of cytoskeletal proteins and neurotransmitters and in their morphology (reviewed in ref. 47). Regional heterogeneity of glial cells may prove to be important for demyelinating diseases where a predilection to affect certain parts of the CNS is common.

III. EFFECTS OF INTERFERONS ON MICROGLIA

Microglia are bone marrow–derived, take residence in the CNS early in life, and resemble blood-borne monocytes/macrophages in most respects (for review see refs. 2, 6, and 48).

Activated microglia and macrophages are prominent cell types in active MS lesions (50) and in inflammatory diseases of the CNS (48). Microglia, however, are not solely mediators of injury. Guilian and colleagues have described microglia-derived proteins which support the growth and survival of neurons and astrocytes (51–53). In this section, we will examine IFNs and their biological effects on ameboid microglia, IFN-mediated induction of NOS as a microglial derived mediator of cytotoxicity, and the induction of MHC antigens.

A. Biological Response of Ameboid Microglia to the IFNs

Cultured microglia can assume many morphologies: ameboid, rod-shaped, and ramified. In response to IFN-γ, ramified microglia revert to the ameboid morphology (54). However, both IFN-γ and IFN-α/β affect the function of microglia; they decrease chemotaxis of microglia in response to zymosan (55), and IFN-γ hinders nonresident macrophage invasion of peripheral nerves undergoing Wallerian degeneration (56). The influence of IFN-γ on microglial motility is clearly relevant to CNS injury and inflammation, where focal expression of IFN-γ may recruit resident microglia and macrophages.

After microglia are primed with the phorbal ester (phorbal myristate acetate [PMA]), both IFN-γ and IFN-α and IFN-β increase superoxide

Table 1 Expression of MHC Antigens by Astrocytes in Response to Interferons

MHC antigen	Species	Cytokine	Effect on astrocyte	Reference
Class I				
polymorphic	Lewis rat	IFN-γ	⇑	28,96
polymorphic	Lewis rat	IFN-γ + neuronal coculture	⇓	28
H2	Mouse	IFN-γ	⇑	33
Class II				
polymorphic	Rat (retina)	IFN-γ	⇑	97
Ia	Lewis rat	IFN-γ	⇑	98
Ia	Rat	IFN-γ + TNF-α	⇑⇑	99
Ia^d	Mouse	IFN-γ + TNF-α	⇑⇑	43
Ia^s	SJL mouse	IFN-γ + IL-1β	⇓	100
Ia	Lewis rat	IFN-γ + Tetraethylammonium	⇓	101
Ia	Lewis rat	IFN-γ + Norepinephrine	⇓	102
Ia	Lewis rat	IFN-γ + ⇑ intracellular cAMP	⇓	103

Molecule	Cells (species)	Inducer		Ref.
OX-6	S104 cells (Lewis Rat)	TGF-β	$\Rightarrow$	104
HLA-DR	Human	IFN-γ	$\Leftarrow\Rightarrow$	105,106
HLA-DR	Human	IFN-γ + IFN-β	$\Leftarrow\Rightarrow$	43
polymorphic	Lewis rat	IFN-γ	$\Leftarrow\Rightarrow$	28
polymorphic	Lewis rat	IFN-γ + neuronal co-culture		28
I-E^k, Ia^d, H2A^k	Mouse	IFN-γ	$\Leftarrow\Rightarrow$	33,43,107
Ia^d, H2A^k	Mouse	IFN-γ + IFN-α or -β	$\Rightarrow$	43,107
CD44/v6 exon	Mouse	IFN-γ/TNF-α	$\Leftarrow$	108
Cell adhesion molecules				
ICAM-1	Human	IFN-γ	$\Leftarrow$	102

anion production and presumably increase cytotoxic function (54, 55). In contrast, IFN-α/β increases IL-1 section, but IFN-γ inhibits IL-1 secretion by microglia (55), pointing to important differences the type I and type II IFNs have on control of immunoregulatory cytokines.

IFN-γ induces cultured microglia to form multinucleated giant cells. Giant cell formation can be inhibited by antibodies directed against leukocyte function associated antigen-1, α-chain (CD11a), and intracellular adhesion molecule (ICAM) (57).

B. Interferon-Induced Nitric Oxide Synthase in Microglia

Rodent microglia express inducible NOS, and IFN-γ is a potent stimulus for this activity (59–63). NOS activity can be detected by the NADPH diaphorase reaction (64,65). In contrast, human microglia express little or no inducible NOS (62,63). Fetal human astrocytes express NOS activity after stimulation with IL-1β or IFN-γ (61). It is interesting that IFN-γ protects both human (66) and murine (67) microglia from infection with the parasite *Toxoplasma gondii*. However, the ability of IFN-γ to protect human microglia from *T. gondii* is independent of nitric oxide–mediated mechanisms (66). In murine microglia, inhibitors of NOS block the protective effects of IFN-γ(67). This raises an important difference between human and rodent microglia and macrophages—human microglia, unlike their rodent counterparts, express little inducible NOS. Glucocorticoids inhibit nitric oxide generation in murine microglia treated with lipopolysaccharide (LPS) and IFN-γ (68).

C. Interferons, Microglia, and the Immune Response

Microglia are central to immune regulation in the brain. Their expression of MHC molecules and Fc receptors enhances immune reactions. In vitro, unstimulated microglia express MHC class I antigens (H2 in mouse, HLA-A, B, C in humans) (69). When stimulated with IFN-γ, they will additionally express class II (Ia) antigens (69–73). IFN-γ administered intravenously to Lewis rats induces class II antigens on microglia, ependyma, and endothelium (70). IFN-γ, TNF-α, or LPS each induce Fc receptors on rat microglia (72). Oddly, when given in combination with either TNF-α or LPS, IFN-γ inhibits Fc receptor expression (72). In contrast, TGF-β, granulocyte-macrophage colony-stimulating factor, dexamethasone, and norepinephrine all inhibit the ability of IFN-γ to induce Fc receptor expression on cultured rat microglia (74,75), which may have therapeutic relevance. IFN-γ-induced MHC class II and FcR expression has functional consequences. IFN-γ–primed microglia induce a significant proliferative response in naive CD4$^+$ and CD8$^+$ T lymphocytes which can be blocked by anti–class II antibodies (72,76,77). When compared with astrocytes, microglia appear to be significantly more competent as antigen-presenting cells and thus are more likely to play a role in the immune response.

Microglia express TNF-α in human brain (78). IFN-γ induces the synthesis of TNF-α in microglia in vitro, and might be expected to induce secretion of TNF-α in vivo. TNF-α has been proposed as an oligodendrocyte toxin (79–81). The effect of type I IFNs on IFN-γ–induced TNF-α secretion is worthy of investigation.

IV. EFFECTS OF INTERFERONS ON OLIGODENDROCYTES

Oligodendrocytes form myelin in the CNS. The oligodendrocyte itself, or the myelin it forms, are the target(s) in MS. It has been proposed by many investigators that the sharp margins noted in MS lesions indicate that myelin internodes are the target in MS. However, primary death of oligodendrocytes and secondary demyelination can also lead to foci of demyelination with sharp margins as in progressive multifocal leukoencephalopathy, a disease caused by primary infection of oligodendrocytes with the papova virus, JC. Little is known about the effects of IFNs on oligodendrocytes. In this section, we will review the effects of IFNs on the survival of oligodendendrocytes and on their ability to induce class I and class II antigens.

A. Interferon-Mediated Induction of Class I and Class II Antigens on Oligodendrocytes

Several in vitro studies have shown that IFN-γ induces class I and/or class II antigens on oligodendrocytes (82–85). However, Noble and colleagues have demonstrated that as oligodendrocyte precursors develop into mature oligodendrocytes, they lose their ability to express class II antigens in response to IFN-γ (86).

ICAM-1 increases lymphocyte adhesion by acting as a ligand for lymphocyte associated antigen (LFA-1) (87,88). IFN-γ increases ICAM expression by cultured oligodendrocytes, suggesting that it could enhance lymphocyte-mediated cytotoxicity against oligodendrocytes (89).

B. Influence of IFNs on Oligodendrocyte Survival

What causes oligodendrocyte injury and demyelination in MS? It has been postulated that oligodendrocyte loss and demyelination in MS is either cell-mediated, antibody-mediated, or cytokine-mediated. However, the mechanism for oligodendrocyte injury in MS remains unclear, and any combination of the above mechanisms or a heretofore undescribed mechanism may be at play. In this section, we will cover the topic of cytokine-mediated oligodendrocyte injury.

We have found that IFN-γ induces the death of cultured oligodendrocytes (20). Forty eight hours after exposure of oligodendrocytes to IFN-γ ~75% of the cells show features of apoptosis. After 4 days of exposure to IFN-γ, most of the oligodendrocytes have begun to demonstrate the late morphological changes of death such as degeneration of processes into vacuoles.

It has been reported that TNF-α, at concentrations of 100 ng/ml, may be toxic to oligodendrocytes (79–81). However, in cultures enriched for oligodendrocytes, with microglia accounting for less than 0.5% of the cells, we found no evidence for TNF-α (100 ng/ml)–induced oligodendrocyte cell death (20). These data imply that injury may be indirectly mediated through other cell types in mixed cultures. In cultures of mature ovine oligodendrocytes, Soliven and Szuchet did not find evidence for TNF-α–mediated oligodendrocyte death (90,91). These investigators have nicely reviewed the data on TNF-α and oligodendrocytes (91).

Although we depleted oligodendrocyte cultures of microglia to approximately 0.5% of the cells, there remained a remote possibility that IFN-γ was acting through a few contaminating microglia. To test this possibility, we performed the following experiments. First, we added equivalent numbers of ameboid microglia to cultures of oligodendrocytes and assessed the viability of oligodendrocytes with and without IFN-γ treatment. There was no significant difference in the percentage of oligodendrocyte killing by IFN-γ in the presence or absence of ameboid microglia (20).

It has been proposed that oligodendrocytes are susceptible to nitric oxide–mediated injury (94). Indeed, rat microglia express inducible NOS in response to cytokines and LPS, as described above. We assessed the second possibility that microglia secreted nitric oxide toxic to oligodendrocytes. We utilized tissue culture inserts with a highly permeable surface which can be placed in close apposition to cells grown in a tissue culture well. Microglia were cultured on inserts which allow free passage of molecules but not cells. They were treated with IFN-γ or control solution for 24 hr and then washed to remove free IFN-γ. Inserts were then placed 1 mm above cultures of oligodendrocytes in the presence of nitric oxide scavengers (reduced hemoglobin, 500 μM), the NOS inhibitor N$^{\omega}$-methyl-L-arginine (500 μM) both during washes as well as coculture, anti–IFN-γ antibodies (200 neutralizing units/ml), or control buffer. After 48 hr of coculture, there was a 30–40% decrease in the number of viable oligodendrocytes in all conditions except with anti–IFN-γ antibodies (20).

Nitric oxide and NOS inhibitors did not reverse oligodendrocyte death. This suggested to us that nitric oxide was not toxic to oligodendrocytes.

Rather, IFN-γ was toxic either by inducing synthesis of IFN-γ in microglia, or it was adhering to microglia and then released during coculture killing of oligodendrocytes by a direct pathway. To assess these possibilities, we perform the same experiments as described above except this time fibroblasts were used in place of microglia. We obtained similar results, suggesting that IFN-γ was adhering to cells on the inserts, since fibroblasts do not synthesize IFN-γ (20).

Oligodendrocytes treated for 18 hrs with IFN-γ exhibited DNA which was degraded into nucleosome-sized (multiples of 200–300 base pairs) fragments and pyknotic nuclei with preservation of the plasmalemma (20). Both are suggestive of apoptosis.

Degraded nuclear DNA of apoptotic cells can also be detected in situ by terminal labeling of the 3'-OH ends of DNA with digoxigenin-dUTP in the presence of terminal deoxynucleotide transferase. Tailed 3'-OH groups are identified with peroxidase-conjugated antibodies directed against digoxigenin and subsequent reaction with DAB and H_2O_2. This method was used to identify apoptotic cells. Staining with a monoclonal antibody against the myelin-oligodendrocyte-glycoprotein (MOG) was used to label oligodendrocytes. Snap-frozen tissue containing four chronic active lesions from four different patients was obtained at autopsies performed between 4 and 12 hrs after death. The advancing margins of chronic active MS plaques, but not unaffected white matter, contain numerous pyknotic, apoptotic nuclei within MOG-labeled cells. The labeled nuclei are not clustered in a contiguous mass of dead cells as in necrosis, but rather are scattered among normal cells throughout the advancing margin of the lesion, a finding consistent with apoptosis. Nuclei in adjacent normal white matter and normal controls do not label with the terminal transferase technique.

A feature of apoptosis is that the dead cells are engulfed by either professional or nonprofessional phagocytes. Prineas and colleagues have reported engulfment of oligodendrocytes by astrocytes within active MS lesions (95).

Thus, we have evidence that IFN-γ induces programmed cell death of oligodendrocytes in vitro, and that there is programmed death of oligodendrocytes in MS plaques. In light of the presence of IFN-γ at the advancing margins of active MS lesions, we speculate that IFN-γ plays a role in the pathogenesis of MS by contributing to oligodendrocyte injury.

V. CONCLUSIONS

The role of the astrocyte in demyelinating diseases is unknown. In the histopathology of MS, reactive astrocytosis is a prominant feature. Work would suggest that IFN-γ and perhaps other cytokines play a role in this cellular reaction by inducing hypertrophy of astrocytes. Class II antigen expression by astrocytes is likely an in vitro rather than an in vivo phenomenon. However, astrocytes produce numerous cytokines which may play a role in both the positive and negative regulation of the immune response. In addition, cytokines and/or reactive oxygen species produced by astrocytes may individually, or in combination, injure oligodendrocytes.

Microglia are the major class II antigen-expressing cell in the CNS. Class II antigen expression on microglia is potentiated by IFN-γ. In addition, microglia may themselves produce IFN-γ, which could act in a autocrine or paracrine fashion, as well as act on other cell types. Rodent experiments (both in vitro and EAE) require cautious interpretation, exemplified by the presence of inducible NOS activity in rodent microglia and its absence in human microglia.

The reasons for oligodendrocyte injury in MS are unknown. Work from our laboratory has shown that there is programmed cell death of oligodendrocytes in MS. Reactive oxygen intermediates may play a role in oligodendrocyte injury and IFN-γ induces the production of these compounds in astrocytes, microglia as well as macrophages, depending on experimental conditions. Our data support a role for IFN-γ in mediating oligodendrocyte injury, but it is likely that a single cytokine alone is not responsible for the marked loss of oligodendrocytes and myelin. Rather, it would seem that multiple cytokines, acting through convergent as well as independent signal transduction pathways, synergistically effect the outcome of oligodendrocyte survival. Other cytokines, such as type I IFNs, may oppose oligodendrocyte injury; exploiting their beneficial effects is a rational but understudied mode for treatment of MS.

REFERENCES

1. Jacobson M. Developmental Neurobiology. 3rd ed. New York: Plenum, 1991.
2. Theele DP, Streit WJ. A chronicle of microglial ontogeny. Glia 1993; 7:5–8.
3. Kandel ER. Nerve cells and behavior. In: Kandel ER, Schwartz JH, Jessell TM, eds. Principles of Neural Science. 3rd ed. Norwalk, CT: Appleton & Lange, 1991.
4. Waxman SG, Ritchie JM, eds. Advances in Neurology. Vol. 31: Demyelinating Diseases: Basic and Clinical Electrophysiology. New York: Raven Press, 1981.
5. McMillian MK, Thai L, Hong J-S, O'Callaghan JP, Pennypacker KR. Brain injury in a dish: a model for reactive gliosis. TINS 1994; 17:138–142.
6. Ling E-A, Wong W-C. The origin and nature of ramified and amoeboid microglia: a historical review and current concepts. Glia 1993; 7:9–18.
7. Traugott U, Lebon P. Multiple sclerosis: Involvement of interferons in lesion pathogenesis. Ann Neurol 1988; 24:243–251.

8. Rubio N, de Felipe C. Demonstration of the presence of a specific interferon-γ receptor on murine astrocyte cell surface. J Neuroimmunol 1991; 35:111–117.

9. Yong VW, Moumdjian R, Yong FP, et al. γ-Interferon promotes proliferation of adult human astrocytes in vitro and reactive gliosis in the adult mouse brain in vivo. *Proc Natl Acad Sci* USA 1991; 88:7016–7020.

10. Balasingam V, Tejada-Berges T, Wright E, Bouckova R, Wee Yong V. Reactive astrogliosis in the neonatal mouse brain and its modulation by cytokines. J Neurosci 1994; 14:846–856.

11. Selmaj KW, Farooq M, Norton WT, Raine CS, Brosnan CF. Proliferation of astrocytes in vitro in response to cytokines: a primary role for tumor necrosis factor. J Immunol 1990; 144:129–135.

12. Benos DJ, McPherson S, Hahn BH, Chaikin MA, Benveniste EN. Cytokines and HIV envelope glycoprotein gp120 stimulate Na^+/H^+ exchange in astrocytes. J Biol Chem 1994; 19:13811–13816.

13. Oka A, Belliveau MJ, Rosenberg PA, Volpe JJ. Vulnerability of oligodendroglia to glutamate: pharmacology, mechanisms, and prevention. J Neurosci 1993; 13:1441–1453.

14. Lee SC, Dickson DW, Liu W, Brosnan CF. Induction of nitric oxide synthase activity in human astrocytes by interleukin-1β and interferon-γ. J Neuroimmunol 1993; 46:19–24.

15. Simmons ML, Murphy S. Roles for protein kinases in the induction of nitric oxide synthase in astrocytes. Glia 1994; 11:227–234.

16. Dawson VL, Dawson TM, Bartley DA, Uhl GR, Snyder SH. Mechanisms of nitric oxide–mediated neurotoxicity in primary brain cultures. J Neurosci 1993; 13:2651–2661.

17. Munöz-Fernandez MA, Fresno M. Involvement of nitric oxide on the cytokine induced growth of glial cell. Biochem Biophys Res Commun 1993; 194: 319–325.

18. Bolanos JP, Peuchen S, Heales JR, Land JM, Clark JB. Nitric oxide–mediated inhibition of the mitochondrial respiratory chain in cultured astrocytes. J Neurochem 1994; 63:910–916.

19. Cannella B, Raine, CS. The adhesion molecule and cytokine profile of MS lesions. Ann Neurol 1995; 37:424–435.

20. Vartanian T, Li Y, Zhao M, Stefansson K. Interferon-γ induced oligodendrocyte death: implications for the pathogenesis of MS. Mol Med (In press).

21. Schmidt B, Stoll G, Toyka KV, Hartung HP. Rat astrocytes express interferon-γ immunoreactivity in normal optic nerve and after nerve transection. Brain Res 1990; 515:347–350.

22. Kiefer R, Kreutzberg GW. Gamma interferon-like immunoreactivity in the rat nervous system. Neuroscience 1990; 37:725–734.

23. Benveniste EN. Inflammatory cytokines within the central nervous system: sources, function, and mechanism of action. Am J Physiol 1992; 263:C1–16.

24. Chung IY, Benveniste EN. Tumor necrosis factor-α production by astrocytes: induction by lipopolysaccharide, IFN-γ, and IL-1β. J Immunol 1990; 144:2999–3007.

25. Chung IY, Norris JG, Benveniste EN. Differential tumor necrosis factor

α expression by astrocytes from experimental allergic encephalomyelitis-susceptible and -resistant rat strains. J Exp Med 1991; 173:801–811.

26. Oropeza RL, Wekerle H, Werb Z. Expression of apolipoprotein E by mouse brain astrocytes and its modulation by interferon-γ. Brain Res 1987; 410–45–51.

27. Low KG, Allen RG, Melner MH. Differential regulation of proenkephalin expression in astrocytes by cytokines. Endocrinology 1992; 131:1908–1914.

28. Tontsch U, Rott O. Intercellular regulation of major histocompatibility complex class I expression in neural cells. Immunology 1993; 80:507–509.

29. Frohman EM, Vayuvegula B, Gupta S, van den Noort S. Norepinephrine inhibits γ interferon–induced major histocompatibility class II (Ia) antigen expression on cultured astrocytes via β2-adrenergic signal transduction mechanisms. Proc Natl Acad Sci USA 1988; 85:1292–1296.

30. Frohman EM, Vayuvegula B, van den Noort S, Gupta S. Norepinephrine inhibits gamma-interferon–induced MHC class II (Ia) intigen expression on cultured brain astrocytes. J Neuroimmunol 1988; 17:89–101.

31. Lee SC, Collins M, Vanguri P, Shin ML. Glutamate differentially inhibits the expression of class II MHC antigens on astrocytes and microglia. J Immunol 1992; 148:3391–3397.

32. Male DK, Pryce G, Hughes CCW. Antigen presentation in brain: MHC induction on brain endothelium and astrocytes compared. Immunology 1987; 60:453–459.

33. Wong GHW, Bartlett PF, Clark-Lewis I, Battye F, Schrader JW. Inducible expression of H-2 and Ia antigens on brain cells. Nature 1984; 310:688–691.

34. Tedeschi B, Barrett JN, Keane RW. Astrocytes produce interferon that enhances the expression of H-2 antigens on a subpopulation of brain cells. J Cell Biol 1986; 102:2244–2253.

35. Uitdehaag BMJ, deGroot CJA, Kreike A, et al. The significance of in-situ antigen expression in the pathogenesis of autoimmune central nervous system disease. J Autoimmun 1993; 6:323–335.

36. Traugott U, Scheinberg LC, Raine CS. On the presence of Ia-positive endothelial cells and astrocytes in multiple sclerosis lesions and its relevance to antigen presentation. J Neuroimmunol 1985; 8:1.

37. Hayes GM, Woodroofe MN, Cuzner ML. Microglia are the major cell type expressing MHC Class II antigens in human white matter. J Neurol Sci 1987; 80:25.

38. Fontana A, Fierz W, Wekerle H. Astrocytes present myelin basic protein to encephalitogenic T cell lines. Nature 1984; 307:273.

39. Dhib-Jalbut S, Kufta CV, Flerlage M, Shimojo N, McFarland HF. Adult human glial cells can present target antigens to HLA-restricted cytotoxic T-cells. J Neuroimmunol 1990; 29:203–211.

40. Fontana A, Erb P, Pircher H, et al. Astrocytes as antigen-presenting cells. Part II: Unlike H-2K–dependent cytotoxic T cells, H-2Ia–restricted T cells are only stimulated in the presence of interferon-γ. J Neuroimmunol 1986; 12:15–28.

41. Takiguchi M, Frelinger JA. Induction of antigen presentation ability in puri-

fied cultures of astroglia by interferon-γ. J Mol Cell Immunol 1986; 2: 269–280.

42. Sedgwick JD, Mobner R, Schwender S, ter Meulen V. Major histocompatibility complex–expressing nonhematopoietic astroglial cells prime only CD8⁺T lymphocytes: Astroglial cells as perpetuators but not initiators of CD4⁺ T cells responses in the central nervous system. J Exp Med 1991; 173:1235–1246.

43. Reder AT, Lascola CD, Flanders SA, Maimone D, Jensen MA, Skias DD, Lancki DW. Astrocyte cytolysis by MHC class II-specific mouse T cell clones. Transplantation 1993; 56:393–399.

44. Massa PT, ver Meulen V, Fontana A. Hyperinducibility of Ia antigen on astrocytes correlates with strain-specific susceptibility to experimental autoimmune encephalomyelitis (EAE). Proc Natl Acad Sci USA 1987; 84: 4219.

45. Borrow P, Nash AA. Susceptibility to Theiler's virus-induced demyelinating disease correlates with astrocyte class II induction and antigen presentation. Immunology 1992; 76:133–139.

46. Johns LD, Babcock G, Green D, et al. Transforming growth factor-β1 differentially regulates proliferation and MHC class-II antigen expression in forebrain and brainstem strocyte primary cultures. Brain Res 1992; 585: 229–236.

47. Wilkin GP, Marriot DR, Cholewinski AJ. Astrocyte heterogeneity. Trends Neurol Sci 1990; 2:43–45.

48. Lassmann H, Schmeid M, Vass K, Hickey WF. Bone marrow derived elements and resident microglia in brain inflammation. Glia 1993; 7:19–24.

49. Kettenmann H, Banati R, Walz W. Electrophysiological behavior of microglia. Glia 1993; 7:93–101.

50. Lumsden CE, in Handbook of Clinical Neurology: The Neuropathology of Multiple Sclerosis 9, 217–309 (Elsevier Science, Amsterdam, 1985).

51. Guilian D, Vaca K, Johnson B. Secreted peptides as regulators of neuron-glia and glia-glia interactions in the developing nervous system. J Neurosci Res 1988; 21:487–500.

52. Guilian D, Vaca K, Corpuz M. Brain glia release factors with opposing actions upon neuronal survival. J Neurosci 1993; 13:29–37.

53. Guilian D. Reactive glia as rivals in regulating neuronal survival. Glia 1993; 7:102–110.

54. Suzumura A, Marunouchi T, Yamamoto H. Morphological transformation of microglia in vitro. Brain Res 1991; 545:301–306.

55. Colton CA, Yao J, Keri JE, Gilbert D. Regulation of microglial function by interferons. J Neuroimmunol 1992; 30:89–98.

56. Bruck W, Friede RL. Activation of macrophages by recombinant interferon-γ has no effect on myelin phagocytosis but hinders invasion of nerves in organ culture. J Neuroimmunology. 1989; 25:47–55.

57. Akiyama H, Ikeda K, Katoh M, McGeer EG, McGeer PL. Expression of MRP14, 27E10, interferon-γ and leukocyte common antigen by reactive microglia in postmortem human brain tissue. J Neuroimmunol 1994; 50: 195–201.

58. Neveu I, Naveilhan P, Menaa C, Wion D, Brachet P, Garabedian M. Synthesis of 1,25-dihydroxyvitamin D_3 by rat brain macrophages in vitro. J Neurosci Res 1994; 38:214–220.

59. Corradin SB, Mauel J, Donini SD, Quattrocchi E, Ricciardi-Castagnoli P. Inducible nitric oxide synthase activity of cloned murine microglial cells. Glia 1993; 7:255–262.

60. Zielasek J, Tausch M, Toyka KV, Hartung H-P. Production of nitrite by neonatal rat microglial cells/brain macrophages. Cell Immunol 1992; 141: 111–120.

61. Chao CC, Hu S, Molitor TW, Shaskan EG, Peterson PK. Activated microglia mediate neuronal cell injury via a nitric oxide mechanism. J Immunol 1992; 149:2736–2741.

62. Peterson PK, Hu S, Anderson R, Chao CC. Nitric oxide production and neurotoxicity mediated by activated microglia from human versus mouse brain. J Infect Dis 1994; 170:457–460.

63. Lee SC, Dickson DW, Liu W, Brosnan CF. Induction of nitric oxide synthase activity in human astrocytes by interleukin-1β and interferon-γ. J Neuroimmunol 1993; 46:19–24.

64. Dawson TM, et al. Nitric oxide synthase and neuronal NADPH diaphorase are identical in brain and peripheral tissues. Proc Natl Acad Sci USA 1988; 88:7797–7801.

65. Hope BT, et al. Neuronal NADPH-diaphorase is a nitric oxide synthase. Proc Natl Acad Sci 1988; 88:2811–2814.

66. Chao CC, Gekker G, Hu S, Peterson PK. Human microglial cell defense against toxoplasma gondii; the role of cytokines. J Immunol 1994; 152: 1246–1252.

67. Chao CC, Anderson WR, Hu S, et al. Activated microglia inhibit multiplication of toxoplasma gondii via a nitric oxide mechanism. Clin Immunol Immunopathol 1993; 67:178–183.

68. Jun C-D, Ryu H, Um J-Y, et al. Involvement of protein kinase C in the inhibition of nitric oxide production from murine microglial cells by glucocorticoid. Biochem Biophys Res Commun 1994; 199:633–638.

69. Suzumura A, Mezitis SGE, Gonatas NK, Silberberg DH. MHC antigen expression on bulk isolated macrophage-microglia from newborn mouse brain: induction of Ia antigen expression by γ-interferon. J Neuroimmunol 1987; 15:263–278.

70. Steiniger B, van der Meide PH. Rat ependyma and microglia cells express class II MHC antigens after intravenous infusion of recombinant gamma interferon. J Neuroimmunol 1988; 19:111–118.

71. Woodroofe MN, Hayes GM, Cuzner ML. Fc receptor density, MHC antigen expression and superoxide production are increased in interferon-gamma–treaed microglia isolated from adult rat brain. Immunology 1989; 68:421–426.

72. Loughlin AJ, Woodroofe MN, Cuzner ML. Regulation of Fc receptor and major histocompatibility complex antigen expression on isolated rat mi-

croglia by tumour necrosis factor, interleukin-1 and lipopolysaccharide: effects on interferon-gamma induced activation. Immunology 1992; 75: 170–175.

73. Frei K, Siepl C, Groscurth P, et al. Antigen presentation and tumor cytotoxicity by interferon-γ–treated microglial cells. Eur J Immunol 1987; 17: 1271–1278.

74. Loughlin AJ, Woodroofe MN, Cuzner ML. Modulation of interferon-γ–induced major histocompatibility complex class II and Fc receptor expression on isolated microglia by transforming growth factor-β1, interleukin-4, noradrenaline and glucocorticoids. Immunology 1993; 79:125–130.

75. Hayashi M, Dorf ME, Abromson-Leeman A. Granulocyte-macrophage colony stimulating factor inhibits class II major histocompatibility complex expression and antigen presentation by microglia. J Neuroimmunol 1993; 48:23–32.

76. Cash E, Rott O. Microglial cells qualify as the stimulators of unprimed CD4+ and CD8+ T lymphocytes in the central nervous system. Clin Exp Immunol 1994; 98:313–318.

77. Williams Jr. K, Ulvestad E, Cragg L, Blain M, Antel JP. Induction of primary T cell responses by human glial cells. J Neurosci Res 1993; 36: 382–390.

78. Griffin WST, Stanley LC, Ling C, et al. Brain interleukin 1 and S-100 immunoreactivity are elevated in Down syndrome and Alzheimer disease. Proc Natl Acad Sci USA 1989; 86:7611–7615.

79. Selmaj K, Raine CS, Farooq M, Norton WT, Brosnan CF. Cytokine cytotoxicity against oligodendrocytes: Apoptosis induced by lymphotoxin. J Immunol 1991; 147:1522–1529.

80. Selmaj KW, Raine CS. Tumor necrosis factor mediates myelin and oligodendrocyte damage in vitro. Ann Neurol 1988; 23:339–346.

81. Louis J-C, Magal E, Takayama S, Varon S. CNTF protection of oligodendrocytes against natural and tumor necrosis factor–induced death. Science 1993; 259:689–692.

82. Suzumura A, Silberberg DH, Lisak RP. The expression of MHC antigens on oligodendrocytes: induction of polymorphic H-2 expression by lymphocytes. J Neuroimmunol 1986; 11:179–190.

83. Hirayama M, Yokochi T, Shimokata K, Iida M, Fujiki N. Induction of human leukocyte antigen-A,B,C and -DR on cultured human oligodendrocytes and astrocytes by human γ-interferon. Neurosci Lett 1986; 72: 369–374.

84. Bergsteinsdottir K, Brennan A, Jessen KR, Mirsky R. In the presence of dexamethasone, γ interferon induces rat oligodendrocytes to express major histocompatibility complex class II molecules. Proc Natl Acad Sci USA 1992; 89:9054–9058.

85. Massa PT, Ozato K, McFarlin DE. Cell type-specific regulation of major histocompatibility complex (MHC) class I gene expression in astrocytes, oligodendrocytes, and neurons. Glia 1993; 8:201–207.

86. Calder VL, Wolswijk G, Noble M. The differentiation of O-2A progenitor cells into oligodendrocytes is associated with a loss of inducibility if Ia antigens. Eur J Immunol 1988; 18:1195–1201.
87. Marlin SD, Springer TA. Purified intercellular adhesion molecule-1 is a ligand for lymphocyte function–associated antigen 1. Cell 1987; 51:813–819.
88. Staunton DE, Marlin SD, Stratowa C, Dustin ML, Springer TA. Primary structure of ICAM-1 demonstrates interaction between members of the immunoglobulin and integrin supergene families. Cell 1988; 52:925–933.
89. Satoh J-K, Kastrukoff LF, Kim SU. Cytokine-induced expression of intercellular adhesion molecule-1 (ICAM-1) in cultured human oligodendrocytes and astrocytes. J Neuropathol Exp Neurol 1991; 50:215–226.
90. Soliven B, Szuchet S, Nelson DJ. Tumor necrosis factor inhibits K^+ current expression in cultured oligodendrocytes. J Membrane Biol 1991; 124: 127–137.
91. Soliven B, Szuchet S. Signal Transduction pathways in oligodendrocytes: Role of tumor necrosis factor-α. Int J Dev Neurosci 1995; 13:351–367.
92. Mauerhoff T, Pujol-Borrell R, Mirakian R, Bottazzo GF. Differential expression and regulation of major histocompatibility complex (MHC) products in neural and glial cells of the human fetal brain. J Neuroimmunol 1988; 18:271–289.
93. Merrill JE. The effect of IL-1 and TNFα on astrocytes, microglia, oligodendrocytes, and glial precursors in vitro. Dev Neurosci 1991; 13:130.
94. Merrill JE, Ignarro LJ, Sherman MP, Melinek J, Lane TE. Microglial cell cytotoxicity of oligodendrocytes is mediated through nitric oxide. J Immunol 1993; 151:2132–2141.
95. Prineas JW, Kwon EE, Goldenberg PZ, Cho E-S, Sharer LR. Interaction of astrocytes and newly formed oligodendrocytes in resolving multiple sclerosis lesions. Lab Invest 1990; 63:624–636.
96. Sun D. Enhanced interferon-γ-induced Ia-antigen expression by glial cells after previous exposure to this cytokine. J Neuroimmunol 1991; 34:205–214.
97. Abu El-Asrar AM, Maimone D, Morse PH, Lascola C, Reder AT. Interferon-γ and tumour necrosis factor induce expression of major histocompatibility complex antigen on rat retinal astrocytes. Br J Opthalmol 1991; 75: 473–475.
98. Fierz W, Endler B, Reske K, Wekerle H, Fontana A. Astrocytes as antigen-presenting cells. I. Induction of Ia antigen expression on astrocytes by T cells via immune interferon and its effect on antigen presentation. J Immunol 1985; 134:3785–3793.
99. Benveniste EN, Sparacio SM, Bethea JR. Tumor necrosis factor-α enhances interferon-γ-mediated class II antigen expression on astrocytes. J Neuroimmunol 1989; 25:209–219.
100. Smith ME, McFarlin DE, Dhib-Jalbut S. Differential effect of interleukin-1β on Ia expression in astrocytes and microglia. J Neuroimmunol 1993; 46: 97–104.
101. Ohira K, Vayuvegula B, Murakami M, et al. Tetraethylammonium, a K^+ channel blocker, inhibits interferon-γ-induced major histocompatibility

class II antigen (Ia) expression and DNA synthesis in rat astrocytes. J Neuroimmunol 1991; 31:43–49.

102. Frohman EM, Frohman TC, Dustin ML, et al. The induction of intercellular adhesion molecule 1 (ICAM-1) expression on human fetal astrocytes by interferon-γ, tumor necrosis factor α, lymphotoxin, and interleukin-1: relevance to intracerebral antigen presentation. J Neuroimmunol 1989; 23: 117–124.

103. Sasaki A, Levison SW, Ting JPY. Differentiatial suppression of interferon-γ–induced Ia antigen expression on cultured rat astroglia and microglia by second messengers. J Neuroimmunol 1990; 29:213–222.

104. Schluesener HJ. Transforming growth factors type β₁ and β₂ suppress rat astrocyte autoantigen presentation and antagonize hyperinduction of class II major histocompatibility complex antigen expression by interferon-γ and tumor necrosis factor-α. J Neuroimmunol 1990; 27:41–47.

105. Yong VW, Yong FP, Ruus TCG, Antel JP, Kim SU. Expression and modulation of HLA-DR on cultured human adult astrocytes. J Neuropathol Exp Neurol 1991; 50:16–28.

106. Pulver M, Carrel S, Mach JP, de Tribolet N. Cultured human fetal astrocytes can be induced by interferon-γ to express HLA-DR. J Neuroimmunol 1987; 14:123–133.

107. Morris AG, Tomkins PT. Interactions of interferons in the induction of histocompatibility antigens in mouse fibroblasts and glial cells. Immunology 1989; 67:537–539.

108. Haegel H, Tolg C, Hofmann M, Ceredig R. Activated mouse astrocytes and T cells express similar CD44 variants. Role of CD44 in astrocytes T cell binding. J Cell Biol 1993; 122:1067–1077.

5

Effects of Interferon on the Central Nervous System

Nachum Dafny

University of Texas Medical School at Houston, Houston Health Science Center, Houston, Texas

Bertha Prieto-Gomez and Cruz Reyes-Vazquez

Universidad Nacional Autónoma de México, Del Cayoacan, Mexico

I. INTRODUCTION

Interferons (IFNs) are a family of proteins that appear in a large variety of vertebrates, from fish to *Homo sapiens*. Interferons were initially characterized for their ability to "interfere" with viral replication (1). They are cytokines and comprise a complex family of endogenous proteins and glycoproteins, (1–6). In vivo IFN is produced at a constant low "physiological" level that must be maintained for correct immune function to occur (4).

Cytokines such as IFN are used to treat various hematological malignancies and infectious diseases and also multiple sclerosis (2,4). Because the cytokines used in immunological therapy are naturally produced in the body, they were thought to be nontoxic (7).

Besides the activation of immunity, IFN produces a broad spectrum of nonimmunological host defenses in the counterreply to infection, including fever, anorexia, and sleep, all of which are central nervous system (CNS) functions (3,8–17). The above features imply that IFN affects central nervous system processes. Although the effects of IFN have been extensively studied in a variety of systems, they have not been studied in the CNS. Until the early 1980s, only a few laboratories (18,19) using behavioral and electrophysiological procedures had investigated whether IFN affects CNS activity.

II. INTERFERON MODULATES BEHAVIOR

The central nervous system side effects associated with IFN are seen during IFN-α therapy; all such side effects are reversed by stopping the IFN treatments (10,20–22). The most debilitating side effects following "low"-dose IFN treatment in cancer patients are fatigue, asthenia, anorexia, and the influenza-like symptoms of fever, chills, headaches, myalgia, somnolence, and lethargy (10,20,21,23–25) (see Chapter 16). In rodents, IFN administration results in a decrease in motor activity and food intake (23,26,27) followed by drowsiness and slowing of electroencephalographic (EEG) activity (20,21,25,28–30). Higher doses of IFN place individuals at risk for developing side effects such as a lack of coordination and photophobia, the loss of taste and smell, impairments of attention, an inability to concentrate, headaches, hallucination, abnormal mood states, emotional problems, frank delirium and psychosis-like behavior, and neurocognitive dysfunctions such as confusion, mental and motor slowing, and expressive dysphasia (7,9,10,20,21,24,30–35), as well as a dysfunction in immediate memory and intellectual ability as measured by three WAIS subtests (see Chapter 6). The psychiatric symptoms elicited by IFN treatment, including fatigue, impaired concentration, anxiety, and depression, all seem to be nonpsychotic (30). On the contrary, IFN may reverse psychotic disease: Psychiatric studies show that IFN has beneficial effects in patients with chronic schizophrenia (36).

Many of these CNS side effects arise from anatomically disparate sites. However, the absence of deficits typical of local posterior cortical lesions, such as in language, speech, expressive dysphasia, reading, writing, calculation, visuognosis, and visual-spatial perception deficits, appear to implicate IFN in frontal lobe and possibly subcortical brain activity (10,11,20–22).

IFN given to healthy volunteers (16,17) slows down activity as assessed by an increased reaction time to stimuli presented at random intervals. In normal rodents, IFN injections depress open-field activity (37,38), and cause weight loss (26,39). The brain areas participating in arousal are the reticular activating system, and those affecting feeding behavior are thought to be in the hypothalamus (40–42). IFN may reach high concentrations in the pons and hypothalamus where the blood-brain barrier is more permeable (43,44).

From the above reports, it is apparent that IFN has remarkable effects on the central nervous system in general, and in particular, IFN affects the hypothalamus, somatosensory, motor, and limbic system sites (28,45). IFN is one of the messengers responsible for the bidirectional communication which links the immune and endocrine systems with the brain (13,45–50).

III. INTERFERON RECEPTOR AND BINDING IN THE CNS

The brain is relatively isolated from the immune system owing to the presence of the blood-brain barrier that limits the penetration of circulating lymphocytes and antibodies (51). High doses of IFN-α (simply referred to as IFN) injections are needed to achieve measurable levels in the cerebrospinal fluid (CSF), but small amounts will penetrate the deep layers of the brain after intrathecal administration (9). However, systemically administered IFN may enter the brain through areas lacking the blood-brain barrier, achieving "significant" concentration only in those sites, whereas failing to penetrate other areas (16,52). IFN reaches "high" concentration in the pons and hypothalamus where the blood-brain barrier is more permeable (3,4,16,43,44).

IFN-α binds to specific IFN receptors in the brain and brain tissue (6,53), and the binding characteristics vary among brain regions. The most frequent binding occurs in hypothalamic sites, and the lowest occurs in the spinal cord (54). The existence of specific IFN receptors and specific binding sites within the central nervous system represent the link between IFN and its effect on neuronal activity.

Moreover, IFN treatment inhibits binding of [^{3}H]-naloxone and enkephalin to rat brain membrane in vitro (55–57). IFN also inhibits dihydromorphine binding in mouse brain homogenates (18). Panchenko et al (57) reported that among the interferon family, only IFN-α preparations actively bind opiate sites on biological membranes. As will be shown, IFN affects a variety of CNS functions, several of which are mediated by opioid receptors.

IV. INTERFERON AND OPIOIDS

IFN-α (IFN) is related both functionally and structurally to regulatory polypeptide hormones. Indeed, polypeptide hormones and IFN share common transmissible pathways of cell activation (18,44,58–62). IFN action requires initial binding to at least one specific receptor site on the cell surface to elicit its effects (53). This binding may share sites common to those of peptide hormones such as adrenocorticotropic hormone (ACTH) and/or melanocyte-stimulating hormone (MSH) (58,59,62). Similarities have been demonstrated among the structures of proopiomelanocortin, ACTH, β-endorphin, and IFN. Other evidence linking IFN with the opioids is provided by experiments showing that lymphocytes stimulated with IFN inducers also produce ACTH and endorphin-like substances. Furthermore, IFNs and endorphins are antigenically similar, suggesting that these peptides have some common structural properties (18,58–60,63,64). Functionally, interferon-α, but not interferon-β or interferon-γ, binds to opiate receptors and shares some pharmacological properties of opioids such as the production of analgesia, reduction in motor activity, and catatonia. These effects are reversed or prevented by the opioid antagonist naloxone (18,58,63,65). Opiate receptor binding of IFN β-1b, which along with most IFN-α subtypes is nonglycosylated, has not been studied.

Opioids exert their effect by binding to specific opiate receptors. Repetitive use of opioids elicits tolerance and dependence (66). Morphine dependence is manifested by an abstinence syndrome when the opioid use is discontinued (66,67). The opiate abstinence syndrome represents a fundamental feature of addiction. Physical dependence (addiction) on opioids can be quantified by the frequency or intensity of the abstinence behaviors observed after abrupt termination of opiate intake or after injection of opiate antagonists such as naloxone (67). The degree of addiction is, therefore, assessed by the intensity of the withdrawal behavior. Since the discovery of endogenous opioids, efforts have been directed toward the identification of active peptide analogues which would prevent tolerance and physical dependence on opioids (68). Endogenous peptides or proteins in the central nervous system may be capable of counteracting the effects of the drug (69). It has been suggested that some endogenous substances are produced and released along with the endogenous opioid in order to prevent the organism from becoming tolerant to, and dependent on, its own morphine-like peptides (70).

When the opiate antagonist naloxone is given prior to IFN treatment, it prevents the analgesia and catatonic behavior produced by IFN given alone (18). This evidence suggests that the effects of IFN on CNS activity are mediated via a number of different mechanisms, some of which may be antagonized by naloxone (65).

The above findings, together with the observations that (1) single injections of morphine into mice reduced the level of serum IFN induced by poly I:C or endotoxin (71,72); (2) IFN receptors are localized in the brain; and (3) IFN is in fact synthesized in the brain, formed the rationale for the following hypothesis: "IFN is the endogenous substance which serves to prevent the development of tolerance and dependence to brain opioids" (46,47). In a series of experiments, IFN was used to reduce the severity of the opioid abstinence syndrome and to prevent the development of physical dependence on opioids (45,48,73–76).

In the initial studies, a single IFN injection was given intraperitoneally (i.p.) to morphine-addicted subjects 1 hr prior to naloxone injection. IFN treatment remarkably decreased the severity of all opioid abstinence behaviors (73,74). Whatever the IFN mechanism is, the striking ability to modify withdrawal behavior in a dosage comparable to that used in clinical therapy suggests that CNS IFN helps maintain homeostasis in the morphine-dependent rodents. In a subsequent experiment (77), a single IFN injection (i.p.) was given prior to chronic morphine treatment (before addiction) and similar results were obtained—it prevented development of dependence. IFN also reduced the severity of opioid withdrawal, indicating that IFN interferes with both the development of physical dependence to morphine and with withdrawal behaviors from morphine. A dose-response experiment using IFN-α and IFN-γ (Fig. 1) demonstrated that IFN-α, and not IFN-γ remarkably reduced the severity of the opiate abstinence syndrome precipitated by naloxone in morphine-dependent rats in a dose-related manner (45,48,77). Studies of IFN-α treatment of human addicts are in progress.

To test the possibility that IFN exerts its effects via opiate receptors, recordings were made from two preparations, the guinea pig ileum (48) and the CNS, using a variety of electrophysiological experiments (evoked-field potentials and single-cell recording) (26,45,47,78–81). The guinea pig ileum preparations reveal the effects of opiates on transmission between autonomic nerves and intestinal smooth muscle (82,83). Opiate receptors are present on the presynaptic neuromuscular endings, and activation of those endings by opiate agonists at the receptor site inhibits the release of acetylcholine (ACh) at the neuromuscular junction (83). Use of this "simple" system has allowed the characterization of various opiate receptors and the study of agonist-antagonist interactions of these receptors (85). Using in vivo rat brain membrane preparations, IFN was shown to inhibit the binding of [^{3}H]naloxone (55). A number of physiological effects of IFN might be explained as a competition between IFN and naloxone for the responsible membrane binding sites. This could be the mechanism of attenuating morphine withdrawal symptoms when IFN is injected systemically 1 hr prior to naloxone in morphine-dependent subjects (55).

In brain slice preparation, IFN elicits both an increase and a decrease in the firing rate recorded from the anterior hypothalamus (AH) and from the ventromedial hypothalamus (VMH). Both responses are blocked by naloxone (85). IFN elicits only excitation in the guinea pig ileum, in cortical neurons, and in some VMH neurons. Naloxone fails to prevent the IFN-induced excitation in the ileum and cortical and VMH neurons (38,86). In some VMH cells, IFN elicits inhibition, but in these neurons, naloxone blocks the IFN effects. These observations in guinea pig ileum and single-cell recordings suggests the IFN action may not be mediated via opiate receptors but rather through IFN receptors (45,48). However, not all possibilities were tested; opiates can act through a number of receptors, and not all of these receptors are blocked by naloxone. Thus, IFN could be acting on an opioid receptor not blocked by naloxone.

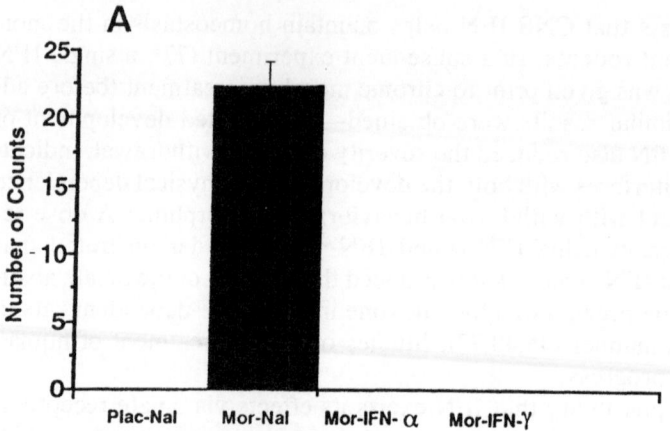

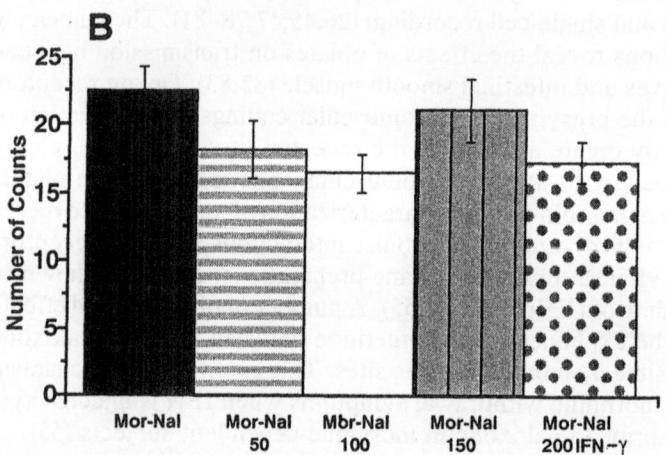

Figure 1 Histograms showing the mean and SE of one abstinence sign (wet dog shake) following naloxone (Nal) injection (1.0 mg/kg i.p.) in placebo (Pla) or morphine (Mor) pellet-implanted rats (100-mg/pellet/animal each group N = 8). Interferon and naloxone were injected 71 and 72 hr after morphine pellet implantation, respectively. In (A), there are four groups; Nal injection (1 mg/kg, i.p.) into Pla pellet-treated animals fails to elicit wet dog shake; Nal in Mor pellet–implanted animals elicits the expected wet dog shake behavior. Interferon-α (IFN-α) or IFN-γ given to Mor-dependent rats failed to elicit abstinence signs. In (B), IFN-γ was

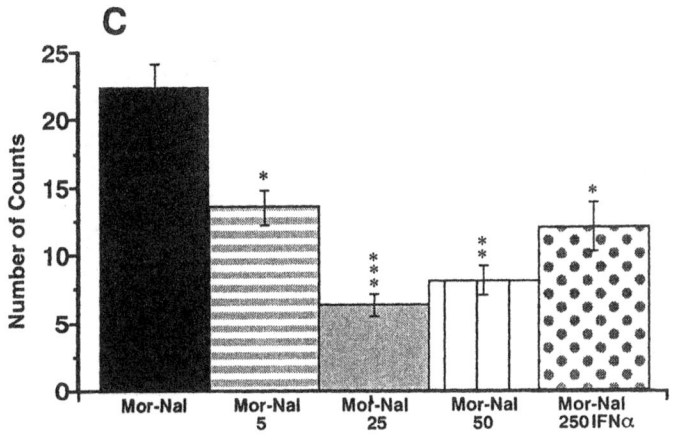

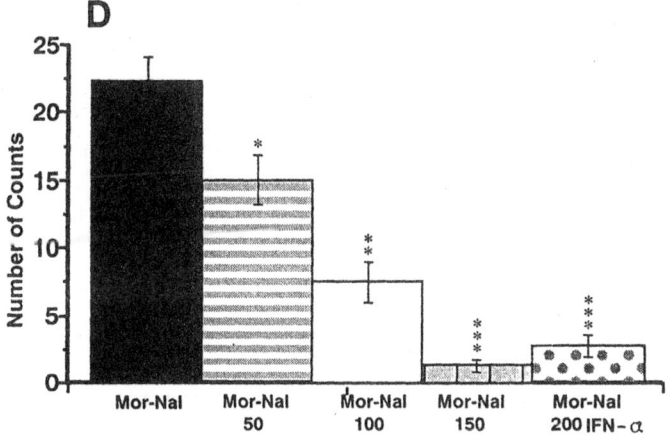

injected i.p. 1 hr prior to naloxone injection. It did not affect withdrawal behavior. The numbers under the columns indicate the International Unit/g/body weight of IFN-γ. In (C), IFN-α was injected i.c.v. 1 hr prior to naloxone injection. It blocked withdrawal behavior, and was most effective at intermediate doses. In (D), IFN-α was injected i.p. 1 hr prior to naloxone. It had a dose-response effect on withdrawal behavior * = $p < .05$; ** = $p < .01$; *** = $p < .001$. The histograms show that only IFN-α injected prior to naloxone to morphine-dependent rats attenuate the severity of the opiate withdrawal signs.

These studies suggest that there are at least three different functional and/or receptor sites for IFN within the CNS: (1) an excitatory site—IFN produces excitation in the neuronal activity which is not antagonized by naloxone (45,81); (2) an inhibitory site—IFN produces reduction in the neuronal activity of naloxone-dependent sites, possibly representing the mu receptor type; and (3) an excitatory site—IFN produces excitation in the neuronal activity which the opiate antagonist naloxone reversed, i.e., naloxone-dependent site, it is possible that this response represents the kappa or delta receptor sites (85). All these findings suggest that IFN modulates some CNS properties through opiate receptors.

V. IMPACT OF INTERFERON ON FEVER AND THERMOSENSITIVE NEURONS

Fever is initiated by activation of thermosensitive neurons located mainly in the preoptic/anterior hypothalamus (PO/AH) by yet unknown mechanisms. Fever is a host defense response to various exogenous pathogenic organisms or their products, such as lipopolysaccharides. It is mediated centrally by endogenous pyrogens which include interferon (87). Interferon-α, when injected intravenously (i.v.) or intracerebroventricularly (i.c.v.) in rabbits, cats, and mice, produces fever which does not involve production of the endogenous pyrogenic substance interleukin-1 (IL-1); therefore, IFN is also an endogenous pyrogen (88,89). The PO/AH area is the most probable site of the pyrogenic actions of IFN (89,90).

IFN-α controls febrile responses by modifying thermosensitive and thermally insensitive neuronal activity in the PO/AH. IFN decreases the neuronal activity of warm-sensitive neurons and increases the activity of cold-sensitive neurons. However, it has no effect on thermally insensitive neurons (8,29,39,85,87,91–94). The IFN effects on single thermosensitive neurons are blocked by the opiate antagonist naloxone (8,85,87,92,93), but not by a dose of sodium salicylate (an antipyrogenic agent) which effectively blocks the neuronal responses to endotoxin and leukocytic pyrogen (IL-1). The fever induced by IFN may be explained, at least in part, by direct effects of IFN on PO/AH thermosensitive neurons, through opiate receptors (93). IFN in the brain appears to produce fever by a two-step mechanism: first by the immediate action on the opioid receptors on thermosensitive PO/AH neurons, and subsequently by the release of prostaglandins, which cause fever (8,87).

VI. INTERFERON MODULATES CNS ELECTRICAL ACTIVITY

A. IFNs Modulate EEG and EEG-like Activity

The behavioral side effects produced by IFN therapy (see Section II) indicate that the sensory, motor, and limbic systems as well as the brain regions such as the hypothalamus, thalamus, and the reticular formation are affected by the drug. Based on these reports, permanent electrodes were implanted in multiple sites to determine function effects of IFNs—in the rat motor and sensory cortices for EEG recording; in the caudate nucleus, which is a subcortical site known to be part of the motor system; in the mesencephalic reticular formation and parafascicular nucleus of the thalamus as representatives of the nonspecific sensory system; in the hippocampus, a representative site of the limbic system; and in the hypothalamus (28). EEG and EEG-like activity were recorded from these structures simultaneously in freely behaving rats before and following single i.p. IFN (150 U/g body weight) injections.

In all the recording sites, single IFN injections elicited high-amplitude, locally synchronized slowing of activity that was independent in multiple sites in the brain (unsynchronized in time). The effects were first observed in the hypothalamus (280 sec after injection), followed by the somatosensory cortex, the hippocampus, the motor cortex, the caudate nucleus, and the parafasciculus nucleus (28). The sleep-inducing effects of IFN are likely to be mediated via the locus coeruleus (63). This brain wave slowing in rodents, without altering other aspects of sleep, is dose-dependent (29,39,65,95,96). IFN given daily (i.p. 150 IU/g body weight) to rats for 3 weeks resulted in an almost flat EEG, yet behaviorally the animals became extremely agitated and aggressive. The EEG returned to a normal pattern 1 week after cessation of IFN (unpublished observation). Similar IFN-elicited sleep also occurs in primates (97) and rabbits (95). EEG slowing also appears in patients treated with IFN (9,11,35,98). The sleep-promoting activity of IFN may be related to the feeling of lassitude and sleepiness that often accompanies viral disease as well as during IFN therapy (95).

B. IFNs Modulate Evoked Field Potentials

Unanesthetized freely behaving rats, implanted previously with permanent electrodes, received single injections of IFN. This potentiated the sensory-evoked potential recorded from the sensory cortex and ventromedial hypothalamus (48). The same treatment in the same animal attenuated

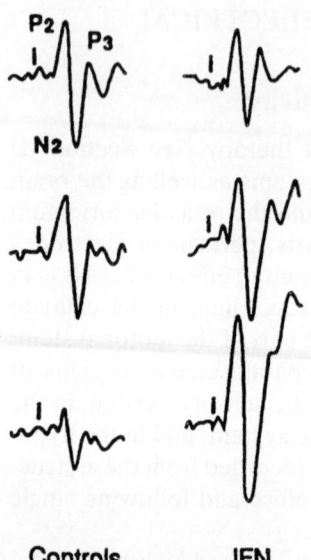

Controls   IFN

Figure 2   Representative averaged (N = 32) sensory-evoked responses recorded from the somatosensory cortex (lower traces), ventromedial hypothalamus (middle traces), and the lateral hypothalamus (upper traces) following IFN-α injection (150 IU/g body weight i.p.) in freely behaving animals previously implanted with permanent electrodes. IFN affects each brain region differently.

the evoked responses recorded from the PO/AH area (Fig. 2). Thus, in some areas of the brain, IFN amplifies the evoked activity, whereas in other structures, it attenuates the evoked activity.

In rat hippocampal slices, IFN reduced the size of short-term potentiation (STP) and suppressed long-term potentiation (LTP) with a dose-dependent character (99). Since STP and LTP are synaptic events (100,101), D'Arcangelo et al (100) suggests that IFN probably affects both pre- and postsynaptic sites.

IFN produced both excitatory effects on CA3 pyramidal cells in recordings from rat hippocampal slice cultures, and decreased evoked inhibitory postsynaptic potential amplitude, which eventually lead to epileptiform bursting (102).

C.   IFNs Modulate Single Neuron Activity

The first report on the effect of IFN on single neuron activity was by Gresser's group (19). IFN enhanced the spontaneous activity of neurons in cerebral and cerebellar cat corticies as well as in rat peripheral nerve cell cultures. These firing rate changes occurred after about 30 min and the excitation lasted for several hours. With repetitive electrical stimulation. IFN treatment caused marked shortening of the latency to the initial evoked activity and an increase in firing rate (19).

Other investigators (26,45–47,49,78–80) used three different sources of IFN-α and one of IFN-γ in in vivo experiments. Four different brain areas were analyzed using multibarrel procedure of single-cell recording and microiontophoretic application of IFNs and other agents. All IFN-α subtypes elicited increases in firing rate in the cerebral cortex and hippocampal neurons in a dose-dependent manner. The majority of the thalamic neurons failed to respond. The ventromedial hypothalamic cells responded in a mixed pattern (i.e., some increased their firing and others decreased their firing rate after IFN-α applications). As the IFN-α dose was increased, some VMH neurons changed their direction of response from an increased firing rate at low doses to decreased firing after high doses. On the other hand, IFN-γ failed to alter the electrical activity of the same cerebral cortex, hippocampus, thalamus, and ventromedial hypothalamus neurons. This observation demonstrated that only IFN-α (and possibly IFN-β) is capable of modulating CNS activity, and that each brain region responds to IFN differently.

Neuronal firing in the (PO/AH) area is also affected by IFN-α. Nakashima et al. (85,93,103) used brain slices and recorded from the PO/AH area and from the ventromedial hypothalamus (VMH) and obtained mixed responses in both regions. IFN caused some cells to increase in activity and others to decrease activity similar to other in vivo experiments (45,78). However, some investigators obtained only decreased activity in PO/AH multiunit activity following central administration of IFN in conscious rats (29,39). In in vitro recording from PO/AH neurons with IFN perfusion experiments (85,87,94), and in antidromic electrophysiologically identified hypothalamic paraventricular nucleus neuron preparation (50), IFN resulted in short-latency decreased firing rates when applied systematically (i.p.) and intacerebroventricularly (i.c.v.). The rapidity of the IFN effect observed by these investigators suggests that the effect of this agent was mediated via membrane-bound receptors.

To affirm whether IFN affects brain activity directly or indirectly, two routes of IFN-α application were used in in vivo experiments: first, a direct local injection into the brain (i.c.v.) and second, systemic (i.v.) application—a potential trigger for a cascade of signals. Recording was obtained from the same amygdala neuron (Fig. 3). The responses obtained were similar, with the only difference being the latency. Thus, IFN applied locally and systemically elicits similar effects on single-amygdala neurons.

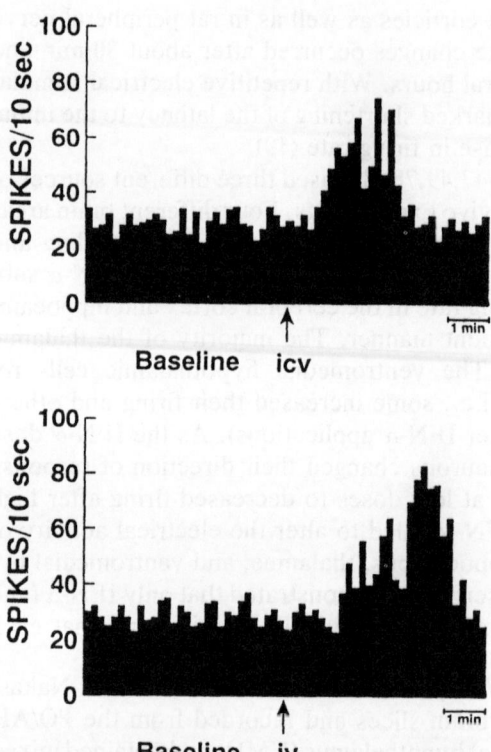

Figure 3 Frequency histogram from one-amygdala neuron. Intracerebroventricular (icv) treatment of 25 IU IFN-α elicits "short"-latency excitatory effects. Intravenous (iv) injection (15 IU/g body weight) 60 min later caused a similar effect and also has a "longer"-latency excitatory effect. The similar response to IFN with these two routes of drug application indicates that IFN-α modulates neuronal activity directly.

All the above reports indicate that IFN directly modulates EEG and EEG-like activity, evoked-field potentials, and single-cell activity.

VII.   INTERFERONS MODULATE FOOD INTAKE AND GLUCOSE-SENSITIVE NEURONS

Patients treated with high doses of IFN display anorexia which results in loss of more than 10% of their body weight (10,20,34,35). A similar decrease in food intake follows IFN treatment in animals (23,26,27,39,104). The major CNS sites participating in control of food intake are the lateral hypothalamus (LH), the paraventricular nucleus (PVN), and the ventromedial hypothalamus (VMH) (40,42,105,106). The VMH may be responsible for the production of the sensation of fullness; that is, it is a "satiety center." The LH is a center involved in initiating feeding and other neuronal activities related to food intake (41,42,98).

The VMH and the LH contain neurons which sense endogenous metabolic parameters, like glucose, and participate in the control of food intake and energy balance (8,41,107). Microiontophoretic application of IFN produced suppression of electrical activity in LH neurons and excitation in VMH neurons (26,45,78). Local application of IFN to specific glucose-responsive cells in the VMH altered neuronal activity in appropriate ways to explain IFN-induced anorexia (8). IFN-induced feeding suppression appears to involve excitation of glucose-sensitive neurons in the VMH (9,95) and inhibition of activity in glucose-sensitive LH neurons. Other cytokines, such as interleukin-1 (IL-1) and tumor necrosis factor (TNF), also inhibit glucose-sensitive neurons in the LH (considered a "hunger center") and suppress feeding (12,104,108). Two-thirds of glucose-sensitive VMH neurons are sensitive to both IFN and IL-1. In the majority of these IL-1–responsive cells, IFN elicited an increase in VMH neuronal activities and suppression in the LH neuronal activity (8,104,107).

Using central (i.c.v.) and systemic (i.p.) IFN-α application, Reyes-Vazquez et al. (26) simultaneously investigated LH neuronal activity and food intake. Rats were treated for 3 weeks with IFN to study whether loss of appetite, one of the major side effects of IFN therapy, was mediated by the operation of IFN on LH neurons. IFN in therapeutic doses elicited a reversible dose-related decrease of both food intake and body weight. The decrease in food intake following IFN injections was correlated with a depression of LH neuronal electrical activity. Since direct brain application (i.c.v.) and systemic (i.p.) IFN treatment caused identical responses, it is possible to postulate that IFN suppresses food intake by a direct action on LH neurons (26).

Recently, using coronal brain slices (350–400 μm thick) containing both the VMH and LH areas and glass microelectrodes, neuronal activity from single neurons was recorded, following both separate and simultaneous glucose and IFN administration. In the LH, glucose perfusion elicits mainly an increased firing rate, whereas in the VMH, glucose perfusion elicits mainly a decreased firing rate (Fig. 4). When IFN was given, most of the LH-responsive cells decreased their activity, whereas most of the VMH neurons increased their activities. A comparison of responses to these two different agents revealed that most of the LH neurons responding to glucose by excitation responded to IFN with decreased firing rate, whereas most VMH neurons with glucose-induced depression were excited by IFN (Fig. 4). Neurons unresponsive to glucose were also unresponsive to IFN treatment. When glucose and IFN were given jointly in the LH, the IFN prevented the excitatory effects of glucose given alone.

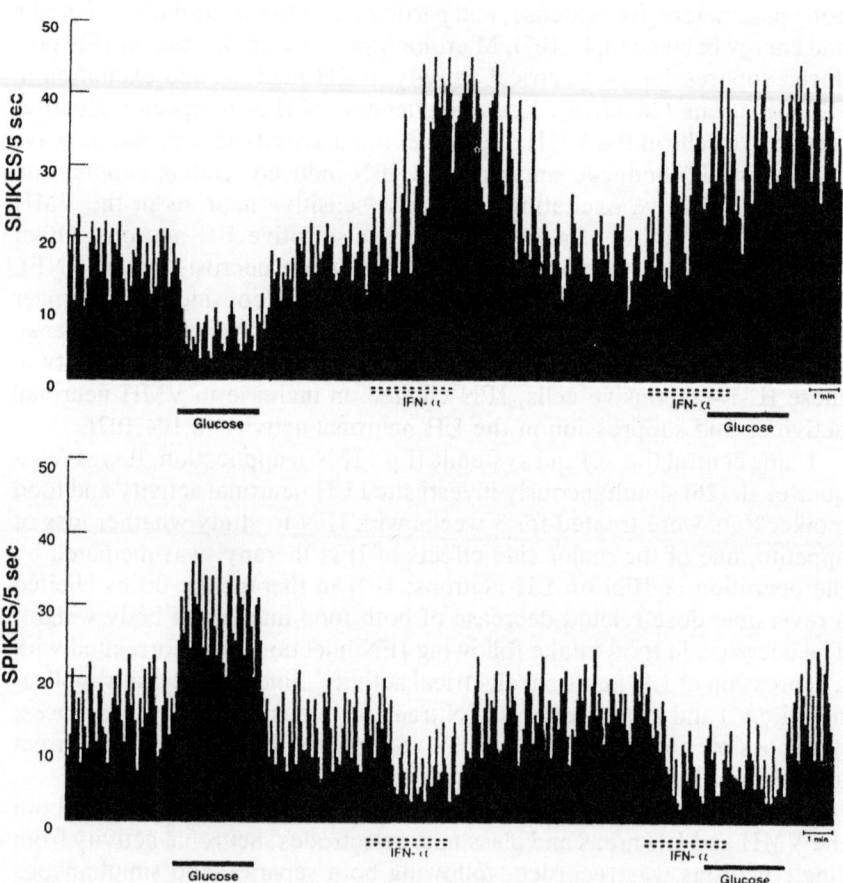

Figure 4 Frequency histograms from representative neurons in lateral hypothalamus (LH) and ventromedial hypothalamus (VMH) following 10 mM glucose and 1500 IU IFN-α applied separately and together. VMH (upper histogram) and LH (lower histogram) neuronal activity are modulated in a push-pull manner in regulating glucose sensitive neurons. Time between treatments is 60 mins.

In the VMH, IFN prevented the depression elicited when glucose was previously given alone (see Fig. 4). These results suggest that IFN, which is endogenously produced by the brain (3–5), is a neurotransmitter involved in feeding regulation.

Hori et al. (8), suggested that cytokine-induced suppression of food intake involves the excitation of glucose-sensitive excitatory neurons in the VMH and the inhibition of glucose-sensitive neurons in the LH. Microiontophoretic application of IFN onto VMH neurons causes excitation (45,78), but it inhibits LH neurons (26). Similarly, morphine as well as glucose has opposing effects on LH and VMH neurons (109,110). The reciprocal interaction between LH and VMH in mechanisms of hunger and satiety has been documented extensively (40,42). It is possible that IFN and opiates affect both VMH and LH in a reciprocal (push-pull) manner in regulating food intake. IFN excites some glucose-sensitive neurons (26) which are also excited by morphine and by endogenous opioid peptides (86). Excitatory responses to microiontophoretic applications of IFN in the VMH, recorded from glucose-sensitive neurons, are also antagonized by naloxone (85,93). Direct interaction of IFN with opioid receptors is a plausible explanation for the observed effects on glucose-sensitive neurons (85,92,93). Collectively, the data suggest that hypothalamic neuronal activity is directly related to the loss of appetite observed during IFN therapy (22).

Several mechanisms in addition to the actions of cytokines on glucose responsive neurons have been suggested for cytokine-induced anorexia. Although cytokines suppress food intake independently of fever, the body temperature increase itself may work to inhibit feeding by modulating the activity of glucose-responsive neurons in the VMH and LH directly (107) or synaptically (103). Immunoregulators such as ILs and IFNs induce sleep (12,28,39,63,65,95,111). Sleep prevents eating, and thus promotes weight loss. Furthermore, in healthy subjects, plasma IFN activity early in the day (at hour 06:00) is negligible, but increases during the day with a peak level at hour 18:00 (112,113). Daily variation in the physiological IFN response is linked to external stimuli such as feeding and/or physical activity (113).

VIII. CONCLUSIONS

Cytokines, including the various forms of interferons, are a group of hormone-like molecules synthesized and secreted by macrophages, monocytes, T lymphocytes, glia, and neurons (8,11,114,115). IFN was initially considered to be solely an antiviral agent. This chapter summarizes evidence to show that IFN is a physiological modulator with multiple effects on CNS neurons, in many cases via opioid receptors. IFN modulates behavior, brain activity, function of temperature and glucose-sensitive neurons, feeding patterns, and opiate activity (46–49,73–77,116–118).

REFERENCES

1. Isaacs A, Lindenmann J. Virus interference. I. The interferon. Proc R Soc London Ser B 1957; 147:258–267.
2. Baron S, Tyring SK, Fleischmann WR Jr, Coppenhaven DH, Niesel DW, Klimpel GR, Stanton GJ, Hughes TK. The interferons: mechanisms of action and clinical applications. JAMA 1991; 266:1375–1376.
3. Bocci V. What are the roles of interferons in physiological conditions? NIPS 1988; 3:201–203.
4. Bocci V. Physicochemical and biologic properties of interferons and their potential uses in drug delivery systems. Crit Rev Ther Drug Carrier Syst 1992; 9:91–133.
5. Marcovitz R, Tsiang H, Hovannesiam AG. Production and action of interferon in mice affected with rabies virus. Ann Virol 1984; 135E:19–33.
6. Pestka S, Langer JA, Zoon KC, Samuel CE. Interferons and their actions. Annu Rev Biochem 1987; 56:727–777.
7. Goldstein D, Laszlo J. The role of interferon in cancer therapy: a current perspective. CA Cancer J Clin 1988; 38:258–277.
8. Hori T, Nakashima T, Take S, Kaizuka Y, Mori T, Katafuchi T. Immune cytokines and regulation of body temperature, food intake and cellular immunity. Brain Res Bull 1991; 27:309–313.
9. Mattson K, Niiranen A, Iivanainen M, Färkkilä M, Bergström L, Holsti LR, Cantell K. Neurotoxicity of interferon. Cancer Treat Rep 1983; 67: 958–961.
10. Meyers CA, Valentine AD. Neurological and psychiatric adverse effects of immunological therapy. CNS Drugs 1995; 3:56–68.
11. Pavol MA, Meyers CA, Rexer JL, Valentine AD, Mattis PJ, and Talpaz M. Pattern of neurobehavioral deficits associated with interferon alfa therapy for leukemia. Neurology 1995; 45:947–950.
12. Plata-Salaman CR. Immunoregulators in the nervous system. Neurosci Behav Rev 1991; 15:185–215.
13. Plata-Salaman CR, Oomura Y, Kai Y. Tumor necrosis factor and interleukin-1β: suppression of food intake by direct action in the central nervous system. Brain Res 1988; 448:106–114.
14. Saphier D, Welch JE, Chuluyan HE. α-Interferon inhibits adrenocortical secretion via μ_1-opioid receptors in the rat. Eur J Pharmacol 1993; 236: 186–194.
15. Shoham S, Davenne D, Cady AB, Dinarello CA, Krueger JM. Recombinant tumor necrosis factor and interleukin 1 enhance slow wave sleep. Am J Physiol 1987; 253:R142–R149.

16. Smith RA, Landel C, Cornelius CE, Revel M. Mapping the action of interferon on primate brain. J Interferon Res 1986; 6(suppl. 1):140.
17. Smith RA, Tyrrell D, Coyle K, Higgins P. Effects of interferon alpha on performance in man: a preliminary report. Psychopharmacology 1988; 96: 414–416.
18. Blalock JE, Smith EM. Human leukocyte interferon (HuIFN-α): potent endorphin-like opioid activity. Biochem Biophys Res Commun 1981; 101: 472–478.
19. Calvet MC, Gresser I. Interferon enhances the excitability of cultured neurons. Nature 1979; 278:558–560.
20. Adams F, Quesada JR, Gutterman JV. Neuropsychiatric manifestations of human leukocyte interferon therapy in patients with cancer. JAMA 1984; 252:938–941.
21. Iivanainen M, Laaksonen R, Niemi ML, Färkkilä M, Bergström L, Mattson K, Niiranen A, Cantell K. Memory and psychomotor impairment following high-dose interferon treatment in amyotrophic lateral sclerosis. Acta Neurol. Scand 1985; 72:475–480.
22. Meyers CA, Scheibel RS, Forman AD. Persistent neurotoxicity of systemically administered interferon-alpha. Neurology 1991; 41:672–676.
23. Crnic LS, Segall M. Behavioral effects of mouse interferons-α and -γ and human interferon-α in mice. Brain Res 1992; 590:277–284.
24. Fent K, Zbinden G. Toxicity of interferon and interleukin. Trends Pharmacol Sci. 1987; 8:100–105.
25. Quesada JR, Talpaz M, Rios A, Kurzrock R, Gutterman JU. Clinical toxicity of interferons in cancer patients: a review. J Clin Oncol 1986; 4:234–243.
26. Reyes-Vazquez C, Prieto-Gomez B, Dafny N. Alpha-interferon suppresses food intake and neuronal activity of the lateral hypothalamus. Neuropharmacology 1994; 33:1545–1552.
27. Segall MA, Crnic LS. An animal model for the behavioral effects of interferon. Behav Neurosci 1990; 104:612–618.
28. Dafny N. Interferon modifies EEG and EEG-like activity recorded from sensory, motor, and limbic system structures in freely behaving rats. Neurotoxicology 1983; 4:235–240.
29. Kidron D, Saphier D, Ovadia H, Weidenfeld J, Abramsky O. Central administration of immunomodulatory factors alters neural activity and adrenocortical secretion. Brain Behav Immun 1989; 3:15–27.
30. McDonald EM, Mann AH, Thomas HC. Interferons as mediators of psychiatric morbidity: an investigation in a trial of recombinant α-interferon in hepatitis-B carriers. Lancet 1987; 21:1175–1177.
31. Born J, Spath-Schwalbe E, Pietrowsky R, Porzsolt F, Fehm HI. Neurophysiological effects of recombinant interferon-γ and -α in man. Clin Physiol Biochem 1989; 7:119–127.
32. Meyers CA, Abbruzzese J. Cognitive functioning in cancer patients: effect of previous treatment. Neurology 1992; 42:434–436.
33. Priestman TJ. Initial evaluation of human lymphoblastoid interferon in patients with advanced malignant disease. Lancet 1980; 2:113–118.

34. Rohatiner AZS, Prior PF, Burton AC, Smith AT, Balkwill FR, Lister TA. Central nervous system toxicity of interferon. Br J Cancer 1983; 47:419–422.

35. Smedley H, Katrak M, Sikora K, Wheeler T. Neurological effects of recombinant human interferon. Br Med J 1983; 286:262–264.

36. Cantell K, Pulkkien E, Eluoso R, Suominen J. Effect of interferon on severe psychiatric diseases. Ann Clin Res 1980; 12:131–132.

37. Dunn AL, Crnic LS. Behavioral effects of repeated injections of interferon-α A/D in Balb/c mice. Brain Behav Immun 1992; 6:355–364.

38. Dunn AL, Crnic LS. Repeated injections of interferon-α A/D in Balb/c mice: behavioral effects. Brain Behav Immun 1993; 7:104–111.

39. Saphier D, Kidron D, Abramsky O, Trainin N, Pecht M, Burstein Y, Ovadia H. Neurophysiological changes in the brain following central administration of immunomodulatory factors. Isr J Med Sci 1988; 24:261–263.

40. Dafny N, Gilman MA, Lichtigfeld FJ. Cholecystokinin induced suppression of feeding in fed, fasting and hypothalamic island rats. Brain Res Bull 1988; 21:225–231.

41. Oomura Y. Chemical and neuronal control of feeding motivation. Physiol Behav 1988; 44:555–560.

42. Schanzer MC, Jacobson ED, Dafny N. Endocrine control of appetite: gastrointestinal hormonal effects on CNS appetite structures. Neuroendocrinology 1978; 25:329–342.

43. Scott GM, Secher DS, Flowers D, Bate J, Cantell K, Tyrrell DAJ. Toxicity of interferon. Br Med J 1981; 282:1345–1348.

44. Smith RA, Norris F, Palmer D, Bernhardt L, Wills RJ. Distribution of alpha interferon in serum and cerebrospinal fluid after systemic administration. Clin. Pharmacol. Ther 1985; 37:85–88.

45. Dafny N, Prieto-Gomez B, Reyes-Vazquez C. Does the immune system communicate with the central nervous system? Interferon modifies central nervous system activity. J Neuroimmunol 1985; 9:1–12.

46. Dafny N. Interferon as a candidate endogenous substance preventing tolerance and dependence to brain opioids. Prog Neuropsychopharmac Biol Psychiatry 1984; 8:351–357.

47. Dafny N. Interferon as an endocoid candidate preventing and attenuating opiate addiction. In: Endocoids. New York: Liss, 1985; 269–276.

48. Dafny N, Lee JR, Dougherty PM. Immune response products alter CNS activity: interferon modulates central opioid function. J Neurosci Res 1988; 19:130–139.

49. Dougherty PM, Dafny N. Interaction of immune cytokines and CNS opioids: a possible interface for stress-induced immune suppression. In: Wybran J, Faith R, McCain HW, Plotnikoff NP, eds. Stress and Immunity. New York: Plenum Press, 1991:173–185.

50. Saphier D, Roerig SC, Ito C, Vlasak WR, Farrar GE, Broyles JE, Welch JE. Inhibition of neural and neuroendocrine activity by α-interferon: neuroendocrine, electrophysiological, and biochemical studies in the rat. Brain Behav Immun 1994; 8:37–56.

51. Darling JJ, Hoyle NR, Thomas DGT. Self and non-self in the brain. Immunol Today 1981; 2:176–181.
52. Wiranowska M, Wilson TC, Thompson K, Prockop LD. Cerebral interferon entry in mice after osmotic alteration of blood-brain barrier. J Interferon Res 1989; 9:355–362.
53. Aguet M. High affinity binding of ^{125}I-labelled mouse interferon to specific cell surface receptors. Nature 1980; 284:459–461.
54. Janicki PK. Binding of human alpha-interferon in the brain tissue membranes of rat. Res Commun Chem Pathol Pharm 1992; 75:117–120.
55. Menzies RA, Patel R, Hall NRS, O'Grady MP, Rier SE. Human recombinant interferon alpha inhibits naloxone binding to rat brain membranes. Life Sci 1992; 50:PL227–PL232.
56. Panchenko LF, Alyab'eva TN, Malinovskaya VV, Balashov AM. α-Interferon–brain opiate receptor interaction. Exp Biol 1987; 46:983–985.
57. Panchenko LF, Alyab'eva TN, Petrichenko OB, Bumialis VV, Balashov AM. Spetsificheskoe sviazyvanie mu- I delta-ligandov opiatny miretseptorami golovnogo mozga krys v prisutstvii reaferona. Biull Eksp Biol Med 1988; 106:307–309.
58. Blalock JE, Smith EM. Human leukocyte interferon: structural and biological relatedness to adrenocorticotropic hormone and endorphins. Proc Natl Acad Sci USA 1980; 77:5972–5974.
59. Blalock JE, Smith EM. Structural and function of interferon (IFN) and neuroendocrine hormones. In: De Maeyer E, Galasso G, Schellekens H, eds. The Biology of the Interferon System. Amsterdam: Elsevier, 1981: 93–99.
60. Blalock JE, Stanton JD. Common pathways of interferon and hormonal action. Nature 1990; 283:406–408.
61. Friedman WJ, Larkfors I. Regulation of NGF expression in rat hippocampal cultures by interleukin-1 and other inflammatory mediators. Soc Neurosci Abstr 1989; 15:953.
62. Smith EM, Blalock JE. Human lymphocyte production of corticotropin and endorphin-like substances: association with leukocyte interferon. Proc Natl Acad Sci USA 1981; 78:7530–7534.
63. De Sarro GB, Masuda Y, Ascioti C, Audino MG, Nistico G. Behavioural and ECoG spectrum changes induced by intracerebral infusion of interferons and interleukin 2 in rats are antagonized by naloxone. Neuropharmacology 1990; 29:167–179.
64. Root-Bernstein RS. 'Molecular sandwiches' as a basis for structural and functional similarities of interferons, MSH, ACTH, LHRH, myelin basic protein, and albumins. FEBS Lett 1984; 168:208–212.
65. Birmanns B, Saphier D, Abramsky O. α-Interferon modifies cortical EEG activity: dose-dependence and antagonism by naloxone. J Neurol Sci 1990; 100:22–26.
66. Jaffe JH, Martin WR. Opioid analgesics and antagonists. In Gilman AG, Rall TW, Nies AS, Taylor P, Goodman LS, eds. The Pharmacological Basis of Therapeutics. 8th ed. New York: Macmillan, 1990; 435–521.

67. Jaffe JH. Drug addiction and drug abuse. In: Gilman AG, Rall TW, Nies AS, Taylor P, eds. The Pharmacological Basis of Therapeutics, 8th ed. New York: Macmillan, 1990:522–523.

68. McCain HW, Lamster IB, Bozzone JM, Grbic JT. β-Endorphin modulates human immune activity via non-opiate receptor mechanisms. Life Sci 1982; 31:1619–1624.

69. Zimmerman E, Krivoy W. Antagonism between morphine and the polypeptides ACTH, ACTH$_{1-24}$, and β-MSH in the nervous system. Prog Brain Res 1973; 39:383–392.

70. Bertolini A, Poggioli R, Fratta W. Withdrawal symptoms in morphine-dependent rats intracerebroventrically injected with ACTH$_{1-24}$ and with β-MSH. Life Sci 1981; 29:249–252.

71. Gober WF, Lefkowitz SS, Hung CY. Effect of morphine, hydromorphine, methadone, mescaline, trypan blue, vitamin A, sodium salicylate, and caffeine on the serum interferon level in response to viral infection. Arch Int Pharmacodyn 1975; 214:322–327.

72. Hung CY, Lefkowitz SS, Geber WF. Interferon inhibition by narcotic analgesics. Proc Soc Exp Biol Med 1973; 142:106–111.

73. Dafny N. Modification of morphine withdrawal by interferon. Life Sci 1983; 32:303–306.

74. Dafny N. Interferon modifies morphine withdrawal phenomena in rodents. Neuropharmacology 1983; 22:647–651.

75. Dafny N, Reyes-Vazquez C. Three different types of α-interferons alter naloxone-induced abstinence in morphine-addicted rats. Immunopharmacology 1985; 9:13–17.

76. Dafny N, Reyes-Vazquez C. Single injection of three different preparations of α-interferon modifies morphine abstinence signs for a prolonged period. Int J Neurosci 1987; 32:953–962.

77. Dafny N, Zielinski M, Reyes-Vazquez C. Alteration of morphine withdrawal to naloxone by interferon. Neuropeptides 1983; 3:453–464.

78. Prieto-Gomez B, Reyes-Vazquez C, Dafny N. Differential effects of interferon on ventromedial hypothalamus and dorsal hippocampus. J Neurosci Res 1983; 10:273–278.

79. Reyes-Vazquez C, Prieto-Gomez B, Dafny N. Novel effect of interferon on the brain: microiontophoretic application and single cell recording in the rat. Neurosci Lett 1982; 34:201–206.

80. Reyes-Vazquez C, Prieto-Gomez B, Georgiades JA, Dafny N. Alpha and gamma interferons effects on cortical and hippocampal neurons: microiontophoretic application and single cell recording. Int J Neurosci 1984; 25: 113–121.

81. Reyes-Vazquez C, Weisbrodt N, Dafny N. Does interferon exert its action through opiate receptors? Life Sci 1984; 35:1015–1021.

82. Kosterlitz HW, Waterfield AA. An analysis of the phenomenon of acute tolerance to morphine in the guinea-pig isolated brain. Br J Pharmacol 1975; 53:131–138.

83. Paton WDM. The action of morphine and related substances on contraction and on acetylcholine output of coaxially stimulated guinea-pig ileum. Br J Pharmacol 1957; 11:119–127.

84. Burks TF. Actions of drugs on gastrointestinal motility. In: Johnson LR, Christensen J, Grossman MI, Jacobson ED, Schultz SG, eds. Physiology of the Gastrointestinal Tract, Vol. 1. New York: Raven Press, 1981:495–516.

85. Nakashima T, Hori T, Kuriyama K, Kiyohara T. Naloxone blocks the interferon-α induced changes in hypothalamic neuronal activity. Neurosci Lett 1987; 82:332–336.

86. Ono T, Oomura Y, Nishino H, Sasaki K, Muramoto K, Yano I. Morphine and enkephalin effects on hypothalamic glucosensitive neurons. Brain Res 1980; 185:208–212.

87. Blatteis CM, Xin L, Quan N. Neuromodulation of fever: Apparent involvement of opioids. Brain Res Bull 1991; 26:219–223.

88. Dinarello CA. Interleukin-1. Ann NY Acad Sci 1988; 546:122–132.

89. Dinarello CA, Bernheim HA, Duff GW, Le HV, Nagabhushan TL, Hamilton NC, Coceani F. Mechanisms of fever induced by recombinant human interferon. J Clin Invest 1984; 74:906–913.

90. Ackerman SK, Hochstein HD, Zoon K, Browne W, Rivera E, Elisberg B. Interferon fever: absence of human leukocytic pyrogen response to recombinant α-interferon. J Leukocyte Biol 1984; 36:17–25.

91. Dantzer R, Satinoff E, Kelley KW. Cyclosporine and alpha-interferon do not attenuate morphine withdrawal in rats but do impair thermoregulation. Physiol Behav 1987; 39:593–598.

92. Kuriyama K, Hori T, Mori T, Nakashima T. Actions of interferon-α and interleukin-1β on the glucose-responsive neurons in the ventromedial hypothalamus. Brain Res Bull 1990; 24:803–810.

93. Nakashima T, Hori T, Kuriyama K, Matsuda T. Effects of interferon-α on the activity of preoptic thermosensitive neurons in tissue slices. Brain Res 1988; 454:361–367.

94. Shibata M, Blatteis CM. Differential effects of cytokines on thermosensitive neurons in guinea pig preoptic area slices. Am J Physiol 1992; 261: R1096–R1103.

95. Krueger JM, Dinarello CA, Shoham S, Davenne D, Walter J, Kubillus S. Interferon alpha-2 enhances slow-wave sleep in rabbits. Int J Immunopharmacol 1987; 9:23–30.

96. Saphier D, Kidron D, Ovadia H, Weidenfeld J, Abramsky O, Burstein Y, Pecht M, Trainin N. Preoptic area (POA) multiunit activity (MUA) and cortical EEG changes following intracerebroventricular (ICV) administration of α-interferon (IFN), thymic humoral factor (THF), histamine (HIS), and interleukin-1 (IL-1). Rev Clin Basic Pharmacol 1987; 6:265–278.

97. Reite M, Laudenslager M, Jones J, Crnic L, Kaemingk K. Interferon decreases REM latency. Biol Psychiatry 1987; 22:104–107.

98. Morley JE. Neuropeptide regulation of appetite and weight. Endocrinol Rev 1987; 8:256–287.

99. D'Arcangelo G, Grassi F, Ragozzino D, Santoni A, Tancredi V, Eusebi F. Interferon inhibits synaptic potentiation in rat hippocampus. Brain Res 1991; 564:245–248.

100. Bliss TVP. Maintenance is presynaptic. Nature 1990; 346:698–699.

101. Gustafsson B, Wingström H. Physiological mechanisms underlying long-term potentiation. Trends Neurosci 1988; 11:156–162.

102. Muller M, Fontana A, Zbinden G, Gähwiler BH. Effects of interferons and hydrogen peroxide on CA3 pyramidal cells in rat hippocampal slice cultures. Brain Res 1993; 619:157–162.

103. Nakayama T, Yamamoto K, Ishikawa Y, Imai K. Effects of preoptic thermal stimulation on the ventromedial hypothalamic neurons in rats. Neurosci Lett 1981; 26:177–181.

104. Plata-Salaman CR. Immunomodulators and feeding regulation: a humoral link between the immune and nervous system. Brain Behav Immun 1989; 3:193–213.

105. Tempel DL, Kim T, Liebowitz SF. The paraventricular nucleus is uniquely responsive to the feeding stimulatory effects of steroid hormones. Brain Res 1993; 614:197–204.

106. Dafny N, Jacobson ED. Gastrointestinal hormones and neural interaction with the central nervous system. Experientia 1975; 31:658–659.

107. Hori T, Kuriyama K, Nakashima T. Thermal responsiveness of neurons in the ventromedial nucleus of hypothalamus. J Physiol Soc Jpn 1988; 50:619.

108. Kow LM, Pfaff DW. Actions of feeding-relevant agents on hypothalamic glucose-responsive neurons in vitro. Brain Res Bull 1985; 15:509–513.

109. Kerr FWL, Triplett JN Jr, Beeler GW. Reciprocal (push-pull) effects of morphine on single units in the ventromedian and lateral hypothalamus and influences on other nuclei: with a comment on methadone effects during withdrawal from morphine. Brain Res 1974; 74:81–103.

110. Prieto-Gomez B, Reyes-Vazquez C, Dafny N. Microiontophoretic application of morphine and naloxone in rat hypothalamus neurons. Neuropharmacology 1981; 23:1081–1089.

111. Färkkilä M, Iivanainen M, Härkönen M, Laakso J, Mattson K, Niiranen A, Larsen TA, Cantell K. Effect of interferon-γ on biogenic amine metabolism, electroencephalographic recordings, and transient potentials. Clin Neuropharmacol 1988; 11:63–67.

112. Bocci V, Paulesu L, Muscettola M, Viti A. The physiologic interferon response. VI. Interferon activity in human plasma after a meal and drinking. Lymphokine Res 1985; 4:151–158.

113. Paulesu L, Muscettola M, Bocci V, Viti A. Daily variations of plasma interferon levels in the rat. IRCS Med Sci 1985; 13:993–994.

114. Farrar WL, Hill JM, Harel-Bellan A, Vinocour M. The immune logical brain. Immunol Rev 1987; 100:361–378.

115. Larsson I, Landstrom LE, Larner E, Lundgren E, Miorner H, Strannegard O. Interferon production in glia and glioma cell lines. Infect Immun 1978; 22:786–789.

116. Dougherty PM, Aronowski J, Samorajaski T, Dafny N. Opiate antinociception is altered by immunomodification: the effect of interferon, cyclosporine and radiation-induced immune suppression upon acute and long-term morphine activity. Brain Res 1986; 385:401–404.
117. Dougherty PM, Harper C, Dafny N. The effect of alpha-interferon, cyclosporine A and radiation-immune suppression on morphine-induced hypothermia and tolerance. Life Sci 1986; 39:2191–2197.
118. Dougherty PM, Pearl J, Krajewski KJ, Pellis NR, Dafny N. Differential modification of morphine and methadone dependence by interferon-α. Neuropharmacology 1987; 26:1595–1600.

6

Neuropsychological Effects of Interferon Therapy

Neil H. Pliskin and Anthony T. Reder

The Brain Research Institute, The University of Chicago, Chicago, Illinois

Diane S. Goldstein

The University of Chicago, Chicago, Illinois

I. INTRODUCTION

Interferon (IFN) was first described by Isaacs and Lindenmann in 1957 (1), who noted the antiviral and immunomodulatory properties of this protein. Three decades of interferon research have revealed clinical benefit for multiple diseases, including cancer, herpes zoster, hepatitis B, subacute sclerosing panencephalitis (SSPE), and multiple sclerosis (MS). Research on the clinical and neurological effects of the IFN has been promising and has increased dramatically over the past 15 years, resulting in the recent approval by the US Food and Drug Administration (FDA) in July of 1993 for IFN-β-1b in the treatment of relapsing-remitting MS (2,3).

Adverse systemic, neuropsychiatric, and neurotoxic alterations are common with IFN treatment. Hematological changes, hair loss, arthralgias/myalgias, and manifestation of influenza-like symptoms are most common. These side effects have been found in IFN-α recipients with MS (4–11), cancer (12–23), amyotrophic lateral sclerosis (ALS) (24–27), hepatitis B (28,29), acquired immunodeficiency syndrome (AIDS)–related Kaposi's sarcoma (30,31), SSPE (32), and normal individuals (33). Loss of appetite (12–14,17–22,27), cardiac changes (13,18,31,34–41), and death (34,37,38,41,42) have additionally been reported in some of these populations. Affective and behavioral changes reported in the literature include loss of libido (12), depression (8,12,19,23,29,31,43,44), anxiety (12,43,44), irritability (12,21,26,30,43,45), and general reduction in physical activity (8,12,16,17,21,25,26).

Of particular interest in this chapter, however, are the neurotoxic side effects reflecting central nervous system (CNS) involvement. Changes noted on encephalography (EEG) (16,22,24,25,43,45–48) in visual (24,46), auditory (24), and brainstem evoked potentials (25,46), slowing on electro-neuromyography (16), and confusion (15,18,21,22,24,28,33,48–50) have been reported. More recently, studies have quantified the cognitive effects of treatment with IFN through the use of neuropsychological testing. This chapter reviews the neurocognitive effects of IFN reported thus far in the literature.

To date, there are multiple neuropsychological investigations into the effects of IFN-α and IFN-β but none with IFN-γ. We separated this chapter into two sections, discussing separately the investigations which have used *natural* versus *recombinant* IFN. This decision was based on findings that contaminants within natural IFNs may elicit adverse side effects which do not accompany the use of recombinant proteins (see Chapter 11). A second important discrimination relates to *dosage*, which affects the severity of the IFN-induced changes (see Chapters 3, 7, and 16). A final discrimination we considered related to *type* of IFN (e.g., α and β). Each section provides a chronological account and critical review of the research completed to date. We then provide a description of our own work evaluating the effects of IFN β-1b on cognition in MS and consider the role of IFN in enhancing learning as suggested by some studies.

A major theme of this chapter centers around methodological difficulties which are present in many of the investigations. Specifically, lack of control groups (12,17,25,43,49,53), nonrandom assignment to groups (or failure to report all details on how subjects were chosen for testing) (8,17,26,43,53), failure to report the equality of groups on baseline cognitive performance (8,26,53), and comparison of subjects receiving different treatment dosages (25,26,43) affect our ability to evaluate conclusions of "cognitive decline," "reversible decline," or "lack of cognitive decline" described with IFN treatment. Although we recognize the practical difficulties involved in doing clinical drug trial research, we also found many controllable methodological flaws that further affected the validity of these investigations. For example, many studies used sample sizes that were too small to obtain adequate statistical power to measure change (when statistics were conducted) (8,26,49), failed to report all tests utilized (12,17,49) or to include all performance scores in publications (8,12,17,25,43,49,53), and provided little control for practice effects (i.e., through the use of alternate forms of tests) (8,12,17,25,26,43,49,53). Fur-

Table 1 Summary of Methodological Difficulties in the Neuropsychology Literature on IFN Treatment

Authors	Lack of control group	Nonrandom assignment to groups	Unequal baseline cognitive performance	Variable dosages within the sample or variable Rx duration	Sample size too small for numbers of variables used in statistical analysis	Failure to report all tests used	Performance scores not reported	Alternate test forms not used to control for practice effects	No statistics conducted	Multiple comparisons without correction[b]
Mattson, 1984 (16)	✓	✓[a]	✓[a]	✓			✓	✓	✓	
Adams, 1984 (12)	✓					✓	✓	✓	✓	
Iivanainen, 1985 (25) [includes Farkkila, 1984 (24)]	✓			✓			✓	✓	✓	
Niiranen, 1988 (17)	✓	✓[a]		✓		✓	✓	✓	✓	
Liberati, 1990 (49)	✓				✓	✓	✓	✓		✓
Meyers, 1991 (43)	✓	✓[a]		✓			✓	✓[a]	✓	
Poutiainen, 1993 (26)		✓	✓	✓	✓			✓	✓	✓
Durelli, 1994 (8)		✓[a]	✓[a]		✓		✓	✓		✓

[a] Not reported/insufficient information.
[b] When statistics conducted

ther, statistics were not always performed on the existing data (12,17,25,43,53) or reported on all data (26). Table 1 contains a summary of the methodological difficulties found in these studies. Taking these methodological variations into account, treatment with IFN, with two exceptions (8,49), has been associated with adverse changes in neurocognitive status.

II. NATURAL INTERFERONS

A. Interferon-α

1. Low Dosage ($1-5 \times 10^6$ IU)

In 1984, Adams et al. (12) reported cognitive changes associated with IFN-α in 10 patients with renal cell carcinoma (3×10^6 IU given daily for at least 1 month, total duration unspecified). Neuropsychological assessment included measures of concentration and cognitive flexibility (Trail making Test Parts A and B from the Halstead-Reitan Neuropsychological Test Battery), visuospatial and visuoconstructional skills (Bender-Gestalt Test), and general intellectual functioning (three unspecified Wechsler Adult Intelligence Scale [WAIS] subtests). After conducting a baseline assessment, subjects were reevaluated 1 week and 1 month after initiation of treatment.

The investigators provide a chart of symptom frequency, tabulating the total combined number of subjects who complained of symptoms, or revealed performance deficits on testing, across the three evaluation points (i.e., combined subjective deficit and objective deficit, respectively). Treatment with IFN-α was associated with memory problems, impaired concentration, slowed thinking, construction dyspraxia and visuospatial disorientation, and cognitive inflexibility. Additional cognitive symptomatology included speech arrest, thought blocking, and feelings of unreality. The majority of complaints and performance deficits were noted by the first week, and most difficulties continued throughout the first month of treatment.

2. Medium Dosage ($6-7 \times 10^6$ IU)

In 1984, Mattson et al. (51) assessed the cognitive effects of two different treatment regimens of IFN-α in patients with small cell lung cancer. Nine patients received an initial high-dose regimen (800×10^6 IU) given intravenously over 5 days, followed by a medium-dose regimen (6×10^6 IU) given three times a week by intramuscular (i.m.) injection until disease progression (treatment duration ranging 5–42 weeks across patients). Six patients patients received only a medium-dose regimen (6×10^6 IU) given by i.m. injection until disease progression (treatment duration ranging 1–17 weeks across patients).

The investigators first reported the effects of neurotoxicity (16), and a later publication provided a more detailed description of the neuropsychological sequelae associated with IFN treatment (17). Additionally, the earlier report provided more details on IFN administration; the 800×10^6 dosage was a cumulative one, beginning with 100×10^6 IU for 2 days, followed by 200×10^6 IU for 3 days. Half of the patients (n = 4) were unable to tolerate the full 800×10^6 IU regimen, and they received variable dosages ranging from 425 to 700×10^6 IU. Additionally, the interim between the conclusion of high-dose therapy and the commencement of medium-dose therapy ranged up to 2 weeks across patients. Finally, it is unclear whether the 1984 paper simply added subjects to the already existing subject pool from the earlier paper (n = 8) or began with new subjects. In either case, interpretation of results is hampered owing to lack of detail on extent of purification of IFN and dosage.

Neuropsychological assessment of four patients (one from the combined high- and medium-dosage regimen, three from the medium-dose–only regimen) included the first four items from the Wechsler Memory Scale (WMS; Information, Orientation, Mental Control, and Logical Memory), and drawing tasks and modified items of the Luria battery measuring visuospatial, visuoconstructional, reading, writing, and calculation skills. Patients were tested daily for 14 days, weekly for 4 weeks, and monthly until disease progression. A comprehensive test battery (including the WAIS subtests in addition to the above tests) was given at baseline and days 5 and 30. The investigators report that declines were seen in Logical Memory performance, visuoconstructional skills, finger-tapping speed, and psychomotor behavior. They add that both regimens produced similar declines in cognitive performance but along different time courses. The greatest changes in the combined high- and medium-dosage regimen occurred between the 8th and 10th days (several days after changing dosages from high to medium levels), whereas the most notable changes in the medium-dosage–alone regimen occurred between the 3rd and 4th weeks.

In addition to the methodological issues noted in Table 1, the investigators' comments regarding the effects of IFN dosage on the degree of cognitive dysfunction need clarification. According to the figures presented (depicting Logical Memory performance in one patient from each treatment regimen, representativeness and method of selection unspecified), the baseline performances are equivalent and the impairment noted in each subject during the treatment regimens is also equivalent. However, the kinetics of dysfunction differed. In the patient receiving the combined high- and medium-dosage regimen, neuropsychological dysfunction appeared and resolved to baseline levels within a 4-day period, whereas dysfunction gradually appeared over a period of 22 days in the patient receiving the medium-dosage–only regimen, and took 2 months to return to the baseline performance level. Further performance declines, although not as severe, were noted in both patients after recovery from the first deficits, indicating a fluctuating cognitive status throughout treatment in both regimens.

Overall, this study was valuable in understanding that neuropsychological changes occur in patients receiving various IFN treatment regimens. Thus far, it seems that the cognitive effects are similar between low- and medium-dosage regimens in type and severity but seem to differ in their time course (e.g., in onset and resolution).

In 1988, Niiranen et al. (17) reported on findings from nine patients with small cell lung cancer who received IFN-α. Initial high dosage was 880×10^6 IU given by continuous intravenous infusion for 5 days, followed by a medium-dosage of 6×10^6 IU given by i.m. injection three times a week until disease progression. Four patients were unable to tolerate the planned regimen owing to adverse systemic side effects, and IFN was subsequently discontinued. One patient received daily neuropsychological evaluation, including several WMS subtests (Orientation, Mental Control, Word Span, Digit Span forward and backward, Logical Memory), and Luria's subtests including those measuring visual and spatial perception, visuoconstructional drawings, speech, reading, writing, and calculation. A comprehensive battery (including Tapping and the WAIS Information, Similarities, and Picture Completion subtests in addition to the above tests) was given at baseline and days 5 and 30.

The investigators report findings from one patient at baseline, days 1–10, and 15 (day 30 not reported). Performance scores are not provided, but a severity rating was applied to all scores (normal, moderately disturbed, or severely disturbed). There was no appearance of cognitive disturbance until day 4, when moderate impairments were noted in visual and spatial perception and calculation. This finding is similar to that previously described by Mattson et al. (16). The above-mentioned functions became severely impaired over the next week, returned to moderate impairment by day 10, and were normal by day 15. Other cognitive functions showed similar impairment patterns, with the majority of impairment occurring after high-dose infusion had been discontinued; again suggesting a delayed adverse effect on cognition.

3. High-Dosage ($>8 \times 10^6$ IU)

In 1985, Iivanainen et al. (25) reported on the neuropsychological results of seven patients with ALS treated with high-dose IFN-α, who had been previously described in a preliminary report by Farkkila et al. (24) in 1984. As the 1985 report contained considerably more detail on neuropsychological results, we combine the findings here to facilitate interpretation of results. Patients received an initial high-dosage regimen of 100×10^6 IU by continuous intravenous infusion for 2 days, followed by 4 days of an additional high-dosage regimen of 200×10^6 IU. Because of adverse systemic side effects, IFN was discontinued in two patients and several others received dosage reductions. As a result, patients received variable cumulative doses of IFN, ranging from 250 to 950×10^6 IU over 6 days. A low-dose maintenance regimen was initially planned for 2 months following high-dose infusion; however, only one patient made it to the maintenance protocol owing to adverse side effects associated with the high-dose treatment.

Neuropsychological evaluation consisted of two batteries. The extended battery, administered at baseline and days 6 and 20, included several WAIS subtests (Information, Similarities, and Picture Completion), WMS subtests (Orientation, Mental Control, Digit Span forward and backward, Logical Memory, and Visual Reproduction), Tapping, and Luria's subtests, including those measuring voluntary movements, visual and spatial perception, visuoconstructional drawings, speech, reading, writing, and calculation. The abbreviated battery, administered on days 4, 8, 12, and 15, excluded the WAIS subtests, Luria's voluntary movement subtests, one subtest from tasks of visual and spatial perception (recognition of familiar objects), and speech tests.

Only the presence or absence of performance change across measures is reported. Findings indicated changes in orientation (details not provided), concentration, memory, psychomotor speed, constructional praxis, and mental speed, with no changes in intellectual functioning (WAIS subtests). The appearance of deficits followed a pattern consistent with other investigations; impairment began on day 4, peaked between days 6 and 8, and resolved by day 12. Severity of performance across patients, however, was quite variable and peaked at different times. As with many investigations, patterns of performance over time should be interpreted liberally, given the repeated use of tests without alternate forms which could lead to a practice effect. One patient revealed motor perseveration, and one revealed handwriting changes including micrographia. EEG slowing was inconsistent with changes in cognition.

In 1993, Poutiainen et al. (26) reported the first controlled study on the cognitive effects of high-dose IFN-α. In this single-blind study of 21 patients with the spinal form of amytrophic lateral sclerosis, 16 patients were assigned to a treatment group and 5 to a placebo group (subjects were randomly assigned to groups, but for ethical reasons, a smaller group size was chosen for the placebo condition). Treatment subjects received a cumulative high-dose regimen of 800×10^6 IU by continuous intravenous infusion over 5 days. Neuropsychological evaluation included WMS sub-tests (counting backwards from 20 to 1, serial 3s, Digit Span backwards, Logical Memory), Stroop Naming and Interference scores, Luria's Copy-ing a Cube, and Signature Writing. Patients were evaluated at baseline and days 5 and 8. Because of severe side effects and refusal by several patients to complete all three evaluations, six subjects were lost to the study. Fifteen subjects (12 treatment, 3 placebo) were thus included in analyses. Results indicated significant performance declines between baseline and day 5 in Logical Memory, Calculation, and Signature Writing (time in seconds). Additionally, following discontinuation of IFN (compar-ison between days 5 and 8), there was improvement on all tasks.

In addition to methodological difficulties noted in Table 1, the conclu-sion that performance declines were reversible is problematic. Slight im-provements were noted between days 5 and 8. However, on most every test given, day 8 performances were still below baseline. It is possible that the effects of treatment are in fact reversible, but the interim period between discontinuation of IFN on day 5 and reevaluation on day 8 was too short to allow for further recovery of function. Additionally, perfor-mance dropped on several measures in the control group: WMS Counting 20–1 (decline from baseline to day 5), WMS Serial 3s (from day 5 to 8), WMS Digit Span backwards (from days 5 to 8), Logical Memory (from baseline to day 5), and Calculation (from day 5 to 8). Thus, the conclusions made by the investigations regarding the effects of IFN on cognition should be considered preliminary.

B. Interferon-β

1. Medium Dosage

In 1990, Liberati et al. (49) reported neuropsychological findings from 22 patients with various types of cancer treated with human IFN-β at a dos-age of 6×10^6 IU through intravenous infusion for 7 days on alternate weeks for a total of three cycles. Maintenance therapy was continued at the same dosage twice a week for 24 weeks. A neuropsychological battery consisting of WAIS Digit Span, Raven's Progressive Coloured Matrices, a Geometrical Shape Cancellation task, constructional apraxia tests (un-specified), measures of long-term verbal memory and verbal fluency was administered at baseline, 1 week following initial induction therapy, and 1 week following cessation of maintenance therapy. Changes in neuro-psychological performance were considered to have occurred if at least three performance scores from either evaluation point fell 1.5 standard deviations from baseline scores.

Highlighting the difficulties associated with this type of research, 21 patients were available at the second evaluation and 9 at follow-up. Results indicated that there were no declines in neuropsychological performance but rather a significant improvement was noted on both attentional tasks (Digit Span and Geometrical Shape Cancellation) between the baseline and second evaluations. However, analyses on the 10 patients who completed all three evaluations indicated only trends toward improvement.

In addition to the methodological difficulties with this study described in Table 1, it is unclear how many evaluations patients actually received. Three evaluation points are initially described, but a table provided indicates an additional four evaluation points on two tests (Digit Span and Geometrical Shape Cancellation) given between the baseline and second evaluation. Further, because no control group was provided, it is difficult to say whether apparent performance improvements or lack of performance declines could not be accounted for by practice alone. Nevertheless, none of the marked adverse cognitive changes described in IFN-α treatment were seen in this population.

Natural IFN-α is a mixture of IFN-α subtypes. Natural IFN-α, and possibly IFN-β, can also contain protein contaminants and other cytokines (see Chapter 11). Even small amounts of other bioactive molecules could synergize with IFNs to produce adverse effects on cognition. Thus, to reduce costs and side effects, recombinant IFNs have been developed.

III. RECOMBINANT INTERFERONS

A. Interferon-α

1. Low Dosage

In the only study we are aware of which monitored cognitive status for extended periods following any IFN therapy, Meyers et al. (43) retrospectively reported on the cognitive status of 14 patients with cancer, who had been referred for neuropsychological evaluation because of persistent neurobehavioral side effects following IFN-α treatment termination. Dosage of IFN varied across patients (ranging from 3 to 20 × 10^6 IU, two method of delivery unspecified), as did schedule of administration (daily, n = 3 or triweekly, n = 9, 2 unspecified) and duration of treatment with IFN-α-2a and IFN-α-2b (ranging from 40 days to 3 years, average 55 weeks); IFN α-2a and IFN α-2b were used. The interim period between termination of treatment and neuropsychological evaluation also varied, ranging from 18 days to 27 months (average 28 weeks). The neuropsychological battery was additionally variable across patients, as selection of tests was based on age, medical status, and referral question. Subjects received various tests from the following selection: WAIS-R, Dementia Rating Scale, Verbal Selective Reminding Test, WMS Logical Memory,

Nonverbal Selective Reminding Test, Benton Visual Retention Test, Booklet Category Test, Wisconsin Card Sorting Test, Trail making Test Part A and B, Multilingual Aphasia Examination, Line Bisection, Grip Strength Tapping, and Grooved Pegboard. No pretreatment baseline assessment was obtained, nor was an assessment conducted while patients were receiving their treatment regimen.

All patients had cognitive dysfunction; 10 patients showed a "frontal subcortical" pattern, with impairments noted in memory, motor functioning, problem solving and cognitive flexibility, whereas the remaining 4 patients revealed a more general cognitive impairment across all tests, particularly in information-processing speed and reasoning ability.

The severity of cognitive impairment could not be entirely explained by the severity of acute neurotoxicity from IFN. For example, four of the six patients (67%) who suffered severe acute neurotoxic effects also revealed severe residual cognitive impairments following treatment termination, and 25% of those suffering mild neurotoxicity also had cognitive impairment (severity not indicated). Duration of treatment was additionally not strongly related to cognitive deficits. Some subjects with mild impairment had been treated for several years, whereas others with more severe impairment had received shorter regimens, although the variable time period between treatment cessation and evaluation across subjects is an important confound. Similar interpretive difficulties exist with the effects of dosage and administration schedule on severity of neurocognitive dysfunction; subjects receiving high-dose or daily injections fared worse than those with lower dosages and less frequent administration. Additionally, although the investigations note that no patients received "other therapy with associated neurotoxicity" between treatment cessation and neuropsychological evaluation, it is later reported that four patients were taking antidepressants or neuroleptics, medications which may have adverse effects on cognition (52).

A follow-up neuropsychological evaluation was conducted on 4 of the 14 patients, who were all equivalent in age, type of disease, and initial severity of impairment. Two patients showed improvement relative to their initial assessment, whereas two showed performance declines. The investigations note that the two patients who showed improvement were those with the shortest interval between treatment termination and neuropsychological evaluation. The two patients who showed performance declines had been off the IFN regimen for a greater period of time (4 and 8 months, respectively). Interim periods between treatment cessation and evaluation varied across patients, as did the dosage, schedule of administration, and duration of treatment. The investigators do not speculate on why apparent improvements may initially be seen following termination of IFN treatment or why apparent declines may take place over time. However, effects from the natural progression of cancer may have altered the neurocognitive status of these patients. Moreover, cancer itself can produce changes in cognition. Thus, the conclusion that cognitive impairment persists following cessation of IFN treatment, a finding contrary to that widely noted in the literature (Poutiainen et al. [26] may be an exception), should be considered preliminary.

2. High Dosage

In the only study thus far to assess the cognitive effects of recombinant high-dose IFN-α during treatment, Durelli et al. (8) reported on the neurological and physiological outcome of patients with relapsing-remitting MS following a high-dose regimen of 9×10^6 IU by i.m. injection every other day for 6 months. Twelve patients were treated, while eight received placebo. Patients received neuropsychological evaluations prior to receiving treatment, 3 months into treatment, and at 6 months, when IFN treatment was terminated. The following tests were given: WMS, Benton Visual Retention Test, and the Bender-Gestalt Test. Unfortunately, the investigators do not provide a detailed account of the results of data analyses, including performance scores. They report, however, that both 3- and 6-month performance scores did not show any change from baseline. It is not indicated whether this refers only to the treatment group or to the placebo group as well. The implications of these findings are great, given that studies to date using natural and recombinant IFN-α had consistently reported adverse effects on neurocognitive function.

B. Interferon-β

1. Low and High Dosage

We (53) examined the longitudinal neuropsychological function of 30 patients with MS via serial assessment in order to determine if there is an effect of long-term IFN β-1b treatment on cognition. Nine patients received high-dose IFN β-1b (8×10^6 IU), 8 low-dose IFN β-1b (1.6×10^6 IU) given subcutaneously, and 13 placebo. All subjects underwent a brief neuropsychological evaluation and magnetic resonance imaging (MRI) on 1 day, 2 years after entry into the trial. Two years later (i.e., 4 years into the clinical trial), all subjects were reevaluated neuropsychologically and MRI was repeated (Fig. 1). The test battery included Logical Memory and Visual Reproduction subtests of the WMS Forms I and II, Trial making Test Part B, Stroop Color Word Test, the Purdue Pegboard, and Beck Depression Inventory (BDI).

An improvement in delayed visual memory was found between the second and fourth years of treatment in the high-dose group (WMS Visual

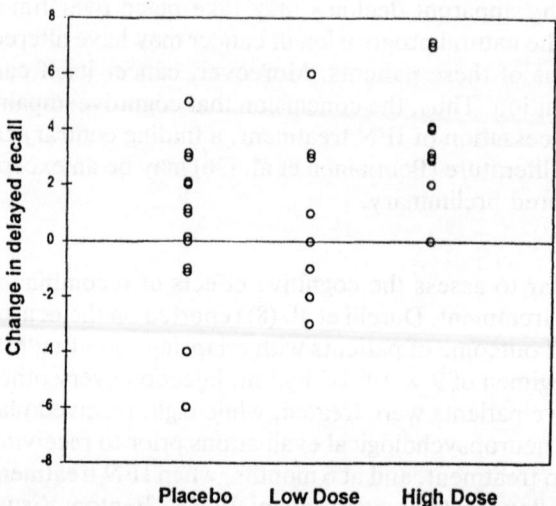

Figure 1 Change in visual reproduction—delayed recall over 2 years of IFN β-1b therapy.

Reproduction–Delayed Recall; $P < .003$). The placebo and low-dose groups did not change significantly (Table 2; see Fig. 1). Moreover, no significant differences between groups were found in age, education, estimated Full Scale IQ, or depression rating at time of initial assessment. This improvement is surprising in light of the IFN-induced cognitive deficits seen in many of the studies above.

The total cohort improved significantly between the first and second assessment on WMS Visual Reproduction–Immediate Recall (F = 25.84 [1,27] $P < .001$) and Stroop Word Reading (F = 5.35 [1,27] $P < .03$) performances, probably indicating practice effects. In contrast, the total cohort declined significantly between the first and second assessment on Purdue Pegboard dominant hand (DH) performance (F = 4.29 [1,27] $P < .05$), reflecting diminished motor speed and dexterity over time in patients with MS, a manifestation of the disease process. This decline was comparable for all three groups. No changes on the Stroop Test or WMS Logical Memory were observed.

We were concerned that changes in Pegboard performance might confound interpretation of improved delayed visual memory performance given the motoric component to the task. However, when Purdue Pegboard performance was covaried with Visual Reproduction–Delayed Recall, the finding of improved performance in the high–dose IFN β-1b group

Table 2 Neuropsychological Test Results During IFN β-1b Therapy

	Placebo		Low Dose		High Dose			
Test	2 year assessment mean (SD)	4 year assessment mean (SD)	2 year assessment mean (SD)	4 year assessment mean (SD)	2 year assessment mean (SD)	4 year assessment mean (SD)	F	P
WMS VR Delay[a]	7.6 (3.2)	8.0 (3.4)	5.8 (1.8)	7.6 (3.3)	5.3 (4.1)	9.1 (3.5)	4.15	<.03[b]
WMS VR Imm.[c]	7.7 (3.5)	9.3 (2.6)	6.8 (2.2)	9.6 (2.7)	6.4 (3.3)	9.9 (2.4)	25.84	<.001[d]
Stroop W (T)[e]	41.9 (6.1)	44.2 (7.8)	44.6 (11.6)	47.1 (9.7)	40.2 (10.4)	43.0 (6.5)	5.35	<.03[d]
Pegs DH[f]	11.0 (2.2)	9.8 (3.5)	9.9 (3.6)	9.0 (4.0)	8.9 (4.0)	8.1 (4.5)	4.29	<.05[d]
Trails B (T)	41.1 (8.2)	41.2 (10.8)	40.9 (15.7)	39.9 (13.0)	32.8 (8.0)	38.0 (3.4)	1.96	<.14
WMS LM Imm.[g]	19.7 (5.5)	19.5 (4.5)	16.1 (4.7)	16.8 (5.1)	16.8 (8.0)	18.7 (4.5)	.089	ns
WMS LM Del.[h]	15.7 (5.8)	15.1 (5.1)	12.6 (5.7)	12.4 (5.6)	12.8 (9.8)	12.1 (7.1)	.090	ns
Stroop C (T)[i]	42.2 (6.6)	42.8 (7.6)	40.5 (7.1)	43.3 (7.6)	42.0 (10.3)	43.4 (9.9)	.242	ns
Stroop CW (T)[j]	40.3 (10.0)	42.9 (9.8)	40.4 (9.3)	45.5 (5.8)	42.9 (11.5)	44.4 (8.9)	.334	ns
Stroop I (T)[k]	46.5 (8.1)	49.2 (7.9)	51.1 (3.4)	49.4 (7.7)	51.4 (9.3)	49.9 (6.1)	.508	ns
Pegs NDH[l]	9.5 (3.0)	9.5 (2.5)	8.9 (2.6)	8.5 (2.0)	8.0 (4.7)	7.1 (3.3)	.685	ns
Pegs B[m]	8.2 (2.5)	7.8 (2.8)	6.9 (2.2)	6.5 (2.4)	6.7 (3.0)	5.8 (3.4)	.097	ns
BDI[n]	6.3 (4.5)	9.0 (6.7)	8.2 (5.7)	11.2 (10.1)	9.6 (6.4)	8.6 (5.2)		ns

[a] Wechsler Memory Scale Visual Reproduction. [b] Interaction effect. [c] Wechsler Memory Scale Visual Reproduction Immediate. [d] Main effect over time. [e] Stroop-Word. [f] Pegs Dominant Hand. [g] Wechsler Memory Scale Logical memory Immediate. [h] Wechsler Memory Scale Logical Memory Delayed. [i] Stroop Color. [j] Stroop Color-Word. [k] Stroop Interference. [l] Pegs Nondominant Hand. [m] Pegs Both. [n] Beck Depression Inventory. (T) = T score; mean of 50, SD of 10. (B) = both hands.

remained significant (F = 4.25 [2,26] $P < .03$), indicating that motoric performance did not account for the improvement. Further, no relationship was found between BDI and Visual Reproduction–Delayed Recall ($r = -.27$), indicating that self-ratings of depression did not account for the changes in test performance. Moreover, BDI score did not relate to any of the other neuropsychological measures examined.

Trails B is a measure of visual scanning speed, motor speed, and simultaneous attention. Subjects in the low-dose and placebo groups showed, on average, unchanged performance over time on Trails B, whereas those in the high-dose drug group improved, although the difference was not significant ($P < .14$). The difference between groups again argues against a practice effect as an explanation for these results. Study of a larger sample (thereby increasing statistical power) or of a longer treatment interval should determine whether Trails B can provide a valid measure of improving cognitive performance in patients with MS.

IFNs reduce the number of active lesions and the total MRI lesion load. Prior to beginning the drug trial, the high-dose group demonstrated a greater total lesion area on MRI than the other two groups, but over time the situation reversed. High-dose IFN β-1b prevented further accu-

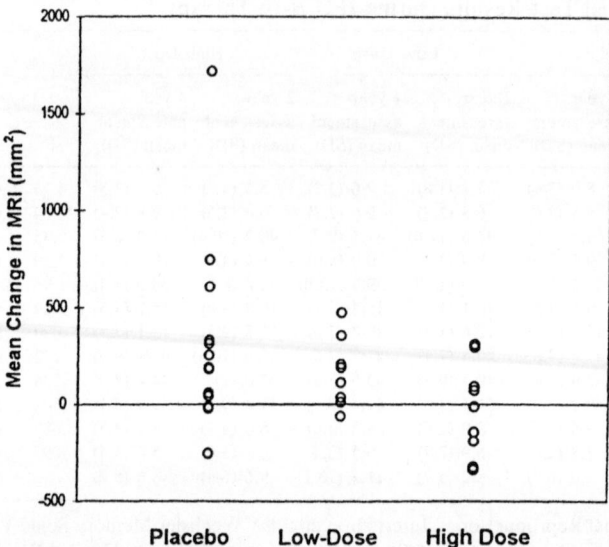

Figure 2 Change in mean MRI lesion area over 4 years of IFN β-1b therapy.

mulation of MRI disease burden accumulation, whereas burden increased in the placebo (by 36%) and the low-dose groups (28%; Fig. 2).

ANCOVA was performed to determine if neuropsychological performance changes remained after changes in MRI were factored out. MRI change scores served as covariates for all groups. Controlling for MRI changes, the Visual Reproduction–Delayed Recall finding remained significant (F = 3.34 [2,25] P < .05), indicating that the cognitive benefit was not simply from a decrease in lesions seen on MRI. The effects for Visual Reproduction–Immediate Recall (F = 24.01 [1,25] P <.001) and Stroop Word-Reading (F = 10.96 [1,25] P < .003) also remained significant, confirming the likelihood of improved performance from practice effects. In contrast, changes in Pegboard DH performance lost significance, suggesting there is a relationship between dominant hand speed/dexterity and MRI-measured disease burden.

Results suggest that treatment with high-dose IFN β-1b improves delayed visual memory performance. Practice effects cannot explain the improvement, nor can changes in motor performance or level of depression account for it. Lesion burden was greater in the placebo group than in the high-dose IFN β-1b–treated group 4 years into the trial, but improved delayed visual memory remained significant in the high-dose–treated group even when changes in lesion area on MRI were factored out. Although the lack of a baseline neuropsychological measurement and the small sample size are important confounds in this study, the results are promising.

How and why IFN β-1b reduces MS attack frequency is not known, and the same holds for cognitive improvement. One possibility might be a direct effect of IFN β-1b on neuronal function, but this seems unlikely given the failure to find IFN β-1b in the circulation following its subcutaneous administration and the limited permeability of the normal blood-brain barrier to IFNs (see p. 155). Since improved cognition was observed late, it is possible that improved visual memory reflects delayed immune system or structural changes (see below, this page). Measures of cognition in MS patients correlate, but not robustly, with disease burden (54,55,56,57) on MRI, a measure of prior activity. Cognitive dysfunction in MS may relate to current inflammatory activity as much as to the effects of prior activity. IFN β-1b decreases new inflammation in the CNS drastically as measured by serial MRI scans at 6-week intervals (58). CNS-invading inflammatory cells release cytokines, and cytokines affect neuronal function, sometimes adversely (59). It is possible that the effect of IFN β-1b on cognition relates to its anti-inflammatory properties. With decreased inflammation, intra-CNS cytokine release might be expected to fall, and this would favorably affect cognition.

2. Is There a Selective Effect of IFN β-1b on Visual Memory?

Improved delayed visual memory as a consequence of treatment with IFN β-1b is intuitively surprising. The WMS Visual Reproduction subtest is a novel task which can be dually (i.e., visual and verbal) encoded but with little reliance on overlearned skills. Hence, this novel encoding task may be quite sensitive to changes in brain function. Indeed, changes in visual memory performance have long-term prognostic significance over as many as 16–22 years for development of dementia (60). Although some investigators have suggested that WMS Form II Visual Reproduction (administered by us during the second assessment) is easier than Form I Visual Reproduction (61,62), this would not explain why improvement was seen over time in the high-dose IFN β-1b group alone. We suggest that the WMS Visual Reproduction subtest should be considered for inclusion in future treatment studies of MS populations.

Could there be a selective effect of IFN β-1b on visual systems? The neuroanatomy of MS lesions offers one suggestion. Demyelinating lesions in MS are scattered throughout the white and gray matter. However, MS plaques have a predilection for periventricular areas of the brain. The median longitudinal fasciculus (MLF) courses next to the aqueduct of Sylvius, which connects the third and fourth ventricles. Lesions of the

MLF cause internuclear ophthalmoplegia, one of the most characteristic and common signs of MS.

The visual radiations are also periventricular along much of their length. After they leave the lateral geniculate nucleus, they pass around the lateral ventricles (temporal and occipital horns) on their way to the visual cortex. From there, visual input leaves the striate cortex and must again pass along the ventricles on the way to memory areas of the medial temporal lobes, as well as to frontal eye fields and oculomotor nuclei of the brainstem. Thus, visual pathways pass the ventricle twice before they are encoded into visual memory. In a related phenomenon, lesions in the corpus callosum are associated with impaired visual-spatial ability (62a). The large number of fibers coursing over an extensive area of brain, however, is likely to prevent devastating lesions from single MS plaques. We hypothesize this extensive periventricular course is often damaged by MS plaques, and that IFN-β therapy causes improvement by reducing plaque size and plaque inflammation.

3. Does IFN-β Directly Enhance Learning and Cognition in MS?

IFN β-1b reduces active MS plaques by 80% (see Chapter 15) and therefore must block CNS inflammation. Many inflammatory cytokines (e.g., interleukins [IL-1, IL-6], IFN-γ, and tumor necrosis factor [TNF]) cause lethargy, fever, or interfere with cognition. IFN could subdue the anticognitive consequences of inflammation. (This assumes that any adverse effects of IFN-β itself have subsided.) Second, IFN-β, or cytokines it induces such as leukemia inhibitory factor (LIF), could promote remyelination and repair (see Chapter 7). Finally, IFN-β alters neuronal function and may be directly involved in learning and conditioning.

4. IFN and Conditioning

Could IFN-β be involved in learning? IFN-β does appear to enhance conditioning. Classical conditioning is a model of learning and memory. To most people, conditioning implies overt behavioral responses. For example, a dog drools when a bell rings (the conditioned stimulus [CS]) after the bell has been paired with an unconditioned stimulus (UCS) that induces salivation (Pavlovian conditioning). Other models condition eye blinking and taste aversion. Conditioning, however, can also affect less obvious internal events such as immune responses [antibody production, graft rejection, DTH, and natural killer (NK) cell function] (63). Potential problems with the latter paradigms are (1) a direct effect of IFN on immunocyte function; (2) indirect IFN effects though demargination, leukocyte homing, or leukopenia; and (3) "compensatory conditioning," where tolerance to a drug develops so that the CS, when presented before the drug, actually enhances tolerance (64).

Polyinosinic:polycytidylic acid (pIC), a form of double-stranded RNA which mimics a viral infection, induces secretion of IFN-α (80% of total) and IFN-β (20%), which in turn enhance NK function. If pIC (the UCS) is paired with the odor of camphor (the CS), the two become linked immunologically. Later, camphor odor alone is able to augment NK activity (65). Purified murine IFN-β (10,000 U), but not IFN-α, can replace pIC as the CS. Is this truly conditioning? A CNS component (i.e., conditioning) is likely because (1) injection of small quantities of IFN-β (10–100 U; note, 1000 U causes death) into the cisterna magna also boosts NK function and augments the effect of pIC; (2) these low doses of IFN-β have no effect given intravenously or subcutaneously; (3) infusion of low dose IFN-β, into the cisterna magna, paired with camphor, also leads to a conditioned response; (4) IFN-β does not leak out of the cisterna magna into the periphery; and (5) rabbit anti–IFN-a/β injected into the cisterna magna prevents conditioning by pIC/camphor (66). Thus, in mice, IFN-β (and not IFN-α) is a CNS mediator of memory.

Olfactory conditioning of immune memory, which requires IFN-β, is only one of many types of learning. Memory traces are laid down in various parts of the brain, including the medial temporal lobe (declarative/explicit memory of events and facts; formation of memory), the striatum (skills, habits), neocortex (priming—enhanced identification of recent events; permanent memory storage), and amygdala and cerebellum (simple classic conditioning) (68). Is IFN-β involved here also?

This model is, in many ways, far removed from IFN-β–induced cognitive improvements in MS. However, low levels of IFN-β may penetrate the CNS through circumventricular organs and through the inflamed MS blood-brain barrier (see Chapters 3 and 14). Central neuronal pathways are necessary to generate the IFN-β/camphor–conditioned response; that is, association of CS and UCS. IFN-β is a signal to central pathways and may be the UCS (67). Depletion of central catecholamines blocks the CS/UCS association. In addition, monosodium glutamate, which destroys the arcuate nucleus in neonatal rats, prevents the association phase of conditioning. This suggests that CNS adrenocorticotropin (ACTH) or β-endorphin pathways (non-HPA) are also involved in conditioning and may interact with IFN-β.

Thus, IFN-β potentially improves the neuropsychological function in MS through multiple pathways. Possible mechanisms include direct actions on neurons involved in learning, or indirect effects such as reduction of inflammatory cytokines or induction of remyelination.

IV. SUMMARY

With several exceptions, most studies using natural interferon preparations have documented significant adverse effects on verbal memory, concentration, mental speed, psychomotor speed, cognitive flexibility, visuo-spatial processing, constructional praxis, speech, reading, writing, calculation, orientation, and general intellectual functioning. A second group of studies report declines in circumscribed areas of cognitive functioning in the context of otherwise stable intellectual functioning. Some investigators describe a frontal-subcortical pattern of deficits. In general, these declines have been dose related and largely transient, although this was not true in all cases. Natural IFN preparations contain protein contaminants and other cytokines which likely contribute to neurocognitive dysfunction. Recombinant IFNs have been developed that minimize cognitive side effects, and recent studies into the cognitive effects of recombinant IFN-β are quite encouraging and reflect possible therapeutic benefit. Neuropsychological assessment is proving to be an important outcome measure in IFN research.

REFERENCES

1. Isaacs A, Lindenmann, J. Virus interference I. The interferon. Proc R Soc Lond (Biol) 1957; 147:258–273.
2. The IFNB Multiple Sclerosis Study Group. Interferon-beta-1b is effective in relapsing-remitting multiple sclerosis. I. Clinical results of a multicenter, randomized, double-blind, placebo-controlled trial. Neurology 1993; 43: 655–661.
3. Paty DW, Li DK, the UBC MS/MRI Study Group, and the IFNB Multiple Sclerosis Study Group. Interferon beta-1b is effective in relapsing-remitting multiple sclerosis. II. MRI analysis results of a multicenter, randomized, double-blind, placebo-controlled trial. Neurology 1993; 43:662–667.
4. Camenga DL, Johnson KP, Alter M, et al. Systemic recombinant α-2 interferon therapy in relapsing multiple sclerosis. Arch Neurol 1986; 43: 1239–1246.
5. AUSTIMS Research Group. Interferon-α and transfer factor in the treatment of multiple sclerosis: a double-blind, placebo-controlled trial. J Neurol Neurosurg Psychiatry 1989; 52:566–574.
6. Knobler RL, Panitch SL, Braheny JC, et al. Systemic alpha-interferon therapy of multiple sclerosis. Neurology 1984; 34:1273–1279.
7. Ruutiainen J, Panelius M, Cantell K. Toxic effects of interferon administered intrathecally. Br Med J 1983; 286:940.
8. Durelli L, Bongioanni MR, Cavallo R, et al. Chronic systemic high-dose recombinant interferon alfa-2a reduces exacerbation rate, MRI signs of disease activity, and lymphocyte interferon gamma production in relapsing-remitting multiple sclerosis. Neurology 1994; 44:406–413.
9. Kastrukoff LF, Oger JJ, Hashimoto SA, et al. Systemic lymphoblastoid interferon therapy in chronic progressive multiple sclerosis. I. Clinical and MRI evaluation. Neurology 1990; 40:479–486.

10. Panitch HS, Hirsch RL, Haley AS, et al. Exacerbations of multiple sclerosis in patients treated with gamma interferon. Lancet 1987; 1:893–895.

11. Panitch HS, Hirsch Schindler J, et al. Treatment of multiple sclerosis with gamma interferon: exacerbations associated with activation of the immune system. Neurology. 1987; 37:1097–1102.

12. Adams F, Queseda JR, Gutterman JU. Neuropsychiatric manifestations of human leukocyte interferon therapy in patients with cancer. JAMA 1984; 252:938–941.

13. Cohen MC, Huberman MS, Nesto RW. Recombinant Alpha$_2$ interferon-related cardiomyopathy. Am J Med 1988; 85:549–551.

14. Gutterman JU, Fine S, Queseda JR, et al. Recombinant leukocyte A interferon: pharmacokinetics, single-dose tolerance and biologic effects in cancer patients. Ann Intern Med 1982; 96:549–556.

15. Laaksonen R, Niiranen A, Iivanainen M, et al. Dementia-like, largely reversible syndrome after cranioirradiation and prolonged interferon treatment. Ann Clin Res 1988; 20:201–203.

16. Mattson K, Niiranen A, Iivanainen M, et al. Neurotoxicity of interferon. Cancer Treat Rep 1983; 67:958–961.

17. Niiranen A, Laaksonen R, Iivanainen M, et al. Behavioral assessment of patients treated with alpha-interferon. Acta Psychiatr Scand 1988; 78: 622–626.

18. Priestman TJ. Initial evaluation of human lymphoblastoid interferon in patients with advanced malignant disease. Lancet 1980; 2:113–118.

19. Queseda JR, Swanson DA, Trindade A, et al. Renal cell carcinoma: Antitumor effects of leukocyte interferon. Cancer Res 1983; 43:940–947.

20. Rohatiner AZ, Prior PF, Burton AC, et al. Central nervous system toxicity of interferon. Br J Cancer 1983; 47:419–422.

21. Sherwin SA, Knost JA, Fein S, et al. A multiple-dose phase I trial of recombinant leukocyte A interferon in cancer patients. JAMA 1982; 248:2461–2466.

22. Smedley H, Katrak M, Sikora K, et al. Neurologic effects of recombinant human interferon. Br Med J 1983; 286:262–264.

23. Talpaz M, Kantarjian HM, McCredie K, et al. Hematologic remission and cytogenetic improvement induced by recombinant human interferon alpha A in chronic myelogenous leukemia. N Engl J Med. 1986; 314:1065–1069.

24. Farkkila M, Iivanainen M, Roine R, et al. Neurotoxic and other side effects of high-dose interferon in amyotrophic lateral sclerosis. Acta Neurol Scand 1984; 69:42–46.

25. Iivanainen M, Laaksonen R, Niemi M-L, et al. Memory and psychomotor impairment following high-dose interferon treatment in amyotrophic lateral sclerosis. Acta Neurol Scand 1985; 72:475–480.

26. Poutiainen E, Hokkanen L, Niemi M-L, et al. Reversible cognitive decline during high-dose α-interferon treatment. Pharmacol Biochem Behav 1994; 47:901–905.

27. Smith RA, Norris F, Palmer D, et al. Distribution of alpha interferon in serum and cerebrospinal fluid after systemic administration. Clin Pharmacol Ther 1985; 37:85–88.

28. Dooley JS, Davis GL, Peters M, et al. Pilot study of recombinant human α-interferon for chronic type B hepatitis. Gastroenterology 1986; 90:150–157.
29. Hoofnagle JH, Peters M, Mullen KD, et al. Randomized controlled trial of a four month course of recombinant human alpha interferon in patients with chronic type B hepatitis 1985; 5:1033.
30. DeWit R, Schattenkerk JK, Boucher CA, et al. Clinical and virological effects of high-dose recombinant interferon-A in disseminated AIDS-related Kaposi's sarcoma. Lancet 1988; 2:1214–1217.
31. Lane HC, Kovacs JA, Feinberg J, et al. Anti-retroviral effects of interferon-A in AIDS-associated Kaposi's sarcoma. Lancet 1988; 2:1218–1222.
32. Maimone D, Grimaldi LM, Incorpora G, et al. Intrathecal interferon in subacute sclerosing panencephalitis. Acta Neurol Scand 1988; 78:161–166.
33. Scott GM, Secher DS, Flowers D, et al. Toxicity of interferon. Br Med J 1981; 282:1345–1348.
34. Oldham RR. Toxic effects of interferon. Science 1983; 219:902.
35. Cooper MR, Fefer A, Thompson J, et al. Alpha-2–interferon/melphalan/prednisone in previously untreated patients with multiple myeloma: a phase I–II trial. Cancer Treat Rep 1986; 70:473–476.
36. Deyton LR, Walker RE, Kovacs JA, et al. Reversible cardiac dysfunction associated with interferon alpha therapy in AIDS patients with Kaposi's sarcoma. New Engl J Med 1989; 321:1246–1249.
37. Dickson D. Deaths halt interferon trials in France. Science 1982; 218:772.
38. Foon KA, Sherwin SA, Abrams PG, et al. Treatment of advanced non-Hodgkin's lymphoma with recombinant leukocyte A interferon. N Engl J Med 1984; 311:1148–1152.
39. Grunberg SM, Kempf RA, Itri LM, et al. Phase II study of recombinant alpha interferon in the treatment of advanced non-small cell lung carcinoma. Cancer Treat Rep 1985; 69:1031–1032.
40. Martino S, Ratanatharathorn V, Karanes C, et al. Reversible arrhythmias observed in patients treated with recombinant alpha2 interferon. J Cancer Res Clin Oncol 1987; 113:376–378.
41. Sarna G, Figlin R, Callaghan M. α (human leukocyte)–Interferon as treatment for non-small cell carcinoma of the lung: a phase II trial. J Biol Response Mod 1983; 2:343–347.
42. Budd GT, Bukowski RM, Miketo L, et al. Phase-I trial of ultrapure human leukocyte interferon in human malignancy. Cancer Chemother Pharmacol 1984; 12:39–42.
43. Meyers CA, Scheibel RS, Forman AD. Persistent neurotoxicity of systemically administered interferon-alpha. Neurology 1991; 41:672–676.
44. McDonald EM, Mann AH, Thomas HC. Interferons as mediators of psychiatric morbidity: an investigation in a trial of recombinant α-interferon in hepatitis B. Lancet 1987; 2:1175–1177.
45. Suter CC, Westmoreland BF, Sharbrough FW, et al. Electroencephalographic abnormalities in interferon encephalopathy: a preliminary report. Mayo Clinic Proc 1984; 59:847–850.
46. Born J, Spath-Schwalbe E, Pietrowsky R, et al. Neurophysiological effects

of recombinant interferon-gamma and -alpha in man. Clin Physiol Biochem 1989; 7:119–127.

47. Cantell K, Mattson K, Niiranen A, et al. Neurotoxicity of interferon. Read before the Third International Congress of Interferon Research, Miami, FL, Nov 1–3, 1982.

48. Rohatiner AZ, Prior PF, Burton AC, et al. Central nervous system toxicity of interferon. Br J Cancer 1983; 47:419–422.

49. Liberati AM, Biagini S, Perticoni G, et al. Electrophysiological and neuropsychological functions in patients treated with interferon-β. J Interferon Res 1990; 10:613–619.

50. Denicoff KD, Rubinow DR, Papa MZ, et al. The neuropsychiatric effects of treatment with interleukin-2 and lymphokine-activated killer cells. Ann Int Med 1987; 107:293–300.

51. Mattson K, Niiranen A, Laaksonen R, Cantell K. Psychometric monitoring of interferon neurotoxicity. Lancet 1984; 1:275–276.

52. Hindmarch, I. Instrumental assessment of psychomotor functions and the effects of psychotropic drugs. Acta Psychiatr Scand 1994; 380(suppl.):49–52.

53. Pliskin NH, Hamer DP, Goldstein DS, Towle VL, Reder AT, Noronha A, Arnason BGW. Improved delayed visual memory function in multiple sclerosis patients receiving interferon beta-1b. Neurology. In press.

54. Rao SM, Leo GJ, Bernardin L, Unverzagt F. Cognitive dysfunction in multiple sclerosis. I. Frequency, patterns, and prediction. Neurology 1991; 41: 685–691.

55. Pozzilli C, Passafiume D, Bernardi S, et al. SPECT, MRI and cognitive dysfunction in multiple sclerosis. J Neurol Neurosurg Psychiatry 1991; 54: 110–115.

56. Rao SM, Leo GJ, Haughton VM, St. Aubin-Faubert P, Bernardi BS. Correlation of magnetic resonance imaging with neuropsychological testing in multiple sclerosis. Neurology 1989; 39; 161–166.

57. Ron MA, Callanan MM, Warrington EK. Cognitive abnormalities in multiple sclerosis: a psychometric and MRI study. Psychol Med 1991; 21:59–68.

58. Stone LA, Frank JA, Albert PS, et al. The effect of interferon-β on blood-brain barrier disruptions demonstrated by contrast-enhanced magnetic resonance imaging in relapsing remitting multiple sclerosis. Ann Neurol 1995; 37:611–619.

59. Arnason BGW, Reder AT. Interferons and multiple sclerosis. Clin Neuropharm 1994; 17:495–547.

60. Zonderman AB, Giambra LM, Arenberg D, Resnick SM, Costa PT Jr. Changes in immediate visual memory predict cognitive impairment. Arch Clin Neuropsychol 1995; 10:111–123.

61. Schultz EE Jr, Keesler TY, Friedenberg L, Sciara AD. Limitations in equivalence of alternate subtests for Russell's Revision of the Wechsler Memory Scale: causes and solutions. J Clin Neuropsychol 1984; 6:220–223.

62. Keesler TY, Schultz EE Jr, Sciara AD, Friedenberg L. Equivalence of alternate subtests for the Russell Revision of the Wechsler Memory Scale. J Clin Neuropsychol 1984; 6:215–219.

62a. Ryan L, Clark CM, Klonoff H, Li D, Paty D. Patterns of cognitive impairment in relapsing-remitting multiple sclerosis and their relationship to neuropathology on magnetic resonance images. Neuropsychology 1996; 10: 176–193.

63. Coussons-Read ME, Dykstra LA, Lysle DT. Pavlovian conditioning of morphine-induced alterations of immune status: evidence of opioid receptor involvement. J Neuroimmunol 1994; 55:135–142.

64. Dyck DG, Driedger SM, Nemeth R, Osachuk TAG. Conditioned tolerance to drug-induced (poly I:C) natural killer cell activation: effects of drug-dosage and context-specificity parameters. Brain Behav Immun 1987; 1:251–266.

65. Solvason HB, Ghanta VK, Hiramoto RN. Conditioned augmentation of natural killer cell activity: independence from nociceptive effects and dependence on interferon-β. J Immunol 1988; 140:661–665.

66. Solvason HB, Ghanta VK, Hiramoto RN. The identity of the unconditioned stimulus to the central nervous system is interferon-β. J Neuroimmunol 1993; 45:75–82.

67. Hiramoto R, Ghanta V, Solvason HB, et al. Identification of specific pathways of communication between the CNS and NK cell system. Life Sci 1993; 53:527–540.

68. Hsueh C, Chen S, Ghanta VK, Hiramoto RN. Expression of the conditioned NK cell activity is β-endorphin dependent. Brain Res 1995; 678:76–82.

7

The Effects of Interferon-β on Cytokines and Immune Responses

Peter Rieckmann

University of Würzburg, Würzburg, Germany

I. INTRODUCTION

Since the initial observations more than 10 years ago that type I interferons (IFNs) have some beneficial effect on the relapse rate in patients with multiple sclerosis (MS) (1), there has been a multifacetted discussion on how these polypeptides might interfere with the immunopathological process underlining the disease (reviewed in ref. 2). This issue is currently being addressed in many editorials and reviews, which comment on the results of two recent multicenter clinical trials in relapsing-remitting MS with recombinant forms of IFN-β, which significantly reduced the relapse rate (3,4).

Although the debate has not come to a definite conclusion about whether the immunomodulatory capacities or the antiviral properties of this cytokine are important for its beneficial effect on the clinical course of MS, there is strong evidence that the former is of major impact. Attenuation of viral infections is a property of both IFN types, but the results of an aborted trial with IFN-γ, which induced an increased relapse rate, argues against a prominent antiviral mode of action (5). On the other hand, it is known that many effects of IFN-γ on the immune system are counteracted by IFN-α or IFN-β. For example, IFN β-1b suppresses the production of IFN-γ in response to antigenic stimulation, antagonizes the immunostimulatory actions of IFN-γ on cells of the immune and nervous system, and enhances the deficient suppressor activity of blood mononuclear cells in MS patients (6).

The major emphasis of this chapter therefore focuses on the effects of the different types of interferons on the immune system with relevance to MS. These effects include (1) the cellular sources of IFNs; (2) regulation of IFN production by cytokines, inflammatory signal molecules, and natural stimuli; (3) IFN control of cell growth and differentiation; (4) IFN effects on expression of major histocompatibility complex (MHC) proteins, adhesion molecules, and activation antigens; (5) effects on immune responses and cytokine production; and (6) IFNs as costimulatory molecules in antigen presentation and immune cell activation.

Most of the data which are presented here are derived from in vitro experiments and can only partly reflect the complex situation of an interactive cytokine network present in vivo. In addition, one has to consider that ongoing immune reactions within the body are compartmentalized, and therefore important local factors are not likely to be present in measurable amounts in the peripheral blood circulation. For example, after the subcutaneous application of 8 million units of IFNβ-1b, this cytokine is not detectable in the blood. Moreover, all IFNs do not cross the blood-brain barrier in significant amounts (7). Therefore, it seems likely that most of the therapeutic IFN effects are indirect and mediated by IFN-induced products released from the injection site.

II. CELLULAR SOURCES OF INTERFERONS AND REGULATION OF PRODUCTION

The members of the IFN type I superfamily represent the classic interferons and consist of IFNα-1 (at least 16 subtypes), IFNα-2, and IFN-β. IFN-α subtypes were designated "leukocyte" IFN and IFN-β subtypes "fibroblast" IFN. The type II IFN, IFN-γ, is also called "immune" IFN. There are different cellular sources for IFNs, but there is some overlap of production of type I IFNs. Many different cell types can produce IFN-α and/or IFN-β. The predominant form of IFN produced by white blood cells (especially monocytes-macrophages and B lymphocytes) is IFN-α, but the proportion of interferon subtypes produced by a cell population can vary depending on cell type and stimulation conditions (Table 1) and (8). In general, IFN-α is the predominant form produced, followed by IFN-β and then IFN-γ (Table 1).

A. Monocytes-Macrophages

Although monocytes are relatively inactive cells in the blood, they can, as participants in inflammatory reactions, rapidly be recruited to sites

Table 1 Immune Cells Involved in the Pathogenesis of MS and Their Cytokines Profile

Immune cell		Major cytokines produced
CD4$^+$ T cells	Th1	IL-2, IFN-γ, LT, TNF-α, GM-CSF
	Th2	IL-4, IL-5, IL-6, IL-10, IL-13, TNF-α, GM-CSF
CD8$^+$ CD28$^-$ T cells (Ts)		IL-4, IL-10, TGF-β, IFN-α/β, IFN-γ
Monocytes/macrophages		IL-1, IL-6, IL-9, IL-10, IL-12, IL-15, TNF-α, TGF-β, IFN-α/β, GM-CSF
B cells		IL-1, IL-4, IL-6, IL-10, IL-12, IL-14, IFN-α, LT, TGF-β, TNF-α
Fibroblasts		IL-15, IFN-β, TGF-β, TNF-α, GM-CSF
NK cells		IFN-γ, IL-1, IL-5, TNF-α

of infection or autoimmune inflammation, where they become important producers of cytokines. Type I IFNs are produced by different cells of the monocyte-macrophage lineage. Viruses and doubled-stranded RNA stimulate interferon production, as well as production of other cytokines (Table 2) (9). In addition, viral envelope glycoproteins can induce IFN in monocytes (10). Treatment of cultured human macrophages with recombinant gp120 of the human immunodeficiency virus type 1 (HIV-1) results in the upregulation of IFN-β mRNA production and an increased antiviral

Table 2 Induction of IFN-β Production in Human Cells

Physiological stimuli	In vitro induction
Free nucleic acid	Nucleic acid
Double-stranded (ds) RNA	LPS (gram-negative bacteria)
Whole virus (e.g., subcutaneous application)	Measles virus
Viral envelope proteins (e.g., HIV-1 gp120)	Newcastle virus (NCDV)
Protozoa	Herpes simplex virus (HSV)
Mycoplasmas	Sendai virus (SV)
Mycobacteria	Double-stranded RNA
Gram-negative bacteria	Poly I:C
IFN-β (autocrine/paracrine)	Vitamin D3
TNF-α	
M-CSF	
IL-1	
IL-2	
IFN-γ	

state to vesicular stomatitis virus (11). In addition, when 7-day cultured macrophages are infected with HIV-1 (strain Ba-L) in the presence of an antibody to IFN-β, a significant increase in HIV-1 p24 release is detected, suggesting an inhibitory effect of this cytokine on HIV-1 production. Finally, protozoa, mycoplasmas, mycobacteria (12), and lipopolysaccharide (LPS) from gram-negative bacteria are also potent inducers of IFN-α/β in monocytes-macrophages (13). In murine peritoneal and human differentiated macrophages, LPS induces the secretion of predominantly IFN-β in amounts almost comparable to those induced by infection with Newcastle disease virus, which is a potent laboratory virus strain commonly used in IFN research (14). This effect is dependent on the availability of protein kinase C, as staurosporine inhibits the accumulation of IFN-β mRNA.

Several growth factors and cytokines promote interferon production in monocytes. There is evidence that interleukins (ILs) IL-1, IL-2, and tumor necrosis factor-α (TNF-α) stimulate IFN-β release from activated human macrophages (15), and that IFN-γ is an important mediator of IFN-α/β production in murine splenic macrophages (16). IFN-β itself is an autocrine-paracrine factor in the induction of macrophage cytocidal activation. The antiviral activity of inflammatory macrophages induced by polyinosinic polycytidylic acid (poly I:C) is dependent on autocrine IFN-β production (17). Exposure of unprimed mouse bone marrow macrophages to a triggering concentration of poly I:C alone fails to induce IFN-β expression (18). However, when macrophages are first primed with IFN-β, poly I:C dramatically increases the expression of IFN-β mRNA. This "priming" effect of IFNs for monocyte activation may have important implications for their biological activity in immune responses involved in autoimmunity. For example, MS patients treated with IFN-β may be less prone to propagating viral infections. On the other hand, priming of monocytes could lead to increased inducible cytokine production by monocytes, which may explain some of the side effects during IFN-β treatment, such as fever, flu-like syndromes, and temporary worsening of neurological symptoms.

Type I interferons regulate differentiation and function of monocytes-macrophages in a complex interaction with other cytokines. For example, the TNF-α–induced cytocidal activity of HEp-2 cells (19) and the differentiating effect of TNF-α on the mouse myeloid leukemic cell line M1 (20) are largely dependent on autocrine-paracrine IFN-β production. Endogenous type I IFNs are also involved in the hydroxyvitamin D_3-induced differentiation of the human promonocytic cell line U937 (21). Regarding function, antiproliferative activity of splenic macrophages, which play a key role in the regulation of chronic pertubations of the hematopoietic system (e.g., in cancer, graft versus host disease, and chronic viral infections) is mediated by autocrine IFN-β production (22). Type I IFNs also regulate synthesis of monocytes products. Nitric oxide production in mouse peritoneal macrophages is inhibited by a monoclonal antibody specific for IFN-β (23). Macrophage colony-stimulating factor (M-CSF) stimulates the release of both IFN-α and IFN-β from murine bone marrow macrophages (24). Moreover, IL-3 and granulocyte-macrophage colony-stimulating factor (GM-CSF) are potent inducers of IFN-α in human blood monocytes (25).

Little is known about the differential regulation of IFN-α and IFN-β production in monocytes. There are experimental data that poly I:C induces more IFN-β than IFN-α (26). Different patterns of mRNA expression for IFN-α and IFN-β were also observed in human monocytes after stimulation with Herpes simplex virus (HSV) or Sendai virus (SV) (27). SV-induced IFN-α production is inhibited by cycloheximide, whereas IFN-β transcription does not require de novo synthesis of intracellular protein(s) (28). There is also a dramatic drop in IFN-α secretion by HIV-infected monocytes, yet IFN-β secretion in response to multiple stimuli remains intact (29). This suggests that there is a stimulus-specific control of IFN-α and IFN-β production in monocytes.

B. T Lymphocytes

In contrast to type I interferons, which can be produced in limited amounts by most cells, IFN-γ production is restricted to activated T cells and natural killer (NK) cells. Among the different types of T lymphocytes, the CD4$^+$ Th1 phenotype and CD8$^+$CD28$^-$ T cells are the major IFN-γ producers. CD8$^+$CD28$^-$ T suppressor cells also produce significant amounts of type I interferons. From long-term clones of murine T cells, the concept of functionally different CD4$^+$ T cells has been established (30). Such clones tend to produce either IFN-γ, IL-2, LT, and low amounts of TNF-α (Th1 type) or IL-4, IL-5, IL-6, IL-10, and IL-13 (Th2 type). However, these subsets also produce a common set of cytokines, including IL-3 and GM-CSF. Th1 clones, particularly through their ability to produce IFN-γ and LT, are well suited to induce enhanced microbicidal activity in macrophages (through enhanced cellular immunity and delayed-type hypersensitivity), whereas the Th2 clone products mediate B-cell help for the development of antibody-producing cells (31).

The molecular process that leads to the development of these T-cell subsets remains undefined. However, it is generally believed that evolution of a particular subset of antigen-specific T cells depends on the nature of the antigen-presenting cell, the presence of specific accessory (costimulatory) molecules, and cytokines. The differentiation of CD4$^+$ T cells is mutually regulated by IL-12 and IFN-γ (which induce the Th1 type) and IL-4 (which induces the Th2 type) in conjunction with IL-2. Activated macrophages are the main producers of IL-12. Treatment of BALB/c mice with IL-12 significantly enhances IFN-γ production by T cells (32). IFN-γ in turn causes the differentiation of Th1 cells and inhibits the generation of Th2 cells. This priming effect of IL-12 for IFN-γ production occurs during antigen presentation to the T cell. This paracrine pathway was recently described as the "immunological synapse", because it takes place at an intimate contact between the two cells (31). Of interest, mononuclear blood cells from MS patients spontaneously secrete excessive levels of IL-12, causing high levels of IFN-γ in vitro (33).

Until recently, there was no consensus as to whether CD4$^+$ T-cell subsets represented distinct cellular populations or a cellular continuum, or whether subset phenotypes were stable (a result of cell differentiation) or transient (a result of cellular activation). Although the concept of two functionally different CD4$^+$ T-cell types is derived from experimental work with long-term murine T-cell clones, there is considerable evidence that this distinction is also important in the pathogenesis of certain microbial diseases in humans (34,35) and in autoimmune phenomenona, such as insulin-dependent diabetes mellitus (36), experimental allergic encephalomyelitis (37,38), or MS (39,40).

The immunomodulatory effect of IFN-γ, particularly its role as a cytokine response modifier, has been well established. In contrast, type I IFNs act predominantly as antiviral and antiproliferative cytokines. Yet type I IFNs also have important immune effects, which usually antagonize IFN-γ.

In general, IFN-γ is induced by treatments which lead to lymphocyte activation. The physiological stimulus for T-cell activation is antigen, presented by an antigen-presenting cell in association with MHC molecules to the antigen-specific T-cell receptor/CD3 complex on T cells. Organ-specific antigens, which may be relevant in the pathogenesis of MS (i.e., myelin basic protein and proteolipid protein) or of myasthenia gravis (acetylcholine receptor) can induce IFN-γ production in peripheral blood mononuclear cells (PBMCs) from patients (41,42). Under experimental conditions, antigen is often replaced with nonspecific T-cell activators; for example, the mitogens concavalin A (ConA) or phytohemagglutinin (PHA). Increased IFN-γ production is observed in PHA-stimulated T-cell clones derived from the cerebrospinal fluid (CSF) of patients with MS (43). Pharmacological stimuli, like phorbol myristate and calcium ionophore, are also potent inducers (44). IFN-γ is usually induced together with IL-2 (45). T-cell–derived IL-2 and monocyte-derived IL-1, hydrogen peroxide (46), nitric oxide (47), and leukotrienes (LTB4, LTC4, and

LTD4) (48) all exert a positive regulatory influence on the generation of IFN-γ (49). These feedback loops contribute to the high levels of IFN-γ production observed after T-cell activation.

Stimulation of T cells results in the induction of IFN-γ mRNA. This is first detectable by 6–8 hr, peaks by 12–24 hr, and declines thereafter. Protein secretion occurs immediately after synthesis. It can be detected in cell culture supernatants 8–12 hr after stimulation and reaches peak levels after 18–24 hr. In contrast, IFN-γ is rarely seen in the circulation after immunological stimulation. This apparent discrepancy between in vitro and in vivo levels of fluid phase IFN-γ (a phenomenon which is also present with many other cytokines) is most likely due to the rapid removal of this cytokine from the circulation by IFN-γ receptors that are abundantly expressed on most cells in the body (see chapters on interferon receptors and signal transduction [Chapters 1 and 2] and reviews in refs. 50 and 51).

IFN-γ production by mitogen-activated T cells is decreased by pretreatment with IFN-β, which may be of importance for the therapeutic effect of this cytokine in MS (52). On the other hand, IFN-α increases the frequency of IFN-γ–producing CD4$^+$ T cells (53), which might indicate some dissociation of type I IFN effects on T-cell activation. In addition, viral infection of T cells stimulates IFN production. For example, the tat protein of HIV-1 transactivates the IFN-α2 gene in transfected T cells (54), and blood mononuclear cells can be induced to secrete IFN-α if cocultivated with HIV-infected monocytes (55). Interestingly, there is evidence that antiretroviral nucleoside analogues exert potent immunomodulatory activity and directly induce IFNs in T cells from uninfected mice (56). Virus-induced type I IFNs could potentially regulate secretion of IFN-γ and other cytokines.

C. Natural Killer Cells

Natural killer (NK) cells probably function as an early defense line against viruses, because they are able to kill virus-infected cells without resorting to clonal proliferation of memory cells, as required with cytotoxic T lymphocytes (CTLs). NK cells are also capable of directly killing tumor cells. In both cases, their activity is MHC unrestricted, preventing escape by viruses and tumor cells which have downregulated MHC class I molecules. NK cells can be activated by various stimuli (e.g., viruses, bacterial products, poly I:C, and mitogens) to secrete IFN-γ. For example, stimulation of CD16$^+$ NK cells with *Staphylococcus aureus* causes significant production of IFN-γ, which is further enhanced by IFN-α. This response could not be observed in T cells (57). In CB-17 SCID mice, which completely lack T and B cells, NK cells are the major source for IFN-γ production after infection with *Listeria monocytogenes* (58). Other cytokines, like IL-1, IL-6, IL-12, and TNF-α, are potent inducers of IFN activity in NK cells (summarized in ref. 59). Thus, the IFN-γ produced by NK cells may represent the host's first-line defense against microbial pathogens that are susceptible to killing by activated macrophages. Both direct cytocidal effects of NK cells and the NK-mediated priming of macrophages are involved in this defense.

In addition to the above-mentioned cell types, there have been reports that the predominant IFN-α–producing cell in the blood induced by HSV-1 (60) is a low-density, nonphagocytic, HLA-DR+ cell which lacks most of the typical surface markers for T and B cells, monocytes, or NK cells and is highly enriched in the dendritic cell population. These cells produce IFN-α rapidly after viral induction, do not require prior sensitization, and do not exhibit immunological memory. Like NK cells, they are therefore a component of natural or innate immunity (61). The physiological importance of these cells is supported by observations in patients with HIV-1 infection showing that deficient IFN-α production in response to HSV-1 is associated with poor prognosis and progression to opportunistic infections (62). Although there are no data on the frequency of these cells in patients with MS, it can be hypothesized that they, together with NK cells, play a role in the immunoregulatory events associated with the increased relapse rates after common viral upper respiratory infections (63,64).

D. B Lymphocytes

There are several reports describing the production of IFN-α by B cells on appropriate stimulation (65–67). However, the purity of the cell preparations was not always absolute and small amounts of contaminating cells (e.g., monocytes) may have contributed to the IFN levels measured in the supernatants of activated B-cell cultures. In more convincing experiment, polyclonal stimulation of purified B cells with *Staphylococcus aureus* Cowan strain-1 (SAC) and IL-2, as well as anti-IgM treatment, induces IFN-α transcription and release after 12–24 hr (68). In addition, some human B-cell tumor lines are capable of producing low amounts of IFN-α constitutively, which is further enhanced by treatment with virus (e.g., Sendai virus) (69) or stimulation with HIV gp120 (our unpublished observation).

E. Fibroblasts

The heterogeneity of type I IFNs led to attempts to define their source of production and their designation as α ("leukocyte") and β ("fibroblast")

IFNs. Fibroblasts and other nonhematopoietic cells often produce IFN-β as the only or predominant type of IFN (8). As in other cell types, viruses, and their constituents, especially double-stranded RNAs, are potent inducers of IFN-β in fibroblasts. For example, human dermal fibroblasts regulate nonspecific host defenses against viruses, and their antiviral activity is mediated by cytokine-activated IFN-β release (70). Infection of diploid fibroblasts with several laboratory viral strains, as well as with measles or rubella virus, concomitantly induces production of IFN-β, GM-CSF, and IL-6 (71). Bacterial infection is similarly effective in stimulating IFN production by fibroblasts. The virus-induced production of IFN-β by fibroblasts has been linked to the activation of NF-κB, a nuclear factor involved in the transcriptional control of many cytokines (72).

Recently, type I IFNs were detected in human trophoblasts of first-trimester placental explants. These IFNs were induced by treatment with ConA and also IL-2, which is probably one of the physiological stimuli for IFN-τ secretion (73,74). The role of trophoblast IFNs (IFN-τ) during pregnancy and their role in the control of the immunological silencing against the fetus and possible effects on MS exacerbations during pregnancy remains to be elucidated (see Chapter 17).

There are other cell types which can contribute to the pool of circulating type I IFNs (e.g., endothelial cells and epithelial cells), but as far as in situ and in vitro stimulation studies are concerned, they produce only limited amounts of these cytokines. (For detailed information about this issue, see ref. 13.)

As immune responses are controlled by various genes (e.g., the HLA locus on chromosome 6), there is an ongoing discussion and intensive research as to whether mutations in immune-response genes determine the susceptibility of individuals to certain autoimmune diseases. For example, the TNF2 allele in conjunction with HLA-DR3 is associated with insulin-dependent diabetes mellitus (75). PBMCs from HLA-DR2$^+$ MS patients (this MHC allele is overrepresented in the MS population) produce less IFN-α in response to certain viruses (76), but others have found normal values (77). To date, there are no conclusive data on a genetic predisposition to produce IFNs in response to antigenic stimulation.

III. BIOLOGICAL ACTIVITIES OF INTERFERONS

The overall mechanism of action of IFN-β in MS has not been fully elucidated. However, the binding of IFN-β to receptors present on most human cells induces the production of a variety of well-characterized products that can be measured in vivo and in vitro (e.g., increased serum levels of soluble IL-2 receptor, β_2-microglobulin, neopterin, and increased cellular 2′,5′-oligoadenylate synthetase). Changes in these proteins can be observed after subcutaneous application of 8 MIU IFN β-1b at 24–48 hours (see Chapter 3). Intramuscular injection of IFN β-1a increases neopterin levels for more than five days (J. Alam, personal communication, 1995). Although the functional pathways of these and other interferon-induced products are not fully understood, it is believed that they are the key mediators of the antiproliferative, antiviral, and immunomodulatory effects of IFN-β. With respect to the rationale of IFN-β as a treatment for relapsing-remitting MS, there are probably other factors which are important for the reduction of the inflammatory disease activity. Initial data from our group demonstrated that in MS patients receiving s.c. IFN-β, mRNA for TGF-β, IL-4, and IL-10 is induced in blood mononuclear cells (our unpublished observation).

A. Regulation of Cell Growth and Differentiation

High levels of circulating IFNs can be induced after viral infection or immune stimulation, but there is still uncertainty about the physiological significance of low levels of IFN present in localized areas of certain tissues (78). Even at low concentrations, IFN-γ is a potent regulator of differentiation of monocytes-macrophages and B cells. IFNs prolong different phases of the cell cycle. They counteract the effects of certain growth factors (e.g., platelet-derived growth factor [PDGF] or fibroblast growth factor [FGF]) and are therefore viewed as "negative growth factors." These effects on cell growth and differentiation led to the first therapeutic applications of IFNs in certain malignancies of the hematopoeitic system more than a decade ago.

Initial studies revealed that the sensitivity of cells in culture to the antiproliferative effect of IFNs varies greatly. The antiproliferative effects cannot be ascribed to a single event. Type I and type II IFNs reduce protooncogene mRNA expression, especially expression of c-*myc* (79,80). In addition, they downmodulate growth factor receptors on susceptible cells (81) and—especially IFN-γ—increase the expression of the growth-inhibitory cytokine TNF-α (82). These effects can be enhanced by retinoids, and the combined use of both substances is proposed in certain malignancies to alleviate some of the side effects of retinoids and to increase therapeutic effectiveness (83).

In addition to the antiproliferative effects, retinoids exert immunomodulatory and anti-inflammatory functions by reducing IFN-γ–induced TNF-α and nitric oxide production by murine peritoneal macrophages (84). Retinoids are potent inducers of the immunosuppressive cytokine

TGF-β (85), which plays an important role during remission in experimental autoimmune encephalitis (EAE) (86) and MS (87).

B lymphocytes can frequently be detected in brain lesions of MS patients, and oligoclonal IgG present in the CSF is a diagnostic hallmark of this disease (89). IFNs affect human B-cell maturation (88). IFN-γ induces kappa light chain transcription in pre-B cells (90). In general, the influence of IFN-γ on B cells depends on the state of B-cell activation—whether the B cell is committed to isotype switch, or whether other B-cell–activating factors are present. For example, IFN-γ is a potent inhibitor of LPS-induced IgM secretion (91), and it can be a cofactor in the switch of B cells to IgG2$_a$ secretion (92). IFN-γ also acts as a late inhibitor of B-cell differentiation by blocking immunoglobulin secretion and interfering with effective splicing of nuclear μ chain mRNA (93). This inhibitory activity depends on prior B-cell activation (94). Late-stage, activated, immunoglobulin-containing B-cells, and to a lesser degree plasma cells, are an important constituent of the typical CSF cytology in MS patients (95). These findings suggest a major role of IFN-γ in the pathophysiology of MS (96).

The importance of IFN-γ in the in vivo regulation of B cells may be illustrated by situations in which—owing to a depletion of CD4$^+$ T cells—IFN-γ production is reduced. For example, in transplant recipients who receive cyclosporin or anti–T cell antibodies, and in patients with advanced acquired immunodeficiency syndrome (AIDS), there is reduced IFN-γ production and increased polyclonal B-cell activation (35). Therefore, it was hypothesized that IFN-γ is an important homeostatic regulator of polyclonal B-cell responses. Whether polyclonal B-cell activation during immunomodulatory (IFN-γ antagonizing) therapy of MS plays a role in remyelination remains to be elucidated.

These findings indicate that the different in vitro effects of IFNs on cell proliferation and differentiation depend on the local cytokine environment, the cell type, and the state of cellular activation. To determine the in vivo properties of IFNs, it is therefore important to look for changes of these parameters in patients under treatment with IFN. IFN β-1b treatment of patients with relapsing-remitting multiple sclerosis has no effect on intrathecal IgG synthesis or oligoclonal bands in the cerebrospinal fluid (J. B. Peter, personal communication, 1995). This could be due to the low availability of this cytokine to the central nervous system (CNS), because IFN-β does not cross the blood-brain barrier in significant amounts (7).

On the other hand, treatment with IFN-α, as well as IFN-β, can induce high titers of neutralizing antibodies in the circulation, and these immunoglobulins may sometimes affect the clinical response (see Chapters 3, 13, 19, and 20). Particularly, aggregates of unstable interferon preparations are highly immunogenic and can induce neutralizing antibodies (S. Goelz, personal communication, 1995). Also, of interest is the fact that type I IFNs can induce autoantibody production in vivo. In one trial with IFN-α for autoimmune hepatitis, antinuclear antibodies were detected in 33% of patients, whereas anti–smooth muscle antibodies occurred in 65%, and anti–parietal cell antibodies in 10% (97). These undesired autoimmune responses should be taken into consideration when a patient on IFN develops treatment failure or otherwise unexplained organ dysfunctions.

B. Effects on Other Cytokines and on Immune Functions

IFNs are potent immunomodulators, and with impact to MS, modulate different steps of T-cell–mediated autoimmune reactions. IFN-γ and IFN-β have sometimes opposite effects on repair mechanisms, T-cell activation, lymphocyte migration, inflammatory reactions, and immune suppression (for a review, see ref. 2).

The production of cytotoxic factors for microbicidal and tumoricidal processes as well as tissue damage by macrophages (e.g., from secreted cathepsin B and nitric oxide [NO·]) is regulated by IFNs. IFN-γ is the only cytokine reported to be capable of inducing NO· production by itself (98). IFN-α/β and TNF-α augment LPS-induced NO· production (23). On the other hand, cytokines like TGF-β, IL-4, IL-10, or prostaglandin E2 inhibit inducible NO production in activated macrophages (99,100). These cytokines regulate the activity of inducible NO· synthase (NOS). Recently, inducible NOS was detected in active lesions of MS brains (101) and in rats after the induction of EAE (102). Pretreatment of macrophages with IFN β-1b blocks the induction of cathepsin activity, suggesting that IFN β-1b might block IFN-γ–induced macrophage cytotoxic functions.

During the development of inflammatory and immune responses, IFN-γ is induced together with TNF-α, a cytokine with strong demyelinating properties (103). Once released, each is capable of enhancing the other's production (104), and these cytokines control important steps during the inductive and effector phase of immune responses. IFN-γ induces TNF-α production in macrophages via transcriptional control and increased mRNA stability (105); and it enhances the expression of TNF receptors on a variety of different cell types (82). In addition, mice lacking the IFN-γ receptor produce less TNF-α than normal littermates after challenge with LPS (106). TNF-α and macrophages are important cofactors for IFN-γ production in SCID mice (107). The effects of interferons on macrophages are usually dependent on the availability of other cytokines. IFN-γ can be regarded as a priming factor, augmenting IL-12 effects (107a), and inducing IL-2 receptor expression on monocytes and thereby making them susceptible to the effects of IL-2 (108). These effects of IFN-γ on IL-2 can be counteracted by low concentrations of IFN-α/β. IFN-γ and TNF-α are both important during the development of new lesions in MS patients, as they act synergistically on the activation of lymphocytes, the upregulation of adhesion and MHC molecules, and the recruitment of activated lymphocytes to the CNS (109).

TNF-α is also an important cofactor for IFN-γ production in NK cells (107). In turn, both cytokines synergize with IL-1 and IL-4 to promote the expression of overlapping sets of cell surface molecules on the vascular endothelium that play an important role in the transmigration of leukocytes to the site of inflammation (110). The induction of adhesion molecules on cerebral endothelial cells is a prerequisite for autoreactive T cells to enter the brain (111).

Synthesis of both TNF-α and IFN-γ is suppressed by IL-4 (112), IL-10 (113), IL-13 (114), TGF-β (115), and IFN-β (116), whereas IFN-γ, and to some extent TNF-α, production is stimulated most effectively by IL-2 (117) and IL-12 (118). These important cytokine interactions are reflected by in vivo changes of cytokine mRNA expression in PBMCs from patients with relapsing-remitting MS. Significant increases of TNF-α, lymphotoxin (LT), and to some extent IFN-γ mRNA expression, are observed 4–6 weeks prior to a relapse, whereas TGF-β and IL-10 mRNA expression is reduced at the same time (87).

The effects of IFN-β on cytokine secretion are less clear. IFN-γ–induced secretion of IL-1β, IL-6, and TNF-α in resting human monocytes is not inhibited by IFN-β, whereas the same concentrations of IFN-β inhibit IFN-γ–induced monocyte surface molecule expression (119). Interestingly, IFN-β induces IL-10 and TGF-β, two cytokines with immunosuppressive potential and beneficial effects on the clinical course and histopathological changes in EAE (120). Therefore, regulation of these cytokines is required for a well-tuned cytokine network, favoring a beneficial outcome of inflammatory and immune reactions for the host. For example, endogenously produced IFN-β can regulate T-cell activation. IL-2, TNF-α, and LT induce endogenous IFN-β production by macrophages (121). IFN-β in turn inhibits T-cell proliferation and profoundly suppresses IFN-γ, LT, and TNF-α release in mitogen-activated blood mononuclear cells (52,122,123) but not in resting and IFN-γ–stimulated monocytes (119). Another study demonstrated that IFN β-1b induces IL-10 mRNA in human mononuclear blood cells, which in turn may suppress secretion of inflammatory cytokines and inhibit immune responses in MS (124). Human IFN-α-AD therapy also induces circulating IL-LRa, an immunoinhibitor, in mice (124a).

Results of binding studies suggest that some of the antagonistic effects of IFN-β on the action of IFN-γ may be attributed to the ability of IFN-β to decrease the binding affinity of the IFN-γ receptor, to enhance the internalization and degradation of IFN-γ, and to compete weakly with IFN-γ for binding to its receptor on the surface of cells (50,104). Although different receptors for type I and type II IFNs have been cloned (see Chapter 1), the IFN-α/β and IFN-γ multisubunit receptor complexes have structural homology and are considered to represent a distinct cytokine receptor family. Interestingly, sufficient signal transduction via the IFN-γ receptor requires the activation of two cytoplasmic tyrosine kinases, JAK 1 and JAK 2, whereas IFN-β action is JAK 1 and TYK 2 dependent (see Chapters 1 and 2). Therefore, one may consider these receptors and kinases as possible targets for immunotherapy.

In addition to these in vitro effects, subcutaneous administration of IFN β-1b to normal volunteers induces β_2-microglobulin, HLA-DR, and HLA-DQ expression on blood lymphocytes, enhanced NK cell activity, and increases serum neopterin levels 24 hr postdose (summarized in ref. 125). In addition, IFN β-1b therapy inhibits IFN-γ secretion by PBMCs from MS patients after an initial induction and reduces the ability of PBMCs isolated from these subjects to express mRNA for TNF-α, LT, and IFN-γ (Rieckmann et al., submitted). Higher serum levels of neopterin and β_2-microglobulin are observed in healthy volunteers after intramuscular injection of IFN β-1a compared with subcutaneous application (J. Alam, personal communication, 1995). This suggests that the route of application may have important implications for the immunomodulatory capacities of IFN-β treatment.

Other type I IFNs have related effects. During a pilot trial with systemic high-dose recombinant IFN-α-2a in patients with relapsing-remitting MS, a significant reduction of lymphocyte IFN-γ and TNF-α production was observed (see Chapter 12 and ref. 126), but no effect was seen on TGF-β and IL-4 production (127). Studies are clearly warranted to compare the immunoregulatory capacities of natural fibroblast IFN, recombinant *Escherichia coli*–derived IFN β-1b, and the Chinese hamster ovarian-derived IFN β-1a on immune cells in vitro as well as after subcutaneous or intramuscular application. From these studies, one may hope to obtain information about the relevant biological activity of IFNs responsible for their immunomodulatory effect in MS therapy.

Interestingly, although the major effects of IFN-γ at physiological concentrations are proinflammatory, at high concentrations IFN-γ itself inhibits Th1 cell proliferation and induces monocytes to produce latent TGF-β (128). This negative feedback loop may contribute to the restriction of an inflammatory response. It can be argued that a defect in this regulatory

process is involved in extensive inflammation with consecutive tissue destruction seen in many T-cell–mediated autoimmune diseases. TGF-β_1,
produced by CD8$^+$ T cells, Th2 cells, B cells, endothelial cells, and activated monocytes, downregulates IFN-γ gene expression and markedly
inhibits IFN-γ production by Th1 cells. In addition, TGF-β inhibits DTH
responses, MHC class II molecule expression, and cellular adhesion to
activated endothelium, and it directly inhibits the release of IL-1, TNF,
and hydrogen peroxide from activated macrophages. These dose-dependent and opposite effects of IFN-γ in vitro may explain some of the discrepancies which have indicated that IFN-γ can either be of benefit in
EAE or enhance disease activity (109) (and see Chapter 9). Another cytokine, GM-CSF, stimulates monocyte proliferation, and is inhibited in vitro
by type I and type II IFNs (129). GM-CSF could also provide an efficient
negative feedback signal for inflammatory reactions.

Monocyte-derived chemotactic proteins, so-called chemokines, facilitate the extravasation of leukocytes to inflamed tissues. These proteins
are induced by IFN-γ (strong inducer) and IFN-β (weak inducer), whereas
Th2 cytokines such as IL-4 reduce expression of chemokines (130,131).
These findings may be of functional importance, because chemokines regulate blood-brain barrier function (132). A possible role for chemokines
as mediators of inflammatory cell migration into the CNS has been proposed, but there are no conclusive data on chemokines in MS pathology
(133).

C. Neuroendocrine Effects of Interferons

Immune cell activation is also regulated via the neuroendocrine axis. Several neuropeptides influence immune reactions and can be produced by
cells of the immune system (134). Conversely, proinflammatory cytokines,
like IL-1, IL-6, and TNF-α, are potent inducers of corticotropin-releasing
factor (CRF) from the hypothalamus (135). CRF causes release of adrenocorticotropin (ACTH), which directly inhibits preactivated lymphocytes.
ACTH also elevates cortisol, a potent inhibitor of IL-1 and TNF synthesis
by macrophages and of IL-2, IFN-γ, and LT synthesis by Th1 cells. High
doses of IFNs are known to elevate cortisol levels, but IFN-β concentrations used in clinical MS trials were without effect on circulating cortisol
levels (136).

Developmentally regulated IFN production by trophoblasts suggests a
physiological mechanism for this cytokine (e.g., to prevent a return to
ovarian cyclicity and rejection of the embryo) (137) (see also Chapter
17). As graft rejection is mainly a delayed-type hypersensitivity (DTH)
response, the immunological acceptance of the histocompatibility-mis-

matched fetus is dependent on effective DTH suppression. TGF-β_2, which is secreted by cells of the pregnant uterus, has potent immunosuppressive properties in the amniotic fluid. Both cytokines may play a role in the reduced Th1-type response in pregnant women and in the lowered relapse rate in female MS patients during pregnancy (138). A recent study demonstrated that plasma from pregnant women inhibit the generation of IFN-γ–producing cells in MS (139). To date, however, there are no reports on longitudinal analysis of cytokine expression in MS patients during pregnancy.

D. Regulation of Cell Surface Proteins by Interferons

In addition to their eminent role within the cytokine network, IFNs exert a variety of direct effects on the expression of surface molecules involved in transcellular signaling and cellular communication. The best-characterized molecules known to be regulated by IFNs are the major histocompatibility antigens (MHC). These molecules are expressed on a variety of antigen-presenting cells and are divided into two classes (MHC class I and MHC class II). Processed antigen presented to T cells is associated with MHC molecules. CD4$^+$ T cells recognize their antigen presented by MHC class II molecules, whereas CD8$^+$ T cells see their antigen presented by MHC class I antigens. By different processing pathways, CD4$^+$ and CD8$^+$ T cells can respond to different epitopes present on an antigen (2,140).

All IFNs are able to increase MHC molecule expression, but IFN-γ is the most potent in augmenting MHC class I molecules on different cell types and is usually the only IFN to induce MHC class II expression on lymphoid cells (141). MHC class II molecule density increases on monocytes during relapses of MS. This expression is further augmented by the addition of IFN-γ (142), and this sensitization by IFN-γ may potentiate inflammation and disease progression. There is evidence that type I IFNs in vitro counteract this IFN-γ–induced MHC class II expression on monocytes (143,143a). To complicate matters, under certain culture conditions, both IFN-α and IFN-β are able to upregulate MHC class II molecules on different cell types in the absence of IFN-γ (144). These differences of cytokine activity argue for an environment-dependent regulation of their effects. MHC class II expression on cells of the CNS is an important issue in autoimmune demyelination (145,146), because it allows autoantigen presentation within the brain and further enhances the activation of invading T cells. As can be seen in Table 3, there are other mechanisms besides the regulation of MHC class II molecule expression which may be responsible for the beneficial effects of IFN-β in MS. The opposite effects of IFN-

Table 3 Differential Effects of IFN-β and IFN-γ on Immune Responses Related to MS

Parameter	Effect of IFN-γ	Effect of IFN-β
MHC class I expression	+ + +	+ +
MHC class II expression	+ + +	±
IL-1 production	+ +	?
IL-2 production	+ +	+
IL-2 receptor expression	+ +	− −
IL-4 production	−	?
IL-10 production	− −	±
IL-12 production	+ +	?
TNF-α production	+ +	∓
LT production	+	− −
TGF-β production	+	+
GM-CSF production	+ +	− −
IFN-γ production	+	− −
IFN-β production	+	+ +
PGE$_2$ production	±	−
"Priming" of monocytes	+ + +	+ +
NO· and O$_2$⁻ production	+ +	±
Adhesion molecule expression	+ + +	− −
Recruitment of T cells into CNS	+ +	−
CD14 expression	+ +	−
Activation of macrophages	+ +	±
B-cell differentiation	+	±
T-cell proliferation	+ +	−
CD8 suppressor function	∓	+ +
Cytotoxic T-cell function	+ +	+ +

+ weak; + + moderate; + + + strong induction; − weak; − − moderate; − − − strong inhibition; ? effect unknown.

γ and IFN-β on cytokine production, T-cell activation, adhesion molecule expression, and cellular trafficking suggest that type I IFNs can reverse many of the proinflammatory effects of IFN-γ.

Cellular adhesion molecules are important membrane proteins involved in intercellular communication during immune reactions. During contact between antigen-presenting cells and antigen-specific T cells, these molecules deliver important costimulatory signals for activation (110). In addition, cellular adhesion molecules regulate the traffic of inflammatory cells across the endothelium and are expressed in active plaques of patients with MS (147). Proinflammatory cytokines, like TNF-α, IL-1, and IFN-γ, are released by activated cells and synergize to upregulate adhesion molecules on the endothelial cell surface. Two members of the immuno-globulin superfamily of adhesion molecules, intercellular adhesion mole-cule-1 (ICAM-1) and vascular cell adhesion molecule-1 (VCAM-1), are induced by IFN-γ on monocytes, T cells, endothelial cells, astrocytes, microglia, and oligodendrocytes (116,148,149,150,151). IFNs recruit T cells into lymphoid organs, and this phenomenon may be an explanation for the lymphopenia observed in patients under IFN therapy (152).

Fc receptors, present on lymphocytes and monocytes-macrophages, mediate the opsonizing effects of immunoglobulins, and are regulated by IFNs. A recent study demonstrated that IFN-γ–induced ICAM-1 and Fc receptor expression on accessory cells is inhibited by oligonucleotides which interfere with the IFN-γ–mediated transcriptional signal molecules of both genes (153). IFNs mainly induce the expression of FcγR-I. This receptor binds IgG$_{2a}$, which is activated by IFN-γ via isotype shifting and strongly fixes complement (92), allowing rapid lysis of target cells.

CD28 is another important molecule in T-cell activation. It provides a potent costimulatory signal for cytokine production to the cells after bind-ing to its ligand B7. IFN-γ is a potent inducer of B7 and ICAM-1 on human monocytes; this expression is inhibited by the addition of IL-10 (154). In general, the effects of IFN-γ on costimulatory molecule and Fc receptor expression enhance immune responses.

The role of IFN-β the regulation of adhesion and costimulatory mole-cule expression has not been extensively studies. Our own data indicate that IFN β-1b reduces lectin-stimulated expression of ICAM-1 on mono-nuclear blood from normal donors and patients with MS (our unpublished observation). Others have demonstrated that IFN-β inhibits the IFN-γ–in-duced expression of VLA-4, an adhesion protein (143a), and the ligand for CD2. LFA-3 is present on freshly isolated normal human monocytes and is important in costimulation of antigen-specific T cells during antigen presentation (155). Another direct effect of IFN-β is the reduction of CD14 expression on monocytes (155). This molecule is involved in macrophage-monocyte activation and LPS-induced TNF release. Overall, IFN-β dow-nmodulates costimulatory molecule expression and thereby reduces im-mune responses.

Furthermore, on human T cells, IFN-β-1a inhibits surface expression of IL-2 and transferrin receptors and the protein CD2 (156), but type I interferons may increase the adhesion function of CD2 (2). These altera-tions result in an overall antiproliferative effect of IFN-β on CD4$^+$ T cells, and they affect both Th1 and Th2 functions. In contrast, CD8$^+$ cytotoxic T cells, which coexpress the CD28 antigen on their surface, are positively regulated by all IFNs. MHC class I is upregulated on cytotoxic T cells cultivated in the presence of interferons and cytolytic function is en-hanced.

Another CD8$^+$ subtype lacks CD28 expression and has been assigned suppressor functions. Suppressor function is reduced during MS relapses and recovers during remissions. In addition, it is persistently low in chronic progressive MS (157). IFN-α and IFN-β restore suppressor cell function to normal levels in vitro as well as in vivo (158). This ability may be linked to the beneficial effects in MS seen with type I IFN therapy. CD8$^+$ cells produce cytokines involved in cell-mediated suppression (e.g., IL-4, TGF-β, IL-10, and IFN-α/β). The regulation of these cytokines by IFNs has been described earlier in this chapter.

Another important immunoregulatory molecule whose expression in macrophages is affected by IFNs, is prostaglandin E2 (PGE$_2$). Its production is strongly inhibited by IFN-γ, but it can be enhanced by IL-1 and phosphodiesterase inhibitors like pentoxifylline (159). PGE$_2$ reduces IL-2, IFN-γ, and LT production by Th1 cells (160) and activates CD8$^+$ suppressor T cells (161). In vitro, PGE$_2$ release from monocytes is reduced early in MS attacks (162), and PGE analogues effectively suppress EAE (163). Type I IFNs have only marginal effects on PGE$_2$ production in freshly isolated human monocytes (164). As PGE$_2$ and IFN-β exert similar immunoregulatory effects, but are differently regulated, they might potentiate each other when used in combination.

Some of the controversial results obtained with the administration of IFN-γ in EAE (165) (see Chapter 9) can be due to the phase of the disease, the site of IFN administration (which has an impact on the unselective recruitment of activated T cells), and the effect of IFN-γ on the destruction of Th1 cells (166). For example, systemic IFN-γ given at the time of induction of EAE may protect the animals by diverting cells into irrelevant sites of the lymphoid system and inducing killing of disease-inducing, antigen-specific Th1 cells before they even have reached their target organ. On the other hand, if IFN-γ is administered to MS patients, in whom disease-specific T cells are already present in the brain, the proinflammatory cascade may be amplified within the central nervous system and thereby cause increased inflammation and release of demyelinating substances.

E. Conclusions

There are various steps during the development of cell-mediated immunity which are differentially regulated by type I and type II IFNs. The opposing effects of these cytokines (summarized in Table 2) on lymphocyte activation, cellular migration, tissue destruction, suppression of inflammatory responses, and repair mechanisms favor IFN-β and IFN-α as immunologically active drugs which counteract many of the major steps involved in the pathogenesis of MS. The observed clinical benefits of IFN-β treatment in MS may be attributed to its in vivo immunomodulatory activities, such as:

Suppression of IFN-γ production in response to (auto)antigenic stimulation

Antagonism of the immunostimulatory and inflammatory actions of IFN-γ on cells of the immune and nervous system

Enhancement of deficient suppressor T cell activity in the blood of MS patients

REFERENCES

1. Jacobs LD, O'Malley, Freeman A, Akes R. Intrathecal interferon reduces exacerbations of multiple sclerosis. Science 1981; 214:1026–1028.
2. Arnason BGW, Reder AT. Interferons and multiple sclerosis. Clin Neuropharmacol 1994; 17:1–53.
3. Paty DW, Li DKB, Group UMS, Group IFN-β MSS. Interferon beta-1b is effective in relapsing-remitting multiple sclerosis: II. MRI analysis results of a multicenter, randomized, double-blind, placebo-controlled trial. Neurology 1993; 43:662–667.
4. Jacobs LD, Cookfair DL, Rudick RA, Herndon RM, Richert JR, Salazar AM, et al. Intramuscular interferon beta-1α for disease progression in relapsing multiple sclerosis. Ann Neurol 1996; 39:285–294.
5. Panitch HS, Bever CJ. Clinical trials of interferons in multiple sclerosis. What have we learned? J Neuroimmunol 1993; 46:155–164.
6. Arnason BGW. Editorial: Interferon beta in multiple sclerosis. Neurology 1993; 43:641–643.
7. Smith RA, Norris F, Palmer D, Bernhardt L, Wills RJ. Distribution of interferon in serum and cerebrospinal fluid after systemic administration. Clin Pharmacol Ther 1985; 37:85–88.
8. Burke DC, Shuttleworth J. The control of interferon alpha and interferon beta gene expression. In: Friedman RM, ed. Interferon. Vol. 3. Mechanisms of Production and Action. New York, Elsevier 1984:85–111.
9. Field AK, Tytell AA, Lampson GP, Hilleman MR. Inducers of interferons and host resistance. II. Multistranded synthetic polynucleotide complexes. Proc Natl Acad Sci USA 1967; 58:1004–1010.
10. Capobianchi MR, Facchini J, di Marco P, Antonelli G, Dianzani F. Induction of alpha interferon by membrane interaction between viral surface and peripheral blood mononuclear cells. Proc Soc Exp Biol Med 1985; 178: 551–556.
11. Gessani S, Puddu P, Varano B, Borghi P, Conti L, Fantuzzi L, Belardelli F. Induction of beta interferon by human immunodeficiency virus type 1 and its gp120 protein in human monocytes-macrophages: role of beta interferon in restriction of virus replication. J Virol 1994; 68:1983–1986.

12. Bermudez LE. Infection of "Nonprofessional" phagocytes with mycobacterium avium complex. Clin Immunol Immunopathol 1991; 61:225–235.
13. De Mayer E, De Mayer-Guignard J. Interferons and Other Regulatory Cytokines. New York: Wiley, 1988.
14. Gessani S, Belardelli F, Pecorelli A, Puddu P, Baglioni C. Bacterial lipopolysaccharide and gamma interferon induce transcription of beta interferon mRNA and interferon secretion in murine macrophages. J Virol 1989; 63: 2785–2789.
15. Cleveland MG, Lane RG, Klimpel GR. Enhanced interferon-alpha/beta and defective IFN-gamma production in chronic graft versus host disease: A potential mechanism for immunosuppression. Cell Immunol 1987; 110: 120–130.
16. Huang S, Hendriks W, Althage A, Hemmi S, Bluethmann H, Kamijo R, Vilček J, Zinkernagel RM, Aguet M. Immune responses in mice that lack the interferon-gamma receptor. Science 1993; 259:1742–1745.
17. Pyo S, Gangemi JD, Ghaffer A, Mayer EP. Poly I:C–induced anti-herpes simplex virus type 1 activity in inflammatory macrophages is mediated by induction of interferon-beta. J Leukocyte Biol 1991; 50:479–487.
18. Riches DWH, Underwood GA. Expression of interferon-β during the triggering phase of macrophage cytocidal activation: Evidence for an autocrine/paracrine role in the regulation of this state. J Biol Chem 1991; 266: 24785–24792.
19. Shemer AY, Wallach D, Sarov I. Reversion of the antichlamydial effect of tumor necrosis factor by tryptophan and antibodies to beta interferon. Infect Immun 1989; 57:3484–3490.
20. Onozaki K, Urawa H, Tamatani T, Iwamura Y, Hashimoto T, Baba T, Suzuki H, Yamada M, Yamamoto S, Oppenheim JJ, Matsushima K. Synergistic interactions of interleukin-1, interferon-beta, and tumor necrosis factor in terminally differentiating a mouse myeloid leukemic cell line (M1). J Immunol 1988; 140:112–119.
21. Testa, U, Ferbus D, Gabbianelli M, Pascucci B, Boccoli G, Louache F, Thang MN. Effect of endogenous and exogenous interferons on the differentiation of human monocyte cell line U937. Cancer Res 1988; 48:82–88.
22. Stout RD, Suttles J. Evidence for involvement of TNF-alpha in the induction phase and IFN-β in the effector phase of antiproliferative activity of splenic macrophages. Cell Immunol 1992; 139:363–374.
23. Zhang X, Alley EW, Russell SW, Morrison DC. Necessity and sufficiency of beta interferon for nitric oxide production in mouse peritoneal macrophages. Infect Immun 1994; 62:33–40.
24. Moore RN, Larsen HS, Horohov DW, Rouse BT. Endogenous regulation of macrophage proliferative expansion by colony-stimulating factor–induced interferon. Science 1984; 223:178–181.
25. Cederblad B, Alm GF. Interferons and the colony-stimulating factors IL-3 and GM-CSF enhance the IFN-alpha response in human blood leucocytes induced by herpes simplex virus. Scand J Immunol 1991; 34:549–555.

26. Seghal PB, Gupta SL. Regulation of the stability of poly(I):poly(C) induced human fibroblast interferon mRNA: selective inactivation of interferon mRNA and lack of involvement of 2'5'-oligo(A) synthetase activation during shut-off of interferon production. Proc Natl Acad Sci USA 1980; 77: 3849–3893.

27. Gobl AE, Funa K, Alm GV. Different induction pattern of mRNA for IFN-alpha and -beta in human mononuclear leukocytes after in vitro stimulation with Herpes simplex virus-infected fibroblasts and Sendai virus. J Immunol 1988; 140:3605–3609.

28. Gobl AE, Cederblad B, Sandberg K, Alm GV. Interferon-α but not -β genes require de novo protein synthesis for efficient expression in human mono-cytes. Scand J Immunol 1992; 35:177–185.

29. Gendelman HE, Friedman RM, Joe S, Baca LM, Turpin JA, Dveksler G, Meltzer MS, Dieffenbach C. A selective defect of interferon alpha produc-tion in human immunodeficiency virus-infected monocytes. J Exp Med 1990; 172:1433–1442.

30. Mossman TR, Cherwinski H, Bond MW, Giedlin MA, Coffman RI. Two types of murine helper T cell clone. I. Definition according to profiles of lymphokine activities and secreted proteins. J Immunol 1986; 136: 2348–2357.

31. Paul WE, Seder RA. Lymphocyte responses and cytokines. Cell 1994; 76: 241–251.

32. Heinzel FP, Schoenhut DS, Rerko RM, Rosser LE, Gately MK. Recombi-nant IL-12 cures mice infected with Leishmania major. J Exp Med 1993; 177:1505–1509.

33. Balachov KE, Smith DR, Khoury SJ, Hafler DA, Weiner HL. Defective regulation of T-cell receptor–mediated IFN-gamma production by Th2-type cytokines in multiple sclerosis. Neurology 1995; 45(suppl 4):A384.

34. Powrie F, Coffman RL. Cytokine regulation of T-cell function: potential for therapeutic intervention. Immunol Today 1993; 14:270–274.

35. Clerici M, Shearer GM. A Th1-Th2 switch is a critical step in the etiology of HIV infection. Immunol Today 1993; 14:107–111.

36. Liblau RS, Singer SM, McDevitt HO. Th1 and Th2 CD4$^+$ T cells in the pathogenesis of organ-specific autoimmune diseases. Immunol Today 1995; 16:34–38.

37. Baron JL, Madri JA, Ruddle NH, Hashim G, Janeway CJ. Surface expres-sion of alpha 4 integrin by CD4 T cells is required for their entry into brain parenchyma. J Exp Med 1993; 177:57–68.

38. Miller SD, Karpus WJ. The immunopathogenesis and regulation of T - cell-mediated demyelinating diseases. Immunol Today 1994; 15:356–361.

39. Brod SA, Benjamin D, Hafler D. Restricted T cell expression of IL-2/IFN-γ mRNA in human inflammatory diseases. J Immunol 1991; 147:810–815.

40. Weber F, Meinl E, Drexler K, Czlonkowska A, Huber S, Fickenscher H, Müller-Fleckenstein I, Fleckenstein B, Wekerle H, Hohlfeld R. Transfor-mation of human T cell clones by herpesvirus saimiri: intact antigen recogni-

tion by autonomously growing myelin basic protein-specific T cells. Proc Natl Acad Sci USA 1993; 90:11049–11053.

41. Link J, Söderström M, Ljungdahl A, Höjeberg B, Olsson T, Xu Z, Fredrikson S, Wang ZY, Link H. Organ-specific autoantigens induce interferon-gamma and interleukin-4 mRNA expression in mononuclear cells in multiple sclerosis and myasthenia gravis. Neurology 1994; 44:728–734.

42. Olsson T, Zhi WW, Höjeberg B, Kostulas V, Yu-Ping J, Anderson G, Ekre HP, Link H. Autoreactive T lymphocytes in multiple sclerosis determined by antigen-induced secretion of interferon-γ. J Clin Invest 1990; 86:981–985.

43. Benvenuto R, Paroli M, Buttinelli C, Franco A, Barnaba V, Fieschi C, Balsano F. Tumor necrosis factor-alpha and interferon-gamma synthesis by cerebrospinal fluid-derived T cell clones in multiple sclerosis. Ann NY Acad Sci 1991; 341–346.

44. Gajewski TF, Schell SR, Nau G, Fitch FW. Regulation of T-cell activation: differences among T cell subsets. Immunol Rev 1989; 111:79–110.

45. Hardy KJ, Manger B, Newton M, Stobo JD. Molecular events involved in regulating human interferon-gamma gene expression during T cell activation. J Immunol 1987; 138:2353–2358.

46. Munakata T, Semba U, Shibuya Y, Kuwano K, Akagi M, Arai S. Induction of interferon-γ production by human T cells stimulated by hydrogen peroxide. J Immunol 1985; 134:2449–2455.

47. Ianaro A, O'Donnell CA, Di-Rossa M, Liew FY. A nitric oxide synthase inhibitor reduces inflammation, down-regulates inflammatory cytokines and enhances interleukin-10 production in carrageenin-induced oedema in mice. Immunology 1994; 82:370–375.

48. Johnson HM, Torres BA. Leukotrienes: positive signals for regulation of gamma-interferon production. J Immunol 1984; 132:413–416.

49. Le J, Lin JX, Henriksen-DeStefano D, Vilcek J. Bacterial lipolpolysaccharide-induced interferon-gamma production: roles of interleukin 1 and interleukin 2. J Immunol 1986; 136:4525–4530.

50. Farrar MA, Schreiber RD. The molecular cell biology of interferon-γ and its receptor. Ann Rev Immunol 1993; 11:571–611.

51. Langer JA, Pestka S. Interferon receptors. Immunol. Today 1988; 9: 393–400.

52. Noronha A, Toscas A, Jensen MA. Interferon β decreases T cell activation and interferon γ production in multiple sclerosis. J Neuroimmunol 1993; 46:145–154.

53. Brinkmann V, Geiger T, Alkan S, Heusser C. Interferon α increases the frequency of interferon γ-producing human CD4⁺ T cells. J Exp Med 1993; 178:1655–1663.

54. Bednarik DP, Mosca JD, Babu N, Raj K, Pitha PM. Inhibition of human immunodeficiency virus (HIV) replication by HIV-trans-activated alpha2-interferon. Proc Natl Acad Sci USA 1989; 86:4958–4962.

55. Gendelman HE, Baca LM, Kubrak CA, Genis P, Burrous S, Friedman RM, Jacobs D, Meltzer MS. Induction of interferon alpha in peripheral blood-

mononuclear cells by human immunodeficiency virus (HIV)-infected mono-cytes: restricted antiviral activity of the HIV-induced interferons. J Immunol 1992; 148:422–430.

56. Del Gobbo V, Foli A, Balzarini J, EDC, Balestra E, Villani N, Marini S, Perno CF, Calio R. Immunomodulatory activity of 9-(2-phosphonyl-methoxyethyl)adenine (PMEA), a potent anti-HIV nucleotide analogue, on in vivo murine models. Antiviral Res 1991; 16:65–75.

57. Yoshihara R, Shiozawa S, Fujita T, Chihara K. Gamma interferon is produced by human natural killer cells but not T cells during Staphylococcus aureus stimulation. Infect Immun 1993; 61:3117–3122.

58. Wherry JC, Schreiber RD, Unanue ER. Mechanism of interferon-gamma production by natural killer cells in scid mice. FASEB J 1990; 4:A1701.

59. Reiter Z, Rappaport B. Dual effects of cytokines in regulation of MHC-unrestricted cell mediated cytotoxicity. Crit Rev Immunol 1993; 13:1–34.

60. Sandberg K, Matsson P, Alm GV. A distinct population of nonphagocytic and low level CD4+ null lymphocytes produce IFN-alpha after stimulation by herpes simplex virus-infected cells. J Immunol 1990; 145:1015–1020.

61. Feldman SB, Ferraro M, Zheng HM, Patel N, Gould-Fogerite S, Fitzgerald-Bocarsly P. Viral induction of low frequency interferon-alpha producing cells. Virology 1994; 204:1–7.

62. Howell D, Feldman S, Kloser P, Fitzgerald-Bocarsly P. Decreased frequency of natural interferon producing cells in peripheral blood of patients with the acquired immune deficiency syndrome. Clin Immunol Immunopathol 1994; 71:223–230.

63. Sibley WA, Bamford CR, Clark K. Clinical viral infections and multiple sclerosis. Lancet 1985; 2:1313–1315.

64. Allen I, Brankin B. Pathogenesis of multiple sclerosis—the immune diathesis and the role of viruses. J Neuropathol Exp Neurol 1993; 52:95–105.

65. Capobianchi M, Malavasi F, DiMarco P, Dianzani F. Differences in the mechanism of induction of interferon-alpha by herpes simplex virus and herpes-simplex virus-infected cells. Arch Virol 1988; 103:219–229.

66. Wiranowska-Stewart M, Stewart W. Determination of human leukocyte populations involved in production of interferons alpha and gamma. J Interferon Res 1981; 1:233–244.

67. Weigent DA, Langford MP, Smith EM, Blalock JE, Stanton GJ. Human B lymphocytes produce leukocyte interferon after interaction with foreign cells. Infect Immun 1981; 32:508–512.

68. Kehrl JH, Miller A, Fauci AS. Effect of tumor necrosis factor α on mitogen-activated human B cells. J Exp Med 1987; 166:786–791.

69. Ferbas JJ, Toso JF, Logar AJ, Navratil JS, Rinaldo CRJ. CD4+ blood dendritic cells are potent producers of IFN-α in response to in vitro HIV-1 infection. J Immunol 1994; 152:4649–4662.

70. Van Damme J, GO. Interaction of interferons with skin-reactive cytokines: from interleukin-1 to interleukin-8. J Invest Dermatol 1990; 95:90S–93S.

71. Van Damme J, Schaafsma MR, Fibbe WE, Falkenburg JHF, Opdenakker G, Billiau A. Simultaneous production of interleukin 6, interferon-beta and

colony-stimulating activity by fibroblasts after viral and bacterial infection. Eur J Immunol 1989; 19:163–168.

72. Lenardo MJ, Fan CM, Maniatis T, Baltimore D. The involvement of NF-κB in beta-interferon gene regulation reveals its role as widely inducible mediator of signal transduction. Cell 1989; 57:287–294.

73. Mathiesen GA, Toth FD, Juhl C, Ladritsen NN. Purification and initial characterization of human placental trophoblast interferon induced by polyriboinosinic polyribocytidylic acid. J Gen Virol 1990; 71:3061–3066.

74. Tao YX, Cao YQ. Modulation of interferon secretion by concanavalin A and interleukin-2 in first trimester placental explants in vitro. J Reprod Immunol 1993; 24:201–212.

75. Pociot F, Wilson AG, Nerup J, Duff GW. No independent association between a tumor necrosis factor-alpha promotor region polymorphism and insulin-dependent diabetes mellitus. Eur J Immunol 1993; 23:3050–3053.

76. Salonen R, Ilonen J, Reunanen M, Salmi A. Defective production of interferon-γ associated with HLA-DW2 antigen in stable multiple sclerosis. J Neurol Sci 1982; 55:197–206.

77. Tovell DR, McRobbie IA, Warren KG, Tyrell DLJ. Interferon production by lymphocytes from multiple sclerosis and non-MS patients. Neurology 1983; 33:640–643.

78. Bocci V. The physiological interferon response. Immunol Today 1985; 6:7–9.

79. Knight EJ, Anton ED, Fahey D, Friedland BK, Jonak GJ. Interferon regulates c-myc gene expression in Daudi cells at the post-transcriptional level. Proc Natl Acad Sci USA 1985; 82:1151–1154.

80. Einat M, Resnitzky D, Kimchi A. Close link between reduction of c-myc expression by interferon and, G0/G1 arrest. Nature 1985; 313:597–600.

81. Pfeffer LM, Donner B, Tamm I. Interferon-alpha down-regulates insulin receptors in lymphoblastoid (Daudi) cells. Relationship to inhibition of cell proliferation. J Biol Chem 1987; 262:3665–3670.

82. Aggarawal BB, Eessalu TE, Has PE. Characterization of receptors for human tumour necrosis factor and their regulation by gamma interferon. Nature 1985; 318:665–667.

83. Roth AD, Abele R, Alberto P. 13-cis-retinoic acid plus interferon-alpha: a phase II clinical study in squamous cell carcinoma of the lung and the head and neck. Oncology 1994; 51:84–86.

84. Metha K, McQueen T, Tucker S, Pandita R, Aggarwal BB. Inhibition by all-trans-retinoic acid of tumor necrosis factor and nitric oxide production by peritoneal macrophages. J Leukoc Biol 1994; 55:336–342.

85. Dickens TA, Colletta AA. The pharmacological manipulation of members of the transforming growth factor beta family in the chemoprevention of breast cancer. Bioassays 1993; 15:71–74.

86. Kuruvilla AP, Shah R, Hochwald GM, Liggitt HD, Palladino MA, Thorbecke GJ. Protective effect of transforming growth factor β1 on experimental autoimmune diseases in mice. Proc Natl Acad Sci USA 1991; 88:2918–21.

87. Rieckmann P, Albrecht M, Kitze B, Weber T, Tumani H, Broocks A, Lüer W, Helwig A, Poser S. Tumor necrosis factor-α messenger RNA expression in patients with relapsing-remitting multiple sclerosis is associated with disease activity. Ann Neurol 1995; 37:82–88.

88. Sidman CL, Marshall JD, Shultz LD, Gray PW, Johnson HM. Gamma interferon is one of several direct B cell-maturing lymphokines. Nature 1984; 309:801–804.

89. Bansil S, Cook SD, Rohowsky-Kochan C. Multiple sclerosis: immune mechanism and update on current therapies. Ann Neurol 1995; 37(suppl 1): S87–S101.

90. Briskin M, Kuwabara MD, Sigman DS, Wall R. Induction of kappa transcription by interferon-gamma without activation of NF-κB. Science 1988; 258:1036–1037.

91. Cowdery JS, Fleming AL. In vivo depletion of CD4 T cells increases B cell sensitivity to polyclonal activation: the role of interferon-γ. Clin Immunol Immunopathol 1992; 62:72–78.

92. Snapper CM, Peschel C, Paul WE. IFN-γ stimulates IgG2a secretion by murine B cells stimulated with bacterial lipopolysaccharide. J Immunol 1988; 140:2121–2127.

93. Chen U. Analysis of cell proliferation and μ-RNA procesing during activation of mouse B cells by anti-μ and T lymphokines. Mol Immunol 1990; 27: 1249–1257.

94. Abed NS, Chace JH, Fleming AL, Cowdery JS. Interferon-gamma regulation of B lymphocyte differentiation. Cell Immunol 1994; 153:356–366.

95. Rieckmann P, Weber T, Felgenhauer K. Class differentiation of immunoglobulin-containing cerebrospinal fluid cells in inflammatory diseases of the central nervous system. Klin Wochenschrift 1990; 68:12–17.

96. Olsson T. Cytokines in neuroinflammatory disease: role of myelin autoreactive T cell production of interferon-γ. J Neuroimmunol 1992; 40:211–218.

97. Mayet WJ, Hess G, Gerken G. Treatment of chronic type B hepatitis with recombinant alpha-interferon induces autoantibodies not specific for autoimmune chronic hepatitis. Hepatology 1989; 10:24–28.

98. Drapier JC, Wietzerbin J, Hibbs JJ. Interferon-gamma and tumor necrosis factor induce the L-arginine-dependent cytotoxic effector mechanism in murine macrophages. Eur J Immunol 18:1587–1592.

99. Oswald IP, Wynn TA, Sher A, James SL. NO as an effector molecule of parasite killing: modulation of its synthesis by cytokines. Comp Biochem Physiol Pharmacol Toxicol Endocrinol 1994; 108:11–18.

100. Alleva DG, Burger CJ and Elgert KD. Tumor-induced regulation of suppressor macrophage nitric oxide and TNF-α production. Role of tumor-derived IL-10, TGF-β, and prostaglandin E_2. J Immunol 1994; 153:1674–1686.

101. Bö L, Dawson TM, Wesselingh S, Mörk S, Choi S, Kong PA, Hanley D, Trapp BD. Induction of nitric oxide synthase in demyelinating regions of multiple sclerosis brains. Ann Neurol 1994; 36:778–786.

102. Koprowski H, Zheng YM, Heber-Katz E, Fraser N, Rorke L, Fu ZF, Hanlon C, Dietzschold B. In vivo expression of inducible nitric oxide synthase

in experimentally induced neurologic diseases. Proc Natl Acad Sci USA 1993; 90:3024–3027.

103. Selmaj KW, Raine CS. Tumor necrosis factor mediates myelin and oligo-dendrocyte damage in vitro. Ann Neurol 1988; 23:339–346.

104. Sheehan, KCF, Schreiber RD. The synergy and antagonism of interferon-γ and TNF. In: Beutler B, ed. Tumor Necrosis Factors. New York: Raven Press, 1992; 145–178.

105. Collart, MA, Belin D, Vassalli JD, de Kossodo S, Vassalli P. γ Interferon enhances macrophage transcription of the tumor necrosis factor/cachectin, interleukin 1, and urokinase genes, which are controlled by short-lived re-pressors. J Exp Med 1986; 164:2113–2118.

106. Kamijo, R, Le J, Shapiro D, Havell EA, Huang S, Aguet M, Bosland M, Vilček J. Mice lacking the interferon-γ receptor have profoundly altered responses to infection with Bacillus Calmette-Guerin and subsequent chal-lenge with lipopolysaccharides. J Exp Med 1993; 178:1435–1440.

107. Wherry, JC, Schreiber RD, Unanue ER. Regulation of gamma interferon production by natural killer cells in scid mice: roles of tumor necrosis factor and bacterial stimuli. Infect Immun 1991; 59:1709–1715.

107a. Wenner CA, Güler ML, Macatonia SE, O'Garra A, Murphy KM. Roles of IFN-γ and IFN-α in IL-12-induced T helper cell-1 development. J Immunol 1996; 156:1442–1447.

108. Herrmann F, Cannistra SA, Lindemann A, Blohm D, Rambaldi A, Mertels-mann RH, Griffin JD. Functional consequences of monocyte IL-2 receptor expression: induction of IL-1β secretion by IFN-γ and IL-2. J Immunol 1989; 142:139–143.

109. Olsson T. Role of cytokines in multiple sclerosis and experimental autoim-mune encephalomyelitis. Eur J Neurol 1994; 1:7–19.

110. Springer T. Traffic signals for lymphocyte recirculation and leukocyte emi-gration: the multistep paradigm. Cell 1994; 76:301–314.

111. Cannella B, Cross AH, Raine CS. Adhesion-related molecules in the central nervous system. Upregulation correlated with inflammatory cell influx dur-ing relapsing experimental autoimmune encephalomyelitis. Lab Invest 1991; 65:23–31.

112. Peleman R, Wu J, Fargeas C, Delespesse G. Recombinant interleukin 4 suppresses the production of interferon γ in human mononuclear cells. J Exp Med 1989; 170:1751–1756.

113. Fiorentino DF, Zlotnik A, Vieira P, Mosmann TR, Howard M, Moore KW, O'Garra A. IL-10 acts on the antigen-presenting cell to inhibit cytokine production by Th1 cells. J Immunol 1991; 146:3444–3451.

114. Minty A, Chalon P, Derocq JM, Dumont X, Guillemont JC, Kaghad M, Labit C, Leplatois P, Liauzun P, Miloux B, Minty C, Casellas P, GL, Lupker J, Shire D, Ferrara P, Caput D. Interleukin-13 is a new human lymphokine regulating inflammatory and immune responses. Nature 1993; 362:248–250.

115. Tsunawaki S, Sporn M, Ding A, Nethan C. Deactivation of macrophages by transforming growth factor-β. Nature 1988; 334:260–262.

116. Pober JS, Gimbrone MA, Lapierre LA. Overlapping patterns of activation of human endothelial cells by interleukin 1, tumor necrosis factor and immune interferon. J Immunol 1986; 22:219–226.

117. Kasahara T, Hooks JJ, Dougherty SF, Oppenheim JJ. Interleukin-2 mediated immune interferon (IFN-γ) production by human T cells and T cell subsets. J Immunol 1983; 130:1784–1789.

118. Kubin M, Kamoun M, Trinchieri G. IL-12 synergizes with B7/CD28 interaction in inducing efficient proliferation and cytokine production in human T cells. J Exp Med 1994; 180:211–222.

119. Porrini, AM, Reder AT. IFN-γ, IFN-β and PGE1 affect monokine secretion: relevance to monocyte activation in multiple sclerosis. Cell Immunol 1994; 157:428–438.

120. Skias DD, Reder AT. IL-10 inhibits EAE. Neurology 1995; 45(suppl 4): A349.

121. Jacobsen H, Mestan J, Mittnacht S, Dieffenbach CW. Beta interferon subtype 1 induction by tumor necrosis factor. Mol Cell Biol 1989; 9:3037–3042.

122. Noronha A, Toscas A, Jensen MA. IFN-beta modulates immune function: implication for multiple sclerosis. J Immunol 1993; 150:A259.

123. Abu-Khabar KS, Armstrong JA, Ho M. Type I interferons (IFN-α and β) suppress cytotoxin (tumor necrosis factor-α and lymphotoxin) production by mitogen-stimulated human peripheral blood mononuclear cells. J Leukoc Biol 1992; 52:165–172.

124. Shakir S, Byskosh PV, Reder AT. Interferon beta induces interleukin-10 mRNA in mononuclear cells (MNC). Neurology 1994; 44(suppl 2): A211–A212.

124a. Tilg H, Mier JW, Vogel W, et al. Induction of circulating IL-1 receptor antagonists by IFN treatment. J Immunol 1993; 150:4687–4692.

125. Faulds D, Benfield P. Interferon β-1b in multiple sclerosis. Clin Immunother 1994; 1:79–87.

126. Durelli L, Bongioanni MR, Cavallo R, Ferrero B, Ferri R, Ferrio MF, Bradac GB, Riva A, Vai S, Geuna M. Chronic systemic high-dose recombinant interferon alpha-2a reduces exacerbation rate, MRI signs of disease activity, and lymphocyte interferon gamma production in relapsing-remitting multiple sclerosis. Neurology 1994; 44:406–413.

127. Durelli L, Bongioanni MR, Ferrero B, Verdun E, Riva A, Geuna M, Bradac GB, Bergamasco B, Bergamini L. Chronic alpha interferon (IFN-α) treatment for multiple sclerosis (MS) modulates cytokine production rather than antigen presentation. Neurology 1995; 45(suppl 4):A234.

128. Twardzik DR, Mikovits JA, Ranchalis JE, Purchio AF, Ellingsworth L, Ruscetti FW. γ interferon-induced activation of latent transforming growth factor-β by human monocytes. Ann NY Acad Sci 1990; 593:276–284.

129. Klimple GR, Fleischman WR, Klimple KD. Gamma interferon (IFN) and IFNα/β suppress murine myeloid colony formation (CFV-C): magnitude of suppression is dependent upon level of colony stimulating factor (CSF). J Immunol 1982; 129:76–80.

130. Van-Damme J, Proost P, Put W, Arens S, Lenaerts JP, Conings R, Op-

denakker G, Heremans H, Billiau A. Induction of monocyte chemotactic proteins MCP-1 and MCP-2 in human fibroblasts and leukocytes by cytokines and cytokine inducers. J Immunol 1994; 152:5495–5502.

131. Brown Z, Gerritsen ME, Carley WW, Strieter RM, Kunkel SL, Westwick J. Chemokine gene expression and secretion by cytokine-activated human chemoattractant protein-1 and interleukin-8 in response to interferon-gamma. Am J Pathol 1994; 145:913–921.

132. Morita M, Kasahara T, Mukaida N, Matsushima K, Nagashima T, Nishizawa M, Yoshida M. Induction and regulation of IL-8 and MCAF production in human brain tumor cell lines and brain tumor tissues. Eur Cytokine Netw 1993; 4:351–358.

133. Tani M, Ransohoff RM. Do chemokines mediate inflammatory cell invasion of the central nervous system parenchyma? Brain Pathol 1994; 4:135–143.

134. Fabry Z, Raine CS, Hart MN. Nervous tissue as an immune compartment: the dialect of the immune response with the CNS. Immunol Today 1994; 15:218–224.

135. Sapolsky R, Rivier C, Yamamoto G, Plotsky P, Vale W. Interleukin-1 stimulates the secretion of hypothalamic corticotropin-releasing factor. Science 1987; 238:522–524.

136. Reder AT, Lowy MT. Interferon-β treatment does not elevate cortisol in multiple sclerosis. J Interferon Res 1992; 12:195–198.

137. Hansen TR, Imakawa K, Polites HG, Marotti KR, Anthony RV, Roberts RM. Interferon mRNA of embryonic origin is expressed transiently during early pregnancy. J Biol Chem 1988; 263:12801–12804.

138. Altmann DJ, Schneider SL, Thompson DA, Cheng HL, Tomasi TB. A transforming growth factor-β2 (TGF-β2)-like immunosuppressive factor in amniotic fluid and localization of TGF-β2 mRNA in the pregnant uterus. J Exp Med 1990; 172:1391–1401.

139. Dayal A, Ismail MA, Jensen M, Lledo A, Arnason BGW. Pregnancy plasma inhibits interferon gamma-secreting cells in multiple sclerosis. Neurology 1995; 45(suppl 4):A197.

140. Evavold BD, Sloan-Lancaster J, Allen PM. Tickling the TCR: selective T cell function stimulated by altered peptide ligands. Immunol. Today 1993; 14:602–606.

141. Basham TY, Merigan TC. Recombinant interferon-γ increases HLA-DR synthesis and expression. J Immunol 1983; 130:1492–1494.

142. Armstrong MA, Crockard AD, Hawkins SA, McNeill TA. Multiple sclerosis and gamma interferon. Lancet 1987; 1:1369–1370.

143. Panitch HS, Folus JS, Johnson KP. Beta interferon prevents HLA class II antigen induction by gamma interferon in MS. Neurology 1989; 39(suppl 1):171.

143a. Soilu-Hänninen M, Salmi A, Salonen R. Interferon-β downregulates expression of VLA-4 antigen and antagonizes interferon-γ-induced expression of HLA-DQ on human peripheral blood monocytes. J Neuroimmunol 1995; 60:99–106.

144. Ransohoff RM, Tuohy VK, Barna BP, Rudick RA. Monocytes in active

multiple sclerosis: intact regulation of HLA-DR density in vitro despite decreased HLA-DR density in vivo. J Neuroimmunol 1992; 37:169–176.

145. Hartung HP. Immune-mediated demyelination. Ann Neurology 1993; 33: 563–567.

146. Washington R, Burton J, Todd R, Newman W, Dragovic L, Dore-Duffy P. Expression of immunologically relevant endothelial cell activation antigens on isolated central nervous system microvessels from patients with multiple sclerosis. Ann Neurol 1994; 35:89–97.

147. Sobel RA, Mitchell ME, Fondren G. Intercellular adhesion molecule-1 (ICAM-1) in cellular immune reactions in the human central nervous system. Am J Pathol 1990; 136:1309–1316.

148. Alosi F, Borsellino G, Samoggia P, Testa U, Chelucci C, Russo G, Peschle C, Levi G. Astrocyte cultures from human embryonic brain: characterization and modulation of surface molecules by inflammatory cytokines. J Neurosci Res 1992; 32:494–506.

149. Cross H. Immune cell traffic control and the central nervous system. Semin Neurosci 1992; 4:213–219.

150. Wong D, Dorovini-Zis K. Upregulation of intercellular adhesion molecule-1 (ICAM-1) expression in primary cultures of human brain microvessel endothelial cells by cytokines and lipopolysaccharide. J. Neuroimmunol 1992; 39:11–22.

151. Ziesalek J, Archelos JJ, Toyka KV, Hartung HP. Expression of intercellular adhesion molecule-1 on rat microglial cells. Neurosci Lett 1993; 153: 136–139.

152. Westermann J, Persin S, Matyas J, P VDM, Pabst R. IFN-γ influences the migration of thoracic duct B and T lymphocytes subsets in vivo: random increase in disappearance from the blood and differential decrease reappearance in the lymph. J Immunol 1993; 150:3843–3852.

153. Fedoseyeva EV, Li Y, Huey B, Tam S, Hunt CA, Benichou G, Garovoy MR. Inhibition of interferon-gamma-mediated immune functions by oligonucleotides. Suppression of human T cell proliferation by downregulation of IFN-gamma-induced ICAM-1 and Fc-receptor on accessory cells. Transplantation 1994; 57:606–612.

154. Willems F, Marchant A, Delville JP, Gerard C, Delvaux A, Velu T, de Boer M, Goldman M. Interleukin-10 inhibits B7 and intercellular adhesion molecule-1 expression on human monocytes. Eur J Immunol 1994; 24: 1007–1009.

155. Reder AT. IFN-β and IFN-γ modify expression of monocyte surface proteins. J Interferon Res 1991; 11(suppl 1):121.

156. Rudick RA, Carpenter CS, Cookfair DL, Tuohy VK, Ransohoff RM. In vitro and in vivo inhibition of mitogen-driven T-cell activation by recombinant interferon beta. Neurology 1993; 43:2080–2087.

157. Antel J, Bania MB, Reder AT, Cashman N. Activated suppressor cell dysfunction in progressive multiple sclerosis. J. Immunol 1985; 137:137–141.

158. Noronha A, Toscas A, Arnason BGW, Jensen M. IFN-beta augments in vivo suppressor function in MS. Neurology 1994; 44(suppl 2):A212.

159. Endres S, Fulle HJ, Sinha B, Stoll D, Dinarello CA, Gerzer R, Weber PC. Cyclic nucleotides differentially regulate the synthesis of tumour necrosis factor-alpha and interleukin-1 beta by human mononuclear cells. Immunology 1991; 72:56–60.
160. Ferreri NR, Sarr T, Askenase PW, Ruddle NH. Molecular regulation of tumor necrosis factor-alpha and lymphotoxin production in T cells: inhibition by prostaglandin E_2. J Biol Chem 1992; 267:9443–9449.
161. Philips RP, Stein SH, Roper RL. A new view of prostaglandin E regulation of the immune response. Immunol Today 1991; 12:349–352.
162. Dore-Duffy P, Donaldson JO, Koff T, Longo M, Perry W. Prostaglandin release in multiple sclerosis: correlation with disease activity. Neurology 1986; 36:1587–1590.
163. Reder AT, Thapar M, Sapugay AM, Jensen MA. Prostaglandins and inhibitors of arachidonate metabolism suppress experimental allergic encephalomyelitis. J Neuroimmunol 1994; 54:117–127.
164. Boraschi D, Soldateschi D, Tagliabue A. Macrophage activation by interferon: dissociation between tumoricidal capacity and suppressive activity. Eur J Immunol 1982; 12:320–326.
165. Heremans H, Dillen C, Dijkmans A, Grau G, Billiau A. The role of cytokines in various animal models of inflammation. Lymphokine Res 1989; 8: 329–333.
166. Liu Y, Janeway CAJ. Interferon γ plays a critical role in induced cell death of effector T cells: a possible third mechanism of self-tolerance. J Exp Med 1990; 172:1735–1739.

8

The Pathogenetic Role of Interferon-γ in Multiple Sclerosis

Gianvito Martino and Luigi M. E. Grimaldi

San Raffaele Scientific Institute, Milan, Italy

I. BIOLOGICAL FEATURES OF HUMAN INTERFERON-γ

Interferon-γ (IFN-γ) is a type II interferon coded by a gene located on chromosome 12 and comprising three introns and four exons. The exons code for a polypeptide of 166 amino acids, 20 of which constitute the signal peptide (1–3). Although IFN-γ displays no molecular homology with type I IFNs ($\alpha, \beta, \omega, \tau$) and it is only produced by T lymphocytes and natural killer cells, it shares with type I IFNs some important biological activities. IFN-γ is, in fact, a pleiotropic cytokine with antiviral, antibacterial, and antiprotozoal activity (4). Its immunomodulatory properties entail coregulation of macrophage as well as B-cell and T-cell functions (5). IFN-γ exerts its activity by binding to a species-specific glycoprotein cell surface receptor (IFN-γR) encoded by a gene located on chromosome 6. The resulting protein has a 228–amino acid extracellular domain, a 19–amino acid single transmembrane domain, and an intracellular domain of 222 amino acids (6). To be functionally active, the IFN-γR requires at least a species-specific signal-transducing factor (accessory factor 1 or IFN-γ β chain) encoded by a gene on chromosome 21 (7) (see Chapter 1).

The intracellular signals generated by the binding of IFN-γ to its receptor have been extensively studied, and part of the IFN-γ–mediated intracellular signaling cascade is now known. When IFN-γ binds to its own receptor on the cell surface, two receptor-associated protein tyrosine kinases, belonging to the Janus kinase (JAK) family and named JAK 1 and JAK 2, are activated (8,9). The activation of these two kinases induces the phosphorylation of the tyrosine$_{701}$ residue on a latent cytoplasmic protein belonging to the signal transducer and activator of transcription (STAT) family, the so-called STAT1 (10). When phosphorylated, STAT1 acts as a transcription factor, it assembles in homodimers, translocates into the nucleus, and directs transcription of IFN-γ–responsive genes (11). IFN-γ activates the transcription of genes containing a consensus-response element, the IFN-γ activation site (GAS) (consensus sequence: TTNCNNNAA) to which STAT1 binds specifically (12) (see Chapter 2).

Although the signaling cascade generated by IFN-γ has been partially delineated, there are several questions which still need to be answered. The most impelling one is how IFN-γ generates a specific response if many other cytokines are also able to induce JAK2 activation (e.g., interleukin-3 [IL-3], IL-6, ciliary neurotrophic factor) or STAT1 phosphorylation (i.e., platelet-derived growth factor, epidermal growth factor). Since transcription factors act generally as protein complexes, studies aimed at the discovery of new members of the JAK-STAT pathway family should provide answers.

II. MULTIPLE SCLEROSIS AND IFN-γ

Multiple sclerosis (MS) is an immune-mediated demyelinating disease of the central nervous system (CNS) of unknown etiology. Activated T lymphocytes play a central role in the pathogenetic processes leading to demyelination in MS patients (13,14). Different antigens and autoantigens have been proposed as a T-cell targets, but none of them currently satisfies the criteria for being the ultimate antigen of MS (13–15). Moreover, little is known about the first and intermediate events triggering the T-cell activation process preceding the development of MS lesions.

T-cell activation occurs when immune-relevant molecules, present in the extracellular space, bind to specific receptors, and induce an intracellular signaling transduction cascade. This causes upregulation of immediate, intermediate, and late T-cell activation genes (e.g., genes coding for trophic factors) (16). Apart from the essential contribution of the antigenic stimulus, most of the extracellular signals involved in triggering T-lymphocyte growth and differentiation are generated by cytokines (17). Among cytokines which primarily contribute to T-lymphocyte activation leading to MS demyelination, IFN-γ is considered essential (18).

A role for IFN-γ in MS was first suggested by the clinical observation that systemic administration of IFN-γ to MS patients markedly increased the rate of disease exacerbations (19). This effect was attributed to a direct stimulation of lymphocyte proliferation by IFN-γ (20). The importance of IFN-γ in the pathogenesis of MS was subsequently supported by the detection of an increase of circulating IFN-γ levels and mRNA transcripts in peripheral blood lymphocytes (PBLs) prior to and during clinical relapses (21,22). A further (although indirect) clinical evidence of IFN-γ involvement in MS came from recent large IFN-β therapeutic trials conducted in patients with relapsing-remitting MS (23,24). Administration of IFN-β had protective effects on the appearance of CNS lesions detected by magnetic resonance imaging (MRI) (25) and on the clinical course (23,24) of the disease. This benefit has been attributed to the immunological interference of IFN-β on IFN-γ (26). Further evidence of an involvement of IFN-γ in MS derives from morphological studies performed on brains from MS patients showing that areas of demyelination contain IFN-γ (27,28).

What are the biological bases for the deleterious effects of IFN-γ in MS? IFN-γ increases in vitro expression of major histocompatibility complex (MHC) class II molecules on CNS resident cells (29,30) and of adhesion molecules on endothelial cells (31,32). This suggests that IFN-γ might facilitate cell to cell contacts necessary for T-lymphocyte activation and lymphocyte traffic through the blood-brain barrier. IFN-γ also activates monocytes and microglial cells, stimulates them to release cytokines able to damage oligodendrocytes (e.g., tumor necrosis factor-α [TNF-α] [33,34]), and mediates the synthesis of molecules potentially noxious to the myelin sheath, such as nitric oxide metabolites (35). In animals affected by experimental allergic encephalomyelitis (EAE), an animal model of MS, circulating IFN-γ levels (18) and the amount of IFN-γ mRNA transcripts (36) correlate with the gravity of the disease. In addition, T-cell lines sensitized against myelin basic protein (a target autoantigen of EAE) are more effective in passive transfer of the disease when prestimulated with IFN-γ (37).

Despite so many clinical and experimental evidence demonstrating the general effect of IFN-γ, the intracellular mechanisms by which IFN-γ mediates T-lymphocyte activation in MS still remain to be fully elucidated.

III. T-CELL ACTIVATION, INTRACELLULAR CALCIUM, AND IFN-γ

Extracellular signals (mainly represented by cytokines and antigens) ignite T-cell activation which proceeds only in the presence of a sufficient

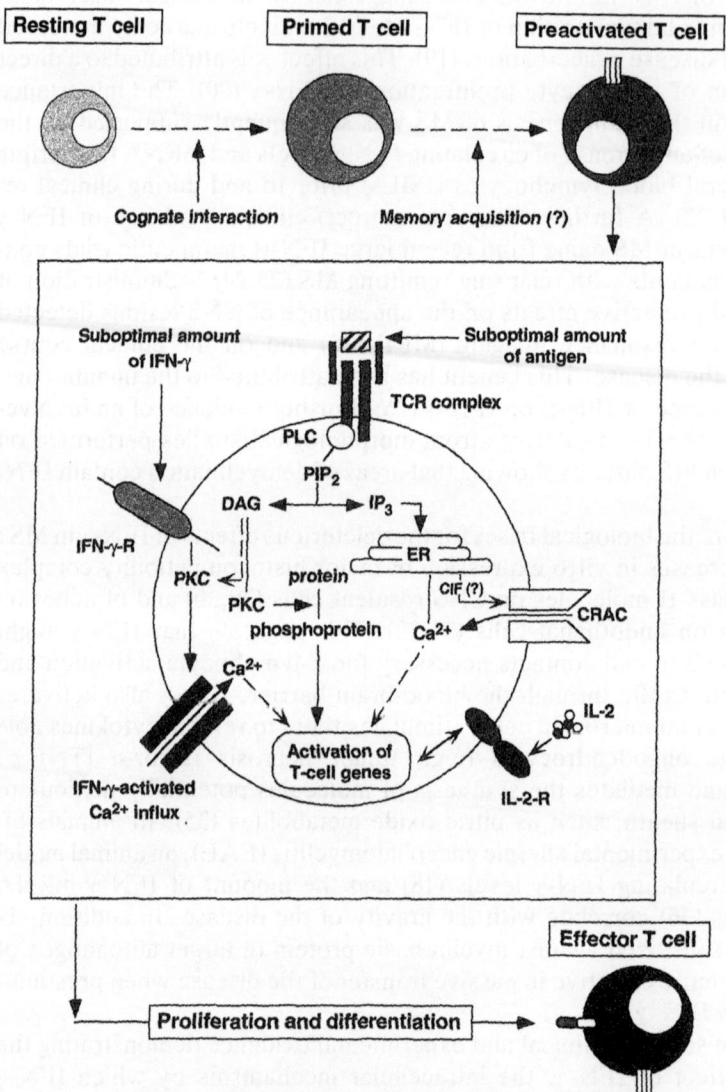

Figure 1 Synopsis of the activation process in T cells from MS patients expressing the IFN-γ–activated Ca²⁺ influx. After priming and acquisition of antigenic memory, T cells expressing the influx proceed to full-blown activation when, along with suboptimal antigenic stimulation (a proposed mechanism to keep memory T cells in a preactivated state [60–62]), even a suboptimal amount of IFN-γ stimulates the IFN-γR. This in turn induces a Ca²⁺ transient through the IFN-γ–acti-

amount of second messengers within the cell cytoplasm. One of the principal second messengers during T-cell activation is calcium (Ca^{2+}) (38). Sustained elevation of intracellular Ca^{2+} ($[Ca^{2+}]_i$) levels are, in fact, required by T cells to generate an intracellular cascade of events leading to T-cell activation and gene transcription (39) (Fig. 1).

The $[Ca^{2+}]_i$ increase in T cells can be generated in two ways: (1) release of Ca^{2+} from intracellular stores, mainly located in the endoplasmic reticulum (ER); or (2) Ca^{2+} entry into cells from outside through plasmalemma channels. After the T-cell receptor (TCR) is stimulated, release of Ca^{2+} from the ER during the activation process is regulated by inositol 1,4,5-trisphosphate (IP_3), which is produced by the hydrolysis of phosphatidyl-inositol-4,5 bisphosphate (PIP_2) induced by phospholipase C (PLC) (40). In turn, IP_3 stimulates IP_3 receptor–enriched ER regions which discharge Ca^{2+}. The release of Ca^{2+} from the ER stores determines the entry of Ca^{2+} from outside the cell through plasmalemmal Ca^{2+} channels (see Fig. 1). This phenomenon, called *capacitative Ca^{2+} entry*, is mainly mediated by the so-called Ca^{2+} release–activated channels (CRAC) (41). These are the only Ca^{2+} channels so far demonstrated on lymphocytes (42–44). Although some hypotheses have been proposed (e.g., a soluble mediator released by the ER, called Ca^{2+}-inducing factor [CIF] [45]), the mechanisms by which Ca^{2+} entry is regulated by Ca^{2+} release from ER-associated intracellular stores are still unclear. When $[Ca^{2+}]_i$ reaches biologically significant levels, it (along with protein kinases upregulated by diacylglycerol [DAG], another product of PIP_2 hydrolysis) triggers protein phosphorylation, which leads to the expression of T-cell activation genes (see Fig. 1) (39).

In conclusion, Ca^{2+} stored in the ER and released via the IP_3 pathway is the major source of Ca^{2+} during T-cell activation. In T lymphocytes from patients with MS, we have recently found evidence of an additional Ca^{2+}-mediated activation pathway which is triggered by IFN-γ and is regulated by a previously undescribed IFN-γ–activated Ca^{2+} influx (46). This novel Ca^{2+}-mediated pathway sheds new light on the mechanisms by which IFN-γ regulates T-cell activation during MS and may explain some of the adverse effects of IFN-γ in MS (19).

---

vated Ca^{2+} influx. This Ca^{2+} transient, coupled with the $[Ca^{2+}]_i$ consistently maintained in the cell cytoplasm by the continuous stimulation of the TCR complex via the IP_3-mediated pathway, causes activation of the T-cell genes necessary for full-blown differentiation and proliferation. T-cell entry into the activation cycle is also reinforced by the parallel induction, owing to the IFN-γR stimulation, of an intracellular transient of PKC which cooperates in the activation (i.e., phosphorylation) of latent cytoplasmic transcription factors.

IV. THE IFN-γ–ACTIVATED Ca^{2+} INFLUX

We found that exposure of T lymphocytes from patients with MS to IFN-γ does not induce Ca^{2+} discharge from intracellular stores or Ca^{2+} entry through the CRAC, but it activates a previously undescribed Ca^{2+} influx (46) (see Fig. 1). This influx, present mostly in CD4$^+$ T lymphocytes from MS patients, shows pharmacological properties different from those of Ca^{2+} channels described so far (42–44), is strongly associated with disease activity (47), and renders T lymphocytes more susceptible to proliferate in response to suboptimal doses of mitogenic stimuli (48). There are important pharmacological, immunological, and clinical correlates of this influx.

A. Pharmacological Properties

The detection and characterization of the IFN-γ–activated Ca^{2+} influx were performed on PBLs from MS patients using the conventional fluorimetric protocol of Grynkiewicz and coworkers (49). The protocol allows measurements of an increase of the $[Ca^{2+}]_i$ level in lymphocytes exposed to IFN-γ by using the Ca^{2+}-binding fluorescent tracer fura-2 (Fig. 2A). To discriminate if the $[Ca^{2+}]_i$ rise measured in MS cells exposed to IFN-γ was due to Ca^{2+} release from intracellular stores or to Ca^{2+} entry from the extracellular milieu, we employed in parallel on the same cell preparations a modification of the Grynkiewicz's protocol, the so-called Ca^{2+}-free Ca^{2+}-reintroduction protocol (50) (Fig. 2B, 2C). This protocol entails the following steps: cells are first bathed in Ca^{2+}-free medium, then are exposed to the Ca^{2+}-releasing agent, and finally Ca^{2+} is reintroduced into the medium. $[Ca^{2+}]_i$ increase is due to release of Ca^{2+} from intracellular stores when it is recorded before Ca^{2+} reintroduction into the medium; $[Ca^{2+}]_i$ increase is due to Ca^{2+} entry from the extracellular milieu when it is measured after Ca^{2+} reintroduction into the medium.

IFN-γ induced a 10–30% $[Ca^{2+}]_i$ increase over the basal level in PBLs from MS patients. The influx shows an initial delay of 10 secs followed by a progressive 2- to 3-min rise, and then a plateau phase maintained for several minutes (see Fig. 2A). Using the Ca^{2+}-free Ca^{2+}-reintroduction protocol we found that the IFN-γ–induced $[Ca^{2+}]_i$ increase was due to a transplasmalemmal Ca^{2+} influx and not to a release of Ca^{2+} from intracellular stores (see Fig. 2B).

Since a transplasmalemmal Ca^{2+} influx was recorded in PBLs from MS patients in response to IFN-γ, we proceded to the pharmacological characterization of the influx by analysing the effects of different Ca^{2+}-releasing agents. All drugs used (Table 1) act on some of the other transplasmalemmal Ca^{2+} influxes so far described: voltage-operated Ca^{2+} channels (VOCCs), second-messenger–operated Ca^{2+} channels (SMOC),

[Ca²⁺]ᵢ nM

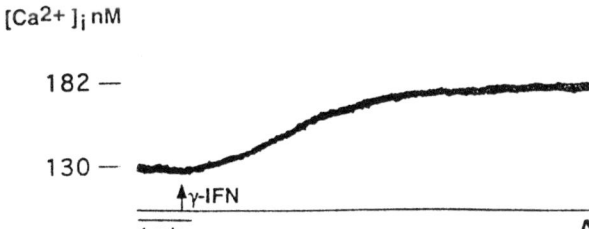

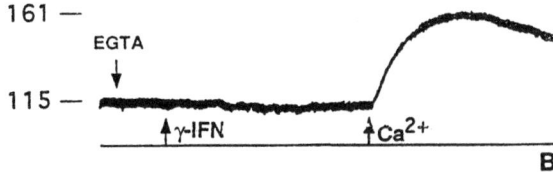

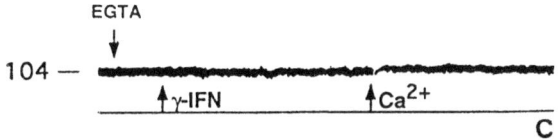

Figure 2 [Ca²⁺]ᵢ increase recorded over a 10-min period in PBLs from a representative MS patient (traces A and B) and from a healthy subject (trace C) exposed to 1 pg/ml of IFN-γ. Trace A represents [Ca²⁺]ᵢ variations induced by IFN-γ in cells processed according to the protocol of Grynkiewicz and coworkers (49); traces B and C were recorded in cell preparations studied according to Ca²⁺-free Ca²⁺-reintroduction protocol (50). Ca²⁺-free medium (traces B and C) were obtained by adding ethylene glycol-bis(β-aminoethylether)*N,N,N',N'*-tetraacetic acid (EGTA). IFN-γ and EGTA where added as indicated by arrows. A [Ca²⁺]ᵢ rise induced by IFN-γ is observed in PBLs from the MS patient (traces A and B) but not in PBLs from the healthy subject (trace C). The [Ca²⁺]ᵢ rise induced by the IFN-γ–activated Ca²⁺ influx is due to an influx coming from outside the membrane, because it occurs only when Ca²⁺ is reintroduced from outside (trace B).

Table 1 Pharmacological Features of the T-Lymphocyte IFN-γ–Activated Ca^{2+} Influx

Drugs	Effect on cationic channels	Effects on the γ-IFN–activated Ca^{2+} influx
SC 38249	Blockage of VOCC, SMOC, CRAC	−
Verapamil	Blockage of VOCC (L-type)	−
Diltiazem	Blockage of VOCC (L-type)	−
ω-Conotoxin	Blockage of VOCC (N-type)	−
Pertussis toxin	Inhibition of G proteins (GOC, VOCC)	−
Forskolin	Activation of adenyl cyclase (VOCC)	−
Na$^+$, Cl$^-$ omission	Blockage of antiporters and cotransporters	−
Mn^{2+}	Permeability to Mn^{2+} (SMOC, CRAC)	−
Staurosporin	Blockage of PKC-dependent channels	+
PMA	Activation of PKC-dependent channels	+
La^{3+}	Blockage of cationic channels	+
KCl	Blockage of cationic channels	+

VOCC, voltage-operated Ca^{2+} channels; SMOC, second-messenger–operated Ca^{2+} channels; CRAC, Ca^{2+} release–activated channels; GOC, G protein-operated Ca^{2+} channels; Mn^{2+}, manganese; La^{3+}, lanthanum; PKC, protein kinase C; PMA, phorbol-12-myristate-13-acetate; KCl, potassium chloride.

and CRAC. The influx we described was insensitive to the imidazole drug SC 38249, a blocker of VOCC, SMOC, and CRAC (50), thus indicating its functional difference with these other channels. Unlike CRAC, the IFN-γ–activated Ca^{2+} influx was impermeable to Mn^{2+}. A second difference with VOCC was its insensitivity to diltiazem, verapamil, and ω-conotoxin, which are specific blockers of the VOCC. Omission of Na$^+$ and Cl$^-$ from the medium did not modify the IFN-γ–induced influx, thus excluding the involvement of neutral cotransporters and antiporters (42,50). Finally, the influx was insensitive to forskolin and pertussis toxin, and therefore G proteins seem not to be involved in the intracellular pathway sustaining its activity (42).

Although the influx was insensitive to most of the drugs used, the La^{3+}-mediated blockage of the influx and its inhibition by KCl-induced depolarization indicate that the influx was probably sustained by a cationic channel (46). We have recently obtained further evidence to support the existence of a specific IFN-γ–activated Ca^{2+} channel by analyzing at a single-cell level, influx-positive T lymphocytes from MS patients by a video-imaging technique (unpublished data). Since protein kinase C (PKC) mediates the intracellular transduction of IFN-γ–dependent stimuli (51), we found, as expected, that the Ca^{2+} influx is inhibited by PKC blockers (i.e., staurosporin) and enhanced by a PKC activator (i.e., phorbol-12-myristate = 13-acetate [PMA]) (46).

B. Clinical and Magnetic Resonance Imaging Studies

To assess whether the IFN-γ–activated Ca^{2+} influx was a distinctive feature of MS, we studied its prevalence in patients with relapsing-remitting definite MS (52) and control patients. The influx was found in 55% of MS patients, but in only 14% of patients with other neurological or active autoimmune diseases, and in 9% of healthy subjects (Table 2).

MS patients were then subdivided according to the clinical phase of the disease (52). Sixty-five percent of the patients in the active group turned out to be influx-positive compared with only 45% of the patents in the clinically stable group (see Table 2) (46). Since influx-positive T lymphocytes were most frequent among the MS patients suffering from

Table 2 Prevalence of the T-Lymphocyte IFN-γ–Activated Ca^{2+} Influx in Patients with MS and in Healthy Controls

Patient groups	No. of patients	No. of IFN-γ–activated Ca^{2+} influx-positive patients (%)
Total MS	67	37 (55)
Clinically active	34	22 (65)
1st week from the onset of a new attack	18	14 (78)
2nd week from the onset of a new attack	7	4 (57)
3rd week from the onset of a new attack	9	4 (44)
Gadolinium-enhanced brain MRI positive	18	13 (72)
Gadolinium-enhanced brain MRI negative	4	2 (50)
Clinically stable	33	15 (45)
Benign	15	5 (33)
Gadolinium-enhanced brain MRI positive	9	5 (55)
Gadolinium-enhanced brain MRI negative	13	5 (38)
Other neurological or active autoimmune diseases	32	4 (14)
Healthy donors	21	2 (9)

MRI, magnetic resonance imaging.

an episode of disease reactivation, they were further grouped according to the time elapsed from the clinical onset of an exacerbation. Almost 80% of the patients tested during the first week after clinical onset were influx positive, a figure that dropped to 57% in the second week, and to 44% in the third week (see Table 2) (46).

Since a strong association was recorded between the influx and clinically active disease, we investigated whether the presence of the influx was temporally associated with the detection of active brain lesions by gadolinium-enhanced brain MRI. The latter technique allows the detection of CNS areas of ongoing inflammation (active lesions) (53), which often develop regardless of the occurrence of signs or symptoms of clinically active disease. Gadolinium-enhancing brain MRI lesions were more frequent in influx-positive (72%) than in influx-negative (47%) MS patients (see Table 2) (47). Furthermore, there was a trend toward a larger average size of enhancing lesions in influx-positive compared with influx-negative MS patients (47). The association between the detection of the influx and clinical and/or MRI evidence of disease activity was further strengthened by the fact that the lowest (30%) prevalence of the influx was detected in a subgroup of 15 MS patients affected by a particularly benign form of the disease (>10 years of disease and an expanded disability status scale [EDSS] score <3) (see Table 2).

Although an association between clinical activity and detection of this new T-lymphocyte Ca^{2+} influx is likely, some of our data seem to contradict a direct relationship between the two phenomena. First, the influx was still detected in 30% of the clinically stable MS patients who lacked gadolinum-enhancing brain MRI lesions. The amount of gadolinium used to enhance CNS lesions by MRI may be crucial in this case. Using a dose of gadolinium (3 mmol/kg) threefold higher than the standard dose, 50% of formerly brain MRI–negative MS patients show enhancing lesions (54). It is possible that the detection of the IFN-γ–activated Ca^{2+} influx may be more sensitive in detecting ongoing brain inflammation than brain MRI using the standard dose of gadolinum (1 mmol/kg), and that lesions seen with high-dose gadolinium may correlate more closely with detection of influx-positive lymphocytes. In the only influx-positive, brain MRI–negative (standard gadolinium dose) stable MS patient in whom the triple dose of gadolinum was used, gadolinium-enhancing lesions were promptly recorded. An alternative explanation is that influx-positive, brain MRI–negative MS patients may harbor spinal cord lesions.

Second, we could not detect any IFN-γ–activated Ca^{2+} influx in 20–30% of clinically active MS patients with positive brain MRI. Two facts are relevant: (1) influx-positive cells do not seem to be long-lasting, as suggested by the progressive decline of influx-positive cells in the first few weeks after the onset of a new attack; and (2) mitogen-stimulated PBLs from patients with MS increase their IFN-γ production 2 weeks before the onset of an exacerbation (in the most benign cases, the increase disappears rapidly, even before the appearance of symptoms) (21). It is therefore possible that the IFN-γ–activated Ca^{2+} influx might have already disappeared by the time of our analysis. It is likely, in fact, that the lymphocyte-activation process begins outside the CNS long before the ensuing inflammation produces the CNS tissue damage that results in a clinically appreciable loss of function (14).

To test this hypothesis, we assessed the presence of the influx in the PBLs of three MS patients every 15 days for approximately 6 months. Gadolinum-enhanced brain MRI scans were performed monthly. There were a total of three clinical attacks. An increase of $[Ca^{2+}]_i$ due to the IFN-γ–activated Ca^{2+} influx always preceded a new clinical attack. The $[Ca^{2+}]_i$ increase peaked between 4 and 45 days before the appearance of clinical manifestations (47). Moreover, when the IFN-γ–activated Ca^{2+} influx was detectable, brain MRI showed active lesions after a single dose of gadolinium in each of these three exacerbations.

C. Immunological Correlates of the IFN-γ–Activated Ca^{2+} Influx

The finding of a new structure on the surface of T lymphocytes of patients with MS and its correlation with clinical events leads to the question of its pathogenetic role in immunoregulation and demyelination. For this reason, we investigated some of the immunological properties of lymphocytes from MS patients carrying the IFN-γ–activated Ca^{2+} influx.

Influx-positive lymphocytes belonged mostly to the $CD4^+$ subset ($CD8^+$ lymphocytes sporadically responded with a weak $[Ca^{2+}]_i$ elevation; B lymphocytes were always influx negative). The influx was triggered by stimulation of the IFN-γR as inferred by its dose-dependent inhibition in PBLs preincubated with a blocking anti–IFN-γR antibody (46). The expression of IFN-γR was, however, per se insufficient to induce the IFN-γ–activated Ca^{2+} influx, since receptor-rich cells from healthy donors (e.g., resting B lymphocytes, phytohemagglutinin [PHA]–stimulated or alloactivated T lymphocytes, the lymphomonocytic cell line U937) did not show the influx (46).

We then investigated the proliferative capacities of influx-positive lymphocytes in response to stimulation with mitogens and/or IFN-γ. Since no studies have been reported on the amount of Ca^{2+} needed to trigger T-cell activation, we first analyzed the overall proliferative capacity of PBLs obtained from healthy subjects in response to various concentrations of an activating stimulus and, in parallel, the associated $[Ca^{2+}]_i$

increase. Resting lymphocytes were stimulated with different concentrations of PHA, a mitogen able to induce T-cell proliferation by triggering the TCR and in turn able to induce $[Ca^{2+}]_i$ accumulation via the IP_3-mediated pathway (see Fig. 1). PHA-induced proliferation and the $[Ca^{2+}]_i$ increase over basal levels were linearly correlated ($r = 0.62$) (Fig. 3A)

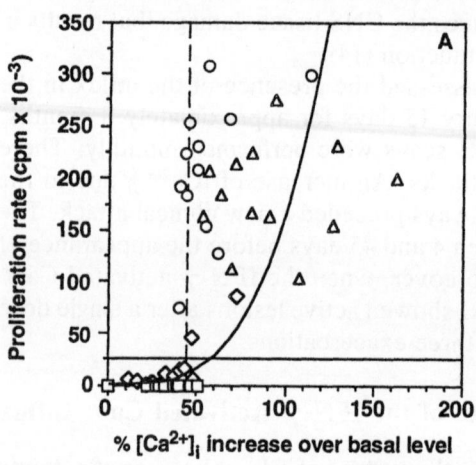

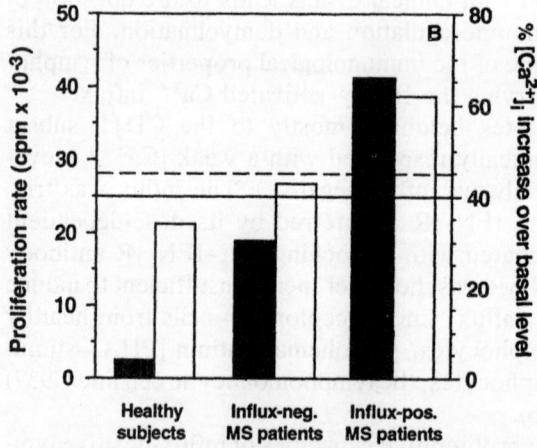

Figure 3 (A) Correlation between proliferation rate expressed in counts per minute (cpm) $\times$ 10^{-3} and percentage of $[Ca^{2+}]_i$ increase over basal level in resting PBLs stimulated with different concentration of PHA (0.1 μg/ml squares; 1 μg/ml diamonds; 10 μg/ml circles; 100 μg/ml triangles). The two phenomena are linearly and significantly correlated ($r = 0.62$). Proliferation significantly starts

(48). The relationship between these two events also indicated that cell proliferation began in lymphocytes only when the $[Ca^{2+}]_i$ level rose by ~45% over basal levels (Fig. 3A). Accordingly, this $[Ca^{2+}]_i$ level rise over baseline was considered as the minimum threshold for T-lymphocyte activation. This finding is also supported by the work of Negulescu and coworkers (39), who found, at a single cell level, that a similar $[Ca^{2+}]_i$ increase over basal is necessary to induce transcription of the nuclear transcription factor of activated T cells (NF-AT), indispensable for IL-2 gene–dependent T-cell activation.

The same parameters were then investigated in PBLs from influx-positive and influx-negative MS patients (48) and the results were compared with those obtained in PBLs from healthy subjects. Cells from normal subjects and MS patients showed no significant differences in the proliferation rate when stimulated with optimal doses of PHA (mitogenic dose: 10 μg/ml). Furthermore, the overall $[Ca^{2+}]_i$ level increase induced by this PHA stimulus was similar in influx-positive and influx-negative cells. However, suboptimal amounts of PHA (1 μg/ml, an amount insufficient to induce proliferation by itself), caused an average $[Ca^{2+}]_i$ increase of ~30% in cells from healthy controls and 40% in cells from MS patients (see Fig. 3B; influx-negative plus influx positive subjects). However, both $[Ca^{2+}]_i$ elevations did not reach the immunological threshold necessary for full-blown activation (>45% of $[Ca^{2+}]_i$ increase over basal level) (see Fig. 3) (48). We attribute the higher responsiveness to suboptimal amounts of PHA of MS cells compared with cells from healthy donors to the preactivated state commonly found in these cells (13,55–57), possibly reflecting an increased responsiveness to (auto)antigens (58,59).

The ability of influx-positive and influx-negative cells from MS patients to proliferate and accumulate Ca^{2+} were then compared. Since in influx-positive cells IFN-γ generates only a 10–20% increase in $[Ca^{2+}]_i$ levels, it is unlikely that it is able to sustain proliferation by itself (see threshold in Fig. 3A). This is confirmed by the lack of proliferation of influx-positive

---

(cpm > 25×10^{-3}; continuous line) only when the percentage of $[Ca^{2+}]_i$ increase over basal is at least 45% (dashed line). (B) Means of percentage increases of $[Ca^{2+}]_i$ over basal level (blank columns) and proliferation rates (dark columns; expressed in cpm $\times 10^{-3}$) measured in PBLs from healthy subjects and influx-negative and influx-positive MS patients stimulated with 1 μg/ml of PHA. Lines in the panel represent levels of significance of the two parameters measured and correspond to the lines drawn in panel A. Significant proliferation occurs only in influx-positive MS patients where the IP3-mediated $[Ca^{2+}]_i$ elevations induced by a submitogenic dose of PHA (1 μg/ml) is coupled with the $[Ca^{2+}]_i$ increase from the IFN-γ–activated Ca^{2+} influx.

cells stimulated with up to 500 U/ml of IFN-γ alone. To overcome the confounding effect of the IP$_3$-dependent Ca^{2+} release from PHA plus Ca^{2+} entry via the IFN-γ–activated Ca^{2+} influx, experimental conditions were set in which the amount of [Ca^{2+}]$_i$ due to both cellular mechanisms would synergistically cooperate to induce T-cell proliferation (i.e. by stimulating cells with 1 μg/ml of PHA) (48). This dose does not promote proliferation by itself, because it is unable to cause a sufficient increase of [Ca^{2+}]$_i$ ($\gtrsim$45%) in cells from healthy donors or MS patients (see Fig. 3B) (48). However, if this suboptimal PHA stimulation is accompanied by a second stimulus provided by IFN-γ, the proliferation rate of cells expressing the IFN-γ–activated Ca^{2+} influx increases by twofold. Thus, there appears to be a summation of at least two separate sources of Ca^{2+} in influx-positive cells—one provided by the conventional IP$_3$-mediated pathway (PHA; TCR) and the other by the Ca^{2+} influx triggered by IFN-γ (see Fig. 1). The significant association between the two phenomena is bolstered by evidence from analysis of T lymphocytes from two patients followed serially for up to 5 months; all but one of six IFN-γ–dependent [Ca^{2+}]$_i$ elevations corresponded with increased proliferative responses to 1 μg/ml of PHA plus 5 U/ml of IFN-γ.

V. CONCLUSIONS

IFN-γ is a pleiotropic cytokine whose numerous immunomodulatory effects are thought to be essential for the development of the pathological lesions in MS (13–15). The well-characterized CNS effects of IFN-γ (i.e., increase of MHC class II [29,30] and adhesion molecule expression [31,32]), stimulation of macrophage–microglial cells to release cytokines toxic to oligodendrocytes (33,34) or myelinotoxic molecules (35)], are probably not the only mechanisms by which IFN-γ leads to demyelination.

T lymphocytes from the majority of patients with active MS show a transmembrane Ca^{2+} influx activated by IFN-γ. The influx is different from other Ca^{2+} influxes so far described (42,43) and is significantly associated with MS compared with other neurological or active autoimmune diseases (46), and correlates with clinical and radiological evidence of disease activity (47). The influx provides an additional amount of Ca^{2+} to the T lymphocyte [Ca^{2+}]$_i$ pool (48) which seems to be crucial for inducing full-blown activation in preactivated T cells.

How does the T-lymphocyte IFN-γ–activated Ca^{2+} influx fit into current views of the pathogenetic mechanisms leading to demyelination in MS?

Proliferation assays performed on T cells from MS patients have repeatedly demonstrated that preactivated T cells are a common finding in MS

(13,55–59). This finding is also confirmed by our measurements of $[Ca^{2+}]_i$ levels in cells from MS patients exposed to stimuli acting via the TCR complex (e.g., PHA). What is the biological relevance of these cells? After priming, T cells may remain in a long-term memory state even in the apparent absence of specific stimulatory antigens (60,61). These cells are CD44$^+$ and, at least in mice, the majority of them are in the G_1 phase (62), implying that long-term memory cells are not truly resting but are in a semiactivated state, possibly as a result of low level signaling via the TCR. This low-level TCR stimulation does not push cells into the cell cycle but it is sufficient to maintain expression of CD44 and other activation markers (58). If this is the case for MS, it is then conceivable that MS lymphocytes reach full-blown activation even when minimally stimulated.

Myelin autoantigens may sometimes drive MS T cells into a full-blown activation state. The following evidence supports this view: (1) myelin-specific T-cell lines are more easily established from MS patients than from healthy donors (15); (2) primary T cells proliferate at a higher rate in response to myelin antigens than cells from healthy donors (32); and (3) IL-2–responsive T cells specific for myelin basic protein are more frequent in peripheral blood and cerebrospinal fluid of MS patients compared with controls (59). The release of CNS autoantigens into the circulation, as well as other MS-putative (auto)antigens such as heat shock proteins, viral antigens, and superantigens, may well represent the primary event leading to cyclic full-blown activation of preactivated T cells in MS patients. However, our results suggest the existence of at least one alternative non–antigen-specific mechanism (Fig. 4). IFN-γ interaction with its cognate receptor would provide, through the IFN-γ–activated Ca^{2+} influx, a quota of $[Ca^{2+}]_i$ necessary to fully activate T cells and drive them to become effector cells (see Figs. 1 and 4). However activation occurs, MS T cells pass through the blood-brain barrier and finally reach the CNS where they expand clonally and induce demyelination (Fig. 4).

The novel Ca^{2+} influx, induced by IFN-γ in T lymphocytes from MS patients and crucial for T cell differentiation and proliferation, can explain the observation that common viral infections, which are usually associated with systemic production of IFN-γ, often precede clinical relapses in patients with MS (63) (see Fig. 4). Moreover, the increased tendency of influx-positive cells to proliferate in vitro in response to IFN-γ might also explain why lymphocytes from patients with MS undergoing systemic IFN-γ treatment show spontaneous proliferation in culture (20).

Although a possible role of this Ca^{2+} influx in the pathogenetic mechanisms leading to demyelination could be inferred, its biology is speculative. First, the putative Ca^{2+} channel sustaining the influx could be a viral protein expressed on the membrane of infected lymphocytes and operating

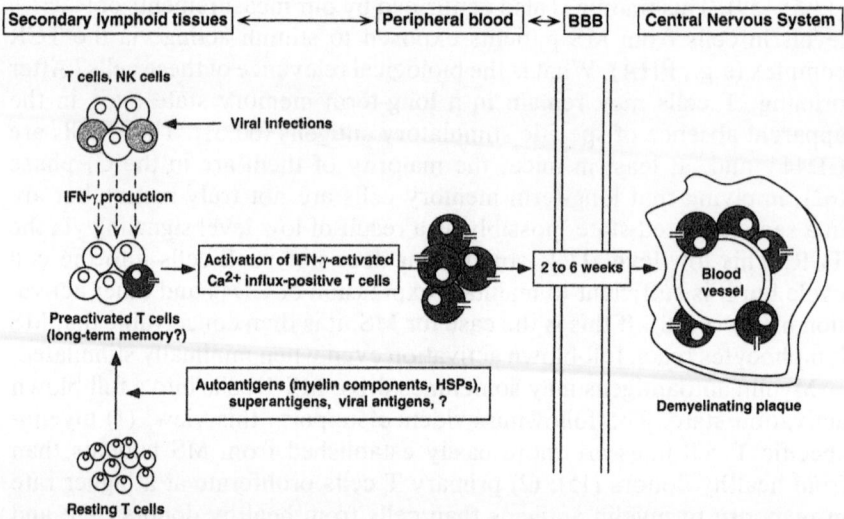

Figure 4 Proposed interplay between IFN-γ–activated Ca²⁺ influx-positive T cells and the pathogenetic mechanisms leading to demyelination in MS. After priming with the "putative" MS (auto)antigen, selected T cells (probably those devoted to the maintaining of the immunological memory) enter in a preactivated state sustained by low-grade stimulation of the TCR and home into secondary lymphoid organs (60–62). At this stage, cells cannot fully activate and become effector but can readily be brought to proliferate by an appropriate antigenic challenge. A cytokine-mediated and antigen-independent "meaningful" challenge is hypothesized in IFN-γ–activated Ca²⁺ influx-positive cells. IFN-γ–activated Ca²⁺ influx-positive cells can, in fact, enter into a full-blown differentiation and proliferation cycle when exposed to IFN-γ (e.g., produced in response to infections). Activated T cells which are also influx-positive can enter the CNS, expand clonally, and induce demyelination through several effector systems (e.g., cytokines, direct cytotoxicity, nitrogen oxide metabolites, gelatinases). BBB, blood-brain barrier; HSPs, heat shock proteins; NK, natural killer.

as a cationic channel. When the M2 capsid protein of the influenza virus is expressed on the membrane of infected cells, it behaves as a channel for monovalent ions (64,65). The cloning of the IFN-γ–activated Ca²⁺ channel will support or exclude this hypothesis. Second, the structure acting as a Ca²⁺ channel might play additional roles in the control of lymphocyte activities. An example comes from the integrin-associated protein (IAP), which is involved in the adhesion process crucial for T-cell activation and also acts as a Ca^{2+} channel (66,67). Third, since it is known that the IFN-γR induces an intracellular signaling cascade only in the presence of accessory factors (7), the receptor in MS may be associated with a membrane factor which transduces an anomalous intracellular signal able to open a usually unresponsive channel (i.e., a channel normally present on T cells but responding to different stimuli).

The finding that the IFN-γ–activated Ca^{2+} influx correlates with active (clinical and MRI) disease, frequently precedes the clinical appearance of new symptoms, and is restricted to $CD4^+$ T lymphocytes (probably the most important lymphocyte subgroup involved in the pathogenesis of MS) supports its value as a cellular marker of disease activity. It may be a valuable marker of the cellular immunological status of MS patients enrolled in clinical trials of therapy for MS. The immunological properties of the influx provide further insights into the cellular mechanisms by which IFN-γ could trigger relapses in MS. Finally, the exuberant responsiveness of influx-positive cells to cytokines and mitogens provides a possible explanation for the observation (63) that common viral infections (usually associated with moderate systemic production of IFN-γ) often precede clinical relapses in patients with MS.

ACKNOWLEDGMENTS

We thank Prof. Nicola Canal and Prof. Giancarlo Comi for their continuous support. We thank Prof. Jacopo Meldolesi and Dr. Emilio Clementi for the fruitful collaboration in the development of this research. We are indebted with Drs. Elena Brambilla and Lucia Moiola for their essential contributions to these investigations. We thank collaborative efforts in providing patients and elaborating clinical data from Drs. Bruno Colombo, Silvia Mammi, Vittorio Martinelli, Marco Rovaris, Mariaemma Rodegher, Antonella Poggi, and the staff of the San Raffaele Multiple Sclerosis Center. We thank Prof. Giuseppe Scotti and Drs. Adriana Campi and Massimo Filippi for helping in MRI data collection and interpretation.

This work was in part supported by the Associazione Italiana Sclerosi Multipla (AISM) and the Italian Research Council (CNR).

REFERENCES

1. Gray PW, Goeddel DV. Structure of the human immune interferon gene. Nature 1982; 298:859–863.
2. Gray PW, Leung DW, Pennica D, Yelverton E, Najarian R, Simonsen CC, Derynck R, Sherwood PJ, Wallace DM, Berger SL, Levinson AD, Goeddel

DV. Expression of human immune interferon cDNA in E. coli and monkey cells. Nature 1982; 295:503–508.

3. Naylor SL, Sakaguchi AY, Shows TB, Law ML, Goeddel DV, Gray PW. Human immune interferon gene is located on chromosome 12. J Exp Med 1983; 157:1020–1027.

4. Trinchieri G, Perussia B. Immune interferon: a pleiotropic lymphokine with multiple effects. Immunol Today 1985; 6:131–136.

5. De Maeyer E, De Maeyer-Guignard J. Interferons. In: Thomson A, ed. The Cytokine Handbook. San Diego: Academic Press, 1994:265–288.

6. Aguet M, Dembic Z, Merlin G. Molecular cloning and expression of the human interferon-γ receptor. Cell 1988; 55:273–280.

7. Soh J, Donnelly RJ, Kotenko S, Mariano TM, Cook JR, Wang N, Emanuel S, Schwartz B, Miki T, Pestka S. Identification and sequence of an accessory factor required for activation of the human interferon gamma receptor. Cell 1994; 76:793–802.

8. Watling D, Guschin D, Muller M, Silvennoinen O, Witthuhn BA, Quelle FW, Rogers NC, Schindler C, Stark GR, Ihle JN, Kerr IM. Complementation by the protein tyrosine kinase JAK2 of a mutant cell line defective in the interferon-γ signal transduction pathway. Nature 1993; 366:166–170.

9. Muller M, Briscoe J, Laxton C, Guschin D, Ziemiecki A, Silvennoinen O, Harpur AG, Barbieri G, Witthuhn BA, Schindler C, Pellegrini S, Wilks AF, Ihle JN, Stark GR, Kerr IM. The protein tyrosine kinase JAK1 complements defects in interferon-α/β and -γ signal transduction. Nature 1993; 366: 129–135.

10. Shuai K, Strak GR, Kerr IM, Darnell JE. A single phosphotyrosine residue of Stat91 required for gene activation by interferon-γ. Science 1993; 261: 1744–1746.

11. Pellegrini S, Schindler C. Early events in signalling by interferons. Trends Biol Sci 1993; 18:338–342.

12. Shuai K. Interferon-activated signal transduction to the nucleus. Curr Opin Cell Biol 1994; 6:253–259.

13. Reder A, Arnason BGW. Immunology of multiple sclerosis. In: Vinken PJ, Bruyn GW, Klawans HL, and Koetsier JC, eds. Handbook of Clinical Neurology, Vol. 3 (47). Amsterdam: Elsevier, 1985:337–395.

14. Olsson T. Immunology of MS. Curr Opin Neurol Neurosurg 1992; 5:195–202.

15. Martin R, McFarland HF, McFarlin DE. Immunological aspects of demyelinating diseases. Annu Rev Immunol 1992; 10:153–187.

16. Weiss A, Littman DR. Signal transduction by lymphocyte antigen receptors. Cell 1994; 76:263–274.

17. Paul WE, Seder RA. Lymphocyte responses and cytokines. Cell 1994; 76: 241–251.

18. Olsson T. Role of cytokines in multiple sclerosis and experimental allergic encephalomyelitis. Eur J Neurol 1994; 1:7–19.

19. Panitch HS, Hirsch RL, Haley AS, Johnson KP. Exacerbation of multiple sclerosis in patients treated with gamma interferon. Lancet 1987; 1:893–895.

20. Panitch HS, Hirsch RL, Schindler J, Johnson KP. Treatment of multiple sclerosis with gamma interferon: exacerbations associated with activation of the immune system. Neurology 1987; 37:1097–1102.

21. Beck J, Rondot P, Catinot L, Falcoff E, Kirchner H, Wietzerbin J. Increased production of interferon gamma and tumor necrosis factor precedes clinical manifestation in MS: Do cytokines trigger off exacerbations? Acta Neurol Scand 1988; 78:318–323.

22. Link J, Soderstrom M, Olsson T, Hojeberg B, Ljungdahl A, Link H. Increased transforming growth factor-beta, interleukin-4, and interferon-gamma in multiple sclerosis. Ann Neurol 1994; 36:379–386.

23. The IFN-Beta Multiple Sclerosis Study Group. Interferon beta-1b is effective in relapsing-remitting multiple sclerosis. I. Clinical results of a multicenter, ramdomized, double-blind, placebo-controlled trial. Neurology 1993; 43: 655–661.

24. Jacobs LD, Cookfair DL, Rudick RA, Herndon RM, Richert JR, Salazar AM, et al. Intramuscular interferon beta-1α for disease progression in relapsing multiple sclerosis. Ann Neurol 1996; 39:285–294.

25. Paty DW, Li DKB, the UCB MS/MRI study group, and the IFN-beta MS study group. Interferon beta-1b is effective in relapsing-remitting MS: II. MRI analysis results of a multicenter, randomized, double-blind, placebo-controlled trial. Neurology 1993; 43:662–667.

26. Weinstock-Guttman B, Ransohoff RM, Kinkel RP, Rudick RA. The interferons: biological effects, mechanisms of action, and use in multiple sclerosis. Ann Neurol 1995; 37:7–15.

27. Traugott U, Lebon P. Demonstration of α, β and γ interferon in active chronic multiple sclerosis lesions. Ann NY Acad Sci 1988; 540:309–311.

28. Traugott U, Lebon P. Interferon-γ and Ia antigens are present on astrocytes in active chronic multiple sclerosis lesions. J Neuroimmunol 1988; 84: 257–264.

29. Fierz W, Endler B, Reske K, Wekerle H, Fontana A. Astrocytes as antigen presenting cells. I. Induction of Ia antigen expression on astrocytes by T cells via immune-interferon, and its effect on antigen presentations. J Immunol 1985; 134:3785–3793.

30. Cannella B, Raine CS. Cytokines up-regulate Ia expression in organotypic cultures of central nervous system. J Neuroimmunol 1989; 24:239–248.

31. Duijvestijn AM, Schreiber AB, Butcher EC. Interferon-gamma regulates an antigen specific for endothelial cells involved in lymphocyte traffic. Proc Natl Acad Sci USA 1986; 83:9114–9118.

32. Tsukada N, Matsuda M, Miyagi K, Yanagisawa N. Adhesion of cerebral endothelial cells to lymphocytes from patients with multiple sclerosis. Autoimmunity 1993; 14:329–333.

33. Collart MA, Belin D, Vassalli JD, de Kossodo S, Vassalli P. Gamma-interferon enhances macrophage transcription of the tumor necrosis factor/cachetin, interleukin-1 and urokinase genes, which are controlled by short-lived repressors. J Exp Med 1986; 164:2113–2118.

34. Selmaj K, Raine CS. Tumor necrosis factor mediates myelin and oligodendrocyte damage in vitro. Ann Neurol 1988; 23:339–346.
35. Hartung H-P, Jung S, Stoll G, Zielasek J, Schmidt B, Archelos JJ, Toyka KV. Inflammatory mediators in demyelinating disorders of the CNS and PNS. J Neuroimmunol 1992; 40:197–210.
36. Renno T, Lin JY, Piccirillo C, Antel J, Owens T. Cytokine production by cells in cerebrospinal fluid during experimental allergic encephalomyelitis in SJL/J mice. J Neuroimmunol 1994; 49:1–7.
37. McCarron RM, Racke M, Spatz M, McFarlin DE. Cerebral vascular endothelial cells are effective targets for in vitro lysis by encephalitogenic T lymphocytes. J Immunol 1991; 147:503–508.
38. Nisbet-Brown E, Cheung RK, Lee JWW, Gelfand EW. Antigen-dependent increase in cytosolic free calcium in specific human T-lymphocyte clones. Nature 1985; 316:545–547.
39. Negulescu PA, Shastri N, Cahalan MD. Intracellular calcium dependence of gene expression in single T lymphocytes. Proc Natl Acad Sci USA 1994; 91:2873–2877.
40. Berridge M. Inositol trisphosphate and calcium signaling. Nature 1993; 361: 315–325.
41. Putney JW, Bird GSJ. The signal for capacitative calcium entry. Cell 1993; 75:199–201.
42. Tsien RW, Tsien RY. Calcium channels, stores, and oscillations. Annu Rev Cell Biol 1990; 6:715–760.
43. Meldolesi J, Clementi E, Fasolato C, Zacchetti D, Pozzan T. Ca^{2+} influx following receptor activation. Trends Pharmacol Sci 1991; 12:289–292.
44. Sontheimer H. Ion channels in inexcitable cells. Neuroscientist 1995; 1: 64–67.
45. Randriamampita C, Tsien RY. Emptying of intracellular Ca^{2+} stores releases a novel small messenger that stimulates Ca^{2+} influx. Nature 1993; 364: 809–814.
46. Martino G, Clementi E, Brambilla E, Comi G, Meldolesi J, Grimaldi LME. γ-interferon activates a previously undescribed Ca^{2+} influx in T-lymphocytes from MS patients. Proc Natl Acad Sci USA 1994; 91:4825–4829.
47. Martino G, Filippi M, Martinelli V, Brambilla E, Comi G, Grimaldi LME. Clinical and radiological correlates of a novel T lymphocyte γ-interferon–activated Ca^{2+} influx in patients with relapsing-remitting multiple sclerosis. Neurology 1996; 46:1416–1421.
48. Martino G, Moiola L, Brambilla E, Clementi E, Comi G, Grimaldi LME. Interferon-γ induces T lymphocyte proliferation in multiple sclerosis via a calcium-dependent mechanism. J Neuroimmunol 1995; 62:169–176.
49. Grynkiewicz G, Poenie M, Tsien RY. A new generation of Ca^{2+} indicators with greatly improved fluorescence properties. J Biol Chem 1985; 260: 3440–3450.
50. Clementi E, Scheer H, Zacchetti D, Fasolato C, Pozzan T, Meldolesi J. Receptor-activated Ca^{2+} influx: two independently regulated mechanisms

of influx stimulation coexist in neurosecretory PC12 cells. J Biol Chem 1992; 267:2164–2172.

51. Hamilton TA, Becton DL, Somers SD, Gray PW, Adams DO. Interferon-γ modulates protein kinase C activity in murine peritoneal macrophages. J Biol Chem 1985; 260:1378–1381.

52. Poser CM, Paty DW, Scheinberg L, McDonald WI, Davis FA, Ebers GC, Johnson KP, Sibley WA, Silberberg DH, Tourtellotte WW. New diagnostic criteria for MS: guidelines for research protocols. Ann Neurol 1983; 13: 227–231.

53. Katz D, Taubenberger JK, Cannella B, McFarlin DE, Raine CS, McFarland HF. Correlation between magnetic resonance imaging findings and lesion development in chronic, active multiple sclerosis. Ann Neurol 1993; 34: 661–669.

54. Filippi M, Yousry T, Campi A, Kandziora C, Colombo B, Voltz R, Martinelli V, Spuler S, Bressi S, Scotti G, Comi G. Comparison of triple dose versus standard dose gadolinium-DTPA for detection of MRI enhancing lesions in patients with MS. Neurology 1996; 46:379–384.

55. Scolozzi R, Boccafogli A, Tola MR, Vicentini L, Camerani A, Degani D, Granieri E, Caniatti L, Paolino E. T cell phenotypic profiles in the cerebrospinal fluid and peripheral blood of multiple sclerosis patients. J Neurol Sci 1992; 108:93–98.

56. Porrini AM, Gambi D, Malatesta G. Memory and naive CD4$^+$ lymphocytes in multiple sclerosis. J Neurol 1992; 239:437–440.

57. Filippini G, Comi GC, Cosi V, Bevilacqua L, Ferrarini M, Martinelli V, Bergamaschi R, Filippi M, Citterio A, D'Incerti L. Sensitivities and predictive values of paraclinical tests for diagnosing multiple sclerosis. J Neurol 1994; 241:132–137.

58. Matsiota-Bernard P, Roullet E, Regimbeau J, Avrameas S. T cell activation by autoantigens in multiple sclerosis. Autoimmunity 1994; 16:237–243.

59. Zhang J, Markovic-Plese S, Lacet B, Raus J, Weiner H, Hafler DA. Increased frequency of interleukin 2-responsive T cells specific for myelin basic protein in peripheral blood and cerebrospinal fluid of patients with multiple sclerosis. J Exp Med 1994; 179:973–984.

60. Lau LL, Jamieson BD, Somasundaram T, Ahmed R. Cytotoxic T cell memory without antigen. Nature 1994; 369:648–652.

61. Sprent J. T and B memory cells. Cell 1994; 76:315–322.

62. Stout R, Suttles J. T cells bearing the CD44^{hi} "memory" phenotype display characteristics of activated cells in G1 stage of cell cycle. Cell Immunol 1992; 141:433–443.

63. Sibley WA, Bamford CR, Clark K. Clinical viral infections and MS. Lancet 1985; 1:1313–1315.

64. Pinto LH, Holsinger LJ, Lamb RA. Influenza virus M2 protein has ion channel activity. Cell. 1992; 69:517–528.

65. Wang C, Lamb RA, Pinto LH. Direct measurement of the influenza A virus

M2 protein ion channel activity in mammalian cells. Virology 1994; 205: 133–140.

66.   Juliano DL, Haskill S. Signal transduction from the extracellular matrix. J Cell Biol 1993; 268:18427–18430.

67.   Collins TL, Kassner PD, Bierer BE, Burakoff SJ. Adhesion receptors in lymphocyte activation. Curr Opin Immunol 1994; 6:385–393.

9

The Effects of Interferons and Other Cytokines on Experimental Autoimmune Encephalomyelitis

Hubertine Heremans and Alfons Billiau

Rega Institute, University of Leuven, Leuven, Belgium

I. INTRODUCTION

Experimental autoimmune encephalomyelitis (EAE) is a frequently used animal model for inflammatory and demyelinating disease of the human central nervous system (CNS); for example, multiple sclerosis (MS). Various acute and chronic relapsing forms of EAE can be induced actively in many susceptible animal species (monkeys, rats, guinea pigs, mice) by immunization with xenogeneic or allogeneic spinal cord homogenates, myelin basic protein (MBP) and its relevant peptide fragments, or proteolipid protein (PLP), together with one or several immune adjuvants (Freund's, *Mycobacterium* tuberculosis, *Bordetella pertussis*) (reviewed in refs. 1 and 2). EAE can also be induced by adoptive transfer of MBP-specific T cells or T-cell clones (see ref. 1). The chronic progressive and/or relapsing forms of EAE may represent especially relevant models for MS.

Immunological processes are widely accepted to contribute to the pathogenesis of MS and EAE (see ref. 1). The contribution of immunocompetent cells to lesion formation is strongly supported by the presence of numerous inflammatory cells, T lymphocytes, macrophages, and polymorphonuclear cells within perivascular infiltrates and demyelinating areas. It has been suggested that the initial stages of demyelination are caused by these cell types. Brain-invading macrophages and activated

CD4⁺ T helper cells specific for MBP are the main effector cells mediating EAE and involved in myelin destruction (2,3). How these cells gain access to the CNS and how the presence and activity of these cells lead to inflammatory and demyelinating lesions in the CNS is presently poorly understood. Susceptibility to EAE is dependent on class II major histocompatibility complex (MHC) alleles and brain antigens (see ref. 2). T cells confronted with their corresponding antigen in the CNS may cause damage by direct destructive contact with neurons or glial components, or they may locally secrete soluble factors which directly or indirectly are responsible for the damage. In recent years, there has been increasing evidence that the transient and local release of multiple cytokines within the CNS from the invading cell population, as well as from cells residing within the CNS such as astrocytes and microglia (reviewed in ref. 4) may contribute to the initiation of and chronic damage in EAE, and this may also play a role in disease remission.

EAE is a prototypic autoimmune disease produced by Th1-like cells specific for MBP. In animals, two types of murine CD4⁺ T helper subsets have been defined based on their cytokine production patterns and specific functions (reviewed in ref. 5). These are Th1 cells which produce interferon-γ (IFN-γ), lymphotoxin, interleukin-2 (IL-2), and IL-3 and play a major role in the delayed-type hypersensitive (DTH) reaction, and Th2 cells mainly producing IL-4, IL-5, IL-6, and IL-10, which are involved in antibody-mediated responses. Since the Th1 and Th2 subpopulations interact and cross regulate each other's growth and function (reviewed in ref. 6), it is considered likely that the course of autoimmune diseases is influenced by an interplay between Th1 and Th2 cytokines. Analysis of cytokine profiles in the CNS of animals with EAE by mRNA expression and immunocytochemical staining have demonstrated that the onset of the disease is associated with elevated levels of typical Th1 cytokines, IFN-γ, lymphotoxin, and IL-2 (7–10). In contrast, IL-4, a cytokine produced by Th2 cells, appeared transiently later in the course of disease as symptoms began to resolve (9). Recovery from disease seems to be paralleled by a switch from Th1-dominated to Th2-dominated intracerebral cytokine synthesis with a decline in IFN-γ and IL-2 (8,9) and a concomitant rise in IL-10 within the inflammatory focus (8).

However, the effects of individual cytokines are pleiotropic and depend on the cell target type and its activation state. They may have additive, synergistic, or antagonistic effects and can induce the synthesis of one another. Therefore, it seems clear that it will be difficult precisely to dissect the functions of any particular cytokine. Nevertheless, the detection of cytokines in the CNS, their in vitro functions, and their correlation with disease severity as well as the passive transfer of cytokines and their antagonists have helped to generate a picture of balance between disease-promoting and disease-limiting cytokines. In this chapter, the current knowledge of interferons and others cytokines as mediators of EAE is reviewed. For more detailed information on cytokine function, we will refer to the numerous references in exellent review articles.

II. ROLE OF TH1 CYTOKINES IN EAE

The predominance of Th1 cytokines IFN-γ, IL-2, and tumor necrosis factor (TNF) within the CNS early in the disease process (7–10) is typical for a Th1-type immune response and suggests that they are operative as proinflammatory cytokines in EAE.

A. IFN-γ

EAE lesions originate from proliferation and activity of MBP-specific CD4$^+$ lymphocytes of the Th1-like phenotype (see Ref. 2). IFN-γ is one of the cytokines produced by these cells after exposure to antigens or other stimuli. In mice and humans the suppressor-cytotoxic CD8$^+$ subset of T cells and natural killer (NK) cells are also able to produce IFN-γ (reviewed in Ref. 11). In vitro studies have demonstrated that effector T cells from rats previously challenged with MBP in complete Freund's adjuvant produce IFN-γ when cultured in the presence of the protein (12). It has to be noted that IFN-γ production by T and NK cells is regulated by IL-12 (reviewed in Ref. 13), and the generation of CD4$^+$ Th1 cells depends on the coordinate action of IL-12 and IFN-γ (14). Recently, an immunoregulatory role of IL-12 in EAE was demonstrated (15). IL-12 enhanced the in vitro activation of encephalitogenic T cells, and administration of IL-12 following adoptive transfer of PLP–stimulated lymph node cells accelerated EAE, whereas blocking of endogenous IL-12 completely prevented disease progression.

1. Effects of IFN-γ Relevant to the Pathogenesis of EAE

IFN-γ is a cytokine with several immunoregulatory activities (reviewed in Ref. 16) that could in different ways contribute to the pathogenesis of EAE. IFN-γ is known as the most potent inducer of class II MHC antigen expression on various cell types in vitro, including cerebral vascular endothelial cells, astrocytes, and microglia, which in EAE have been shown to play an important role as presenters of MBP antigen to encephalitogenic T cells (reviewed in Ref. 4). In animals with EAE, there is a marked elevation of class II MHC antigen expression. The elevation is mainly on microvascular endothelial cells, but it also occurs on infiltrating macrophages and microglia, probably induced by IFN-γ produced by the invading T cells. Following intracerebral injection of IFN-γ, MHC class II antigen expression increases on microglia and perivascular cells (17). Although class II antigen expression on astrocytes has been conclusively demonstrated in vitro, in vivo studies have generated conflicting results (see Ref. 4). With some exceptions, most studies fail to detect class II antigen-positive astrocytes in the CNS of rats and mice during the disease process. However, class II antigen expression on astrocytes was reported in active MS lesions, indicating that the ability of astrocytes to function as antigen-presenting cells in vivo may only be relevant in certain disease models and may be different between rodents and humans.

IFN-γ also influences production as well as activity of other cytokines (TNF-α, IL-1) (see Ref. 16) and other mediators of inflammation that play an important role in the pathogenesis of EAE (reviewed in Ref. 18). This is of particular importance for mediators released by macrophages and macrophage-like cells such as endothelial cells, astrocytes, and microglia. For instance, production of proteases by these cells is thought to be responsible for destruction of myelin (reviewed in Ref. 19). In addition, IFN-γ synergizes with TNF-α, a cytokine that exerts a disease-promoting effect in EAE (see below), probably by increasing the number of receptors for TNF-α on a variety of different cells (see Ref. 16).

IFN-γ induces molecules on endothelial cells involved in T-cell homing. Adhesion to the endothelial cell wall is a critical step in regulating the recruitment of MBP-specific T cells and the subsequent influx of additional inflammatory cells (monocytes, granulocytes) from the circulation into the CNS. Thus, IFN-γ causes increased lymphocyte adhesion to microvascular endothelial cells derived from the CNS (20,21) and even migration through endothelial cell layers in vitro (22). After intracerebral injection or microinjection of IFN-γ into the lumbosacral spinal cords of rats, an influx of lymphocytes and other inflammatory cells into the CNS was noted (17,23). Increased expression of endothelial adhesion molecules may underly this action of IFN-γ. For instance, IFN-γ upregulates intercellular adhesion molecule-1 (ICAM-1) on brain microvascular endothelial cells in vitro (24,25). There have also been several reports of fluctuating patterns of elevated levels of ICAM-1 and vascular adhesion molecule-1 (VCAM-1) on CNS endothelial cells during EAE, corresponding to periods of clinical disease (7,26,27). Recently, the involvement of IFN-γ in the expression of VCAM-1 in vivo has been demonstrated; anti–IFN-γ antibody treatment inhibits the upregulation of VCAM-1 in a passive-transfer EAE model (28).

Finally, IFN-γ has a profound antiproliferative effect on the Th2 subset of murine CD4$^+$ cells (see Ref. 6), thereby eliminating a key cellular source for IL-4 and IL-10. IFN-γ blocks the production of IL-10 by monocytes (29) and diminishes the ability to produce IL-4 in an immune response (see Ref. 6), thereby reducing or interfering with the merely antiinflammatory properties of these cytokines.

Taken together, these data show that IFN-γ exerts many effects on macrophages, endothelial cells and resident cells of the CNS that suggest a predominantly disease-promoting role of IFN-γ in EAE.

2. IFN-γ Production in EAE

In animals, IFN-γ has been detected in cerebrospinal fluid (CSF) during infections of the CNS but not in noninfectious inflammatory diseases of the CNS, such as EAE (30,31). However, with sensitive methods, individual IFN-γ–secreting cells can be detected in peripheral lymphoid organs and, more intriguingly, in the CNS of animals with acute and passively induced EAE (7–10,32–34). The presence of IFN-γ within the CNS correlated with disease severity and occurred predominantly on inflammatory cells, which is consistent with previous observations correlating disease progression with infiltrations of effector CD4$^+$ T cells, a major source of this cytokine. The highest levels of IFN-γ were observed at the peak of disease activity and during relapses; IFN-γ levels were very low or absent in recovered and refractory animals. It is interesting to note that IFN-γ had persistent expression into the early chronic stages of EAE (8). Persistent local production of IFN-γ could exacerbate the inflammatory lesions, perhaps by contributing to reactive gliosis of astrocytes (35).

3. In Vivo Evidence for the Involvement of IFN-γ in EAE

Since IFN-γ is present in the CNS, and since many facets of the immune system which are influenced by IFN-γ are important in EAE, it is reasonable to expect that IFN-γ would promote EAE. In a single study on patients with MS, systemic treatment with IFN-γ was associated with exacerbated disease symptoms (36). However, in rodents, the effects of IFN-γ have been variable.

Studies done in our laboratory (31) and confirmed by others (37–39) have shown that in rodents, treatment with neutralizing anti–IFN-γ monoclonal antibody (mAb) leads to a significant exacerbation of EAE induced by either active immunization or passive transfer and to increased mortality, even in strains which are relatively resistant to the disease (31,39,40). The disease-enhancing effect is observed only when the MoAb is given early; that is, shortly after immunization or at the time of passive cell transfer but not at later times (31,38,39), indicating that the effect of anti–IFN-γ MoAb is exerted early in the induction phase of the disease. In addition, IFN-γ receptor knockout mice are more susceptible to induction of EAE than their wild-type littermates (H. Heremans et al., unpublished data; 39a). These results indicate that IFN-γ is indeed produced during the development of EAE and plays a disease-limiting rather than a disease-promoting role as was expected from in vitro studies.

The enhancing effect of anti-IFN-γ is consistent with the observation that, in mice, exogenously administered IFN-γ ameliorates the actively-induced EAE reaction (31). This protective role is not observed when EAE is induced using the passive T cell transfer protocol (39). In rats, systemic administration of IFN-γ does not change the disease course of EAE, whereas intracerebral injection of IFN-γ shortly before the onset of clinical signs resulted in a complete suppression of clinical signs (37). These findings again support the notion that IFN-γ plays a disease-limiting role early in the development of EAE.

4. Mechanisms Involved

The exact mechanisms by which IFN-γ exerts its suppressive action have as yet not been unraveled. Several explanations are possible for the disease-limiting effect of IFN-γ. It is tempting to speculate that IFN-γ has a dual role, as revealed by studies on inflammation in non-CNS tissue (41). At the local level IFN-γ may promote inflammation, whereas at the systemic level, it may act in an anti-inflammatory fashion. This two-sided effect of IFN-γ has also been suggested for EAE (31). It is possible that systemically administered antibodies do not cross the blood-brain barrier (BBB) and hence may not neutralize endogenous IFN-γ secreted by activated T cells in the CNS. Therefore, the antibodies may only counteract the systemic anti-inflammatory activity of IFN-γ with the net result of enhanced EAE.

Some in vitro and in vivo functions of IFN-γ suggest that systemic IFN-γ may serve as a physiological regulator of a suppressor mechanism in EAE. The abrogation of this regulatory mechanism by anti-IFN-γ administration might cause a more severe form of EAE. For instance, IFN-γ may facilitate the induction of T suppressor cells by antigen-presenting cells in vitro (42,43). T helper cells can be functionally inactivated, possibly through the influence of T suppressor cells (reviewed in ref. 43). It has also been demonstrated that IFN-γ can induce Th1 cell death in the absence of costimulatory cells (44,45). The CNS may lack costimulatory factors and allow apoptosis. A relationship between increased MHC class II antigen expression and suppression of EAE has also been suggested (37). Furthermore, IFN-γ is a potent activator of macrophages (see ref. 16). Macrophages are able to exert a suppressive action on the immune system (46), and IFN-γ can inhibit macrophage-induced antigen-specific T-cell proliferation (47,48). IFN-γ is also a potent inducer of nitric oxide (NO) (see ref. 16). Recently, an immunosuppressive role for NO produced by infiltrating macrophages during EAE has been reported (49). Macrophages isolated from CNS cell suspensions of rats with EAE produced large amounts of NO, whereas in vivo treatment with an antibody to NO synthetase, either intraperitoneally or intracerebrally, resulted in a marked aggravation of the disease. IFN-γ may also affect secretion of other cytokines implicated in EAE. IFN-γ has been reported to be required for release of the active form of transforming growth factor-β (TGF-β) from human monocytes (50). On the other hand, TGF-β downregulates IFN-γ production by T effector cells (51). It is therefore tempting to speculate that a feedback regulatory loop exists between IFN-γ and TGF-β, and that neutralization of IFN-γ may prevent TGF-β release. Finally, IFN-γ downregulates the induction of IL-8 by IL-1 and IL-2 in monocytes, and as such may act as a repressor of neutrophil chemotaxis in EAE (52). An altered trafficking of immune cells caused by IFN-γ acting on endothelial cells has also been suggested (see ref. 53). Systemic IFN-γ could allow non–Ag-specific extravasation of activated T cells into peripheral tissues and blunt brain inflammation, whereas anti–IFN-γ antibodies would lower adhesion molecule expression at irrelevant sites and favor homing into the CNS.

A clear-cut explanation for the contrasting effect of IFN-γ treatment in MS patients compared with EAE is not available. The discrepancy may be due to differences in dosage, treatment schedules, or timing. It may be connected to the fact that these patients had already undergone some overt clinical episodes and were in remission at the time of IFN-γ treatment. Further experimentation is required to determine the molecular mechanisms responsible for the seemingly contradictory roles of IFN-γ in EAE and MS.

B. IL-2

IL-2, a primary product of stimulated Th1 cells, not only acts as an autocrine growth factor but is also implicated in the proliferation of B cells, NK cells, macrophages, and oligodendrocytes (reviewed in ref. 54). The biological effects of IL-2 are mediated through its binding to the high-affinity IL-2 receptor (IL-2R) expressed on these various cell types. IFN-γ is an inducer for IL-2R on monocytes and macrophages.

Numerous reports support the idea that an endogenously hyperactivated or hyperactive IL-2/IL-2R system is involved in a series of immunological reactions that lead to autoimmune tissue injury (reviewed in ref. 55). As for EAE, it has been demonstrated that IL-2 is produced by encephalitogenic T cells (56). After intracerebral injection of IL-2, the BBB is disrupted and inflammatory cells are recruited to the site of injection

(57). Analysis of the cells infiltrating the CNS in animals with EAE showed that a large proportion of them bear the IL-2 receptor (58). A marked upregulation of IL-2R together with other cell surface molecules has been correlated with potent encephalitogenicity (59). Furthermore, analysis of intracerebral cytokine production during the acute exacerbation phase of EAE reveals a predominance of IL-2 and IFN-γ synthesis (7,8,10,33). IL-2 is an important stimulus for expression of inflammatory cytokine genes such as IL-1 and TNF in mononuclear phagocytes (60–62). Thus, secretion of IL-2 by activated lymphocytes recruited at the inflammatory site can control effector and regulatory functions of monocytes and may contribute to neutrophil recruitment by stimulating IL-8 secretion by monocytes (52). In addition, it has been suggested that IL-2 produced locally in CNS lesions may negatively affect the proliferation potential of oligodendrocytes and thus have an impact on whether remyelination and repair or gliosis and scar formation predominate (63).

A striking demonstration of the role of IL-2 in EAE was revealed by in vivo application of IL-2 or IL-2R antagonists. Treatment of rodents with antibodies directed against IL-2 (38) or IL-2R (64,65) blocked the development of EAE from passive transfer of MBP-specific T cells, but the antibodies failed to affect actively induced EAE. It was suggested that the discrepancy in therapeutic efficiency could be due to a different intensity of IL-2R expression on in vitro and in vivo activated MBP-specific T cells (65). Furthermore, IL-2–PE40, a chimeric protein which selectively kills proliferating IL-2R–bearing lymphocytes is effective in suppressing actively and passively induced EAE (66). Collectively, these studies imply a critical disease-promoting role of IL-2 in EAE.

C. TNF-α/Lymphotoxin

TNF-α and lymphotoxin (LT, TNF-β) are genetically and functionally related cytokines with pleiotropic biological effects (reviewed in refs. 67 and 68). The involvement of TNF in inflammatory, infectious, and certain autoimmune diseases is well documented.

In recent years, there is also increasing evidence implicating TNF-α and LT in the pathogenesis of MS and EAE. TNF-α is mainly produced by activated antigen-presenting cells, including microglia and astrocytes (see ref. 4), and it is present in these cells during EAE (69), whereas TNF-β (LT), primarily produced by activated Th1 lymphocytes, is expressed both by these Th1 cells and also microglia within the CNS white matter (70). In vitro, both cytokines cause myelin damage and death of oligodendrocytes (71,72). Encephalitogenicity of MBP-reactive T-cell clones is positively correlated with TNF secretion (73). Furthermore, T cells isolated from the CNS during active EAE exhibit a greater capacity to secrete TNF than T cells isolated from the peripheral organs during active disease (74). The different susceptibility of rat strains to develop EAE has been ascribed to differential TNF-α gene expression in astrocytes (75).

Evidence that LT/TNF play a role in the pathogenesis of EAE also comes from several in vivo studies. TNF-α has been identified in active EAE lesions (7,9,33), where it could contribute to chronic damage associated with reactive gliosis and demyelination by destruction of oligodendrocytes and myelin (71,72,76). Administration of exogenous TNF-α was found to augment actively induced EAE (77), whereas polyclonal and monoclonal TNF-α and β-specific antibodies or TNF antagonists, when administered systematically in multiple doses prior to disease onset, significantly inhibited disease progression of both passively transferred and actively induced EAE (69,78,79). A therapeutic effect was evident even when the antibody was administered after the onset of clinical signs, further indicating an important role for TNF in pathogenic effector mechanisms of EAE (69). A recent report has found that the incidence of relapses was decreased by weekly administration of anti–TNF-α MoAb to animals with CREAE induced by adoptive transfer (80). In most studies, however, clinical EAE develops rapidly following the cessation of antibody therapy (69,79), suggesting that immunotherapy does not exert an effect through generalized, long-term immunosuppression. Probably TNF secretion and activity is localized mainly in the CNS, as suggested by the detection of TNF in lesions within the CNS of animals with EAE (7,9,33,69). Also, intracranial administration of neutralizing MoAb is significantly more effective than systemic administration in inhibiting clinical signs of EAE (69).

The precise mechanisms by which anti-TNF therapy affects EAE and the relative involvement of TNF-α and TNF-β during EAE is currently unknown. TNF-α induces breakdown of the BBB (81) and causes the appearance of lesions typical of EAE following direct injection into the CNS (23). Although TNF exhibits a variety of proinflammatory effects (see ref. 67), it may particularly influence vascular permeability (82) and leukocyte extravasation through upregulation of leukocyte-endothelial adhesion molecules (ELAMs). TNF-α causes increased adhesiveness of the endothelial cell surface for leukocytes by inducing synthesis of ELAM-1 (83) and is the most potent inducer of ICAM-1 expression by rat astrocytes (84). In addition, microinjection of TNF-α into the spinal cord of rats is followed by expression of ICAM-1 on vascular endothelium and by accumulation of leukocytes at the injection site (85). Moreover, treatment with anti-TNF MoAb inhibits the upregulation of adhesion molecules expressed by the CNS vessels induced during adoptively transferred EAE

(28) and markedly reduces leukocyte infiltration into the CNS (28,79). TNF may also be involved in demyelination either directly (69) or indirectly by inducing the production of proteases (see ref. 19).

III. ROLE OF TH2 CYTOKINES IN EAE

In animals with EAE, the recovery phase is characterized by decreased expression of the Th1 cytokines, IL-2 and IFN-γ, and a concomitant upregulation of IL-4 and IL-10 in brain lesions (7–9), implicating a Th2 response as participating in suppressing inflammation of the CNS.

A. IL-6

IL-6 is a cytokine produced by a variety of cells, including monocytes, endothelial cells, activated T cells, fibroblasts, astrocytes, and microglia under a variety of circumstances, but in particular after stimulation by cytokines, bacterial LPS, or viral infections. The molecule affects the function of various cells and tissues (reviewed in ref. 86). It is a potent inducer of proliferation, activation, and differentiation of B and T cells. Hence, IL-6 can be inferred to play a role in the development of the reactive T cells responsible for lesion formation in EAE, and in antigen recognition by B cells producing antibodies. IL-6 is also involved in the regulation of production of acute phase proteins by hepatocytes (reviewed in ref. 87). These proteins appear in the circulation in various pathological conditions, especially as a result of extensive tissue damage, infection, or autoimmunity. Despite extensive investigation, their full significance remains largely a matter of speculation. The general assumption is that they serve to dampen tissue damage by counterregulating proinflammatory mediators. For instance, the acute-phase proteins include a variety of protease inhibitors (e.g., tissue inhibitors of proteases, plasminogen activator inhibitors). In addition, IL-6 may exert anti-inflammatory effects through its ability to inhibit production of other cytokines, such as TNF, an effect that occurs in vitro as well as in vivo (88). Finally, IL-6 also acts as a secretagogue for anterior pituitary hormones, including adrenocorticotropin (ACTH) (89). Via this pathway, it may enhance production of glucocorticoids, which exert an overall immunosuppressive and anti-inflammatory effect.

IL-6 is well known to appear in the circulation during almost every inflammatory condition of infectious and noninfectious nature, including autoimmunity (30). Increased levels of IL-6 have been found in the CNS of animals suffering from EAE associated with disease onset but not in their sera or spleens (90). These findings are indicative of local production of IL-6 in the CNS during EAE. Indeed, detailed immunohistology and polymerase chain reaction (PCR) analysis of CNS tissue from animals at the peak of the disease have shown increased expression of IL-6 (7,8). In contrast, little if any IL-6 has been detected in the CSF of MS patients (91,92). Possible explanations for this discrepancy between EAE and MS could be that IL-6 is only produced in MS when the disease is initiated or during exacerbations. Which cells do produce IL-6 within the CNS is at yet unclear, but possible candidates are either the infiltrating mononuclear cells (7) or resident neural cells. In this respect, it has been shown that virus-infected astrocytes can secrete IL-6 (93), and that cytokines present in the CNS during EAE, including IFNγ, IL-1β, and TNF-α, exert a strong inducing signal for IL-6 in primary rat astrocytes (75,94). Considering the effect of IL-6 on B cells, the increased production of IL-6 in EAE could explain the finding of raised Ig levels in the CSF of animals with EAE.

Taking into account the increased levels of IL-6 in the CNS of mice with developing EAE and the multiple biological effects this cytokine may exert, one can expect it to be involved in the disease process. However, whether it has a net in vivo proinflammatory or anti-inflammatory effect is difficult to predict. In a recent study, systemic administration of neutralizing antibodies to IL-6 reduced the development of actively induced as well as adoptively transferred EAE in mice (95), suggesting that IL-6 may promote the pathology in EAE. The reduction of EAE was paradoxically associated with elevated levels of IL-6 activity in the CSF and sera. In analogy with other experimental models of inflammatory conditions (96), the increased levels of IL-6 in sera and CNS are most probably due to delayed elimination and accrued accumulation of endogenous IL-6 as complexes with the injected antibody (97,98). Hence, it appears that treatment with anti–IL-6 antibody can result in increased and more prolonged exposure to endogenous IL-6. The protective effect of anti–IL-6, as noted in EAE, could indicate that endogenous IL-6 exerts a disease-limiting effect. If this hypothesis is correct, one can expect treatment with the cytokine itself to be beneficial in EAE. Although studies to that effect are as yet not available, a recent study reported that administration of recombinant human IL-6 suppresses demyelination in a murine model of MS induced by Theiler's murine encephalomyelitis virus (99).

One of the possible mechanisms by which IL-6 may exert a downregulating effect in EAE is by inducing potent and specific proteinase inhibitors. IL-6 increases synthesis of potent tissue inhibitors of metalloproteases (TIMPs) (100). Reduced extracellular proteolysis might limit the production of encephalitogenic peptides.

B. IL-4 and IL-10

IL-4 is a cytokine with marked immunoregulatory effects on B cells, T cells, and mononuclear phagocytes. It can affect numerous functions of mononuclear phagocytes in both a positive and a negative way (reviewed in ref. 101). IL-4 downregulates Th1 functions in mice and is a critical factor for the generation of Th2-like cells in vitro and in vivo (see ref. 6). Thus, the production of IL-4 during the course of an inflammatory autoimmune disease may induce or enhance Th2 cells and prevent the tissue-damaging effects of autoreactive Th1 cells. This concept is supported by the in vitro observation that CD4$^+$ T cells from animals recovered from EAE produce IL-4, but not IL-2 and IFN-γ, in response to a determinant associated with EAE effector cells. This suggests that T effector function may be regulated by IL-4 secreted by CD4$^+$ T suppressor cells (102). In addition, a Th2-type cell clone, recognizing epitopes within the encephalitogenic region of myelin proteolipid protein and producing IL-4 after stimulation, did not induce any signs of EAE, in contrast to an encephalitogenic Th1 cell clone which produced IL-2 and IFN-γ (103).

Involvement of IL-4 in EAE has been demonstrated by the detection of IL-4 within the CNS during the course of EAE, but some reports seem to be contradictory. In mice, IL-4 expression was very low or absent in the CNS during early disease, with a predominance of IFN-γ and IL-2 (9). Peak levels of IL-4 occurred during the acute phase of the disease, whereas stabilization of the clinical signs and the recovery phase were characterized by a rapid decline in expression of IL-4 together with IFN-γ and IL-2 (8). In contrast to these data, Khoury et al. (7) found that in rats IL-4 expression was absent at the peak of the disease but appeared in the target organ of recovering animals, whereas staining for inflammatory cytokines diminished. The differences in time course of IL-4 expression in the target organ may be a reflection of differences in animal strains and in disease models used. Recently, a therapeutic effect of IL-4 on EAE was reported (104). IL-4 treatment in mice with EAE resulted in an amelioration of clinical disease, diminished demyelination, and reduced gene expression of the inflammatory cytokines TNF-α and IL-2 in the CNS. In addition, T-cells from IL-4–treated animals showed a marked increase in IL-4 production on antigenic stimulation, and MBP-reactive T cells lost their encephalitogenicity after in vitro priming with IL-4. The investigators suggest that the therapeutic effect of IL-4 is related to the induction or enhancement of MBP-specific Th2-like cells in the treated animals. Probably, IL-4 also modulates disease activity by antagonizing the effects of pathogenic Th1 cytokines, such as IFN-γ, thereby inhibiting the production of inflammatory mediators, such as TNF-α or IL-1, by CNS macrophages or glial cells. IL-4 can antagonize many of the effects induced by

IFN-γ on both B cells (see ref. 101) and macrophages (e.g., 105,106). EAE-attenuating effects comparable to those reported for IL-4 can be observed after application of IL-13 (P600) (107), another typical Th2 cytokine with functions that overlap those of IL-4 (108). However, in mice which are deficient in IL-4 production and suffer from a profound disturbance of Th2 cell generation, the clinical course of EAE was not significantly different from that in control animals (109), indicating that Th2 cells and IL-4 alone do not mediate the immunosuppressive effect. Probably in their absence other immunosuppressive cytokines such as IL-10 and TGF-β take over their role.

IL-10, originally defined as a cytokine synthesis inhibitor factor, is also a product of activated Th2 cells, B cells, and macrophages. Current data favor the idea that IL-10 inhibits antigen-specific proliferation of Th1 cells by blocking synthesis of IFN-γ and/or antagonizing its activating effect on antigen-presenting cells by inhibiting production of TNF-α, IL-1, and IL-12 (reviewed in refs. 110 and 111). IL-10 may also indirectly enhance Th2 cell growth, as the decrease in IFN-γ levels should reduce their inhibitory effects on Th2 cell growth (see ref. 6). The known functions of IL-10 raise the possibility that IL-10 may act as a suppressor factor in certain T-cell–mediated autoimmune diseases or as an anti-inflammatory agent.

IL-10 is selectively upregulated in brain lesions of EAE-affected animals in the recovery phase. Levels of IL-10 correlate well with both the resolution of clinical symptoms and concomitant waining of Th1-like cytokine expression (8). In vitro, IL-10 can efficiently deactivate the two main effector cell populations in EAE; that is, encephalitogenic MBP-specific T cells and macrophages. IL-10 suppresses IFN-γ–induced MHC class II antigen upregulation in rat peritoneal macrophages and totally abrogates TNF production by encephalitogenic MBP-specific T lymphocytes (112). When administered systemically during the induction phase of the disease, IL-10 significantly suppresses the clinical course of EAE in rats (112). These in vivo effects of IL-10 administration are consistent with the ability of IL-10 to block the secretion of cytokines by activated macrophages and are probably due to an enhancement of Th2-like immune response.

Taken together, the findings suggest that in situations of Th1 cell–mediated autoimmune disease, recovery is associated with the activation of IL-4–secreting and IL-10–secreting Th2-type cells. The Th2 cells in turn regulate Th1 cells and thereby inhibit secretion of proinflammatory cytokines.

IV. ROLE OF NON–Tʜ CELL–RELATED CYTOKINES IN EAE

Some cytokine expression patterns in vivo do not fit the simple Th1/Th2 dichotomy. Although these two cytokine patterns are often found in strong responses, additional cytokines have been identified. One such example is EAE in which several other cytokines such as IFN-α/β, TGF-β, IL-1, and chemokines are produced and hence are implicated in the disease process.

A. IFN-α/β

Over the past few years, clinical trials have shown IFN-β to be beneficial in the treatment of MS. Many different cells can produce type I interferons (IFN-α or INF-β, or both). IFN-α is a product mainly of lymphocytes. IFN-β can be produced by virtually any cell infected with virus or given another appropriate stimulus. In addition, several growth factors and cytokines induce the synthesis of IFN-α and IFN-β (reviewed in ref. 113). For example, IL-2 induces the production of murine IFN-α/β in mouse bone marrow cells. IFN-γ can also act as an inducer of IFN-α or IFN-β.

In animals, studies have shown that IFN-α/β can exert a downregulating effect on the development of EAE. In rats both the active form of EAE and the adoptively transferred disease are inhibited by both natural and highly purified IFN-α/β administered during the induction phase (114,115,116). A similar effect has been reported to occur in EAE induced in SJL/J mice (31,116a). In these studies, inhibition was obtained by systemic treatment or by adding the IFN to the cultures before transfer. In addition, infection of mice with lactic dehydrogenase virus, known to act as an inducer of IFN-α/β, had a similar inhibitory effect (31,117). Human IFN-β, on the contrary, had no effect when similarly tested in the rat model, probably due to the known species specificity of IFNs (115). Recently, low doses of orally administered natural IFN-α/β have been shown to suppress clinical relapses and diminish inflammation in a murine model for chronic relapsing EAE (118) (see Chapter 10). In contrast, studies with intracerebrally injected IFN were inconclusive. Highly purified rat IFN-α/β was not effective in preventing or ameliorating the disease process in rats (119), whereas natural fibroblast-derived IFN had a beneficial effect (115). This discrepancy may possibly have been due to the fact that the natural rat IFN used was of low purity and may therefore have contained several other cytokines (see Chapter 11).

Although IFN-α/β has antiviral activity, and since viral infections are a common trigger for exacerbation in MS, there is little current support for the proposition that the beneficial effect of IFN-β results from attenuating viral infections. The downregulating effect of IFN-α/β in EAE may therefore stem from the immunomodulatory properties of this type of IFN. Among these properties are its ability to inhibit IFN-γ secretion by activated lymphocytes. Suppression of relapses by IFN-α/β correlates with decreased concavallin A (ConA)–stimulated IFN-γ secretion in spleen cells (118), and IFN-β limits IFN-γ production by activated lymphocytes from both MS patients and controls (120). IFN-α/β also antagonizes the effects of IFN-γ on macrophages. In this respect, IFN-β inhibits class II MHC antigen expression on the surface of antigen-presenting cells in vitro, such as macrophages and astrocytes (121,122). Thus, IFN-β lessens the capacity for antigen presentation to T cells and so might be expected to attenuate T-cell responses. T-cell proliferation in response to antigen presentation is a prominent feature of the induction phase of immune reactions. T-cell proliferation in vitro is inhibited by IFN-α β (118,120). Thus, in EAE and MS, IFN-β may curtail immune activation by decreasing T-cell proliferation, by blocking IFN-γ production, and by counteracting the peripheral actions of circulating IFN-γ directly. IFN-β may also lessen tissue damage by inhibiting release of TNF-α and LT (123), molecules reported to be toxic to oligodendrocytes (71,72). Finally, IFN-β may keep in check ongoing immune response by restoring T suppressor cell function. Human IFN-β augments suppressor cell activity in MS, at least in vitro (124,125). Alternatively, IFN-β may induce secretion of suppressor factors such as IL-10 or TGF-β (also see Chapter 7).

B. TGF-β

TGF-β belongs to a family of cytokines secreted by various cell types, including antigen-activated lymphocytes, macrophages, astrocytes, and microglia. It exhibits profound proinflammatory and anti-inflammatory activities (reviewed in ref. 126).

Accumulating evidence suggests that TGF-β may be another important molecule in the natural recovery from EAE. T suppressor cells that regulate recovery of rats from EAE secrete TGF-β (51). Moreover, long-term MBP-specific T-cell lines not only lose the ability to transfer EAE but actually secrete a suppressor factor that inhibits T-cell proliferation and can passively transfer protection to naive mice subsequently immunized with MBP (127,128). TGF-β was also found to be present in inflammatory lesions in the CNS during EAE both at the peak of disease activity and in the early remission phase (129,130), and TGF-β is expressed de novo in brains of recovering animals (7).

Several in vivo studies have shown that small amounts of TGF-β reduce the incidence and severity of EAE in both acute and adoptive EAE (80,129,131,132) even when given during ongoing disease. TGF-β also abrogates the ability of encephalitogenic T cells to transfer EAE in naive animals (132). The protection is accompanied by a marked reduction of inflammation and demyelination in the CNS (129,132). In addition, when TGF-β is given to mice with chronic relapsing disease after the expression of clinical signs or during remission, the severity and occurrence of relapses is drastically reduced (131,132). On the other hand, administration of anti–TGF-β leads to a worsening of the clinical course of acute EAE with more extensive pathological lesions (80,130,133), and treatment during remission accelerates and increases the severity of relapses (80). Although, in general, TGF-β has a suppressive effect on EAE, Weinberger et al. (134) found that TGF-β potentiated the encephalitogenic capacity of PLP-specific T cells to transfer EAE and to induce a more extensive demyelination in the spinal cord. Some of the discrepancies could be explained by the assumption that the effect of TGF-β may vary according to the differentiation state of the responding T cells (132), the dose, and contact time used (134). The effects of TGF-β may follow a biphasic dose-response curve, with lower doses enhancing and higher doses inhibiting disease potential (see ref. 126).

A number of mechanisms have been proposed to explain the involvement of TGF-β in disease remission. First, in view of its inhibitory effect on T-cell proliferation (see ref. 126), TGF-β may inhibit the development of autoantigen-specific T cells. TGF-β inhibits Ag-specific proliferation of MBP-specific T-cell lines or sensitized T cells (135) and reduces the capacity of these cells to transfer EAE in rats and mice (80,132). Second, TGF-β can also interfere with adhesion of lymphocytes and neutrophils to blood vessel endothelia (136,137), thereby possibly inhibiting the entry of effector cells into the CNS. In this respect, TGF-β counteracts the effects of IFN-γ, TNF-α, and IL-1 all of which increase the adhesiveness of the endothelial cell. Third, TGF-β may protect against the induction of EAE by antagonizing the production of IFN-γ, TNF-α, TNF-β, IL-1, and IL-2 as well as some of their effects, thereby interfering with inflammatory processes inside the CNS. In vitro, exogenous TGF-β modulates the production of cytokines (see ref. 126); it downregulates the production of IFN-γ (51) and TNF-α/LT (138) by effector cells that mediate EAE. In addition, TGF-β has downregulating effects on MHC class II antigen expression by IFN-γ and TNF-α (see refs. 126 and 139) and on CNS endothelial cells during EAE (132). Exposure of host endothelial cells, microglia, and astrocytes to TGF-β could render these cells resistant to IFN-γ–induced MHC class II molecule upregulation and subsequently affect antigen presentation to T cells. TGF-β may also decrease CNS tissue damage by deactivating IFN-γ–induced macrophage activation (see refs. 126 and 140) and inhibiting natural as well as IFN-γ–induced cytotoxicity of microglia toward oligodendrocytes, as was shown in vitro (141). Finally, TGF-β also induces TIMP and represses the formation of metalloproteinases (see ref. 19).

Taken together, it is possible that the secretion of TGF-β by lymphocytes in an acute EAE lesion eventually leads to a remission by downregulating class II molecules and by changing the cytokine profiles of infiltrating cells and surrounding glia. This could suppress proliferation of the invading cells and promote recovery from inflammation, thus leading to a clinical remission.

C. IL-1

IL-1α and IL-1β are produced by a variety of cells, including activated macrophages, endothelial cells, microglial cells, and astrocytes (reviewed in refs. 142 and 143). IL-1 exerts a wide range of immunoregulatory functions on cells, organs, and the whole body, and it is implicated in the host response to inflammatory reactions, including those in the CNS. Many of these effects are mediated by other cytokines induced by IL-1. It stimulates numerous cell types, including astrocytes, to produce various cytokines such as IL-6, TNF-α, several chemokines, and IL-1 itself (see refs. 4, 142 and 143). In addition, IL-1 and TNF share several biological properties and synergize in a number of phenomena.

The implication of IL-1 in EAE stems from the fact that it is found within the CNS during the disease process, that inhibition of IL-1 activity can prevent CNS inflammation, and that its in vitro biological activities are concordant with a possible role in EAE. IL-1 acts on endothelial cells to promote leukocyte adhesion by stimulating the expression of several adhesion molecules (25). It also increases expression of ICAM-1 on astrocytes, which could facilitate the ability of these cells to function as antigen-presenting cells (84). Furthermore, guinea pigs with chronic EAE have elevated levels of IL-1 in the CSF (144), and IL-1 is distributed throughout the CNS of rats and mice with EAE (7,8,33,145). Kennedy et al. (8) reported that IL-1 mRNA levels were elevated very early in the disease course and persisted into the chronic phase. Within the CNS, infiltrating macrophages as well as resident astrocytes, microglia cells, and possibly neurons are the source of IL-1 (145,146,147). Local production of IL-1α may contribute to reactive gliosis of astrocytes (148). In experimental animals, a deleterious role has been ascribed to IL-1α. IL-1 enhances the in vitro activation of encephalitogenic T cells, thereby enhancing adoptive transfer of EAE (149). Treatment of rats with soluble mouse IL-1R, and IL-1 antagonist, reduced EAE, whereas administration of exogenous IL-1α enhanced the severity of actively induced disease (150). These data suggest that IL-1 initiates or promotes inflammation within the CNS.

D. Chemokines

Besides the already known chemotactic factors released by platelets (e.g., platelet factor 4 and β-thromboglobulin), numerous additional chemoattractant cytokines of low molecular weight, collectively designated as chemokines, have been discovered during the past decade. These factors are the product of two related gene families preferentially active on granulocytes (C-X-C chemokines: e.g., IL-8, granulocyte chemotactic proteins [GCPs] IP-10) or monocytes (C-C chemokines: e.g., monocyte chemotactic proteins [MCPs], JE = mouse MCP-1 [JE/MCPs], macrophage inflammatory protein [MIP] (reviewed in ref. 151). However, the activating effects of chemokines extend to other cells, such as basophils, eosinophils, and distinct subsets of lymphocytes. In addition, some of them have lymphocyte adhesion-inducing properties. Members of the chemokine superfamily are mainly produced by activated macrophages. However, many other cells are also good producers of these molecules, including endothelial cells, astrocytes, and fibroblasts. Disease-promoting cytokines such as IFN-γ, IL-1, and TNF-α are prominent inducers of chemokines (see ref. 151).

Chemokines regulate cell motility and allow the immune system selectively to attract different types of leukocytes into the injured sites of the body. It should be mentioned that besides their chemotactic activity, the chemokines also contribute to inflammatory tissue damage. Attracted macrophages and lymphocytes release proteinases or release latent metalloproteases that are subsequently activated (see ref. 19). For instance, IL-8 stimulates the production of gelatinase B from granulocytes. This proteinase cascade can directly lead to enzymatic demyelination. The leukocyte-attractant and activating properties of the chemokines make them logical candidates for involvement in the pathogenesis of chronic inflammatory or autoimmune processes.

A few publications during the past 2 years have demonstrated the expression of chemokines in CNS of animals with EAE. Khoury et al. (7) first demonstrated an increased IL-8 expression in animals with EAE. The expression of IL-8 correlates well with the presence of neutrophils in the inflammatory infiltrates. More recently, accumulation of mRNA for IP-10, an IFN-γ–induced mouse chemokine and JE/MCP-1 (152,153)) were shown to occur in the CNS of mice and rats at the onset of EAE and disappeared at disease resolution. Within the inflamed CNS, many cell types may be the source of these factors, inflammatory infiltrates as well as cells endogenous to the CNS are candidates. In this regard, a recent study has shown that astrocytes are the major source of mRNAs encoding for IP-10 and MCP in mice (152). It is possible that IFN-γ, which is one of the potent inducers of these chemokines (see ref. 151) and is produced within the meningeal and inflammatory EAE lesions by activated lymphocytes and macrophages (7–10,33), accounts for the extensive activation of chemokine expression by astrocytes.

V. CONCLUSIONS

Although these studies suggest that chemokines produced locally within the CNS are the main attractants for inflammatory cells into the affected sites, a causal relationship between the presence of cytokines and pathological conditions has so far not been shown. More work is required to assess their actual pathological role in EAE. The use of inhibitory antibodies or chemokine-specific antagonists could be of considerable utility.

NOTE ADDED IN PROOF

On page 221 the possible role of inducible NO synthase as a mediator of IFN-γ effects in EAE is briefly mentioned. Since submission of this chapter, additional information has become available in the literature. Unfortunately, the evidence remains controversial. In adoptively transferred EAE in SJL/J mice, aminoguanidine, an inhibitor of the inducible NO synthetase (iNOS), was found to ameliorate disease parameters (154). With other NOS inhibitors, L-NAME and L-NMMA, used in the rat model reported results are contradictory (155,156).

REFERENCES

1. Martin R, McFarland HF, McFarlin DE. Immunological aspects of demyelinating diseases. Ann Rev Immunol 1992; 10:153–187.
2. Zamvil SS, Steinman L. The T lymphocyte in experimental allergic encephalomyelitis. Annu Rev Immunol 1990; 8:579–621.
3. Dijkstra CD, De Groot CJA, Huitinga I. The role of macrophages in demyelination. J Neuroimmunol 1992; 40:183–188.
4. Benveniste EN. Inflammatory cytokines within the central nervous system: sources, function, and mechanism of action. Am J Physiol 1992; 263: C1–C16.
5. Street NE, Mosmann TR. Functional diversity of T lymphocytes due to secretion of different cytokine patterns. FASEB J 1991; 5:171–177.
6. Seder RA, Paul WE. Acquisition of lymphokine-producing phenotypes by CD4+ T cells. Annu Rev Immunol 1994; 12:635–673.
7. Khoury SJ, Hancock WW, Weiner HL. Oral tolerance to myelin basis protein and natural recovery from experimental autoimmune encephalomyelitis are associated with downregulation of inflammatory cytokines and differential upregulation of transforming growth factor β, interleukin 4, and prostaglandin E expression in the brain. J Exp Med 1992; 176:1355–1364.
8. Kennedy MK, Torrance DS, Picha KS, Mohler KM. Analysis of cytokine mRNA expression in the central nervous system of mice with experimental autoimmune encephalomyelitis reveals that IL-10 mRNA expression correlates with recovery. J Immunol 1992; 149:2496–2505.

9. Merrill JE, Kono DH, Clayton J, Ando DG, Hinton DR, Hofman FM. Inflammatory leukocytes and cytokines in the peptide-induced disease of experimental allergic encephalomyelitis in SJL and B10.PL mice. Proc Natl Acad Sci USA 1992; 89:574–578.

10. Renno T, Lin YJ-Y, Piccirillo C, Antel J, Owens T. Cytokine production by cells in cerebrospinal fluid during experimental allergic encephalomyelitis in SJL/J mice. J Neuroimmunol 1994; 49:1–7.

11. Young HA, Hardy KJ. Interferon-γ: producer cells, activation stimuli, and molecular genetic regulation. Pharmacol Ther 1990; 45:137–151.

12. McDonald AH, Swanborg RH. Antigen-specific inhibition of immune interferon production by suppressor cells of autoimmune encephalomyelitis. J Immunol 1988; 140:1132–1138.

13. Brunda MJ. Interleukin-12. J Leukoc Biol 1994; 55:280–288.

14. Schmitt E, Hoehn P, Huels C, Goedert S, Palm N, Rüde E, Germann T. T helper type 1 development of naive CD4+ T cells requires the coordinate action of interleukin-12 and interferon-γ and is inhibited by transforming growth factor-β. Eur J Immunol 1994; 24:792–798.

15. Leonard JP, Waldburger KE, Goldman SJ. Prevention of autoimmune encephalomyelitis by antibodies against interleukin 12. J Exp Med 1994; 181: 381–386.

16. Farrar MA, Schreiber RD. The molecular cell biology of interferon-γ and its receptor. Annu Rev Immunol 1993; 11:571–711.

17. Sethna MP, Lampson LA. Immune modulation within the brain: recruitment of inflammatory cells and increased major histocompatibility antigen expression following intrathecal injection of interferon-γ. J Neuroimmunol 1991; 34:121–132.

18. Hartung HP, Jung S, Stoll G, Zielasek J, Schmidt B, Archelos JJ, Toyka KV. Inflammatory mediators in demyelinating disorders of the CNS and PNS. J Neuroimmunol 1992; 40:197–210.

19. Opdenakker G, Van Damme J. Cytokine regulated proteases in autoimmune diseases. Immunol Today 1994; 15:103–107.

20. Hughes CCW, Male DK, Lantos PL. Adhesion of lymphocytes to cerebral microvascular cells: effects of interferon-γ, tumor necrosis factor and interleukin-1. Immunology 1988; 64:677–681.

21. Issekutz TB. Effects of six different cytokines on lymphocyte adherence to microvascular endothelium and in vivo lymphocyte migration in the rat. J Immunol 1990; 144:2140–2146.

22. Oppenheimer-Marks N, Ziff M. Migration of lymphocytes through endothelial cell monolayers: augmentation by interferon-γ. Cell Immunol 1988; 114: 307–323.

23. Simmons RD, Willenborg DO. Direct injection of cytokines into the spinal cord causes autoimmune encephalomyelitis-like inflammation. J Neurol Sci 1990; 100:37–42.

24. Fabry Z, Waldschmidt MM, Hendrickson D, Keiner J, Love-Homan L, Takei F, Hart MN. Adhesion molecules on murine brain microvascular

endothelial cells: expression and regulation of ICAM-1 and Lgp 55. J Neuro-immunol 1992; 36:1–11.

25. McCarron RM, Wang L, Racke MK, McFarlin DE, Spatz M. Cytokine-regulated adhesion between encephalitogenic T lymphocytes and cerebro-vascular endothelial cells. J Neuroimmunol 1993; 43:23–30.

26. Cannella B, Cross AH, Raine CS. Upregulation and coexpression of adhesion molecules correlate with relapsing autoimmune demyelination in the central nervous system. J Exp Med 1990; 172:1521–1523.

27. Lindsey JW, Steinman L. Competitive PCR quantification of CD4, CD8, ICAM-1, VCAM-1 and MHC class II mRNA in the central nervous system during development and resolution of experimental allergic encephalomyeli-tis. J Neuroimmunol 1993; 48:227–234.

28. Barten DM, Ruddle NH. Vascular adhesion molecule-1 modulation by tumor necrosis factor in experimental allergic encephalomyelitis. J Neuro-immunol 1994; 51:123–133.

29. Chomarat P, Rissoan M-C, Banchereau J, Miossec P. Interferon-γ inhibits interleukin 10 production by monocytes. J Exp Med 1993; 177:523–527.

30. Frei K, Leist TP, Meager A, Gallo P, Leppert D, Zinkernagel RM, Fontana A. Production of B cell stimulatory factor-2 and interferon-γ in the central nervous system during viral meningitis and encephalitis. J Exp Med 1988; 163:449–453.

31. Billiau A, Heremans H, Vandekerckhove F, Dijkmans R, Sobis H, Meu-lepas E, Carton H. Enhancement of experimental allergic encephalomyelitis in mice by antibodies against IFN-γ. J Immunol 1988; 140:1506–1510.

32. Mustafa MI, Diener P, Höjeberg B, Van der Meide P, Olsson, T. T cell immunity and interferon-γ secretion during experimental allergic encephalo-myelitis in Lewis rats. J Neuroimmunol 1991; 31:165–177.

33. Baker D, O'Neill JK, Turk JL. Cytokines in the central nervous system of mice during chronic relapsing experimental allergic encephalomyelitis. Cell Immunol 1991; 134:505–510.

34. Stoll G, Müller S, Schmidt B, Van Der Meide P, Jung S, Toyka KV, Hartung HP. Localization of interferon-γ and Ia-antigen in T cell line-mediated ex-perimental autoimmune encephalomyelitis. Am J Pathol 1993; 142: 1866–1875.

35. Yong VW, Moumdjian R, Yong FP, Ruijs TCG, Freedman MS, Cashman N, Antel JP. γ-Interferon promotes proliferation of adult human astrocytes in vitro and reactive gliosis in the adult mouse brain in vivo. Proc Natl Acad Sci USA 1991; 88:7016–7020.

36. Panitch HS, Hirsch RL, Haley AS, Johnson KP. Exacerbation of multiple sclerosis in patients treated with gamma interferon. Lancet 1987; 1:893–894.

37. Voorthuis JAC, Uitdehaag BMJ, De Groot CJA, Goede PH, Van Der Meide PH, Dijkstra CD. Suppression of experimental allergic encephalomyelitis by intraventricular administration of interferon-gamma in Lewis rats. Clin Exp Immunol 1990; 81:183–188.

38. Duong TT, St Louis J, Gilbert JJ, Finkelman FD, Strejan GH. Effect of

anti–interferon-γ and anti–interleukin-2 monoclonal antibody treatment on the development of actively and passively induced experimental allergic encephalomyelitis in the SJL/J mouse. J Neuroimmunol 1992; 36:105–115.

39. Lublin FD, Knobler RL, Kalman B, Goldhaber M, Marini J, Perrault M, D'Imperio C, Joseph J, Alkan SS, Korngold R. Monoclonal anti–gamma interferon antibodies enhance experimental allergic encephalomyelitis. Autoimmunity 1993; 16:264–374.

39a. Ferber IA, Brocke S, Taylor-Edwards C, et al. Mice with a disrupted IFN-γ gene are susceptible to the induction of experimental autoimmune encephalomyelitis (EAE). J Immunol 1996; 156:5–7.

40. Duong TT, Finkelman FD, Singh B, Strejan GH. Effect of anti–interferon-γ monoclonal antibody treatment on the development of experimental allergic encephalomyelitis in resistant mouse strains. J Neuroimmunol 1994; 53: 101–107.

41. Heremans H, Dijkmans R, Sobis H, Vandekerckhove F, Billiau A. Regulation by interferons of the local inflammatory response to bacterial lipopolysaccharide. J Immunol 1987; 138:4175–4179.

42. Noma T, Dorf ME. Modulation of suppressor T cell induction with interferon-γ. J Immunol 1985; 135:3655–3660.

43. Mueller DL. Do tolerant T cells exist? Nature 1989; 339:513–514.

44. Liu Y, Janeway Jr CA. Interferon γ plays a critical role in induced cell death of effector T cell: a possible third mechanism of self-tolerance. J Exp Med 1990; 172:1735–1739.

45. Zeine R, Owens T. Loss rather than downregulation of CD4 + T cells as a mechanism for remission from experimental allergic encephalomyelitis. J Neuroimmunol 1993; 44:193–198.

46. Thepen T, Van Rooijen N, Kraal G. Alveolar macrophage elimination in vivo is associated with an increase in pulmonary immune response in mice. J Exp Med 1989; 170:499–509.

47. McKernan NL, Blank KJ, Spitalny GL, Murasko DM. Inhibition of macrophage-induced antigen-specific T-cell proliferation by interferon-γ. Cell Immunol 1988; 114:432–430.

48. Duong TT, Finkelman FD, Strejan GH. Effect of interferon-γ on myelin basic protein-specific T cell line proliferation in response to antigen-pulsed accessory cells. Cell Immunol 1992; 145:311–323.

49. Ruuls SR, Van Der Linden S, Huitinga I, Dijkstra CD. Immunosuppressive role for nitric oxide in experimental allergic encephalomyelitis. Clin Exp Immunol 1996; 103:467–474.

50. Twardzik DR, Mikovits JA, Ranchalis JE, Purchio AF, Ellingsworth L, Ruscetti FW. γ-interferon-induced activation of latent transforming growth factor-β by human monocytes. Ann NY Acad Sci 1990; 593:276–284.

51. Karpus WJ, Swanborg RH. CD4 + suppressor cells inhibit the function of effector cells of experimental autoimmune encephalomyelitis through a mechanism involving transforming growth factor-beta. J Immunol 1991; 146: 1163–1168.

52. Gusella GL, Musso T, Bosco MC, Espinoza-Delgado I, Matsushima K,

Varesio L. IL-2 up-regulates but IFN-γ suppresses IL-8 expression in human monocytes. J Immunol 1993; 151:2725–2732.

53. Arnason BGW, Reder AT. Interferons and multiple sclerosis. Clin Neuropharmacol 1994; 17:495–547.

54. Ruscetti FW. Interleukin 2. In: Oppenheim JJ, Shevach EM, eds. Immunophysiology. Oxford University Press, 1990:46–66.

55. Kroemer G, Wick G. The role of interleukin 2 in autoimmunity. Immunol Today 1989; 10:246–251.

56. Ando D, Clayton J, Kono D, Urban J, Sercarz EE. Encephalitogenic T cells in the B10.PL model of experimental allergic encephalomyelitis (EAE) are of the Th-1 lymphokine subtype. Cell Immunol 1989; 124:132–143.

57. Watts RG, Wright JL, Atkinson LL, Merchant RE. Histopathological and blood-brain barrier changes in rats induced by an intracerebral injection of human recombinant interleukin 2. Neurosurgery 1989; 25:202–208.

58. Sedgwick J, Brostoff S, Mason D. Experimental allergic encephalomyelitis in the absence of a classical delayed-type hypersensitivity reaction. Severe paralytic disease correlates with the presence of interleukin 2 receptor-positive cells infiltrating the central nervous system. J Exp Med 1987; 165:1058–1075.

59. Kira J-I, Itoyama Y, Goto I. Generation of CD4+ blastoid cells showing marked upregulation of CD4, class I and II MHC, and IL-2R molecules is required for the expression of potent encephalitogenicity. Cell Immunol 1989; 123:264–275.

60. Strieter RM, Remick DG, Lynch JP III, Spengler RN, Kunkel SL. Interleukin-2 induced tumor necrosis factor-alpha (TNF-α) gene expression in human alveolar macrophages and blood monocytes. Am Rev Respir Dis 1989; 139:335–342.

61. Kovacs EJ, Brock B, Varesio L, Young HA. IL-2 induction of IL-1β mRNA expression in human monocytes. J Immunol 1989; 143:3532–3537.

62. Narumi S, Finke JK, Hamilton TA. Interferon γ and interleukin 2 synergize to induce selective monokine expression in murine peritoneal macrophages. J Biol Chem 1990; 265:7036–7041.

63. Sanetto RP, Altman A, Knobler RL, Johnson HM, De Vellis J. Interleukin 2 mediates the inhibition of oligodendrocyte progenitor cell proliferation in vitro. Proc Natl Acad Sci USA 1988; 83:9221–9225.

64. Hayosh NS, Swanborg RH. Autoimmune effector cells. IX. Inhibition of adoptive transfer of autoimmune encephalomyelitis with a monoclonal antibody specific for interleukin 2 receptors. J Immunol 1987; 138:3771–3775.

65. Engelhardt B, Diamantstein T, Wekerle H. Immunotherapy of experimental autoimmune encephalomyelitis (EAE): differential effect of anti-IL-2 receptor antibody therapy on actively induced and T-line mediated EAE of the Lewis rat. J Autoimmun 1989; 2:61–73.

66. Beraud E, Lorberboum-Galski H, Chan CC, Fitzgerald D, Pastan I, Nussenblatt RB. Immunospecific suppression of encephalitogenic-activated T-lymphocytes by chimeric cytotoxin IL-2-PE40. Cell Immunol 1991; 133:379–389.

67. Beutler B, Cerami A. The biology of cachectin, a primary mediator of the host response. Annu Rev Immunol 1989; 7:625–655.
68. Paul N, Ruddle N. Lymphotoxin. Annu Rev Immunol 1989; 6:407–438.
69. Baker D, Butler D, Scallon BJ, O'Neill JK, Turk JL, Feldman M. Control of established experimental allergic encephalomyelitis by inhibition of tumor necrosis factor (TNF) activity within the central nervous system using monoclonal antibodies and TNF receptor-immunoglobulin fusion proteins. Eur J Immunol 1994; 24:2040–2048.
70. Selmaj K, Raine CS, Cannella B, Brosnan CF. Identification of lymphotoxin and tumor necrosis factor in multiple sclerosis lesions. J Clin Invest 1991; 87:949–954.
71. Selmaj KW, Raine CS. Tumor necrosis factor mediates myelin and oligodendrocyte damage in vitro. Ann Neurol 1988; 23:339–346.
72. Selmaj K, Raine CS, Farooq M, Norton WT, Brosnan CF. Cytokine cytotoxicity against oligodendrocytes. Apoptosis induced by lymphotoxin. J Immunol 1991; 147:1522–1529.
73. Powell MB, Mitchell D, Lederman J, Buckmeier J, Zamvil SS, Graham M, Ruddle NH, Steinman L. Lymphotoxin and tumor necrosis factor-alpha production by myelin basic protein specific T cell clones correlates with encephalitogenicity. Int Immunol 1990; 2:539–544.
74. Hershkoviz R, Mor F, Gilat D, Cohen IR, Lider O. T cells in the spinal cord in experimental autoimmune encephalomyelitis are matrix adherent and secrete tumor necrosis factor alpha. J Neuroimmunol 1992; 37:161–166.
75. Chung IY, Norris JG, Benveniste EN. Differential TNF-α expression by astrocytes from experimental allergic encephalomyelitis susceptible and resistant strains. J Exp Med 1991; 173:801–811.
76. Selmaj KW, Farooq M, Norton WT, Raine CS, Brosnan CF. Proliferation of astrocytes in vitro in response to cytokines. A primary role for tumor necrosis factor. J Immunol 1990; 144:129–135.
77. Kuroda Y, Shimamoto YJ. Human tumor necrosis factor-α augments experimental allergic encephalomyelitis in rats. J Neuroimmunol 1991; 34: 159–164.
78. Ruddle NH, Bergman CM, McGrath KM, Lingenheld EG, Grunnet ML, Padula SJ, Clark RB. An antibody to lymphotoxin and tumor necrosis factor prevents transfer of experimental allergic encephalomyelitis. J Exp Med 1990; 172:1193–1200.
79. Selmaj K, Raine CS, Cross AH. Anti-tumor necrosis factor therapy abrogates autoimmune demyelination. Ann Neurol 1991; 30:694–700.
80. Santambogio L, Hochwald GM, Saxena B, Leu CH, Martz JE, Carlino JA, Ruddle NH, Palladino MA, Gold LI, Thorbecke GJ. Studies on the mechanisms by which transforming growth factor-β (TGF-β) protects against allergic encephalomyelitis: antagonism between TGF-β and TNF. J Immunol 1993; 151:1116–1127.
81. Kim KS, Wass CA, Cross AS, Opal SM. Modulation of blood-brain barrier permeability by tumor necrosis factor and antibody to tumor necrosis factor in the rat. Lymphokine Cytokine Res 1992; 11:293–298.

82. Brett JH, Gerlach P, Nawroth P, Steinberg S, Godman G, Stern D. Tumor necrosis factor/cachectin increases permeability of endothelial cell monolayers by a mechanism involving regulatory G proteins. J Exp Med 1989; 169:1977–1991.

83. Bevilacqua MP, Pober JS, Mendrick DL, Cotran RS, Gimbrone MA Jr. Identification of an inducible endothelial-leukocyte adhesion molecule. Proc Natl Acad Sci USA 1987; 84:9238–9242.

84. Shrikant P, Chung IY, Ballestas ME, Benveniste EN. Regulation of intracellular adhesion molecule-1 gene expression by tumor necrosis factor-α, interleukin-1β, and interferon-γ in astrocytes. J Neuroimmunol 1994; 51: 209–220.

85. Willenborg DO, Simmons RD, Tamatani T, Miyasaka M. ICAM-1-dependent pathway is not critically involved in the inflammatory process of autoimmune encephalomyelitis or in cytokine-induced inflammation of the central nervous system. J Neuroimmunol 1993; 45:147–154.

86. Van Snick J. Interleukin-6: an overview. Annu Rev Immunol 1990; 8: 253–278.

87. Baumann H, Gauldie J. The acute phase response. Immunol Today 1994; 15:74–80.

88. Aderka D, Le J, Vilček J. IL-6 inhibits lipopolysaccharide-induced TNF production in cultured human monocytes, U937 cells, and in mice. J Immunol 1989; 143:3517–3523.

89. Naitoh Y, Fukata J, Tominaga T, Nakai Y, Tamai S, Mori K, Imura H. Interleukin-6 stimulates the secretion of adrenocorticotropic hormone in conscious freely moving rats. Biochem Biophys Res Commun 1988; 155: 1459–1463.

90. Gijbels K, Van Damme J, Proost P, Put W, Carton H, Billiau A. Interleukin-6 production in the central nervous system during experimental autoimmune encephalomyelitis. Eur J Immunol 1990; 20:233–235.

91. Maimone D, Gregory S, Arnason BGW, Reder AT. Cytokine levels in cerebrospinal fluid and serum of patients with multiple sclerosis. J Neuroimmunol 1991; 32:67–74.

92. Hauser SL, Doolittle TH, Lincoln R, Brown RH, Dinarello CA. Cytokine accumulations in CSF of multiple sclerosis patients: frequent detection of interleukin-1 and tumor necrosis factor but not interleukin-6. Neurology 1990; 40:1735–1739.

93. Rubio N, Sierra A. Interleukin-6 production by brain tissue and cultured astrocytes infected with Theiler's murine encephalomyelitis virus. Glia 1993; 9:41–47.

94. Benveniste EN, Sparacio SM, Norris JG, Grenett HE, Fuller GM. Induction and regulation of interleukin-6 gene expression in rat astrocytes. J Neuroimmunol 1990; 30:201–212.

95. Gijbels K, Brocke S, Abrams JS, Steinman L. Effect of anti–interleukin-6 treatment on experimental autoimmune encephalomyelitis (abstr). Neurology 1993; 43(suppl 2):A412. Gijbels K, Brocke S, Abrams JS, Steinman L. Administration of neutralizing antibodies to interleukin-6 (IL-6) reduces

experimental autoimmune encephalitis and is associated with elevated levels of IL-6 bioactivity in central nervous system and circulation. Mol Med 1995; 1:795–805.

96. Heremans H, Dillen C, Put W, Van Damme J, Billiau A. Protective effect of anti–interleukin (IL)–6 antibody against endotoxin, associated with paradoxally increased IL-6 levels. Eur J Immunol 1992; 22:2395–2401.

97. Lu Z, Brochier J, Wijdeness J, Brailly H, Bataille R, Klein B. High amounts of circulating interleukin (IL)-6 in the form of monomeric immune complexes during anti–IL-6 therapy. Towards a new methodology for measuring overall cytokine production in human in vivo. Eur J Immunol 1992; 22: 2818–2824.

98. Martens E, Dillen C, Put W, Heremans H, Van Damme J, Billiau A. Increased circulating interleukin-6 (IL-6) activity in endotoxin-challenged mice pretreated with anti–IL-6 antibody is due to IL-6 accumulated in antigen-antibody complexes. Eur J Immunol 1993; 23:2026–2029.

99. Rodriguez M, Pavelko KD, McKinney CW, Leibowitz JL. Recombinant human IL-6 suppresses demyelination in a viral model for multiple sclerosis. J Immunol 1994; 153:3811–3821.

100. Lotz M, Guerne P-A. Interleukin-6 induces the synthesis of tissue inhibitor of metalloproteinases-1/erythroid potentiating activity (TIMP-1). J Biol Chem 1991; 266:2017–2020.

101. Paul WW. Interleukin-4: a prototypic immunoregulatory lymphokine. Blood 1991; 77:1859–1870.

102. Karpus WJ, Gould KE, Swanborg RH. CD4$^+$ suppressor cells of autoimmune encephalitis respond to T cell receptor–associated determinants on effector cells by interleukin-4. Eur J Immunol 1992; 22:1757–1763.

103. Van der Veen RC, Kapp JA, Trotter JL. Fine specificity in the recognition of an encephalitogenic peptide by T helper 1 and 2 cells. J Neuroimmunol 1993; 48:221–226.

104. Racke MK, Bonomo A, Scott DE, Cannella B, Levine A, Raine CS, Shevach EM, Röcken M. Cytokine immune deviation as a therapy for inflammatory autoimmune disease. J Exp Med 1994; 180:1961–1966.

105. Gautam S, Tebo JM, Hamilton TA. IL-4 suppresses cytokine gene expression induced by IFN-γ and/or IL-2 in murine peritoneal macrophages. J Immunol 1992; 148:1725–1730.

106. te Velde AA, Huijbens RFJ, Heije K, de Vries JE, Figdoe CG. Interleukin-4 (IL-4) inhibits secretion of IL-1β, tumor necrosis factor α, and IL-6 by human monocytes. Blood 1990; 76:1392–1397.

107. Cash E, Minty A, Ferrara P, Caput D, Fradelizi D, Rott O. Macrophage-inactivating IL-13 suppresses experimental autoimmune encephalomyelitis in rats. J Immunol 1994; 153:4258–4267.

108. Zurawski G, De Vries J. Interleukin 13, an interleukin 4-like cytokine that acts on monocytes and B cells, but not on T cells. Immunol Today 1994; 15:19–26.

109. Liblau R, Brocke S, Steinman L, McDevitt H. L'encephalomyélite autoimmune expérimentale chez les souris déficientes en interleukine-4. Les straté-

gies thérapeutiques dans la sclérose en plaques, Multiple Sclerosis 1995;1 (supplement).

110. Mosmann TR. Properties and functions of interleukin-10. Adv Immunol 1994; 56:1–26.

111. Moore KW, O'Garra A, de Waal-Malefyt R, Vieira P, Mosmann TR. Interleukin 10. Annu Rev Immunol 1993; 11:165–190.

112. Rott O, Fleischer B, Cash E. Interleukin-10 prevents experimental allergic encephalomyelitis in rats. Eur J Immunol 1994; 24:1434–1440.

113. De Maeyer E, De Maeyer-Guignard J. Interferons. In: Thomson A, ed. The Cytokine Handbook, 2nd ed. London: Academic Press, 1994:265–288.

114. Abreu SL. Suppression of experimental allergic encephalomyelitis by interferon. Immunol Commun 1982; 11:1–7.

115. Hertz F, Degheni R. Effect of rat and β-human interferons on hyperacute experimental allergic encephalomyelitis in rats. Agents Actions 1985; 16: 397–403.

116. Abreu SL, Tondreau J, Levine S, Sowinski R. Inhibition of passive localized experimental allergic encephalomyelitis by interferon. Int Archs Allergy Immunol 1983; 72:30–33.

116a. Yu M, Nishiyama A, Trapp BD, Tuohy VK. Interferon-β inhibits progression of relapsing-remitting experimental autoimmune encephalomyelitis. J Neuroimmunol 1996; 64:91–100.

117. Inada T, Mims CA. Infection in mice with lactic dehydrogenase virus prevents development of experimental allergic encephalomyelitis. J Neuroimmunol 1986; 11:53–56.

118. Brod SA, Burns DK. Suppression of relapsing experimental autoimmune encephalomyelitis in the SJL/J mouse by oral administration of type I interferons. Neurology 1994; 44:1144–1148.

119. Abreu SL, Thampoe I, Kaplan P. Interferon in experimental autoimmune encephalomyelitis: intraventricular administration. J Interferon Res 1986; 6:627–632.

120. Noronha A, Toscas A, Jensen MA. IFN-β decreases T cell activation and IFN-γ production in MS. J Neuroimmunol 1993; 46:145–153.

121. Ling PD, Warren MK, Vogel SN. Antagonistic effect of interferon-beta on the interferon-gamma–induced expression of Ia antigen in murine macrophages. J Immunol 1985; 135:1857–1863.

122. Ransohoff RM, Devajyothi C, Estes ML. Interferon-beta specifically inhibits interferon-induced class II major histocompatibility complex gene transcription in a human astrocytoma cell line. J Neuroimmunol 1991; 33: 103–112.

123. Abu-Khabar KS, Armstrong JA, Ho M. Type I interferons (IFN-α and IFN-β) suppress cytotoxin (tumor necrosis factor-α and lymphotoxin) production by mitogen-stimulated human peripheral blood mononuclear cells. J Leukoc Biol 1992; 52:165–172.

124. Noronha A, Toscas A, Jensen MA. Interferon beta augments suppressor cell function in multiple sclerosis. Ann Neurol 1990; 27:207–210.

125. Noronha A, Toscas A, Jensen MA. Contrasting effects of alpha, beta, and

gamma interferons on non-specific suppressor function in multiple sclerosis. Ann Neurol 1992; 31:103–106.

126. Derynck R. Transforming growth factor-beta. In: Thomson A, ed. The Cytokine Handbook, 2nd ed. London: Academic Press, 1994:319–342.

127. Barzaga-Gilbert ME, Skeen MJ, Chou CHJ, Fritz RB. Suppressive activity of long-term myelin basic protein-specific SJL T cell lines. J Neuroimmunol 1989; 23:241–247.

128. Huang SK, Sriram S. Spontaneous development in vitro of a myelin basic protein–specific suppressor T cell line. J Neuroimmunol 1989; 25:177–183.

129. Johns LD, Flanders KC, Ranges GE, Sriram S. Successfull treatment of experimental allergic encephalomyelitis with transforming growth factor-$\beta1$. J Immunol 1991; 147:1792–1796.

130. Racke MK, Cannella B, Albert P, Sporn M, Raine CS, McFarlin D. Evidence of endogenous regulatory function of transforming growth factor-$\beta1$ in experimental allergic encephalomyelitis. Int Immunol 1992; 4:615–620.

131. Kuruvilla AP, Shah R, Hochwald GM, Liggitt HD, Palladino MA, Thorbecke GJ. Protective effect of transforming growth factor beta 1 on experimental autoimmune disease in mice. Proc Natl Acad Sci USA 1991; 88: 2918–2921.

132. Racke MK, Dhib-Jalbut S, Cannella B, Albert PS, Raine CS, McFarlin DE. Prevention and treatment of chronic relapsing experimental allergic encephalomyelitis by transforming growth factor-$\beta1$. J Immunol 1991; 146: 3012–3017.

133. Johns LD, Sriram S. Experimental allergic encephalomyelitis: neutralizing antibody to TGF-beta 1 enhances the clinical severity of the disease. J Neuroimmunol 1993; 47:1–7.

134. Weinberger AD, Whitman R, Swain SL, Morrison WJ, Wyrick G, Hoy C, Vandenbark AA, Offner H. Transforming growth factor-β enhances the in vivo effector function and memory phenotype of antigen-specific T helper cells in experimental autoimmune encephalomyelitis. J Immunol 1992; 148: 2109–2117.

135. Schluesener HJ, Lider O. Transforming growth factors β_1 and β_2: cytokines with identical immunosuppressive effects and a potential role in the regulation of autoimmune T cell function. J Neuroimmunol 1989; 24:249–258.

136. Gamble JR, Vadas MA. Endothelial cell adhesiveness for human T lymphocytes is inhibited by transforming growth factor-$\beta1$. J Immunol 1991; 146: 1149–1154.

137. Cai JP, Falanga V, Chin Y-H. Transforming growth factor-β regulates the adhesive interactions between mononuclear cells and microvascular endothelium. J Invest Dermatol 1991; 97:169–174.

138. Stevens DB, Gould KE, Swanborg RH. Transforming growth factor-$\beta1$ inhibits tumor necrosis factor-α/lymphotoxin production and adoptive transfer of disease by effector cells of autoimmune encephalomyelitis. J Neuroimmunol 1994; 77:77–83.

139. Schluesener HJ. Transforming growth factor $\beta1$ and $\beta2$ suppress rat astrocyte autoantigen presentation and antagonize hyperinduction of class II

major histocompatibility complex antigen expression by interferon-γ and tumor necrosis factor-α. J Neuroimmunol 1990; 27:41–47.

140. Ding A, Nathan CF, Graycar J, Derynck R, Stuehr DJ, Srimal S. Macrophage deactivating factor and transforming growth factors-β1, -β2, and -β3 inhibit induction of macrophage nitrogen oxide synthesis by IFN-γ. J Immunol 1990; 145:940–944.

141. Merrill JE, Zimmerman RP. Natural and induced cytotoxicity of oligodendrocytes by microglia is inhibited by TGF-β. Glia 1991; 4:327–331.

142. Dinarello C. Interleukin-1 and interleukin-1 antagonism. Blood 1991; 77: 1627–1652.

143. Dinarello C. Interleukin-1. In: Thomson A, ed. The Cytokine Handbook, 2nd ed. London: Academic Press, 1994:31–56.

144. Symons JA, Bundick RV, Suckling AJ, Rumsby MG. Cerebrospinal fluid interleukin 1-like activity during chronic relapsing experimental allergic encephalomyelitis. Clin Exp Immunol 1987; 68:648–654.

145. Bauer J, Berkenbosch F, Van Dam AM, Dijkstra CD. Demonstration of interleukin-1 beta in Lewis rat brain during experimental allergic encephalomyelitis by immunocytochemistry at the light and ultrastructural level. J Neuroimmunol 1993; 48:13–21.

146. Guilian D, Baker TJ, Shih L-CN, Lachman LB. Interleukin 1 of the central nervous system is produced by ameboid microglia. J Exp Med 1986; 164: 594–604.

147. Hetier E, Ayala J, Denèfle P, Bousseau A, Rouget P, Mallat M, Prochiantz A. Brain macrophages synthesize interleukin-1 mRNAs in vitro. J Neuroscience Res 1988; 21:391–397.

148. Guilian D, Woodward J, Young DG, Krebs JF, Lachman LB. Interleukin-1 injected into mammalian brain stimulates astrogliosis and neovascularization. J Neurosci 1988; 8:2485–2490.

149. Mannie MD, Dinarello, CA, Paterson PY. Interleukin 1 and myelin basic protein synergistically augment adoptive transfer activity of lymphocytes mediating experimental autoimmune encephalomyelitis in lewis rats. J Immunol 1987; 138:4229–4235.

150. Jacobs CA, Baker PE, Roux ER, Picha KS, Toivola B, Waugh S, Kennedy MK. Experimental autoimmune encephalomyelitis is exacerbated by IL-1 alpha and suppressed by IL-1 receptor. J Immunol 1991; 146:2983–2989.

151. Baggiolini M, Dewald B, Moser B. Interleukin-8 and related chemotactic cytokines—CXC and CC chemokines. Adv Immunol 1994; 55:97–179.

152. Ransohoff RM, Hamilton TA, Tani M, Stoler MH, Shick HE, Major JA, Estes ML, Thomas DM, Tuohy VK. Astrocyte expression of mRNA encoding cytokines IP-10 and JE/MCP-1 in experimental autoimmune encephalomyelitis. FASEB J 1993; 7:592–600.

153. Hulkower K, Brosnan CF, Aquino DA, Cammer W, Kulshrestha S, Guida MP, Rapoport DA, Berman JW. Expression of CSF-1, c-fms, and MCP-1 in the central nervous system of rats with experimental allergic encephalomyelitis. J Immunol 1993; 150:2525–2533.

154. Cross AH, Misko TP, Lin RF, Hickey WF, Trotter JL, Tilton RG. Aminoguanidine, an inhibitor of inducible nitric oxide synthase, ameliorates experimental autoimmune encephalomyelitis in SJL mice. J Clin Invest 1994; 93:
2684–2690.
155. Zielasek J, Jung S, Gold R, Liew FY, Toyka KV, Hartung HP. Administration of nitric oxide synthase inhibitors in experimental autoimmune neuritis
and experimental autoimmune encephalomyelitis. J Neuroimmunol 1995;
58:81–88.
156. Ruuls SR, Van der Linden S, Huitinga I, Dijkstra CD. Aggravation of experimental allergic encephalomyelitis (EAE) by administration of nitric oxide
(NO) synthase inhibitors. Clin Exp Immunol 1996; 103:467–474.

10

Effects of Oral Administration of Type I Interferons on Experimental Autoimmune Encephalomyelitis

Staley A. Brod

University of Texas Medical School at Houston,
Houston Health Science Center, Houston, Texas

I. OVERVIEW OF MULTIPLE SCLEROSIS

Multiple sclerosis (MS) is a chronic demyelinating disease of the central nervous system (CNS), which has been postulated to be a T-cell–mediated autoimmune disease (1). Although the etiology of MS is unknown, most investigators believe that the immune system is intimately involved in the progression of the disease (2). MS is clinically associated with periods of disability (relapse) alternating with periods of recovery (remission) but often leading to progressive neurological disability (3). The lesions in the CNS are similar to the lesions produced by T-lymphocyte delayed-type (DTH) hypersensitivity reactions. Studies of the cellular immune system in tissue compartments have suggested that there is a sequestration of antigen-specific T-cell populations in the cerebrospinal fluid (CSF) (4). A major hypothesis concerning the CNS inflammation is that T lymphocytes are reacting to an (un)identified self-antigen(s) intrinsic to myelin (such as myelin basic protein [MBP] or proteolipid protein [PLP]), and these T lymphocytes damage myelin directly or by activating macrophages and other agents of inflammation. Progression or recurrence of immune damage appears to result from a failure of normal regulatory mechanisms to suppress the immune process in MS (5). We have recently shown that there is a CD3 pathway defect (6) and that secretion of interferon-γ (IFN-γ) was significantly decreased and transforming growth factor-β (TGF-β)

was significantly increased via anti-CD3 mAb in stable relapsing-remitting MS (RRMS) patients compared with controls (7).

II. TYPE I IFNs

In 1957, Isaacs and Lindenmann described a factor (interferon) produced by virus-infected cells with rapid antiviral activity (8). Type I IFNs are composed of two highly homologous proteins, IFN-α (leukocyte IFN) and IFN-β (fibroblast IFN) with similar biological properties (9–10). IFN-α and IFN-β are relatively similar in their actions and interact with the same cell receptor (11). Natural IFNs-α contain 165–166 amino acids with about 80% sequence homology to each other (12–13). IFN activates cellular 2,5-oligoadenylate synthetase (2,5-OAS) (14), β_2-microglobulin (15), or other proteins (IRF-1, PI/eIF-2a protein kinase, Mx, major histocompatibility complex [MHC]) (16), thus providing markers indicating IFN/IFN receptor interaction. IFN-α can also decrease T-cell function and T-cell–dependent antibody production in humans when given parenterally (17).

A. IFNs in Disease and Their Present Parenteral and Oral Therapeutic Use

In view of the immunoregulatory and antiviral properties of the type I IFNs, their response and production has been assessed in autoimmune diseases. Inactive rheumatoid arthritis (RA) is marked by augmented inducibility to an IFN-α stimulus, whereas active RA is associated with low inducibility of peripheral blood lymphocytes (PBLs) to an IFN stimulus and no evidence of IFN production in vivo (18). Patients with active rheumatoid arthritis exhibit a significantly reduced IFN-α/β production compared with normal donors (19). Other autoimmune diseases such as psoriasis and atopic dermatitis show decreased type I IFN production (20–21). Peripheral blood leukocyte (PBLs) in patients with MS show a similar ineffective production of type I IFNs in response to viral or mitogenic stimulus (22–23) which parallels the severity of the disease (24). Defects in natural killer (NK) cell activity and renormalization after IFN-α treatment have also been observed in Sjögren's syndrome (25), type I diabetes mellitus (26), rheumatoid arthritis (18,27), and MS (24,28–29), where NK function is correlated with disease severity, but not by all investigators (30). Human IFN-β reportedly augments suppressor cell function in vitro and in vivo in progressive MS (31–32).

The observed abnormalities of production or response to type I IFN in autoimmune diseases have prompted several small pilot studies using parenteral type I IFNs as therapeutic agents in MS. These studies showed no conclusive results (33–35), a clear trend toward fewer relapses during treatment with IFN (36), and a decreased capacity to synthesize native IFN (37), but were without a clear marker for either MS activity or therapeutic effect (38). Other studies used subcutaneous or intrathecal type I IFN and demonstrated no significant clinical improvement (37,39–41), reduction in relapses (42), stabilization of disease progression (43–44), therapeutic efficacy (45), relationship of IFN treatment to MS disease activity (46), nor an increased number of circulating NK cells (47). More recent studies of parenterally administered human recombinant type I IFNs (hrIFN) in RRMS demonstrate decreased relapses (48) and decreased brain inflammation (49), decreased spontaneous in vitro IFN-γ production (50), and a reduction of progression, relapse rate, and active lesions on MRI (51) (see Chapter 13).

Oral administration of type I IFNs may avoid the inconvenience and side effects of intrathecal and systemic administration and work through a unique and more effective mode of action. Natural human IFN-α has been orally administered at low doses in the treatment of viral disease in animals. The first report suggesting that orally administered IFN could exert a protective effect showed that 500 U IFN/ml protected suckling mice from per os (p.o.) lethal viral challenge (52). Orally administered natural human IFN-α can prevent the experimental development of feline leukemia (53) and bovine *Theileria parva* infection (54). Stanton found that low doses of recombinant hIFN-α A/D (which is highly active on mouse cells (55)) or mouse IFN-α/β given orally in drinking water protected mice from encephalitis and death from intraperitoneal (i.p.) injection of Semliki Forest virus (56). Importantly, this response was biphasic: higher levels of IFN were not protective, nor were high or low i.p. doses protective. Recent studies indicate that systemic IFN effects can be achieved with comparatively very low dose ($\approx$100–1000 U) natural human IFN-α (53,57–59).

The therapeutic effect of oral IFNs may not require transit of intact IFN across the bowel. Proteins which might not survive transit through the alimentary canal may still exhibit immunomodulatory activity via the gut-associated lymphoid tissue (GALT) in the oropharynx and beyond via paracrine activity (60–63). Several early studies on the pharmacokinetics of IFNs delivered by various routes reported that orally administered IFNs failed to appear in the bloodstream (64–66). There are no reports of p.o. administration of IFN peptides or the presence of IFN breakdown products in the lumen of the gut or in the bloodstream, although IFN-α amino acids 9–18 and 26–40 in vitro inhibit antigen receptor–stimulated proliferation or viral activity in human cells (67–68). However, several investigations have shown small but measurable amounts of IFN can be absorbed from the oral pharynx or large intestine in rats (69–70). More recent studies demonstrate that oral administration of low-dose IFN-α in mice (71), dogs (72), green monkeys (73), or humans (74) (see Chapter 3) does not result in detectable levels of IFN-α in the blood in contrast to parenteral administration, nor can its effect be blocked by circulating anti-IFN antibodies in mice (71). The inability to detect p.o. administered IFNs in blood may be due to their modest spillover in a rapidly turning over lymphatic pool (75).

The absence of increases in biological markers (β_2-microglobulin, neopterin, or 2,5-OAS) after p.o. IFN β-administration (74) and their presence with subcutaneous (s.c.) or intravenous (i.v.) IFN-β (76), suggest that p.o. IFN acts through a different mechanism. The neutropenic effect of orally administered IFN can be transferred by injection of blood cells but not by serum from IFN-fed animals to recipient animals or humans (71). Activated monocytes and lymphocytes, by virtue of their circulatory ability, potentially can transfer their biological activities all over the body in the absence of circulating cytokines after contacting IFN or IFN-induced cells in GALT (75,77). Therefore, the evaluation of type I IFN therapy by the oral compared with the parenteral route in experimental autoimmune encephalomyelitis (EAE) may be of relevance for the therapy of early autoimmune disease including RRMS and other chronic non-neurological autoimmune diseases.

III. ORAL IFN IN ACUTE EAE

Acute EAE is a T-cell–mediated inflammatory autoimmune process of the CNS which resembles the human disease multiple sclerosis (78). Acute EAE provides a model to assess the ability of orally administered immunoactive substances to influence the course of an autoimmune disease. However, in spite of the parenteral IFN-β trials in MS, very limited information exists about the effect of type I IFNs on EAE (see Chapter 9). Previous investigators have demonstrated that parenteral TGF-β can decrease clinical disease and inflammation in brain and spinal cord in EAE (79), and that rat natural IFN-α/β decreases the severity of symptoms in rat EAE (80). CD4$^+$ T cells from the spleens of rats that have recovered from EAE inhibit the in vitro production of IFN-γ by effector cells cultured with MBP, and this inhibition can be abrogated by anti–TGF-β_2 antibodies (81). Parenteral (i.v.) rat natural IFN-α/β (10^5 U) can partially suppress acute EAE in male Lewis rats (82) and inhibit passive hyperacute, localized EAE (83) when administered on the same day as inoculation of immunogen. Investigation of cytokine evolution in the CNS during the natural course of EAE suggests that interleukin-2 (IL-2), IL-6, and

IFN-γ mRNA are elevated in acute disease, but during stabilization of symptoms, these cytokines are decreased with increasing IL-10 mRNA levels (84). Therefore, since IFN-β proved useful in MS, an understanding of the mechanism of action of parenterally administered type I IFNs on cytokine profiles would be important and might determine whether an immune response can be inhibited by orally administered cytokines. Recent studies cited above (53–54,57–59,85) indicate that systemic IFN effects can indeed be achieved with natural human IFN-α administered orally. We therefore examined whether the oral administration of such type I IFNs would inhibit the clinical expression of attacks, decrease pathological sequelae, and inhibit inflammatory cytokine IFN-γ secretion in a model of acute autoimmune disease, EAE.

A. Oral Natural Rat IFN-α/β Can Modify Clinical Disease, Inhibit Proliferative Responses, and Decrease Inflammation to GP-MBP

Seven days preceding immunization with MBP (day −7) and for 21 days thereafter (day +14 postimmunization), three groups of Lewis rats were fed either 1000 U mock IFN or 5000 U rat IFN-α/β daily in 0.1 ml phosphate-buffered saline (PBS) (86). All animals were scored for clinical disease until day 16 after immunization (Fig. 1). Results from blinded examination of daily group clinical scores demonstrated significant differences in clinical outcome in the mock-fed versus 5000 U IFN-α/β–fed animals at days 14–16 and in the animals fed 1000 U at day 14 only. Rats treated with 5000 U rat natural IFN-α/β had peak disease that was less severe than in the mock group, and the 5000 U IFN-α/β–treated group recovered more quickly and returned to baseline sooner than the mock-treated group. Rats treated with 1000 U rat natural IFN-α/β had peak disease that was less severe than in the mock group, but neither recovered nor returned to baseline as quickly as the 5000-U fed group. The overall mean cumulative clinical score (area under the curve) of the animals treated with 5000 U rat natural IFN-α was significantly less than mock IFN–fed controls (0.8 ± 0.2, *5000 U* fed vs 1.2 ± 0.2, *mock IFN* fed, *p* < .02). Animals were also examined histologically 16 days following immunization. There were less inflammatory foci in the IFN-α/β–treated compared with the control mock IFN group, although this did not attain statistical significance owing to the small number of spinal cords examined per group (Table 1, *5000 IFN* p.o. vs *mock IFN*, *p* < .06).

Sixteen days after immunization, draining popliteal lymph node concanavallin A (ConA) proliferation was inhibited from 16,209 ± 1,234 cpm from mock-fed animals to 8120 ± 765 cpm in 5000-U IFN-α/β–fed animals

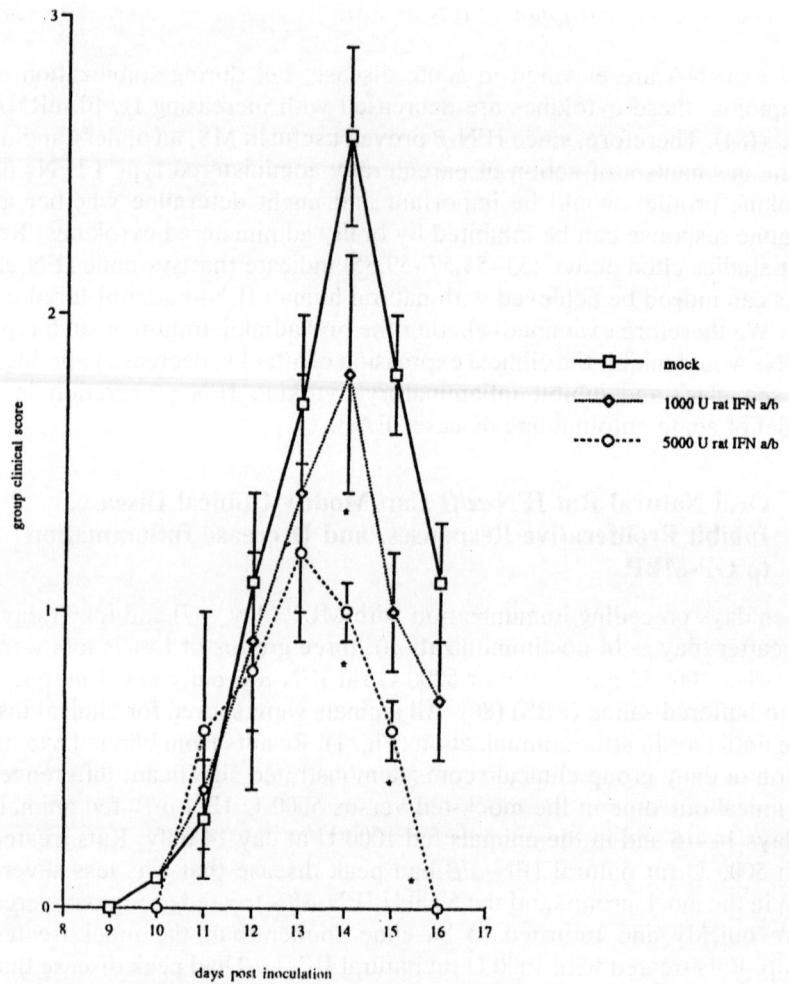

Figure 1 Oral administration of 5000 U rat IFN-α/β inhibits clinical disease in acute EAE. Three groups of six 8- to 10-week-old Lewis rats were immunized with equal parts MBP and CFA (76) and subsequently had attacks beginning by day 9 and followed until day 16. Seven days preceding immunization (day −7) and for 21 days thereafter (day +14), each group of animals were fed either 1000 U mock IFN, or 5000 U rat type I IFN-α/β (Cytimmune rat IFN-α + β, 4 × 10⁵ IRU/ml, Lee Biomolecular Research, Inc., San Diego, CA) daily in 0.1 ml PBS. All animals were scored for clinical disease until day 16 after immunization. Results from blinded examination of daily group clinical scores. Results are expressed as average clinical score for each group on each day of disease postinnoculation ± SEM. Combined data from at least two experiments are shown. *p < .001 between mock IFN and 5000 U IFN-α/β fed–animals on day 14 and between mock IFN and 5000 U IFN-α/β–fed animals on days 14, 15, and 16 by nonpaired t test.

Table 1 Inhibition of Clinical Disease in Rat Acute EAE by Oral Rat Species-Specific and Human Recombinant Type I IFNs Correlates with Decreased Inflammation in Spinal Cord

	Mock	1000 IFN p.o.	5000 IFN p.o.	5000 IFN s.c.
Rat IFN	50 ± 2^a	Not detected	26 ± 2	—
p.o.	(n = 3)		(n = 3)	
hrIFN-α	52 ± 6	62 ± 8	$32 \pm 6^*$	—
p.o.	(n = 7)	(n = 7)	(n = 7)	
hrIFN-α	60 ± 4	—	$40 \pm 10^{**}$	82 ± 12
p.o./s.c.	(n = 5)		(n = 5)	(n = 5)

^{a} Inflammatory foci (>20 inflammatory cells in parenchyma).
* $p < .05$ compared with control; ** $p < .01$ compared with control.

($p < .05$). Draining popliteal lymph node cells from mock and 5000 U–treated animals were stimulated with ionomycin + phorbol myristate acetate (PMA), and demonstrated decreasing proliferation from mock-treated (20,505 cpm $\pm$ 505) to 5000 U–treated (6111 cpm $\pm$ 636, $p < .05$) animals. No consistent differences in MBP or *Mycobacterium tuberculosis hominis* (MT) proliferation between fed and mock-fed animals was demonstrated in draining popliteal lymph node (data not shown). There was also no inhibition in spleen or nondraining mesenteric lymph node responses to ConA or ionomycin/PMA in IFN-treated animals (data not shown).

These data suggest that species-specific type I IFNs can inhibit the severity of acute clinical disease when given at adequate dosages. Inhibition of proliferation from orally administered IFN-α/β could be due to a direct action of IFN which enters the bloodstream through the gut or to and indirect mechanism. We examined whether in vitro type I IFN treatment of draining popliteal lymph node and spleen cells from immunized, but mock-treated, animals would demonstrate effects similar to in vivo treatment. There was no clear inhibitory effect on ConA proliferation in draining popliteal lymph node or spleen cells exposed to IFN in vitro (Fig. 2), in contrast to in vivo IFN oral administration.

B. Modification of Acute Rat EAE by Oral Administration of Human Recombinant IFN-α

Since human type I interferon can show cross-species activity in mice (87), guinea pigs (88), gnotobiotic calves (89), horses and pigs (90), and cats (91–92), we also utilized recombinant human IFN-α (hrIFN-α), a

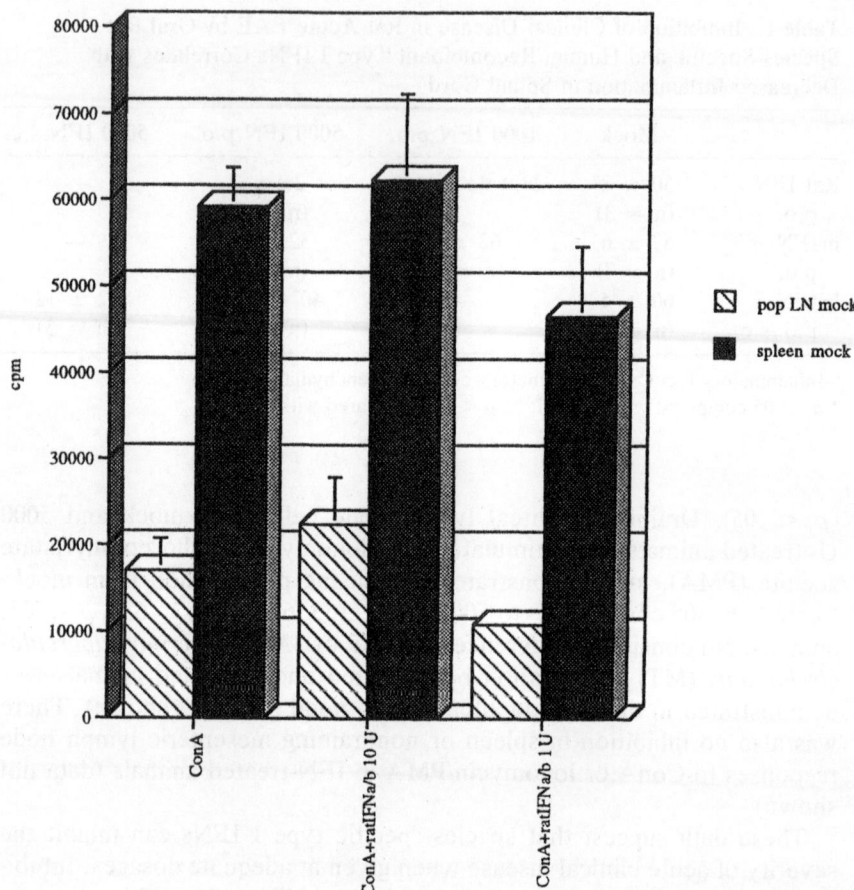

Figure 2 In vitro rat natural IFN-α/β does not inhibit ConA–induced proliferation of mock-fed draining popliteal LN (pop LN) or spleen cells in acute EAE. Following clinical attack, rats were sacrificed, and spleen and draining lymph node cells were pooled and cultured in vitro with ConA $\pm$ 1 or 10 U rat natural IFN-α/β. Cultures were run in triplicate and the results expressed as ΔCPM $\pm$ SEM. Cell preparation and proliferation is as described in ref. 86.

uniform material that would eliminate the possibility that disease was modified by non-IFN rat immunoactive proteins, induced during manufacturing by induction of rat fibroblast cultures with Newcastle disease virus. Recombinant human IFN-α_2 (Schering Pharmaceuticals, Kenilworth, NJ) was used in these experiments. There is a high degree of homology between human and murine type I IFN gene products (93); type I IFNs can induce viral resistance in cultured heterologous cells thus demonstrating transspecies activity (94), and human IFN has been successfully used in cats (53) and pigs (57). In addition, human recombinant IFN-α may also provide more immunosuppression per unit of activity than natural preparations. Since both 1000 and 5000 U natural rat IFN-α/β administered p.o. demonstrated some effectiveness in inhibiting acute disease for 7 days preceding immunization (day -7) and for 21 days thereafter (day $+14$), each group of animals was fed either mock PBS, 1000 U, or 5000 U hrIFN-α daily. Three groups of seven 8- to 10-week old Lewis rats were immunized and subsequently had an attack beginning by day 10 and extending through day 16. All animals were scored for clinical disease until day 16 after immunization.

Results from blinded examination of daily group clinical scores demonstrated significant differences in clinical outcome in the mock-fed versus 5000-U hrIFN-α–fed animals at days 12–15 but not in the animals fed 1000 U (Fig. 3A). Animals fed 5000 U hrIFN-α showed delayed attack onset, decreased severity at peak, and earlier resolution of the attack. The overall mean cumulative clinical score of the animals treated with either PBS control-fed (1.8 $\pm$ 0.2) or 1000 U-fed animals (2.1 $\pm$ 0.3) was significantly greater than 5000 U hrIFN-α (0.5 $\pm$ 0.2; $p < .001$). There was a trend for decreased ConA proliferation in draining popliteal lymph node from 56,209 $\pm$ 5386 cpm in mock PBS–fed animals to 37,438 $\pm$ 8862 cpm in 5000 U IFN-α/β–fed animals ($p < .06$). This suggests that orally administered hrIFN-α can inhibit clinical attacks of EAE in the Lewis rat when administered before inoculation. Following sacrifice 16 days postimmunization, animals were also examined histologically. There were significantly more inflammatory foci in the mock PBS group or 1000 U hrIFN-α–fed group compared with the 5000 U hrIFN-α–fed group (see Table 1, hrIFN-α p.o.).

C. Oral But Not Equivalent Doses of Parenteral Administered hrIFN-α Modifies Clinical Disease

The above data suggest that orally administered hrIFN-α can modify clinical disease and decrease inflammation in spinal cord. Experiments were performed to examine equivalent amounts of orally versus parenterally administered hrIFN-α. Three groups of 10 Lewis rats were immunized and either not treated, fed 5000 U hrIFN-α, or injected with 5000 U hrIFN-α s.c. for 7 days preceding immunization (day -7) and for 21 days thereafter (day $+14$). All animals were scored for clinical disease until day 18

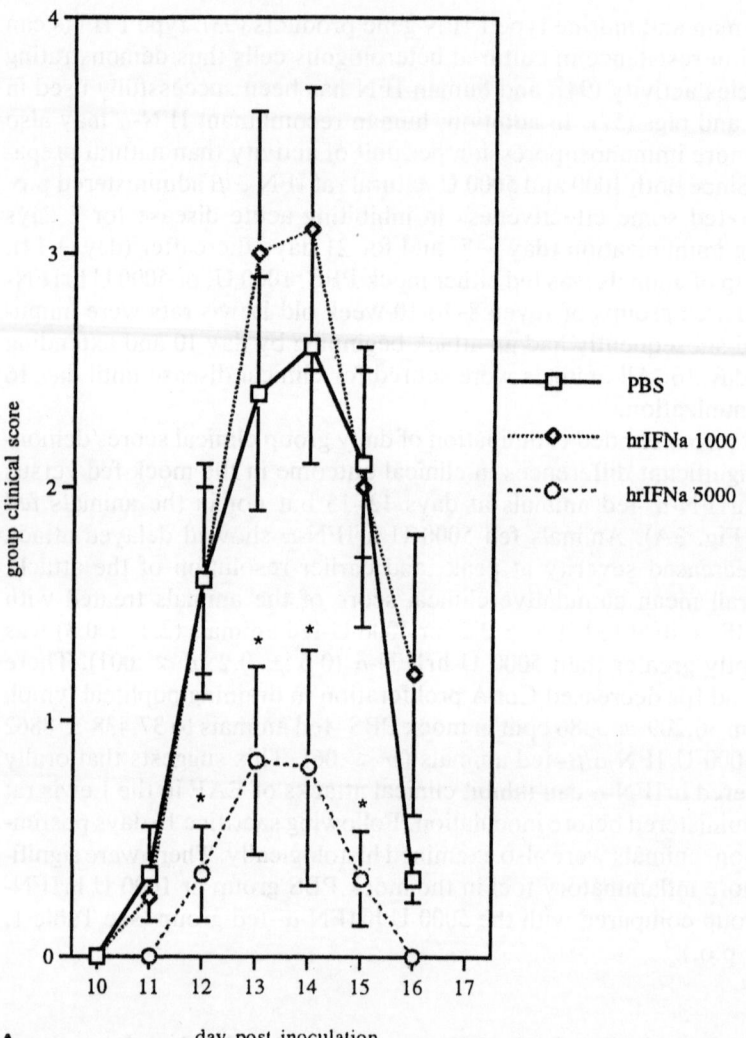

A.

day post inoculation

Figure 3 Oral administration of 5000 U human IFN-α in rat acute EAE, but not s.c. administration, decreases the severity and speeds the recovery of clinical attacks. (A) Dose effect. Three groups of seven Lewis rats were inoculated with MBP and CFA on day 0 and orally administered PBS, 1000 U or 5000 U hrIFN-α (Schering human recombinant IFN-α_{2b}, 3×10^6 IU/ml, Schering Pharmaceuticals, Kenilworth, NJ) daily, starting 7 days preceding immunization (day -7) and for 14 days thereafter (day $+14$). Values represent mean clinical scores for each group of seven animals $\pm$ SEM. Combined data from at least two experiments are shown. *$p < .05$ between mock PBS/1000 U IFN-α–fed versus 5000 unit IFN-

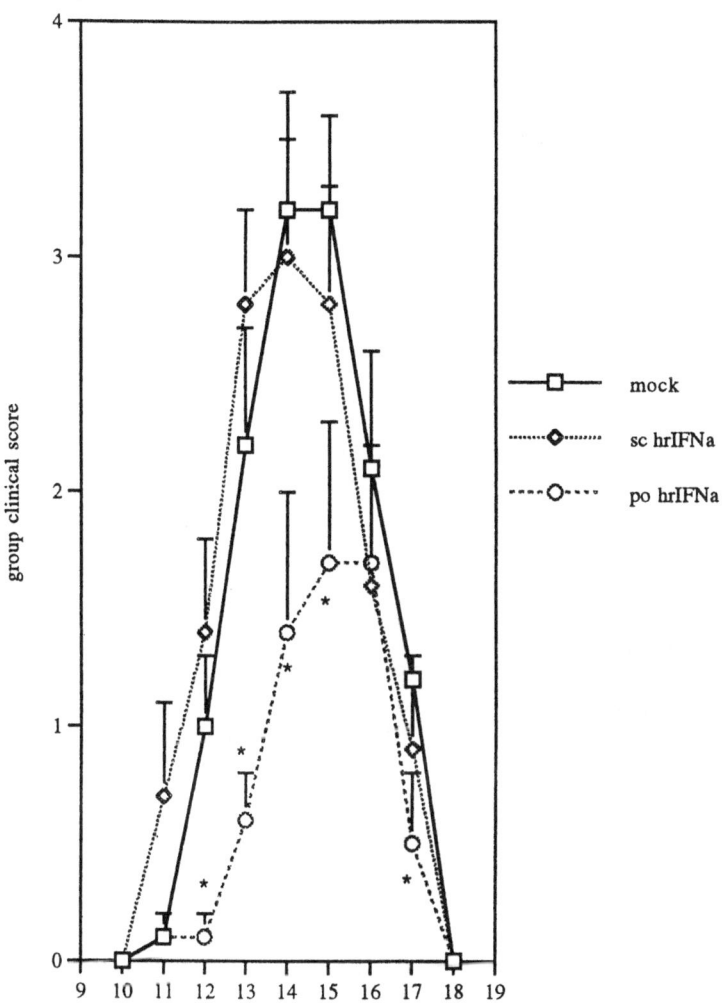

B. day post inoculation

α–fed animals on days 12–15 by nonpaired t test. (B) Oral administration of 5000 U hrIFN-α, not s.c. administration, decreases the severity of clinical attacks. Three groups of 10 Lewis rats were inoculated with MBP and CFA on day 0 and were either untreated, fed 5000 U, or injected s.c. with 5000 U hrIFN-α daily starting 7 days preceding immunization (day -7) and for 21 days thereafter (day $+14$). Values represent mean daily clinical scores for each group of 10 animals $+$ SEM. Combined data from at least two experiments are shown. *$p < .005$ between mock PBS/5000 U s.c. IFN-α versus 5000 U IFN-α–fed animals on days 12–14, $p < .05$ on days 15 and 17 by nonpaired t test.

after immunization. Results from blinded examination of daily group clinical scores demonstrated significant differences in clinical outcome in the mock-fed versus 5000-U hrIFN-α–fed animals at days 12–15 and 17 but not in the animals injected s.c. with 5000 U hrIFN-α (Fig. 3B). Rats treated with oral 5000 U hrIFN-α had a less severe disease at peak of the disease and more rapid recovery compared with the untreated group. Indeed, the untreated and the subcutaneously treated groups had very similar clinical curve scores, suggesting that s.c. hrIFN-α had little or no effect on clinical disease. Overall mean cumulative clinical scores demonstrated significant differences in clinical outcome in the untreated (1.5 ± 0.2) and subcutaneously treated (1.8 ± 0.4) versus fed animals (0.6 ± 0.2; $p < .005$, fed vs untreated/s.c. treated). There was no significant difference between untreated and subcutaneously treated animals. There was no significant difference in draining popliteal lymph node ConA proliferation between untreated and 5000 U subcutaneously treated animals (*untreated*: 30,854 ± 2142 cpm vs *5000 U* s.c.: 38,242 ± 4476 cpm). Eighteen days following immunization, animals were sacrificed and examined histologically. There were significantly more inflammatory foci in the 5000-U subcutaneously treated group and untreated group compared with the 5000-U fed group (see Table 1, hrIFN-α p.o./s.c.).

Experiments using PBS-fed and PBS subcutaneously injected controls demonstrated similar findings. In this case, four groups of six Lewis rats were either fed PBS, injected s.c. with PBS, fed 5000 U hrIFN-α, or injected with 5000 U hrIFN-α s.c. for 7 days preceding immunization (day −7) and for 21 days thereafter (day +14). All animals were immunized on day 0. Animals were scored for clinical disease until day 18 after immunization and sacrificed. Mean cumulative clinical scores were significantly less in hrIFN-α–fed animals (1.0 ± 0.2) compared with PBS-fed animals (2.5 ± 0.4) ($p < .005$). There was no significant difference between mock s.c. (1.7 ± 0.4) and 5000 U hrIFN-α s.c. (2.1 ± 0.4) animals even though subcutaneously treated animals did have higher mean cumulative clinical scores. This suggests that subcutaneously administered hrIFN-α cannot modify the onset of acute clinical disease when given at clinically preventive oral dosages.

D. Orally Administered IFN-α Inhibits the Mitogen-Induced Production of IFN-γ in Draining Popliteal Lymph Nodes

The intensity of disease in EAE has been associated with IFN-γ secretion after ConA stimulation (95). We assessed IFN-γ secretion at 9 days postimmunization and before disease onset, at day 16 during a time point when there was significant clinical difference between mock IFN and 5000 U hrIFN-α–fed animals, and at day 18 postimmunization after clinical attack had subsided. Spleen and draining popliteal lymph node cells from both mock-fed, 5000 U fed hrIFN-α-fed, or 5000 U s.c. hrIFN-α–treated rats were stimulated with ConA (2.5 μg/ml) for 2 days. At day 9 preceding clinical disease, but during the generation of antigen-specific T cells in draining popliteal lymph node, draining popliteal lymph node cells from mock IFN–treated animals demonstrated detectable IFN-γ production, whereas there was no IFN-γ production from 5000 U hrIFN-α–fed animals (Table 2). At day 16, when clinical differences persisted in animals, and at day 18 postimmunization, after clinical attack had subsided, draining popliteal lymph node cells from mock PBS–treated animals continued to demonstrate significantly greater IFN-γ production compared with 5000 U–fed animals (Table 2). There was no difference between mock- and 5000 U–treated spleen cells (data not shown). There were no differences in draining popliteal lymph node IFN-γ secretion between animals subcutaneously mock-treated versus injected subcutaneously treated with 5000 U hrIFN-α. The results show that p.o., not s.c. hrIFN-α, decreased IFN-γ, a mediator of inflammation, in draining popliteal lymph node.

Orally administered type I IFNs, as opposed to identical s.c. doses, can be utilized as modifiers of biological response to MBP in acute EAE in Lewis rats when they are administered before sensitization and clinical attack. Orally administered type I IFNs modify clinical attacks, decrease the number of inflammatory foci in spinal cord, decrease nonspecific proliferation by ConA and ionomycin/PMA, and decrease the production of IFN-γ in draining popliteal lymph nodes. This suggests that IFN-α is more active by the oral route compared with the parenteral route, has definable immunological effects, and confirms that specific cytokines are capable of inhibiting clinical disease when given via the gastrointestinal (GI) tract. Both human recombinant IFN-α and species-specific rat natural IFN worked in our experiments. Natural IFNs are a mixture of 14 separate subspecies, including the IFN-α_2 subtype, which may be only a small

Table 2 Orally Administered Human Recombinant IFN-α Inhibits Mitogen-Induced Production of IFN-γ in Draining Popliteal Lymph Nodes

Day postimmunization	Mock p.o. PBS	5000 p.o. IFN	Mock s.c. PBS	5000 s.c. IFN
9	50 ± 14	Not detected	—	—
16	1,140 ± 6	68 ± 22*	—	—
18	460 ± 60	96 ± 32*	540 ± 80	421 ± 38**

* $p < .05$ compared with mock p.o. PBS control; ** $p < .05$ compared with mock s.c. PBS.

component of the natural type (10). Human IFN shows cross-species activity when used at larger doses (5000 U) compared with rat species-specific type I IFN, which showed some activity at 1000 U p.o. The use of the IFN-α_2 subtype may provide a relative greater amount of inhibitory activity/total units of antiproliferative activity of the most important component for immunosuppression in the rat.

Antiproliferative effects of orally administered IFN were greater in draining popliteal lymph nodes than in nondraining mesenteric lymph nodes (data not shown). Oral administration of IFN-α, as opposed to s.c. administration, inhibited the production of IFN-γ in draining popliteal lymph nodes. Draining popliteal lymph nodes are the natural draining areas for subcutaneously administered antigens and are therefore presumably the reservoir of high frequencies of sensitized MBP-specific T cells. Orally administered cytokines may preferentially affect proliferation and cytokine production at sites of immune activation compared with *equivalent* systemic doses. Inhibition of IFN-γ secretion in an activated regional immune compartment by IFN-α may cause decreased inflammatory effect of MBP-specific cells in the CNS (see also Chapter 7).

IV. ORAL IFN IN CHRONIC EXPERIMENTAL AUTOIMMUNE ENCEPHALOMYELITIS

One major difficulty in treating autoimmune disease in humans is that the immune system has already been sensitized to autoantigen at the time of clinical presentation. An animal model which mimics clinical disease and previous immunological sensitization is useful in the evaluation of potential therapies for human disease. Chronic relapsing experimental autoimmune encephalomyelitis (CREAE) is such a disease, since it is a chronic inflammatory CNS autoimmune process that more closely resembles MS (96–98). After immunization, animals cycle repeatedly through manifest clinical attacks. Therefore CREAE provides an excellent model to test for the modulation of clinical, immunological, and histological sequelae by orally or parenterally administered IFNs.

A. Orally Administered Murine Type I IFNs Can Suppress Clinical Disease and Inflammation and Inhibit Proliferative Responses to MBP

Initial experiments suggested that 1–10 U of orally administered murine type I IFN had an immunological effect, but was not adequate to suppress clinical relapses (data not shown). Therefore, experiments were performed in which two groups of six immunized SJL/J mice (using the method of Brown and McFarlin (99), modified by Miller (100)) were fed mock IFN or 100 U murine natural IFN-α/β three times per week beginning on day 30, following recovery from the first clinical attack. Group clinical scores after the initial attack were not significantly different among the different groups. Clinical relapses began approximately 40 days after inoculation. Clinical scores demonstrated significant differences in outcome in the mock IFN–fed versus 100 U murine natural IFN-α/β–fed animals ($p < .03$; see Fig. 4). Two major relapses occurred in the mock IFN–fed group over the course of 7 weeks with a resultant increased neurological deficit. The oral murine natural IFN-α/β group underwent a delayed single attack without residual neurological deficit. Oral murine natural IFN-α/β blunted the severity and decreased the group score during clinical relapse. Oral administration of IFN-γ has no effect on EAE (unpublished results, S. A. Brod).

ConA activation of draining inguinal lymph node cells was inhibited in animals fed 100 U murine natural IFN-α/β compared with mock IFN–fed (38,095 cpm $\pm$ 3160 vs 88,222 cpm $\pm$ 1910, $p < .05$). Lymph node cells from mock IFN–fed animals tested with MBP generated a robust proliferative response, but that response was profoundly inhibited in murine natural IFN-α/β–fed animals (14,052 cpm $\pm$ 842 vs 448 cpm $\pm$ 50, $p < .05$).

To determine whether there was inhibition to another sensitized antigen, we examined antigen-specific proliferation of draining inguinal lymph node to a second sensitized antigen, MT, a component of mouse spinal cord homogenate (MSCH) inoculum. Lymph node cells from mock IFN–fed animals generated a robust proliferative response to MT, but that response was profoundly decreased in 100-U murine natural IFN-$\alpha/$ β–fed animals (52,401 cpm $\pm$ 857 vs 5214 cpm $\pm$ 808, $p < .05$).

Animals were also examined histologically 65 days following immunization and after clinical relapse. There were significantly fewer inflammatory foci in the IFN-fed group (0.5 $\pm$ 0.1) compared with the mock IFN group (1.8 $\pm$ 1.1) ($p < .05$). The data above suggests that orally administered murine natural type I IFNs can suppress clinical relapse disease, decrease inflammation, and inhibit proliferation to mitogen, MBP, and MT.

B. Suppression of Relapse by Oral IFN-α/β Correlates with Decreased IFN-γ Secretion

The intensity of disease in EAE has been associated with IFN-γ secretion after ConA stimulation of spleen cells (95). Therefore, pooled mouse spleen cells were stimulated from both mock-fed (n = 5) or 100-U–fed (n = 5) murine IFN-α/β with ConA (2.5 μg/ml) at 1 $\times$ 10^6 cells/ml for 2 days, and supernatants were assayed by solid-phase ELISA (IL-2, IL-10,

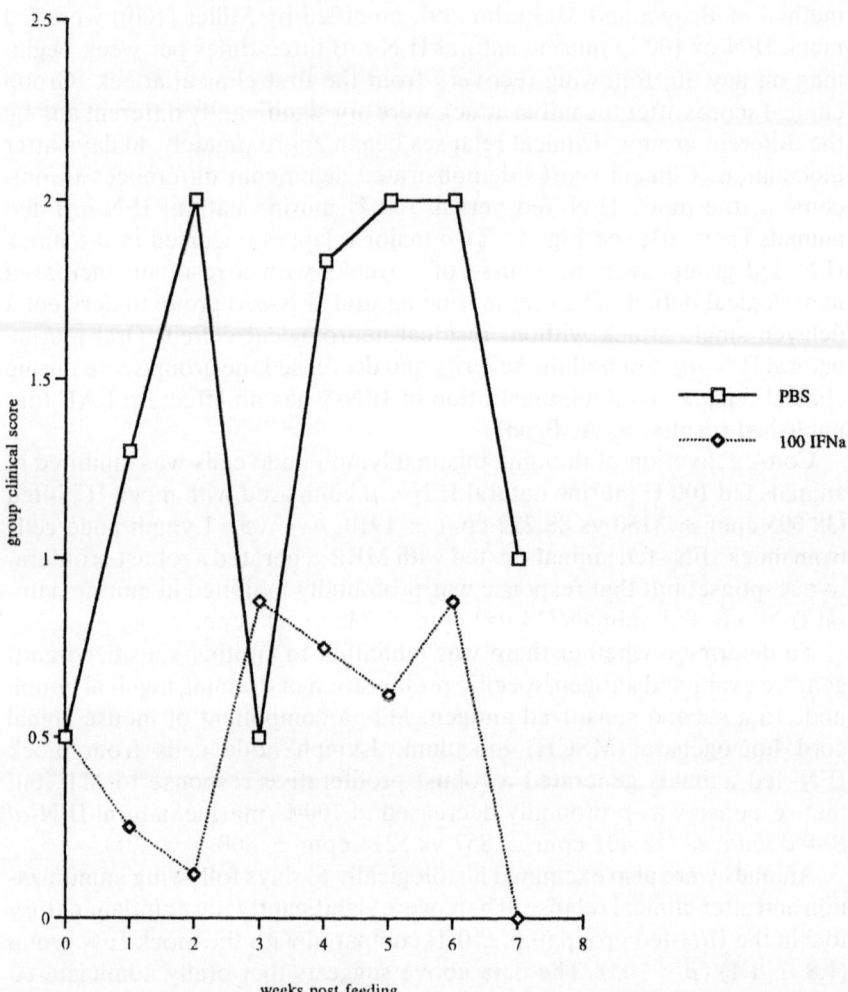

Figure 4 Orally administered murine natural IFN-α/β suppresses clinical relapse in murine CREAE. Two groups of six animals were inoculated and following the first attack were fed either mock IFN or 100 U murine natural IFN-α/β (Cytimmune mouse IFN-α/β, 4 × 10^5 IRU/ml, Lee Biomolecular Research, Inc., San Diego, CA) or mock murine IFN-α/β (Cytimmune <2 IRU/ml, Lee Biomolecular Research, Inc., San Diego, CA. [generated identically to IFN-α/β except cultures are mock induced] three times per week for 7 weeks. One of two representative experiments are shown. SEM is <10% and is not shown.

IFN-γ). Oral murine IFN-α/β consistently decreased IFN-γ, a mediator of inflammation (Table 3, $p < .001$). There was also a decrease in IL-2, a T-cell growth factor, and increased IL-10 production, although these changes did not attain statistical significance (data not shown).

As in the rat system, available natural murine type I IFN are manufactured by viral induction in murine fibroblasts and could contain non-IFN immunoactive proteins responsible for disease modification. Others have found that human IFN-α_1 and IFN-α_2 have 1–50% of antiviral activity in L929 mouse cells compared with human WISH or HEp2 cell lines (55,101–102). Therefore, suppression of actively induced relapses and prevention of adoptive transfer with pure human preparations would eliminate the possibility that non-IFN murine proteins modify disease but might require higher doses relative to murine IFN to show effects. Accordingly, we examined whether the oral administration of hrIFN-α and lower doses of murine species-specific IFN-α would prevent clinical relapses of EAE.

C. Orally Administered hrIFN-α Can Suppress Clinical EAE and Inhibit Proliferative Responses to MBP

Three groups of six SJL/J 6- to 8-week-old female mice that were immunized with MSCH subsequently had an attack beginning by day 16 and ending by day 30. Each group of animals had comparable scores after the initial clinical attack had subsided. On day 30 postimmunization, groups were either mock fed PBS, 100 U human recombinant IFN-α (hrIFN-α), or 100 U hrIFN-α three times per week over the following 5 weeks (103). Mean weekly clinical relapse scores demonstrated significant differences in outcome in the mock PBS–fed versus 100 and 1000 U hrIFN-α–fed animals (Fig. 5). The mock PBS–fed group incurred increasing disease severity over the course of 5 weeks, as shown by increasing neurological deficit (group clinical score) over time. The 1000 U hrIFN-α-fed groups underwent a mild single attack with decreasing neurological deficit. Overall, oral hrIFN-α decreased the group scores during relapse. Thus, orally administered hrIFN-α is active by the oral route and suppresses clinical relapses in mice.

Table 3 Orally Administered Murine IFN-α/β Inhibits Mitogen-Induced Production of IFN-γ in Spleen Cells

	Mock IFN	100 U IFN
Experiment 1	2500 ± 300	1100 ± 200*
Experiment 2	2180 ± 100	247 ± 143*

* $p < .001$ compared with mock IFN control.

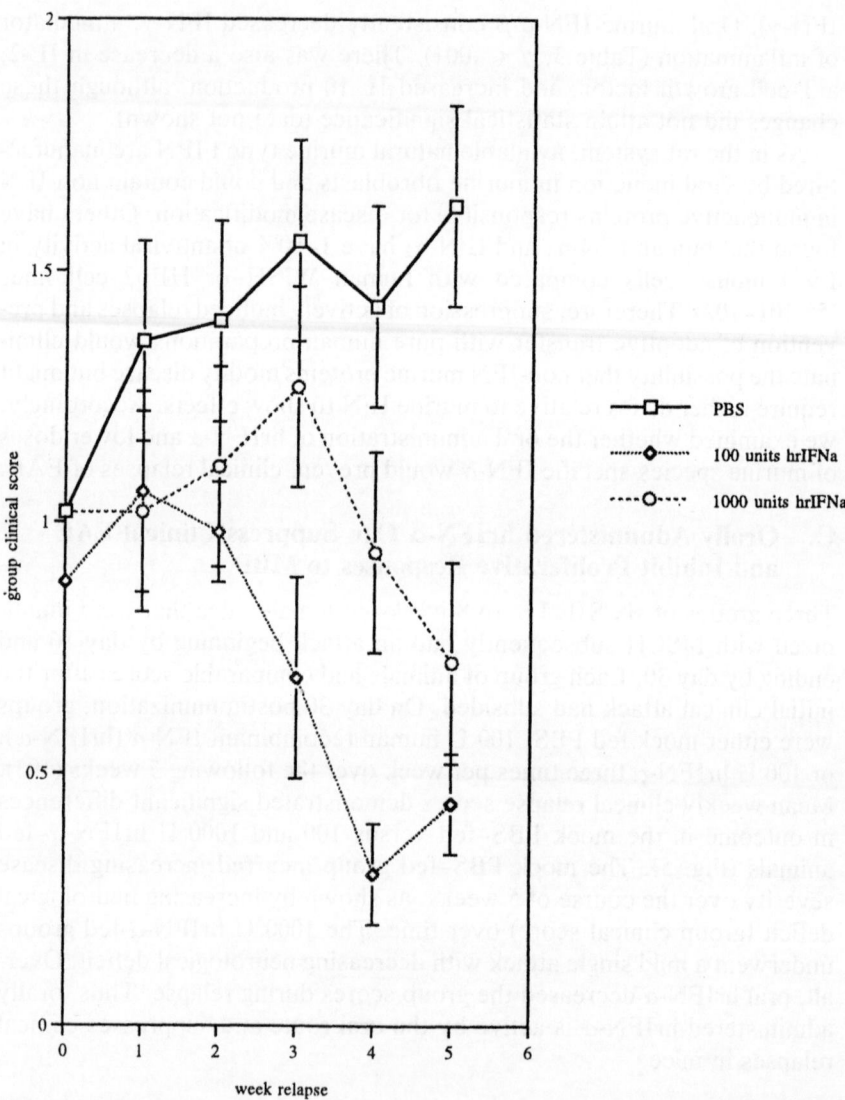

Figure 5 Oral administration of human recombinant IFN-α in murine CREAE suppresses relapses. Three groups of six SJL/J 6- to 8-week-old female mice were immunized as with MSCH in CFA. On day 40 postimmunization, one group was fed PBS, another group 100 U hrIFN-α, and a third group was fed 1000 U hrIFN-α three times per week over the following 5 weeks. All animals were scored by a blinded observer for clinical disease until day 75 pastimmunization. Values represent combined data of two separate experiments of mean weekly group clinical scores $\pm$ SEM (mock PBS-fed vs 100 U for weeks 2–5, $p < .001$; vs 1000 U hrIFN-α–fed animals for weeks 4–5, $p < .01$ by nonpaired t test).

Following clinical relapse, mice were sacrificed, spleen and draining inguinal lymph node cells were pooled into hrIFN-α-fed (n = 6) and mock PBS-fed (n = 6) group, and cells were cultured in vitro to determine antigen-specific T-cell proliferation. There was a significant decrease in proliferation to GP-MBP in draining inguinal lymph nodes of mice fed 1000 U hrIFN-α compared with mock PBS-fed control ($p < .05$), and a decrease in proliferation to GP-MBP and MT in spleen cells of mice fed 100 U hrIFN-α compared with mock PBS-fed animals (see Table 4, experiment 1).

D. Lower Doses of Orally Administered Murine Species-Specific IFN-α Can Suppress Clinical Disease and Decrease Inflammation and Cytokine Secretion

We have previously shown that 100 U of orally administered murine species-specific IFN-α/β (104; also see above) and 100 U of hrIFN-α can

Table 4 Oral IFN-α Inhibits Proliferation to GP-MBP, PLP 139–151, MT, and ConA

Experiment 1			
	GP-MBP LN	GP-MBP spleen	MT spleen
Mock PBS	6105 ± 705	11357 ± 948	14086 ± 1385
100 U hrIFN	3330 ± 595	5841 ± 1846*	8396 ± 948*
1000 U hrIFN	1182 ± 121*	Not done	Not done

Experiment 2		
	Con A spleen	PLP 139–151 LN
Mock PBS	40,822 ± 1803	46187 ± 2836
100 U hrIFN	2406 ± 436*	25966 ± 929*

Experiment 3		
	ConA LN	PLP 139–151 spleen
Mock mIFN	94,770 ± 2783	5360 ± 262
10 U mIFN	31,943 ± 7840*	2166 ± 93*

Experiment 4	
	ConA LN
Mock mIFN	126625 ± 10743
10 U mIFN	85900 ± 7153*

* $p < .05$ compared with mock control.

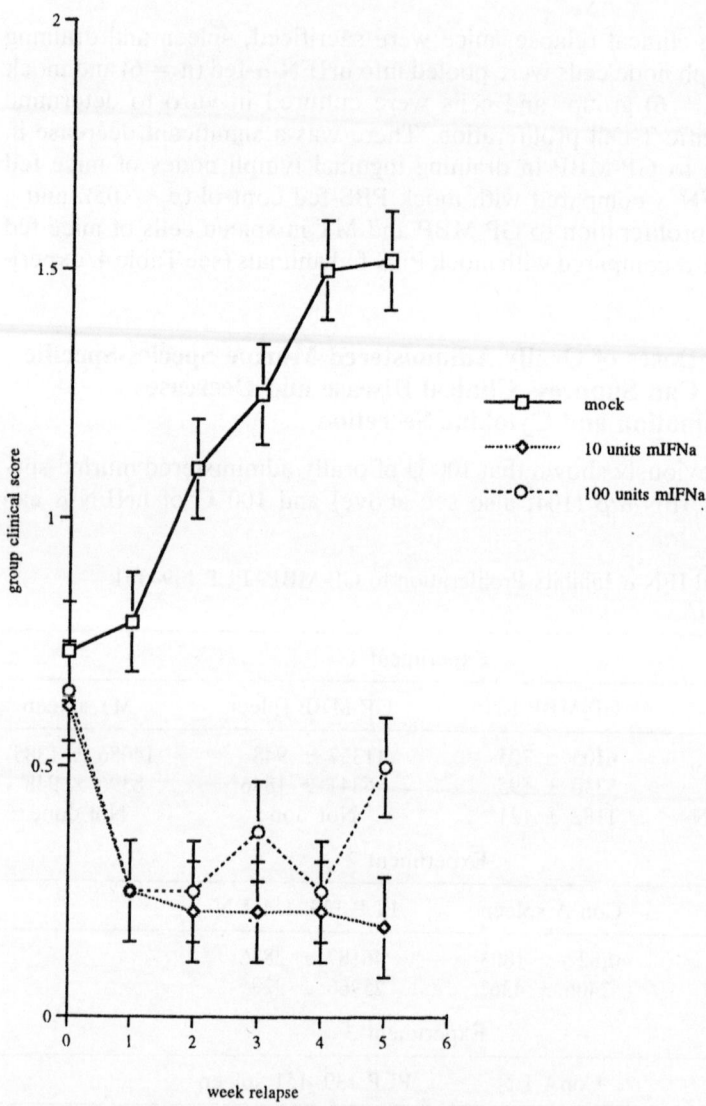

Figure 6 Oral murine species-specific IFN-α suppresses relapses at one-tenth the effective cross-species hrIFN dose. Animals (n = 8/group) were immunized, followed as described in Fig. 4, and treated with 10 U mock mIFN or 100 U mIFN-α. Animals were scored by a blinded observer for clinical disease for 5 weeks after feeding. Values represent combined data of two separate experiments of mean weekly group clinical scores ± SEM (mock IFN–fed vs 10 U mIFN-α–fed animals for weeks 1–5, p < .001; vs 100 U mIFN-α-fed for weeks 1–5, p < .001 by non-paired t test).

suppress clinical relapse attacks (103,105). A dose-response ranging experiment for oral IFN treatment is critical in order to design clinical trials in patients with MS. Therefore, we determined if one-tenth the dose (10 U) of p.o. administered murine species-specific IFN-α (mIFN-α) would suppress relapse attacks. Animals were immunized and after 30 days at the completion of the initial attack were fed with mock murine IFN or 10 or 100 U mIFN-α. The mock IFN–fed group incurred relapse over the course of 5 weeks. Clinical scores demonstrated significant differences in the outcome in the mock mIFN–fed versus 10 and 100 U mIFN-α–fed animals (Fig. 6). Histological examination showed decreased inflammation in animals with decreased clinical scores (*mock IFN*: 2.2 ± 0.1; *10 U mIFN-α*: 0.9 ± 0.4, *p* < .01; *100 U mIFN-α*: 0.8 ± 0.6, *p* < .05). Orally administered mIFN-α is effective at an order of magnitude less than the effective hrIFN dose, which is consistent with data for cross-species antiviral activity (103,105). Phenotyping at the time of sacrifice demonstrated no significant differences in CD3, CD4, or CD8 cell surface expression in pooled lymph node or pooled spleen cells from mock IFN–fed compared with mIFN-α–fed animals in two separate experiments (data not shown). ConA activation of draining popliteal lymph node cells was inhibited in mIFN-α–fed compared with mock IFN–fed animals (see Table 4, experiment 3). There was a significant decrease in proliferation in spleen cells to proteolipid protein (PLP) 139–151 in mice fed 10 U

Table 5 Oral IFN-α Inhibits IFN-γ and IL-2 Secretion

	Experiment 2	
	PLP 139–151: IFN-γ	
Mock PBS	30 ± 2	
100 U hrIFN	12 ± 2*	
	Experiment 3	
	ConA spleen: IFN-γ	ConA: IL-2
Mock mIFN	42 ± 1	112 ± 3
10 U mIFN	14 ± 1*	61 ± 3*
	Experiment 4	
	ConA LN: IFN-γ	
Mock mIFN	26 ± 1	
10 U mIFN	6 ± 1*	

* p < .05 compared with mock control.

mIFN-α compared with mock IFN–fed (see Table 4, experiment 3). ConA-stimulated spleen cells from mIFN-α–fed animals demonstrated decreased secretion of IFN-γ and IL-2 (Table 5, experiment 3) compared with mock IFN–fed animals.

V. ORAL IFN IN ADOPTIVE OR PASSIVE TRANSFER OF EAE

EAE can be adoptively or passively transfered by using in vitro antigen-activated lymph node or spleen cells from actively immunized mice (106) that have been immunized with spinal cord (107). Transfer of disease can also be performed by activation with the mitogens ConA and pokeweed mitogen (108). CREAE in SJL/J mice can be adoptively transferred following the intravenous injection of an MBP peptide 89–100-specific T-cell line (109) or of in vitro PLP-stimulated lymph node cells from SJL/J mice immunized with human myelin PLP (110). The immunodominant epitopes of PLP in the SJL/J mouse are PLP peptides 139–151 and 178–191 (111–113). Treatment of mice with splenocytes coupled with mouse spinal cord homogenate or PLP after immunization with MSCH suppressed the onset and severity of clinical and histological signs of relapsing EAE (114–115). This suggests that PLP is a major encephalitogen in MSCH-induced CREAE in the SJL/J mouse.

A. Activated Donor Cells from Animals Administered hrIFN-α Orally Are Less Effective in Transfering Clinical Disease Compared with Cells from Mock PBS–Fed Mice

Adoptive transfer experiments were performed to determine if activated spleen cells from hrIFN-α–fed animals could transfer disease (103,105). ConA-activated T cells from mock PBS–fed or 100 U hrIFN-α–fed immunized SJL/J mice, followed for 5 weeks after initiation of feeding during relapse, were transferred adoptively i.p. to recipient mice that were then followed for evidence of disease. Mice that received ConA-activated mock PBS-fed T cells had a significant clinical attack starting at day 5, whereas recipients of ConA-activated T cells from hrIFN-α-fed mice had a much less severe clinical attack (Fig. 7). In contrast, ConA-activated spleen cells from animals treated with hrIFN-α in vitro, as opposed to in vivo feeding, did not prevent adoptive disease transfer (data not shown). ConA-induced spleen cell proliferation from mock PBS–fed recipients was significantly greater than in hrIFN-α–fed recipients (see Table 4, experiment 2). Pooled spleen cells from immunized recipients of either mock-fed or 100 U hrIFN-α–fed donor cells were stimulated with PLP 139–151 (10

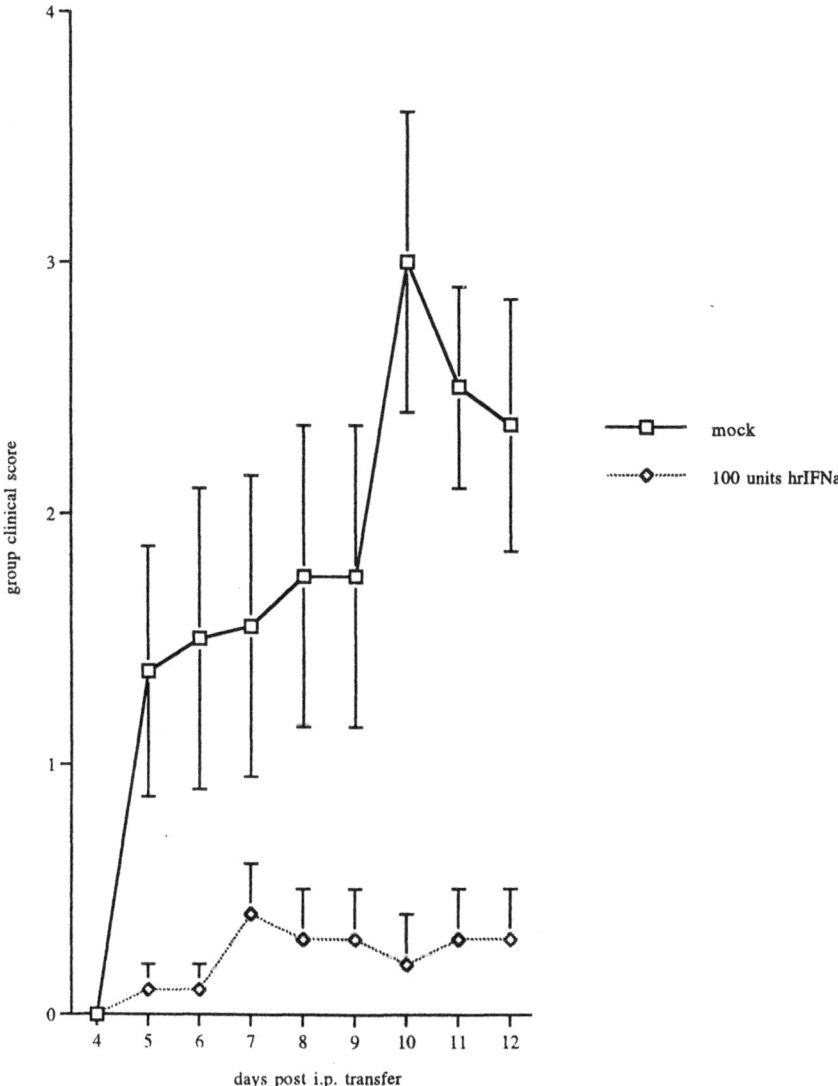

Figure 7 Human recombinant IFN-α–fed animals do not adoptively transfer disease. 10 × 10^6 3-day ConA–activated T cells from mock PBS–fed or 100 U hrIFN-α–fed immunized donor SJL/J mice, which had undergone relapse attacks 5 weeks earlier, were transferred adoptively i.p. to naive SJL/J mice (n = 6, mock donor) (n = 6, 100-U hrIFN-α donor) and followed for evidence of disease. Values represent combined data of two separate experiments of mean group daily blinded clinical scores ± SEM (mock PBS–fed donors vs hrIFN-α–fed donors for days 5–12, *p* < .01 by nonpaired t test).

μg/ml) for 2 days and supernatants were assayed by ELISA. As shown in Table 5, experiment 2, the results combined from two separate experiments demonstrate that cells from oral hrIFN-α–treated donors secrete less IFN-γ, a mediator of inflammation.

Since PLP is the major encephalitogen in the SJL/J mouse (111–115), adoptive transfer experiments were performed to determine if spleen cells from IFN-α–fed animals activated with PLPs 139–151 could transfer disease. CEAE was induced in SJL/J mice with MSCH and complete Freund's adjuvant (CFA). Following recovery, animals were fed mock or hrIFN-α-three times per week for 6 weeks. 10 × 10⁶ of 3-day PLP 139–151–activated T cells from mock-fed or 10-U hrIFN-α–fed SJL/J mice (previously immunized) were adoptively transferred i.p. to nonfed recipient SJL/J mice and followed for evidence of disease (Fig. 8). The recipient mice that received PLP 139–151–activated T cells from a mock-fed donor had a significant clinical attack starting at days 4–5, whereas recipients of PLP 139–151–activated T cells from hrIFN-α–fed donors had a much less severe clinical attack (ConA: 3.0 ± 0.3 *mock IFN* vs 0.5 ± 0.2 *100-U IFN*, p < .01) (PLP 139–151: 1.7 ± 0.2 *mock IFN* vs 0.7 ± 0.1 *100-U IFN*, p < .01). Pooled spleen cells stimulated with PLP 139–151 (10 μg/ml) from recipients of IFN-α–fed donor cells secreted less IFN-γ compared with mock fed (donor *mock IFN*–fed: 30 ng/ml ± 2 donor; *100-U IFN*–fed: 10 ng/ml ± 2, p < .05). There were no changes in IL-2 or IL-4 secretion between mock PBS– and hrIFN-α–fed treated animals (data not shown). Activated cells from IFN-α–fed animals transfer disease less well and secrete less IFN-γ in recipients.

B. Activated Donor Cells from Animals Administered Murine IFN-α Orally Are Less Effective in Transfering Clinical Disease Compared with Cells from Mock Murine IFN–Fed Mice

Adoptive transfer experiments were performed to determine if activated spleen cells from 10 U mIFN-α–fed animals could prevent transfer of disease. ConA-activated mock murine IFN–fed or 10 U mIFN-α–fed T cells from immunized SJL/J mice, obtained 5 weeks after initiation of feeding during relapse, were transferred adoptively i.p. to recipient mice and followed for evidence of disease. Recipient mice of activated mock IFN T cells had significantly more severe clinical attacks starting at day 13 compared with mIFN-α recipients (Fig. 9). ConA-stimulated proliferation of draining lymph nodes was significantly less from mIFN-α recipients than from mock IFN recipients (see Table 4, experiment 4). ConA-induced IFN-γ secretion by lymph node cells was inhibited in mIFN-α compared

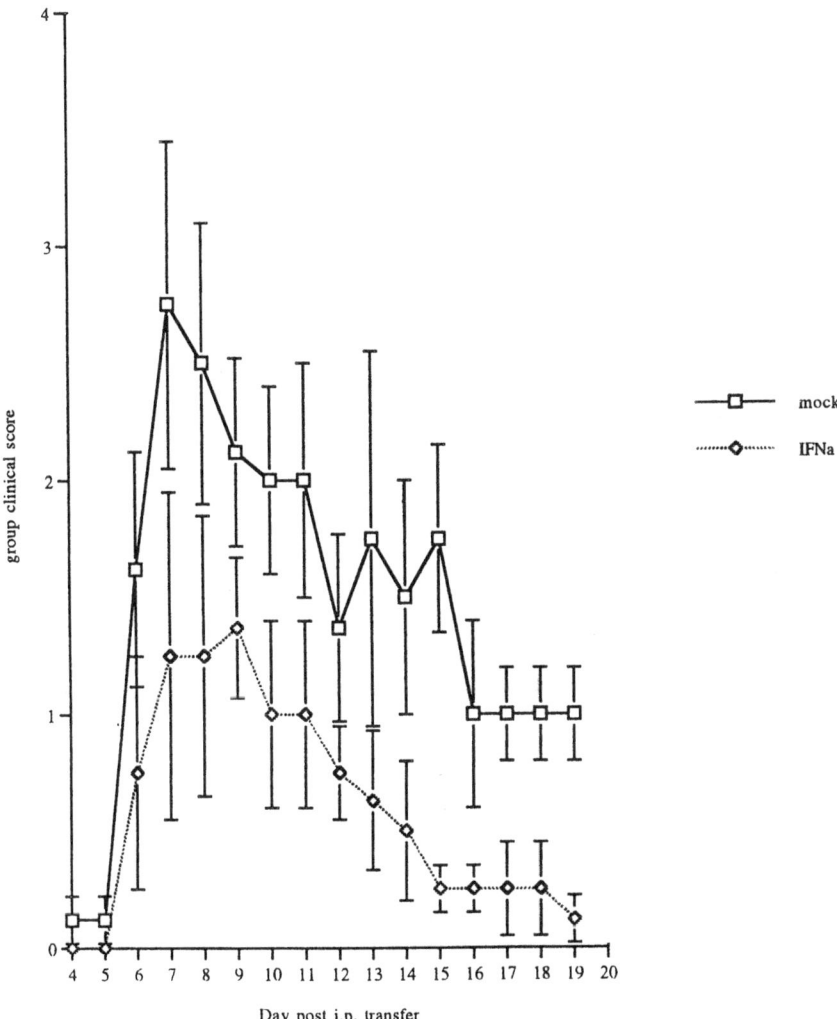

Figure 8 PLP 139–151–activated cells from IFN-α–fed animals do not transfer disease passively. 10×10^6 3-day PLP 139–151–activated T cells from mock-fed or 100 U hrIFN-α–fed immunized SJL/J mice, which had undergone relapse attacks, were adoptively transferred i.p. to previously nonfed immunized SJL/J mice (recipient n = 3, mock donor) (recipient n = 3, 100-U IFN donor) and followed for evidence of disease. Values represent mean group daily blinded clinical scores ± SEM ($p < .05$ by nonpaired t test at days 7–8, 10–11, 14–19).

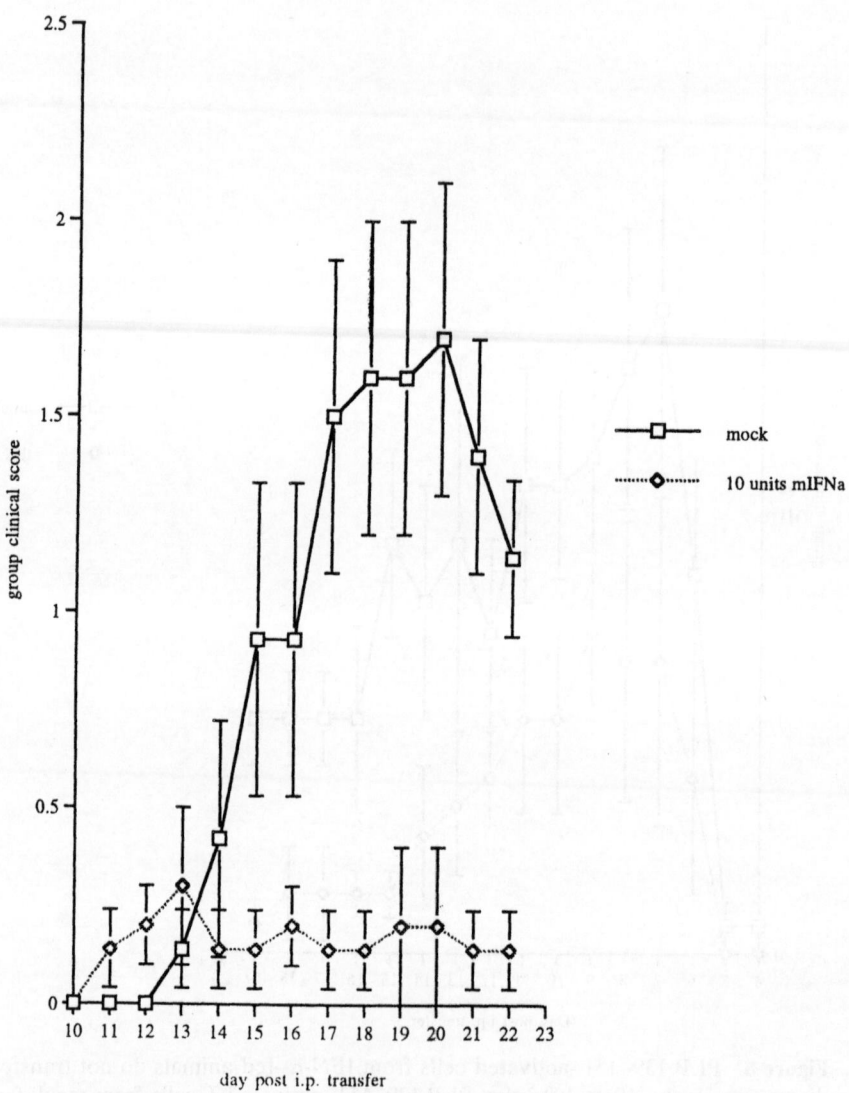

Figure 9 Murine IFN-α–fed animals do not adoptively transfer acute disease. 10 × 10⁶ 3-day ConA–activated T cells from mock IFN–fed or 10 U mIFN-α–fed immunized SJL/J mice that had undergone relapse attacks 35 days earlier were transferred adoptively i.p. to naive SJL/J mice (n = 6, mock IFN donor) (n = 6, 10-U mIFN-α donor) and followed for evidence of disease. Values represent combined data of two separate experiments of mean group daily blinded clinical scores ± SEM (mock IFN recipients vs mIFN-α–treated recipients for days 15–22, $p < .01$ by nonpaired t test).

with mock IFN–recipient animals (see Table 5, experiment 4). However, there was no significant difference in the number of lesions between mock recipients versus mIFN-α recipients (*mock IFN*: 1.8 ± 0.6 [n = 6]; *10-U mIFN-α*: 1.5 ± 0.5 [n = 6]).

VI. DISCUSSION

These data document that orally administered mIFN and hrIFN can suppress relapses and prevent adoptive transfer of EAE. The inhibition of an established and ongoing immune response by oral administration of immunoactive proteins is an important therapeutic issue. Oral administration of myelin proteins improves CREAE and decreases inflammation in rats and guinea pigs (116) and may decrease the severity of attacks in male HLA-DR2$^-$ MS patients and the frequency of MBP-specific T cells in myelin-treated individuals (117). However, in the human trials and animal experiments, there was only partial suppression of clinical or pathological disease, suggesting that other orally administered immunoactive substances may be superior to myelin antigens. Animals administered 100–1000 U hrIFN-α exhibited less severe relapses than mock-fed animals, although 1000 U is marginally less effective compared with 100 U. Animals fed murine species-specific IFN at only 10–100 U had suppressed clinical relapses. Thus, species-specific mIFN-α decreased the overall neurological deficits from baseline values at a dose one order of magnitude less than hrIFN-α. This is consistent with ongoing preliminary experiments that suggests a therapeutic dose-response window with 10–100 U species-specific oral mIFN-α as the optimal dose, and 0.1, 1.0 and 1000 U significantly less effective in suppressing clinical relapse disease in murine CREAE (data not shown).

The immunomodulatory mechanism of orally administered IFN-α may be a decrease in precursor frequency via clonal anergy (transient IFN-induced hyporesponsiveness of encephalitogenic T cells (67–68)) or generation of suppressor factors by T cells. Modulatory effects of ConA-activated lymphocytes on the mitogen responses of normal responder cells can be abrogated by addition of anti–human leukocyte IFN serum in vitro (118), which may prevent the production of inhibitory factors induced by IFN-α; for example, soluble immune response suppressor (SIRS) (119) and macrophage-derived suppressor factor (e.g., TGF-β) by CD8$^+$ T cells (120–121). Peripheral T cells may be required for IFN production after such mitogen stimulation (122). Other cytokines may also be important because both IFN-α and IFN-β stimulate the production of at least 12 new cellular proteins (123). Serum IFN at detectable levels may not be necessary for clinical effect; recent experiments in our laboratory show that 10 U mIFN-α administered parenterally (s.c.), and unlikely to generate significant serum levels, are not clinically efficacious (data not shown), whereas 10 U mIFN-α are effective via oral delivery, and also do not generate significant serum levels. Therefore, type I IFNs may induce suppressor factors inhibiting responses to immunogenic antigens such as MBP and PLP. IFN-α may be an immunomodulatory molecule produced by activated CD8$^+$ T and other immune cells that induces suppressor factors, such as SIRS or other cytokines, which in turn induce hyporesponsiveness to immunized antigens such as MBP and MT.

In the murine system, class II–restricted T helper cells have been separated into two nonoverlapping subsets according to the interleukin gene transcription and secretion (124–127). One subset (Th2) produces IL-4 and IL-5 and uses IL-4 as a growth factor. The other subset (Th1) secretes IL-2 and IFN-γ on stimulation, uses IL-2 as a growth factor, and regulates inflammation and the DTH response via IFN-γ and TNF-α secretion. Inoculation of SJL/J mice with myelin basic protein peptides in EAE can activate pathogenic neuroantigen-specific Th1 T helper cells in vivo (128–129). Th1-like T helper cells can also be demonstrated in human inflammatory diseases, including MS. We have demonstrated, using PHA-derived human T-cell clones, that CD4$^+$ Th1 T-cell clones, expressing IL-2 and IFN-γ, but not IL-4 or IL-5, mRNA, are present in the peripheral blood and CSF immune compartments from patients with MS and Lyme meningoencephalomyelitis (130). Th2 cells, expressing IL-4 and IL-5, but not IFN-γ or IL-2, mRNA, were not found in any patient. This was the first evidence for Th1-like T-cell clones in humans, which may be associated with systemic inflammation. Subsequently, *Borrelia burgdorferi* (131) and *Mycobacterium leprae* (132) antigen-specific Th1-like T-cell subsets have been isolated from patients with Lyme arthritis and tuberculoid leprosy, respectively. Therefore, the inhibition of IFN-γ and IL-2 indirectly by oral IFN-α suggests a functional inhibition of Th1-like T helper cells in EAE and a potential site of intervention at the level of effector T cells in MS (133).

The GALT has multiple types of constituent immune cells. It consists of lymphoid nodules termed Peyer's patches (PP), villi containing epithelial cells and intraepithelial lymphocytes (IEL), and lymphocytes scattered throughout the lamina propria (LP) (134). PP contain T and B lymphocytes, macrophages, dendritic cells, and a germinal center with B lymphocytes. T lymphocytes in PP are predominantly composed of the CD4$^+$ Th1 and Th2 phenotypes, whereas parafollicular cells are both CD4$^+$ and CD8$^+$ (135–136). PP are the site where regulatory cells can be generated (137–139). T cells in lymphoid organs draining from nonmucosal sites such as inguinal lymph nodes secrete IL-2 as the primary T-cell growth factor after activation, whereas T cells from mucosal sites such as PP produce IL-4 (140). This demonstrates that the lymphoid microenvironment can determine the pattern of T-cell responses in different immune organs (141).

An integrin receptor molecule termed lymphocyte high endothelial venule (HEV) adhesion molecule (LPAM-1) can mediate organ-specific adhesion of lymphocytes to specialized HEVs found in PP (142). TGF-β and IL-4 regulate the adhesiveness of PP HEV for lymphocytes on HEVs possibly through LPAM-1 expression (143). IELs are distinct from other lymphocyte populations, because monoclonal antibodies raised against human IEL, termed human mucosal lymphocytes [HML-1, β_7-integrin family], react with virtually all IELs, 40% of LP lymphocytes, but less than 2% of PBLs, suggesting they are specific GALT addressins.

IELs include 75% CD8$^+$ in humans and in mice 40–65% CD8$^+$ T cells. Some IEL CD8$^+$ T cells utilize the $\gamma\delta$ TCR and express the CD8 α chain without the β chain (144). The CD8$^+$ IELs expressing the $\alpha\beta$ TCR are of thymic origin and arrive from nearby PP (145). LP lymphocytes have CD4$^+$/CD8$^+$ ratios resembling PP and PBLs (134). In oral tolerance, antigen-specific regulatory cells migrate to lymphoid organs and suppress immune responses by inhibiting the generation of effector cells (146). Therefore, there are diverse cell populations in the GALT that may potentially become immunoregulatory via p.o. IFN and suppress peripheral immune Th1-like T helper cell function.

Previous studies in the EAE model suggested that orally administered MBP suppressed the afferent limb of the immune response (147–148). This suppression may be mediated by CD8$^+$ T cells (149) and provides organ-specific immune hyporesponsiveness. Cells responsible for prevention of sensitization after intragastric administration of sheep red blood cells have been tracked from PP [2 days] to mesenteric lymph node [4 days] and subsequently to spleen [7 days] (139). These data suggest active and antigen-specific suppression as the mechanism of orally induced tolerance. More recent studies suggest that mucosal derived MBP-specific CD4$^+$ Th2-like T-cell clones which produce TGF-β were able to suppress EAE (150). These data suggest that there are migrating pools of different cell populations originating in the GALT which transfer acquired immunoregulation into the systemic efferent immune system. Moreover, the tolerizing antigen does not need to cause the autoimmune disease; MBP-specific suppressor cells would home to the CNS in MS even if MBP was not the MS antigen.

For oral administration of low doses of IFN to be effective, there should be a fantastic amplification system: IFN-induced activities could be either transferred between adjacent epithelial cells and from these to lymphocytes, or they may be directly transfered from lymphocytes to other cells in other lymphoid sites (151). Subsequent antiviral and immunomodulatory activities could be achieved by either cell-to-cell communication (152) or be transported and generalized by lymphocytes that home via lymph to lymphoid and nonlymphoid organs (153) without having any accompanying side effects due to circulating IFN (63). At their destination, activated cells can release cytokines in a paracrine fashion (154–156) which in turn stimulate either neighboring or circulating cells. This suggests that biological response modifiers [BRM] such as p.o. type I IFNs are drugs that act outside the realm of classic pharmacological parameters (157) and suppress autoimmune disease by activating a unique natural immune system originating in the mucosa that involves cellular communication and amplification. However, it is unknown which cellular element is responsible for immunoregulation in EAE by p.o. IFNs.

Mice receiving T cells adoptively from mIFN-α–fed animals do exhibit inflammation (see above). Others have shown that adoptively transferred myelin oligodendrocyte glycoprotein [MOG] peptide-specific T cells can demonstrate inflammation in the CNS without inducing a neurological deficit (158). We might speculate that oral administration of IFN-α generates immunoregulatory CD8$^+$ T cells via the gut immune system that can traffic to the recipient's peripheral lymphoid system or CNS. These cells would not cause clinical disease, but instead might suppress inflammation by either generating suppressor factors locally in the CNS compartment, or by decreasing responsiveness to immunizing antigens by inhibiting IFN-γ secretion.

These data document that orally administered murine and rat species-specific and human recombinant type I IFNs can inhibit disease and inflammation and decrease proliferation of activated and antigen-specific cells in EAE in mice and rats when administered after or before sensitization. Type I IFNs are active by the oral route and have significant immunological effects at very low dosages, even though they lack a protective matrix to prevent protein digestion. Specific cytokines, in particular type I IFNs, directly delivered to the distal esophagus, stomach, and proximal small intestine [determined experimentally by injecting Evans blue during routine feeding and subsequent sacrifice], are capable of producing immunomodulation, but not tolerance, to previously sensitized antigens. Oral IFN-α therapy in EAE appears to be more effective than equivalent doses of parenteral IFN-α. In vitro IFN did not inhibit ConA proliferation, in contrast to the strong inhibition seen after in vivo p.o. administration. This suggests that route of administration is critical and may determine the immunological mechanism for IFN. In contrast to equivalent s.c. doses, which do not directly act on similar GALT-cell subsets, oral IFN-α may activate immunomodulatory cell populations in the GALT and thereby function by a different mechanism.

Passive immunization provides a method to investigate the mechanism of oral administration of type I IFNs on different cell populations in adoptively transferred disease, eliminating the role of potential "suppressor" antigen-presenting cells in actively immunized animals. Preliminary experiments in our laboratory suggest that i.p. adoptive transfer of ConA-activated splenic T cells from p.o. IFN–treated mice suppresses actively induced EAE. This suggests that p.o. IFN-α actively suppresses effector encephalitogenic T cells. If so, compared with the parenteral route, oral administration of selected cytokines may provide a more effective delivery system to produce organ-blind immunomodulation without tolerance to sensitized antigen, irrespective of haplotypic background, for the treatment of human autoimmune diseases.

Our studies in murine CREAE suggest that an ongoing immune response can be modified by orally administered type I IFNs. The oral administration of biological response modifier (BRMs) such as IFN potentially provides a continuous means of generating immunosuppression of autoreactive T-cell populations. BRMs delivered by the oral route may also provide a means to treat autoimmune diseases such as MS and other chronic nonneurological autoimmune diseases such as rheumatoid arthritis and type I diabetes mellitus by the generation of immunoregulatory cells via the esophageal/gut immune system. The oral route is a convenient drug-delivery system that may allow the use of lower doses of cytokines, minimize side effects, and provide enhanced efficacy via potent immunoregulatory circuits.

Experiments are underway to determine whether actively induced disease can be suppressed by adoptively transferred T-cell subsets from IFN-fed animals [suppression] or whether T cells from IFN animals are unable to transfer disease to naive recipients [anergy]. In light of the results from our animal experiments, we are currently assessing the dose-response effect on phenotypic, immunological, and IFN-induced markers of a wide range of human recombinant IFN-α doses in normal volunteers in preparation for a trial of oral IFN-α in early relapsing-remitting MS patients.

ADDENDUM

We determined whether ingested IFN-α was nontoxic and had biological effects in humans. Ingested hrIFN-α showed no toxicity in normal volunteers or patients with RRMS at doses ranging from 300 to 100,000 units. In subjects with RRMS, a significant decrease in Con A–mediated proliferation and serum soluble intercellular adhesion molecule-1 (sICAM-1), a surrogate measure for disease activity in MS, was found after ingestion of 10,000 and 30,000 units IFN-α. The RRMS subjects also showed decreased IL-2 secretion after ingestion of 10,000 units IFN-α, and decreased IFN-γ, TGF-β, and IL-10 production after ingestion of 30,000 units IFN-α. There was no change in proliferation or secretion of any other cytokine at 100,000 units or change in TNF-α secretion at any drug dose. Therefore, the inhibition of IFN-γ and IL-2 indirectly by ingested IFN-α suggests a functional inhibition of Th1-like T helper cells in EAE and RRMS and a potential site of intervention at the level of effector T cells in MS. The absence of alterations of the relative levels of TNF-α in RRMS suggests that ingested IFN-α may have selective biological effects on different cytokines. Our studies suggest that ingested human IFN-α is a profound biological response modifier in mammals including humans.

ACKNOWLEDGMENT

This work was supported by a grant from the Clayton Foundation.

REFERENCES

1. Hafler DA, Brod SA, Weiner HL. Immunoregulation in multiple sclerosis. Res Immunol 1989; 140:233–239.
2. Hafler DA, Brod SA, Weiner HL. Experimental approaches to specific immunotherapy in multiple sclerosis. In: R Ruduck, A Goodkin eds. Treatment of Multiple Sclerosis: Trial Design, Results, and Future Perspectives. London: Springer-Verlag, 1992:301–308.
3. McFarlin D, McFarland H. Multiple Sclerosis. N Engl J Med 1982; 307: 1183–1188.
4. Waksman B, Reynolds WE. Multiple sclerosis as a disease of immune regulation. Proc Soc Exp Biol Med 1984; 175:282–294.
5. Antel JP, Freedman MS, Brodsovsky S, Francis GS, Duquette P. Activated suppressor cell function in severely disabled patients with multiple sclerosis. Ann Neurol 1989; 25:204–207.
6. Brod SA, Scott M. Defective CD3 mediated proliferation and LPS responsiveness in multiple sclerosis. Autoimmunity 1994; 17:143–148.
7. Brod SA, Khan M, Bright J, Sriram S, Marshall GD, Henninger EM, Kerman RH, Wolinsky JS. Decreased CD3 mediated IFN-γ production in relapsing-remitting multiple sclerosis. Ann Neurol 1995; 37:546–549.
8. Isaacs A, Lindenmann J. Virus Interference. I. The interferon. Proc R Soc Lond (Biol), 1957; 147:258–267.
9. Johnson HM, Baron S. Evaluation of effects of interferon and interferon inducers on the immune response. Pharmacol Ther 1977; 1:349–367.
10. Trotta PP, Narula SK. Interferon genes: In: Baron S, Dianzani F, Stanton GJ, Fleischmann WR, eds. Interferon System. Austin, TX: UT Press, 1987: 137–143.
11. Aguet M, Mogensen KE. Interferon receptors. In: Gresser I, ed. Interferons. Vol. 5. New York: Academic Press, 1983:1–22.

12. Rashidbaigi A, Pestka S. Interferons: Protein structure. In: Baron S, Dianzani F, Stanton GJ, Fleischmann WR, eds. The Interferon System. Austin TX: UT Press, 1987:149–168.
13. Zoon KC. Human interferons: Structure & function In: Interferon 9. London: Academic Press, 1987:1–12.
14. Baglioni C. 2',5'-oligo(A) pathway of interferon action. In: Baron S, Dianzani F, Stanton GJ, Fleischmann WR, eds. The Interferon System. Austin TX: UT Press, 1987:365–371.
15. Dolei A, Ameglio F. Effects of IFN on phenotypic expression by cells. In: Baron S, Dianzani F, Stanton GJ, Fleischmann WR, eds. The Interferon System. Austin TX: UT Press, 1987:271–277.
16. Pestka S, Langer J, Zoon KC, Samuel CE. Interferons and their actions. Ann Rev Biochem 1987; 56:727–777.
17. Balkwill FR. The regulatory role of interferons in the human immune response. In: Taylor-Papadimitriou, ed. Interferons: Their Impact in Biology of Medicine Oxford Medical, 1985:61–80.
18. Hertzog PJ, Emery P, Cheetham BF, MacKay IR, Linnane AW. Interferons in rheumatoid arthritis: alterations of production and response related to disease activity. Clin Immunol Immunopathol 1988; 48:192–201.
19. Seitz M, Napierski I, Augustin R, Hunstein W, Kirchner H. Reduced production of interferon alpha and interferon gamma in leukocyte cultures from patients with active rheumatoid arthritis. Scand J Rheumatol 1987; 16: 257–262.
20. Kapp A, Gillitzer R, Kirchner H, Schopf E. Production of interferon and lymphoproliferative response in whole blood cultures derived from patients with atopic dermatitis. Arch Dermatol Res 1987; 279(suppl: S):55–58.
21. Kapp A, Gillitzer R, Kirchner H, Schopf E. Decreased production of interferon in whole blood cultures derived from patients with psoriasis. J Invest Dermatol 1988; 90:511–514.
22. Hertzog PJ, Wright A, Harris G, Linnane AW, Mackay IR. Intermittent interferonemia and interferon responses in multiple sclerosis. Clin Immunol Immunopathol 1991; 58:18–32.
23. Neighbour PA, Bloom BR. Absence of virus-induced lymphocyte suppression and interferon production in multiple sclerosis. Proc Natl Acad Sci USA 1979; 76:476–480.
24. Maruo Y. Interferon production and natural killer activity of peripheral blood lymphocytes obtained from patients with multiple sclerosis. Hokkaido J Med Sci 1988; 63:521–533.
25. Struyf NJ, Snoeck HW, Bridts CH, De Clerck LS, Stevens WJ. Natural killer cell activity in Sjogren's syndrome and systemic lupus erythematosus: stimulation with interferons and interleukin-2 and correlation with immune complexes. Ann Rheum Dis 1990; 49:690–693.
26. Negishi K, Gupta S, Chandy KG, Waldeck N, Kershnar A, Buckingham B, Charles MA. Interferon responsiveness of natural killer cells in type I human diabetes. Diabetes Res. 1988; 7:49–52.
27. Thoen J, Waalen K, Forre O. Natural killer (NK) cells at inflammatory sites

of patients with rheumatoid arthritis and IgM rheumatoid factor positive polyarticular juvenile rheumatoid arthritis. Clin Rheumatol 1987; 6:215–225.

28. Kastrukoff LF, Morgan NG, Aziz TM, Zecchini D, Berkowitz J, Paty DW. Natural killer (NK) cells in chronic progressive multiple sclerosis patients treated with lymphoblastoid interferon. J Neuroimmunol 1988; 20: 15–23.

29. Vranes Z, Poljakovic Z, Marucic M. Natural killer cell number and activity in multiple sclerosis. J Neurol Sci 1989; 94:115–123.

30. Rice GPA, Casali P, Merigan TC, Oldstone MBA. Natural killer cell activity in patients with multiple sclerosis given alpha interferon. Ann Neurol 1983; 14:333–338.

31. Noronha A, Toscas A, Jensen MA. Interferon beta augments suppressor cell function in multiple sclerosis. Neurology 1990; 27:207–210.

32. Noronha A, Toscas A, Arnason BG, Jensen MA. Interferon beta augments in vivo suppressor function in multiple sclerosis (abstr). Neurology 1994; 2(suppl):212.

33. Fog T. Interferon treatment of multiple sclerosis patients: a pilot study. In: Boese A, ed. Search for a Cause of Multiple Sclerosis and Other Chronic Diseases of the CNS. Weinheim: Verlag Chemie, 1980:491–493.

34. Ververken D, Carton H, Billiau A. Intrathecal administration of interferon in MS patients? In: Karcher D, Lowenthal A, Strosberg AD, eds. Humoral Immunity in Neurological Disease. New York: Plenum Press, 1979: 625–627.

35. Montezuma-de-Carvalho MJ. A treatment for the chronic disabilities of stable multiple sclerosis. Acta Medicotechnica 1983; 31:155–160.

36. Knobler RL, Panitch HS, Braheny SL, Sipe JC, Rice GPA, Huddlestone JR, Francis GS, Hooper CJ, Kamin-Lewis RM, Johnson KP, Oldstone MBA, Merigan TC. Controlled clinical trial of systemic alpha interferon in multiple sclerosis. Neurology 1983; 34:1273–1279.

37. Kamin-Lewis RM, Panitch HS, Johnson KP. Leucocytes from multiple sclerosis patients respond to α- and γ-interferons. J Neuroimmunol 1985; 9:221–227.

38. Panitch HS, Francis GS, Hooper CJ, Merigan TC, Johnson KP. Serial immunological studies in multiple sclerosis patients treated systemically with human interferon alpha. Ann Neurol 1985; 18:434–438.

39. Panitch HS. Systemic alpha-interferon in multiple sclerosis: Long term patient follow-up. Arch Neurol 1987; 44:61–63.

40. Knobler RL. Systemic interferon therapy of multiple sclerosis: the pros. Neurology 1988; 38:58–61.

41. Kastrukoff LF, Oger JJ, Hashimoto SA, Sacks SL, Li DK, Palmer MR, Koopmans RA, Petkau AJ, Berkowitz J, Paty DW. Systemic lymphoblastoid interferon therapy in chronic progressive multiple sclerosis. I. Clinical and MRI evaluation. Neurology 1990; 40:479–486.

42. Jacobs L, O'Malley JA, Freeman A, Ekes R. Intrathecal interferon in multiple sclerosis. Arch Neurol 1982; 39:609–615.

43. Jacobs L, O'Malley JA, Freeman A, Ekes R, Reese PA. Intrathecal interferon in the treatment of multiple sclerosis. Arch Neurol 1985; 42:841–847.
44. Jacobs L, Herndon R, Salazar AM, Reese PA, Freeman A, Josofewicz R, Cuetter A, Husain F, Smith WA, Ekes R, O'Malley JA. Intrathecally administered natural human fibroblast interferon reduces exacerbations of multiple sclerosis, results of multicenter, double-blinded study. Arch Neurol 1987; 44:589–595.
45. Camenga DL, Johnson KP, Alter M, Engelhardt CD, Fishman PS, Greenstein JI, Haley AS, Hirsch RL, Kleiner JE, Kofie, VY, Koski CL, Margulies SL, Panitch HS, Valero R. Systemic recombinant alpha 2 interferon therapy in relapsing multiple sclerosis. Arch Neurol 1986; 43: 1239–1245.
46. Hirsch RL, Johnson KP. Placebo induced enhancement of natural killer cell activity in a double blind trial of recombinant alpha-2 interferon in multiple sclerosis patients. In: Spector NH, ed. Neuroimmunomodulation. Proceedings of the first International Workshop of Neuroimmunomodulation. Bethesda, MD. IWGN, 1985:219–226.
47. Hirsch RL, Johnson KP. The effect of long term administration of recombinant alpha-2 interferon on lymphocyte subsets, proliferation, and suppressor cell function in multiple sclerosis. J Interferon Res 1986; 6:171–177.
48. IFNB MS Study Group. Interferon beta-1b is effective in relapsing-remitting multiple sclerosis. I. Clinical results of a multicenter, randomized, double blind, placebo-controlled trial. Neurology 1993; 43:655–661.
49. IFNB MS Study Group. Interferon beta-1b is effective in relapsing-remitting multiple sclerosis. II. MRI analysis results of a multicenter, randomized, double blind, placebo-controlled trial. Neurology 1993; 43:662–667.
50. Durelli L, Bongioanni MR, Cavallo R, Ferraro B, Ferri R, Ferrio MF, Bradac GB, Riva A, Vai S, Geuna M, Bergnami L, Bergamasco B. Chronic systemic high-dose recombinant interferon alpha-2a reduces exacerbation rate, MRI signs of disease activity, and lymphocyte interferon gamma production in relapsing-remitting multiple sclerosis. Neurology 1994; 44: 406–413.
51. Jacobs L, Cookfair D, Rudick R, Herndon R, Richert J, Salazar A, Fischer J, Granger C, Simon J, Goodkin D, and the MS Collaborative Group. Results of a phase III trial of intramuscular recombinant beta interferon as treatment for multiple sclerosis. Ann Neurol 1994; 36(2):259.
52. Schafer TW, Lieberman M, Cohen M, Came P. Interferon administered orally: protection of neonatal mice from lethal virus challenge. Science 1972; 176:1326–1327.
53. Cummins JM, Tompkins MB, Olsen RG, Tompkins WA, Lewis MG. Oral use of human alpha interferon in cats. J Biol Response Modifiers 1988; 7: 513–523.
54. Young AS, Maritim AC, Karuiki DP, Stagg DA, Wafula JM, Mutugi JJ, Cummins JM, Richards AB, Burns C. Low-dose oral administration of human interferon alpha can control the development of Theileria parva infection in cattle. J Parasitol 1990; 101 (Pt 2):201–209.

55. Streuli M, Hall A, Boll W, Stewart WE, Nagat S, Weisman C. Target cell specificity of two species of human interferon-α produced from Escherichia coli and of hybrid molecules derived from them. Proc Natl Acad Sci USA 1981; 78:2848–2852.

56. Stanton G, Hughes T, Heard H, Georgiades J, Whorton E. Modulation of a natural virus defense system by low concentrations of interferons at mucosal surfaces. J Interferon Res 1990; 10:(S-1)S99.

57. Lecce JG, Cummins JM, Richards AB. Treatment of rotavirus infection in neonate and weanling pigs using natural human interferon alpha. J Mol Biother 1990; 2:211–216.

58. Koech DK, Obel AO, Minowada J, Hutchinson VA, Cummins JM. Low dose oral alpha interferon therapy for patients seropositive for human immunodeficiency virus type I (HIV-I). Mol Biother 1990; 2:91–95.

59. Young AS, Cummins JM. The history of interferon and its use in animal therapy. East Afr Med J 1990; 67(suppl 2):SS31–63.

60. Bocci V. Is interferon effective after oral administration? The state of the art. J Biol Reg Homeostasis Agents 1990; 4:81–83.

61. Bocci V. Catabolism of therapeutic proteins and peptides with implications for drug delivery. Adv Drug Del Rev 1990; 4:149–169.

62. Bocci V. Absorption of cytokines via the oropharyngeal associated lymphoid tissues—Does an unorthodox route improve the therapeutic index of interferon? Clin Pharmacokinet 1991; 21:411–417.

63. Bocci V. Immunomodulators as local hormones: new insights regarding their clinical utilization. J Biol Res Mod 1985; 4:340–352.

64. Cantell K, Pyhala L. Circulating interferon in rabbits after administration by different routes. J Gen Virol 1973; 20:97–104.

65. Hanley D, Wironowska-Stewart M, Stewart II WE. Pharmacology of interferons. I. Pharmacologic distinctions between human leucocyte and fibroblast interferons. Int J Immunopharmacol 1979; 1:219–225.

66. Stewart II WE, Wironowska-Stewart M. Characterization of human interferon types and subtypes. In: Khan A, Hill NO, Dorn GL, eds. Interferon. Properties and Clinical Uses. Dallas: L. Fikes Press, 1980:111–120.

67. Ruegg CL, Strand M. Identification of a decapeptide region of human interferon α with antiproliferative activity and homology to an immunosuppressive sequence of the retroviral transmembrane protein P15E. J Interferon Res 1990; 10:621–626.

68. Waine GJ, Tymms MJ, Brandt ER, Cheetham BF, Linnane AW. Structure-function study of the region encompassing residues 26–40 of human interferon-α4: identification of residues important for antiviral and antiproliferative activities. J Interferon Res 1992; 12:43–48.

69. Paulesu L, Corradeschi F, Nicoletti C, Bocci V. Oral administration of human recombinant interferon-α2 in rats. Int J Pharmaceut 1988; 46: 199–202.

70. Bocci V, Corradeschi F, Naldini A, Lencioni E. Enteric absorbtion of human interferon α and β in the rat. Int J Pharmaceut 1988; 46:199–202.

71. Fleischmann WR, Koren S and Fleischmann CM. Oral administered inter-

ferons exert their white blood cell suppressive effects via a novel mechanism. Proc Soc Exp Biol Med 1992; 201:199–207.

72. Gibson DM, Cotler S, Spiegel HE, Colburn WA. Pharmokokinetics of recombinant leucocyte A interferon following various routes and modes of administration to the dog. J Interferon Res 1985; 5:403–408.

73. Wills RJ, Spiegel HE, Soike KF. Pharmacokinetics of recombinant leucocyte A interferon following IV infusion and bolus, IM, and PO administration to african green monkeys. J Interferon Res 1984; 4:399–409.

74. Witt PJ, Goldstein D, Storer BE, Grossberg SE, Flashner M, Colby CB, Borden EC. Absence of biological effects of orally administered interferon-β_{ser}. J Interferon Res 1992; 12:411–413.

75. Bocci V. Roles of interferon produced in physiological conditions. A speculative review. Immunology 1988; 64:1–9.

76. Goldstein D, Sielaff KM, Storer BE, Brown RR, Datta SP, Witt PJ, Teitlebaum AP, Smalley RV, Borden EC. Human biologic response modification by interferon in the absence of measurable serum concentrations: a comparative trial of subcutaneous and intravenous interferon-β serine. J Natl Cancer Inst 1989; 81:1061–1068.

77. Blalock JE, Baron S, Johnson HM, Stanton GJ. Transmission of interferon-induced activities by cell to cell communication. Tex Rep Biol Med 1982; 41:344–349.

78. Alvord EC, Shaw CM, Huby S, Kies MW. Encephalitogen-induced inhibition of experimental allergic encephalomyelitis: prevention, suppression and therapy. Ann NY Acad Sci 1965; 122:333–345.

79. Johns LD, Flanders KC, Ranges GE, and Sriram S. Successful therapy of experimental allergic encephalomyelitis with transforming growth factor-β_1. J Immunol 1991; 147:1792–1796.

80. Hertz F, Deghenghi R. Effect of rat and β-human interferons on hyperacute experimental allergic encephalomyelitis in rats. Agents Actions 1985; 16:397–403.

81. Karpus WJ, Swanborg RH. CD4+ suppressor cells inhibit the function of effector cells of experimental autoimmune encephalomyelitis through a mechanism involving transforming growth factor-β. J Immunol 1991; 146:1163–1168.

82. Abreu SL. Suppression of experimental allergic encephalomyelitis by interferon. Immunol Commun 1982; 11:1–7.

83. Abreu SL, Tondreau J, Levine S, Sowinski R. Inhibition of passive localized experimental allergic encephalomyelitis by interferon. Int Arch Allergy Appl Immunol 1983; 72:30–33.

84. Kennedy MK, Torrance DS, Picha KS, Mohler KM. Analysis of cytokine mRNA expression in the central nervous system of mice with experimental autoimmune encephalomyelitis reveals that IL-10 mRNA expression correlates with disease. J Immunol 1992; 149:2496–2505.

85. Hutchison VA, Angenend JL, Mok WL, Cummins JM, Richards AB. Chronic recurrent aphthous stomatitis: oral treatment with low dose interferon alpha. Mol Biother 1990; 2:160–164.

86. Brod SA, Scott M, Burns DH. 1994. Modification of acute experimental autoimmune encephalomyelitis in the Lewis rat by oral administration of type I interferons. J Interferon Res. In Press.

87. Tabata Y, Uno K, Yamaoka T, Ikada Y and Muramatsu S. Effects of recombinant alpha interferon gelatin conjugate on in vivo murine tumor cell growth. Cancer Res 1991; 51:5532–5538.

88. Shibita M and Blatteis CM. Human recombinant tumor necrosis factor and interferon affect the activity of neurons in the organum vasculosum lamina terminalis. Brain Res 1991; 562:323–326.

89. Dennis MJ, Thomas LH, and Stott EJ. Effects of recombinant human alpha A interferon in gnotobiotic calves challenged with respiratory syncyntial virus. Res Vet Sci 1991; 50:222–228.

90. Horisberger MA, and Gunst MC. Interferon induced proteins: identification of Mx proteins in various mammalian species. Virology 1991; 180: 185–190.

91. Weiss RC, Cummins JM, Richards AB. Low-dose orally administered interferon alpha treatment for feline leukemia virus infection. J Am Vet Med Assoc 1991; 199:1477–1481.

92. Weiss RC and Oostrom-Ram T. Effects of recombinant human interferon alpha in vitro and in vivo on mitogen induced lymphocyte blastogenesis in cats. J Clin Immunol Immunopathol 1990; 24:147–157.

93. Kawade Y. The interferon system in the mouse. In: Baron S, Dianzoni F, Stanton GJ, Fleischmann WR, eds. The Interferon System. Austin, TX: UT Press, 1987:169–175.

94. Blalock JE, Baron S. Interferon induced transfer viral resistance between animal cells. Nature 1977; 269:422–425.

95. McDonald AH, Swanborg RH. Antigen-specific inhibition of immune interferon production by suppressor cells of autoimmune encephalomyelitis. J Immunol 1988; 140:1132–1138.

96. Raine CS, Stone SH. Animal models for multiple sclerosis: chronic experimental allergic encephalomyelitis in inbred guinea pigs. N.Y. State J Med 1977; 77:1693–1696.

97. Wisniewski HM, Keith AB. Chronic relapsing experimental allergic encephalomyelitis: An experimental model of multiple sclerosis. Ann Neurol 1977; 1:144–148.

98. Feuer C, Prentice DE, Cammisuli S. Chronic relapsing experimental allergic encephalomyelitis in the Lewis rat. J Neuroimmunol. 1985; 10:159–166.

99. Brown AM, McFarlin DE. Relapsing experimental allergic encephalomyelitis in the SJL/J mouse. Lab Invest 1981; 45:278–284.

100. Miller SD, Clatch RJ, Pevear DC, Trotter JL, Lipton HL. Class II restricted T cell response in Theiler's murine emcephalomyelitis virus induced demyelinating disease. J Immunol 1987; 138:3776–3784.

101. Weber H, Valenzuela D, Lujber G, Gubler M, Weissman C. Single amino acid changes that render human IFN-α_2 biologically active on mouse cells. EMBO J 1987; 6:591–598.

102. McInnes M, Chambers PJ, Cheetham BF, Beilharz MW, Tymms MJ. Struc-

ture function studies of interferons-α: amino acid substitutions at the conserved residue tyrosine 123 in human interferons-α. J Interferon Res 1989; 9:305–314.

103. Brod SA, Khan M, Kerman RH, Pappolla M. Oral administration of human or murine IFN-α suppresses relapses and modifies adoptive transfer in experimental autoimmune encephalomyelitis. J Neuroimmunol 1995; 58: 61–69.

104. Brod SA, Burns DH. Suppression of relapsing experimental allergic encephalomyelitis in SJL/J mouse by oral administration of type I interferons. Neurology 1994; 44:1144–1148.

105. Brod SA, Khan M. 1994. Oral administration of human or murine type I interferons suppresses relapses in chronic relapsing EAE. Cytokine 6(5): 567:A169.

106. Lublin, F. Adoptive transfer of murine relapsing experimental autoimmune encephalomyelitis. Ann Neurol 1985; 17:188–190.

107. Whitham RH, Bourdette DN, Hashim GA, Herndon RM, Ilg RC, Vandenbark AA, Offner H. Lymphocytes from SJL/J mice immunized with spinal cord respond selectively to a peptide of proteolipid protein and transfer demyelinating relapsing experimental autoimmune encephalomyelitis. J Immunol 1991; 146:101–107.

108. Peters BA, Hinrichs DJ. Passive transfer of experimental allergic encephalomyelitis in the Lewis rat with activated spleen cells: Differential activation with mitogens. Cell Immunol 1982; 69:175–185.

109. Fallis RJ, Raine CS, McFarlin DE. Chronic relapsing experimental allergic encephalomyelitis in SJL/J mice following the adoptive transfer of an epitope-specific T cell line. J Neuroimmunol 1989; 22:93–105.

110. van der Veen RC, Trotter, JL, Clark HB, Kapp JA. The adoptive transfer of chronic experimental allergic encephalomyelitis with lymph nodes sensitized to myelin proteolipid protein. J Neuroimmunol 1989; 21:183–191.

111. Tuohy VK, Lu Z, Sobel RA, Laursen RA, Lees MB. Identification of an encephalitogenic determinant of myelin proteolipid protein for SJL/J mice. J Immunol 1989; 142:1523–1527.

112. Greer JM, Kuchroo VJ, Sobel RA, Lees MB. Identification and characterization of a second encephalitogenic determinant of myelin proteolipid protein (residues 178–191) for SJL/J mice. J Immunol 1992; 149:783–788.

113. Sobel RA, Tuohy VK, Lu Z, Sobel RA, Laursen RA, Lees MB. Acute experimental allergic encephalomyelitis in the SJL/J mouse induced by a synthetic peptide of myelin proteolipid protein. J Neuropathol Exp Neurol 1990; 49:468.

114. Kennedy MK, Tan L-J, Del Canto MC, Miller SD. Regulation of the effector stages of experimental autoimmune encephalomyelitis via neuroantigen-specific tolerance induction. J Immunol 1990; 145:117–126.

115. Kennedy MK, Tan L-J, Del Canto MC, Tuohy VK, Lu Z, Trotter JL, Miller SD. Inhibition of murine autoimmune encephalomyelitis by immune tolerance to proteolipid protein and its encephalitogenic peptides. J Immunol 1990; 144:909–915.

116. Brod SA, al-Sabbagh A, Sobel RA, Weiner HL. Suppression of relapsing experimental allergic encephalomyelitis in Lewis rats and strain 13 guinea pigs by oral administration of myelin antigens. Ann Neurol 1991; 29: 615–622.

117. Weiner HL, Friedman A, Miller A, SJ Khoury, DM Dawson, DA Hafler. Double blind pilot trial of oral tolerization with myelin antigens in multiple sclerosis. Science 1993; 259:1321–1324.

118. Kadish AS, Tansey FA, Yu GSM, Doyle AT and Bloom BR. Interferon as a mediator of human lymphocyte suppression. J Exp Med 1980; 151: 637–650.

119. Devens BH, Semenuk G, Webb DR. Antipeptide antibody specific for the N-terminal of soluble immune response suppressor neutralizes concavalin A and IFN-induced suppressor cell activity in an in vitro cytotoxic T lymphocyte response. J Immunol 1988; 141:3148–3155.

120. Aune TM, and Pierce CW. Activation of a suppressor T cell pathway by interferon. Proc Natl Acad Sci USA 1982; 79:3808–3812.

121. Schnapper HW, Pierce CW, Aune TM. Identification and initial characterization of Con A and interferon-induced human suppressor factor: evidence for a human equivalent of murine soluble immune response suppressor [SIRS]. J Immunol 1984; 132:2429–2435.

122. Stobo J, Green I, Jackson L and Baron S. Identification of a subpopulation of mouse lymphoid cells required for interferon production after stimulation with mitogens. J Immunol 1974; 112:1589–1593.

123. Weil J, Epstein CJ, Epstein LB, Sedmak JJ, Sabran JL, Grossberg SE. A unique set of polypeptides is induced by gamma interferon in addition to those induced in common with alpha and beta interferon. Nature 1983; 301: 437–439.

124. Mossmann TR, Cherwinski H, Bond MW, Giedlin MA, and Coffman RL. Two types of murine helper T cells. I. Definition according to profiles of lymphokine activities and secreted proteins. J Immunol 1986; 136: 2348–2357.

125. Kim J, Woods A, Becker-Dunn E, and Bottomly K. Distinct functional phenotypes of cloned Ia-restricted helper T cells. J Exp Med 1985; 162: 188–201.

126. Cher DJ Mosmann TR. Two types of murine helper T cell clone. II. Delayed-type hypersensitivity is mediated by Th1 clones. J Immunol 1987; 138: 3688–3694.

127. Boom WH, Liano D, and Abbas AK. Heterogeneity of helper/inducer T lymphocytes II. Effects of interleukin-4 and interleukin-2 producing T cell clones on resting B cells. J Exp Med 1988; 167:1350–1363.

128. Street N, Schumacher JH, Fong TAT, Bass H, Fiorentino DF, Leverach JA, Mosmann TR. Heterogeneity of mouse helper T cells: evidence from bulk cultures and limiting dilution cloning for precursors of Th1 and Th2 cells. J Immunol. 1990; 144:1629–1637.

129. Merrill JE, Kono DH, Clayton J, Ando DG, Hinton DR. Inflammatory leukocytes and cytokines in the peptide-induced disease of experimental

allergic encephalomyelitis in SJL and B10.PL mice. Proc Natl Acad Sci USA 1992; 89:574–578.

130. Brod SA, Benjamin D, Halfer DA. Restricted T cell expression of IL-2/IFN-γ mRNA in human inflammatory disease. J Immunol 1991; 147:810–815.

131. Yssel H, Shanafelt M-C, Soderberg C, Schneider PV, Anzola J, Peltz G. Borrelia burgdorferai activates a T helper type-1 like T cell subset in Lyme arthritis. J. Exp. Med. 1991; 174:593–601.

132. Haanen J, Malefijt R, Res P, Kraakman, EM, Ottenhoff, THM, deVries, RRP, Spits, H. Selection of a human T helper type I-like T cell subset by Mycobacteria. J Exp Med 1991; 174:583–591.

133. Mossman T, Moore KW. The role of IL-10 in crossregulation of Th1 and Th2 responses. Immunol Today 1991; 12:A49–53.

134. Brandtzaeg P. Overview of the mucosal immune system. Curr Top Microbiol Immunol 1989; 146:13–28.

135. Ermak TH, Owen RL. Differential distribution of lymphocytes and accessory cells in Peyer's patches. Anat. Rev. 1986; 215:144–52.

136. Witmer MD, Steinman RM. The anatomy of peripheral lymphoid organs with emphasis on accessory cells: light-microscopy immuno-cytochemical studies of the mouse spleen, lymph node, and Peyer's patch. Am J Anat 1984; 170:465–481.

137. MacDonald TT. Immunosuppression caused by antigen feeding. II. Suppressor T cells mask Peyer's patches B cell priming to orally administered antigen. Eur J Immunol 1983; 13:138–142.

138. Santos LMB, al-Sabbagh A, Londono A, Weiner HL. Oral tolerance to MBP induces TGF-β secreting T cells in Peyer's patch. J Immunol 1993; 150[8,II]: 115A.

139. Mattingly JA. Immunologic suppression after oral administration of antigen. Cell Immunol 1984; 86:45–52.

140. Xu-Amano J, Aicher WK, Taguchi T, Kiyono H, McGhee JR. Selective induction of Th2 cells in murine Peyer's patches by oral immunization. Int Immunol 1992; 4:433–45.

141. Daynes RA, Areneo BA, Dowell TA, Huang K, Dudley D. Regulation of murine cytokine production in vivo. III. The lymphoid tissue microenvironment exerts regulatory influence over T helper function. J Exp Med 1990; 171:979–996.

142. Hu MCT, Crowe DT, Weissman IL, Holzmann B. Cloning and expression of mouse integrin β_p (β_7): a functional role in Peyer's patch-specific lymphocyte homing. Proc Natl Acad Sci USA 1992; 89:8254–8258.

143. Chin YH, Cai JP, Xu XM. TGF-β_2 and IL-4 regulate adhesiveness of Peyer's patch HEV cells for lymphocytes. J Immunol 1992; 148:1106–12.

144. LeFrancois L. IEL of the intestinal mucosa: curioser and curioser. Semin Immunol 1991; 3:99–108.

145. Sydora BC, Mixter PF, Holcombe HR, Eghtesady P, Williams K, Amaral MC, Nel A, Kroenberg M. IELs are activated and cytolytic but do not proliferate as well as other T cells in response to mitogenic stimulation. J Immunol 1993; 150(6):2179–91.

146. Weiner HL, GA Mackin, M Matsui, EJ Orav, SJ Khoury, al-Sabbagh A, Santos L, Sayegh M, Nussenblatt RB, Trentham DE, Hafler DA. Oral tolerance: immunologic mechanisms and treatment of animal and human organ-specific autoimmune diseases by oral administration of autoantigens. Ann Rev Immunol 1994; 12:809–37.

147. Higgins P, Weiner HL. Suppression of experimental autoimmune encephalomyelitis by oral administration of myelin basic protein and its fragments. J Immunol 1988; 140:440–445.

148. Fuller KA, Pearl D, Whitacre CC. Oral tolerance in experimental autoimmune encephalomyelitis: serum and salivary antibody responses. J Neuroimmunol 1990; 28:15–26.

149. Lider O, Santos LMB, Lee CSY, Higgins PJ, Weiner HL. Suppression of experimental autoimmune encephalomyelitis by oral administration of myelin basic protein II. Suppression of disease and in vitro immune responses is mediated by antigen-specific CD8 + T lymphocytes. J Immunol 1989; 142:748–752.

150. Chen Y, Kuchroo VJ, Inobe J-I, Hafler DA, Weiner HL. Regulatory T cell clones induced by oral tolerance: suppression of autoimmune encephalomyelitis. Science 1994; 265:1237–1240.

151. Georgiades JA, Kruzel ML, Seman G. Transfer of antiviral resistance by spleen and blood cells of mice receiving low doses of IFN alpha or gamma. J Interferon Res 1989; 9:S213.

152. Blalock JE, Baron S, Johnson HM, Stanton GJ. Transmission of interferon-induced activities by cell to cell communication. Tex Rep Biol Med 1982; 41:344–349.

153. Butcher EC. The regulation of lymphocyte traffic. Curr Top Microbiol Immunol 1986; 128:85–122.

154. Bocci V. Roles of interferon produced in physiological conditions. Immunology 1988; 64:1–9.

155. Boccoli G, Masciulli R, Ruggeri EM, Carlini P, Giannella G et al. Adoptive immunotherapy of human cancer: the cytokine cascade and monocyte activation following high-dose interleukin 2 bolus treatment. Cancer Res 1990; 50:5795–5800.

156. Dinarello CA, Cannon JG, Wolff SM, Bernheim HA, Beutler B, et al. Tumour necrosis factor (cachectin) is an endogenous pyrogen and induces production of interleukin-1. J Exp Med 1986; 163:1433–1450.

157. Bocci V. Absorption of cytokines via oropharyngeal-associated lymphoid tissues: Does an unorthodox route improve the therapeutic index of interferon? Clin. Pharmacokinet 1991; 21:411–417.

158. Linington C, Berger T, Perry L, Weerth S, Hinze-Selch D, Zhang Y, Li H-C, Lassmann H, Wekerle H. T cells specific for the myelin oligodendrocyte glycoprotein mediate an unusual autoimmune inflammatory response in the central nervous system. Eur J Immunol 1993; 23:1364–1372.

11

Interferon-α in the Treatment of Multiple Sclerosis

Lorne F. Kastrukoff and Joel J.-F. Oger

The University of British Columbia, Vancouver, British Columbia, Canada

I. INTRODUCTION

Recombinant human interferon-β-1b (IFN β-1b; Betaseron) was recently approved for the treatment of relapsing-remitting (RR) multiple sclerosis (MS) based on the results of a multicenter, randomized, double-blind, placebo-controlled trial (1,2). This trial evolved from preliminary studies with IFN-β (3,4) as well as from experience gained from studies with IFN-α in MS. Although the results of the Betaseron trial have immediate implications for the management of RR disease, they also raise important questions. During the studies with IFN-α in MS, much information was gained and a review of the lessons learned has merit not only in designing future clinical trials of IFN in other courses of MS, but also in beginning to understand the mechanisms of action of IFN relevant to MS.

II. THE INTERFERONS

IFN was first identified by Isaacs and Lindenmann in 1957 (5). Originally, it was shown to play a role in interfering with viral replication, but later IFN was also shown to slow cell proliferation and to profoundly affect the immune system (6,7). There are four main classes of IFNs in humans: α, ω (formerly α₂), β, and γ (8). Trophoblast IFN represents a fifth class of IFN that has recently been recognized (9,10) (see Chapter 17).

IFN-α represents a superfamily of related proteins which likely evolved from a common ancestor. There are at least 18 (and possibly more) nonallelic genes, including 4 pseudogenes, clustered on the short arm of chromosome 9. All of the genes lack introns and all code for proteins of 165–166 amino acids. There is extensive homology among these proteins in humans. IFN-ω is coded for by six nonallelic genes, including five pseudogenes, clustered on chromosome 9. These genes also lack introns and code for a 172–amino acid protein. There is between 57 and 63% homology with other human types of IFN-α. Although most cells can make some IFN-α, both classes of IFN are preferentially induced in leukocytes by a variety of agents, including foreign, virus-infected, and tumor cells along with bacterial products and viral envelopes. Both IFN-α and IFN-β share the same receptor, which is present on most cell types. The gene coding for this receptor is located on chromosome 21. Affinity for this receptor and biological activity varies from one IFN-α to another. Once bound to its receptor, transcription of IFN-α and IFN-β activatible genes is mediated through a cascade of events which is discussed in detail in Chapters 1 and 2.

III. CLINICAL TRIALS OF IFN-α IN MS

Clinical trials with IFN-α have been undertaken in both relapsing and progressive disease. Four trials have studied the effect of IFN-α in MS patients with the former and two trials with the latter MS course. The nature of the IFNs used in these trials varied, with some studies using recombinant IFN-α, while others used natural IFN-α. A preliminary trial was also undertaken with polyinosinic acid polycytidylic acid complexed with polylysine in carboxymethyl cellulose (poly I:C/L:C) a potent inducer of IFNs. Although the results of studies with nonrecombinant IFN-α require careful scrutiny because of the potential of "contaminants" to affect both clinical and immunological outcomes, these trials can still provide important information.

A. Clinical Trials of IFN-α in Relapsing MS

1. The first trial was a randomized double-blind placebo-controlled crossover trial designed to test the efficacy of natural IFN-α in relapsing disease. Results were reported by Knobler et al. in 1984 (11). Twenty-four patients (11 male, 13 female) with a mean age of 34 years and an average disease duration of 7.5 years entered the trial. Half the group initially received 5×10^6 IU of the Cantell preparation (12) of natural IFN-α i.m. daily for 6 months followed by a 6-month washout and then

placebo (human serum albumin) for 6 months followed by a 6-month wash-out. In the other half of the study population, placebo was given first and was then followed by IFN. Disease activity was evaluated clinically using the Kurtzke disability status score (DSS) and the Scripps neurological rating scale (NRS). Magnetic resonance imaging (MRI) was not used to assess disease activity. Fewer exacerbations tended to occur during IFN treatment than with placebo, but the difference was not statistically significant ($P = .22$). Severity of exacerbations, measured with the Scripps NRS, was also not significantly different when IFN was compared with placebo.

Finally, treatment with IFN-α did not result in improvement over the 24-month interval as measured by the DSS. Fifteen of the 24 patients had a RR course, whereas 9 had a relapsing-progressive (RP) course. In the RR group, there were significantly fewer relapses with IFN when compared with placebo ($P = .05$). The benefit of IFN in this group may, however, have resulted from two patients who did particularly well and who may have favorably skewed the results in the RR group. There were no severe and few moderately severe attacks in this group. In contrast, the RP group did not benefit from IFN therapy and continued to have relapses throughout the trial. This group also tended to have more severe relapses and to worsen over the course of the trial.

A number of lessons can be learned from this trial. First, it was observed that exacerbation rates fell in both IFN and placebo phases when compared with the prestudy period. This points out the importance of a placebo group. Had they not been included, the entire reduction in exacerbation rate in the active treatment group might have mistakenly been attributed to a treatment effect. Second, using a crossover design appeared to result in a greater reduction in relapses when IFN was given after placebo. This might be explained on the basis of a "learning phenomenon" and would argue against the use of this design in future trials. Third, the small number of patients, the inclusion of patients with two different clinical courses (RR and RP), the relatively short period of treatment, the moderate dose of IFN used in this study, and evaluation of disease activity limited to a clinical signs could negatively influence the chance of identifying any treatment effect other than a profound effect. Fourth, RR patients may respond more favorably to IFN-α then RP patients, and furthermore, subpopulations of patients, some of whom may respond more favorably to IFN than others, might exist in the larger study group. Fifth, the use of a natural IFN preparation has the potential disadvantage of "contaminants" which might affect the clinical outcome and contribute to the side-effect profile of the treatment. Sixth, side effects of the treatment have the potential to unblind the study.

In 1987, Panitch (13) reevaluated 12 of the original 24 patients treated with IFN-α (11). Seven were RR patients and five were RP. Follow-up was 2.5 years after the completion of the original trial. A sustained effect during follow-up was claimed as the exacerbation rate dropped to 0.47/year. Prior to entry into the study, the exacerbation rate had been 1.33/year, whereas during the trial, it was 1.08/year in the first year and 0.75/year in the second. In many of these cases, however, the clinical course had changed. Only five of the original seven patients remained RR; two had developed a RP course. Three of the original five RP patients developed chronic progressive (CP) disease. The design of this trial did not allow for a determination of whether the worsening in clinical course was more likely with IFN then placebo treatment.

2. The second trial, using natural IFN-α in relapsing MS patients, was reported by the AUSTIMS research group in 1989 (14). This was a randomized placebo-controlled double-blind trial to test the efficacy of IFN-α and transfer factor (TF) in patients with relapsing disease. One-hundred and eighty-two patients were entered. Eighty-five percent had MS for less than 10 years and 82% had DSS scores of <4. Entry criteria included either one or more relapses or progression of >1 on the DSS score within the 3 pretrial years. Sixty of the patients received 3×10^6 IU of natural IFN-α s.c. prepared by the method of Cantell and Hirvonen (12). This was administered twice weekly for 2 months, followed by once per week for 10 months, and finally once every 2 weeks for 24 months. Sixty-one patients received placebo and the remainder TF. Disease activity was evaluated clinically using the Kurtzke DSS, functional systems scale (FSS), and the ambulatory status scoring system (ASSS). MRI was not performed in this trial. Of the 182 patients entered, 153 patients completed the trial. Fifty-eight placebo patients, 53 TF-treated patients, but only 42 IFN-treated patients completed the study. No significant difference was observed in exacerbation rates between the three arms of the study. Furthermore, IFN-α did not appear to alter the rate of disease progression.

This study supports several observations made in the previous trial. First, the inclusion of patients with two different clinical courses (55 RR and 5 RP in the IFN-treatment arm), the low dose of IFN used in the trial, and evaluation of disease activity limited to a clinical evaluation might affect the chance of identifying a treatment effect other than a profound effect. Second, a significant dropout rate occurred in the IFN-treated group and could influence the chance of identifying a significant treatment effect. Third, the use of a natural IFN preparation had the potential disadvantage of carrying with it "contaminants" which might affect the clinical outcome and contribute to the side-effect profile of the treatment.

3. The third trial of IFN-α in relapsing MS was reported in 1986 by Camenga et al. (15). This was a randomized placebo-controlled double-blind trial to test the efficacy of recombinant human IFN-α_2 in patients with relapsing MS. Ninety-eight patients (40 male, 58 female) with a range of ages from 20–50 years, a MS duration of <10 years, and two or more attacks in the 2 years preceding entry into the trial were randomized to either a treatment group where they received recombinant IFN-α_2 2 × 10^6 IU s.c. three times a week for 12 months or placebo (mixture of albumin, glycine, and phosphate buffer). Patients were evaluated clinically throughout the trial and for an additional 3 months using the FSS, the Kurtzke expanded disability status score (EDSS), and the MS incapacity scale. MRI was not performed in this study. Of the 98 patients who entered the trial, only two-thirds completed the treatment phase, but dropouts were divided equally between both treatment and placebo groups.

No significant treatment effect was identified on the exacerbation rate or on the severity of the exacerbations. During the first 24 weeks, more placebo than IFN-treated patients appeared to improve. In the second half of the study (months 7–13), both groups appeared to be equal. However, months after the treatment phase, more patients receiving IFN were significantly worse than those receiving placebo ($P = .03$).

Of the 98 patients, 72 had a RR course, whereas 25 had a RP course. Thirty-four of the RR patients received IFN, whereas 38 received placebo. Of the IFN-treated group, 24 remained RR but 9 developed RP and one a CP course. In contrast, of the 38 RR patients who received placebo, 35 remained RR, 2 developed RP, and 1 a CP course. Thirteen of the originally RP patients received IFN, whereas 12 received placebo. Of the IFN-treated group, seven remained RP but six developed CP disease. In contrast, of the 12 RP patients who received placebo, 8 remained RP, whereas 4 developed CP disease. Overall, 16 patients receiving IFN but only 7 receiving placebo developed a more progressive disease following the completion of the trial. It is not clear from this study if this worsening resulted from the IFN, if there was a problem with randomization (there was some reason to believe that the MS was more severe in the IFN-treated group prior to treatment, although the EDSS scores were similar in both groups), a combination of both, or a random event. This trial supported several observations made in previous trials as well as generated new ones. First, as in the trial reported by Knobler (11), exacerbation rates fell in both IFN- and placebo-treated patients when compared with the prestudy period. Second, the inclusion of patients with two different clinical courses (RR and RP), the relatively short period of treatment, the low dose of IFN used in this study (one-sixth of that used in the trial reported by Knobler), and evaluation of disease activity limited to a clinical nature might reduce the chance of identifying a treatment effect. This trial also raised the concern that IFN might have a long-term detrimental effect on MS. Although it is unclear if this was related to IFN or possibly the low dosage of IFN, the patient's clinical course, or a random event, it is in keeping with observations made by Knobler et al. (11) that some MS patients (RP) continue to develop relapses and worsen while being treated with IFN. Unlike the previous studies, this trial used a pure recombinant IFN without contaminating substances.

4. The fourth trial of IFN-α in relapsing MS was recently published by Durelli et al. (16). This was a randomized placebo-controlled double-blind trial to test the efficacy of high-dose recombinant IFN α_{2a} in RR MS. Twenty patients (11 female, 9 male) with clinically definite MS, a mean age of 35 years, an EDSS score less than or equal to 6 at entry, and at least two clinically defined relapses in the 2 years preceding entry into the trial were randomized to a treatment group (12 patients) which received 9×10^6 IU of IFN-α_{2a} i.m. every other day for 6 months or a placebo group (8 patients) (albumin + sodium chloride). Patients were evaluated clinically using Scripps NRS and Kurtzke EDSS scores. Patients were also evaluated with MRI before and after treatment.

A statistically significant reduction in exacerbations in the IFN-treated group was observed over the 6-month period ($P < .03$). Ten of 12 patients receiving IFN and only 2 of 8 patients receiving placebo were free of relapses during the treatment phase. When compared with the relapse rate prior to entry, the IFN-treated group had significantly fewer relapses ($P < .02$), whereas this reduction was not observed in the placebo group. There also appeared to be an effect on the severity of the exacerbations with only one mild and one moderate relapse developing in the IFN group and two mild, three moderate, and three severe relapses in the placebo group. The clinical results were supported by MRI studies where the mean number of active lesions/patient was 0.08 ± 0.08 in the IFN group and 3.37 ± 1.03 in the placebo group ($P < .01$).

Despite the relatively small number of patients and the short time of treatment which could have negatively influenced the outcome of this trial, the study did benefit from a number of design features. These included patients with only RR disease, the availability of MRI along with clinical scales for the evaluation of disease activity, and pure recombinant IFN-α given at high dosage. Side effects of the IFN did have the potential for unblinding this study. The beneficial results reported in this trial suggest that, similar to IFN-β-1b, IFN-α may be of benefit in MS patients with RR disease.

B. Clinical Trials of IFN-α in Chronic Progressive MS

IFN-α in MS patients with CP disease has not been studied as thoroughly as in relapsing disease. Two very early studies did not show any benefit of IFN in MS with this course. Fog, in a pilot trial, reported on the treatment of five MS patients with CP disease (17). Patients received 5 × 10^6 U of natural IFN-α daily for 2 weeks and then 2.5 × 10^6 U daily for 5–15 months. He reported: "in all cases the disease process continued and the patient's clinical status deteriorated." Ruutiainen treated five patients with CP disease with intrathecal IFN-α (Cantell preparation) weekly for 3 months. Although no definite conclusions could be drawn from this trial, treatment did not appear to give rise to improvement (18).

1.   Kastrukoff et al. reported on the effect of lymphoblastoid IFN in patients with CP disease (19). This was a randomized placebo-controlled double-blind trial. One hundred patients (58 female, 42 male) with a mean age of 45 years, a mean disease duration of 14 years, a CP course for at least 6 months, and a Kurtzke EDSS score of 7 or less were randomized to either a treatment arm (50 patients) which received human lymphoblastoid IFN, 5 × 10^6 IU s.c. daily for 6 months or a placebo group (50 patients) (normal saline). Patients were evaluated clinically using the Kurtzke FSS and EDSS along with the incapacity status scale (ISS). MRI was performed prior to entry, at 6 months, and at 24 months in a subgroup of 37 IFN-treated and 31 placebo-treated patients. Fifteen patients receiving IFN and one receiving placebo dropped out of the study.

No significant difference between the two patient groups was identified after 2 years either clinically or by MRI. The placebo group slowly deteriorated over the 2 years and became significantly worse after 2 years. Although not statistically significant, a trend was observed in the IFN-treated group with patients being worse than controls at 1 and 3 months but better at 6 and 18 months. MRI results at 6 months supported the clinical trend. However, the two treatment groups were not homogeneous. In the placebo group, 27 of the 50 CP patients remained stable over the 2-year trial, whereas 23 of these patients deteriorated. This was also seen in the IFN group where 24 patients remained stable, whereas 16 patients deteriorated. However, there were 10 patients in the treated group whose EDSS scores improved at 6 and 18 months and were thought to be responsible for the trend of a benefit from IFN therapy. Thus, there appears to be a subset of patients who respond to IFN. This subset was similar to other study patients except for a higher female/male ratio and a lower EDSS score at entry into the study.

There were several advantages to this study over earlier efforts. These included the ability to evaluate disease activity both clinically and by MRI, the reasonable number of patients that were entered, and patients with a specific course (CP). Disadvantages of this study included the high dropout rate in the treatment arm which could result in a type II statistical error, prominent side effects making blinding difficult, the relatively short treatment time and moderate dosage of IFN which could limit a beneficial effect, and an IFN which contained mostly IFN-α but some IFN-β and also possibly some other "contaminants" which could influence the outcome of the trial.

Three additional points are of note. First, patients who entered the trial were not homogeneous despite the fact that they all had a CP course and had shown deterioration prior to entry. Although many continued to deteriorate in both treatment groups after entry, a significant number showed no evidence of deterioration over the next 2 years. Second, there were two phases to the clinical course in some patients receiving IFN. Patients initially deteriorated, possibly secondary to the induction of IFN-γ (20) but then improved. Had the study been terminated during the initial stages, the secondary improvement would not have been identified. Third, there appeared to be a subset of patients among the larger group of CP patients who may have shown a response to IFN therapy.

2.   The second study of IFN-α in CP MS was reported by Kinnunen et al. (21). This was an open trial where the intent was to treat 10 patients with CP disease to test the efficacy of recombinant IFN-α$_{2b}$. The study was terminated after six patients had been treated. All six patients had MS for an average of 10 years. Although all had RR disease initially, this had evolved into a CP course for 2–3 years prior to entry into the study. Their EDSS scores ranged from 3.5 to 4.5. Patients received recombinant IFN-α$_{2b}$ 3 × 10^6 IU s.c. daily for 6 months. Both clinical evaluation (Kurtzke EDSS) and MRIs were used to monitor disease activity.

Five of the six patients had subjective and objective worsening of their disease. The mean progression index during the period of treatment was significantly higher then prior to entry ($P < .02$). One patient showed no change. MRI confirmed the clinical impression of progression in four patients, showed no change in one, and showed improvement in one (the same patient who showed clinical improvement). The trial was limited by its small size and the fact that it was not blinded nor placebo controlled. Treatment was also given for a short period of time and at a relatively low dose. It did have the advantage of using a pure recombinant IFN-α. When the results are compared with the previous trial, it is of interest that a number of patients worsened during the first 6 months, which is similar to what was observed in that trial. Furthermore, one patient, possibly in a subset of CP patients, appeared to improve both clinically and by MRI, which is similar to the previous trial.

C. Clinical Trial of Poly I:C/L:C in MS

A preliminary trial with I:C/L:C in CP MS was also undertaken (22). Poly I:C/L:C is a potent inducer of IFNs, with IFN-β usually predominating in vivo. Nine patients (five female, four male) with rapidly progressive disease and a disease duration of 2–19 years as well as nine patients (four female, five male) with slowly progressive disease and a disease duration of 5–20 years were entered. DSS scores ranged from 3 to 9. Poly I:C/L:C was given i.v. at a dose of 20 µg/kg initially and then gradually increased to 100 µg/kg. The medication was given weekly for 6–12 weeks followed by bimonthly or monthly treatments for up to 18 months. Patients were evaluated clinically (quantitative neurological examination Kurtzke DSS score, ambulation index) but not by MRI. The administration of poly I:C/L:C induced IFN in the serum with peak levels lasting for 8–12 hr. Levels over 50 IU/ml were induced in 82% of patients and over 500 IU/ml in 15% of patients.

In the rapidly progressive group, four patients improved, one improved but then deteriorated while on treatment, two stabilized, one stabilized for 5 months but then deteriorated, and one continued to deteriorate. In the slowly progressive group, four patients remained stable, four withdrew from the study, and one died unrelated to the study. The small numbers of patients, the lack of controls, and the nonblinded nature of this study made it somewhat difficult to interpret the results, but no clear benefit was identified.

IV. ADVERSE EFFECTS OF IFN-α

Side effects of IFN were identified in all of these trials with the frequency and severity varying with the nature and dosage of the preparation. Throughout these studies, certain side effects were repeatedly observed, suggesting that they may be common to the different preparations of IFN-α. These included, among others, fever and rigors initially, also fatigue, malaise, headaches, myalgias, nausea, anorexia, alopecia, and local injection site reactions. Relative granulocytopenia, lymphopenia, and mild elevations in liver enzymes were also observed in some cases. The adverse effects of IFN are discussed in detail in Chapter 16.

V. SUMMARY OF CLINICAL TRIALS WITH IFN-α IN MS

In summary, there are a number of lessons that can be taken from earlier studies of IFN-α in the treatment of MS. A number of these are related to the design of the clinical trial itself. First, placebo-controlled double-blinded trials are clearly important to prevent inaccurate interpretation of results. The need for placebo controls is documented in the studies of Knobler et al. (11) and Camenga et al. (15) where exacerbation rates fell in both treatment and placebo groups compared with their prestudy rates. In the trial of CP MS reported by Kastrukoff et al. (19), a significant number of patients who had a progressive course prior to entry into the trial stabilized for over 2 years while on placebo. Without the benefit of controls, the decrease in exacerbation rates or the stabilization of progression could be mistakenly interpreted as a beneficial effect of IFN. Second, there is reasonable evidence to suggest that crossover design trials should now be avoided. In the trial reported by Knobler et al. (11), a greater reduction in relapses occurred when active treatment followed after placebo and may reflect a "learning phenomenon." Third, increasing evidence would suggest that most clinical trials in MS would now benefit from evaluating disease activity both clinically and by serial MRIs. Since clinical methods to evaluate disease activity continue to have problems associated with them, confidence in the accuracy of the clinical impression would be enhanced if they were supported by MRI results (16,19,21). Fourth, because of the difficulties in interpreting results from trials where MS patients with different clinical courses are included (11,14,15), future trials should be limited to patients with a single clinical course. Fifth, because of the difficulties in interpreting results from trials where nonrecombinant IFNs were used and there was a potential for "contaminants" to affect the results (11,14,19), trials should use recombinant IFNs wherever possible.

The studies with IFN-α in MS also identified a number of problems which might have affected the results but are difficult to predict and plan for prior to the completion of the trial. The numbers of patients, the length of time the treatment is administered, the dosage of the medication, the problem of patients drop outs, and the problem of side effects unblinding the study are most easily identified once the trial has been completed. Despite the difficulties with predicting outcome, these potential problems must be dealt with in advance. Experience gained from these studies would suggest that there might be subpopulations of patients who would benefit from therapy where others might not (11,19,21). Although the reasons for this are unclear, differences in disease activity or dosage of medication may be important and will have to be considered in future trials.

Finally, the use of IFN in MS in these early trials has shown that there may be an initial worsening of symptoms and clinical course. The studies suggest that this phase is better tolerated in RR disease than in RP or CP disease. As clinical trials begin to study the effect of IFNs on RP and CP disease, it will be important to remember that the potential for initial worsening may be followed by improvement. If the trials are terminated prematurely, the improvement phase could be missed and a potentially valuable therapy lost.

VI. IMMUNE STUDIES IN CLINICAL TRIALS OF IFN-α IN MS

Although IFN-β-1b (Betaseron) is effective in the treatment of RR MS, its mechanism of action remains unknown. Although benefit may be mediated through its antiviral effect, it is more likely that it is mediated through its modulating effects on the immune system (23). IFN-α is known to have a variety of effects on the immune system, many of which may be relevant to MS. It can augment the expression of major histocompatibility complex (MHC) class I antigens throughout the body (24). It can also affect a number of lymphokines. IFN-α is reported to increase interleukin-1 (IL-1) secretion by human monocytes exposed to lipopolysaccharide (LPS) (25) and to induce IL-1 secretion by cultured human monocytes (26). In contrast, IFN-α can cause macrophages to release a potent natural inhibitor of IL-1, IL-1 receptor antagonist (27,28). IFN-α increases IL-2 secretion (29) and antagonizes IL-4–induced suppression of IFN-γ production by peripheral blood CD4$^+$ cells in vitro (30). It will inhibit both granulocyte-macrophage colony-stimulating factor in vitro (31) and the in vitro production of lymphotoxin (LT) by concanavalin A (ConA)–stimulated peripheral blood mononuclear see (PBMCs) (32). IFN-α can inhibit IgE and IgG production by human B cells cultured with IL-4 (33,34). In vitro, IFN-α in low concentration will antagonize the activating effect of IFN-γ on macrophages but in high concentration will activate macrophages by increasing their number and phagocytic activity.

In many cases, immune studies accompanied the clinical trials of IFN-α in MS. These studies focused on the effect of IFN-α on immunoglobulins, cell phenotypes both in the blood and cerebrospinal fluid (CSF), nonspecific suppressor cell function, natural killer (NK) cell function, and IFN synthesis (also see ref. 23 and Chapter 7 for the role of the immune system in MS.) In those cases where IFN was measured in the serum and CSF, it was found to be present only in serum and only in IFN-treated patients (11), suggesting that any effects of IFN-α on the immune system were restricted to its actions in the periphery.

The effect of IFN-α on immunoglobulin synthesis was studied in both relapsing and CP MS patients. In relapsing MS patients treated with natural IFN-α, Panitch et al. (35) reported a dramatic increase in both serum and CSF IgG. Seven of 12 patients had elevations in serum IgG (ranging from 31 to 115%) that were significantly different from controls at 1, 3, and 6 months of therapy. Intrathecal IgG was increased in 6 of the 12 patients. Similar results were reported by Rice et al. (36). In CP disease, Kinnunen et al. (21), using recombinant IFN-α$_{2b}$, also reported an increase in intrathecal IgG synthesis with treatment. In four of six patients, IFN treatment resulted in an increase in intrathecal IgG synthesis, whereas in one patient, it remained unchanged, and it was normal in one patient. In CP MS patients treated with lymphoblastoid IFN, Kastrukoff et al. (37) also observed a significant increase in intrathecal IgG production at 3 months and this remained elevated 6 months after treatment was initiated. Thus, despite different clinical courses, and types and dosages of IFN-α employed, treatment most often resulted in an increase in intrathecal IgG synthesis. Furthermore, results from two studies suggest that a correlation between intrathecal IgG synthesis and clinical course may exist. Panitch et al. (35) observed that in six patients with elevated IgG, only two mild attacks developed. In contrast, 4 of 12 IFN-treated patients whose intrathecal IgG synthesis rates decreased, and 2 of 12 treated patients whose rates remained unchanged, suffered six moderate or severe exacerbations. This would suggest that increased intrathecal IgG synthesis might be beneficial. This unexpected result is supported by observations of Kastrukoff et al. (37). In a subpopulation of 10 IFN-treated patients who improved both clinically and by MRI, there was an early and significant increase in intrathecal IgG synthesis.

In vitro IgG synthesis in response to pokeweed mitogen (PWM) stimulation is a technique frequently applied to the study of mononuclear cells (MNCs) in MS patients. Generally, MNCs in MS secrete more IgG than do cells from healthy controls (38–40). A group of 38 CP MS patients treated in Vancouver similarly had high IgG secretion prior to treatment with lymphoblastoid IFN or placebo (41). In 14 patients who received IFN, IgG synthesis was significantly reduced after 1 week and remained low throughout the treatment phase of the study. Six months after treatment was terminated, PWM-induced IgG synthesis increased to a level similar to that in placebo-treated patients. Since it is known that the effect of IFN on IgG synthesis varies with the type of IFN employed, its concentration, and the timing of its addition in relation to the addition of mitogen or antigen (42–44), differences in results obtained in vitro and in vivo likely can be reconciled on that basis.

Several trials also studied the development of specific antibodies in MS patients receiving IFN-α. The potential to develop neutralizing antibodies to IFN is of obvious concern. In some cases, normal human sera may already contain low-titer autoantibodies to IFN-α (45). Furthermore, a proportion of patients without MS treated with IFN-α have been reported to develop neutralizing antibodies although generally only after prolonged treatment (46,47). In the trial reported by Knobler et al. (11), no specific antibodies to IFN were identified. However, MS patients were treated for only 6 months, and this may have been too early for antibodies to develop. In some trials where patients without MS had been treated with IFN-α for prolonged periods of time, antithyroid antibodies developed (48), and in some patients, these antibodies were associated with thyroid failure (49,50). This was not the case with MS patients, but again the duration of treatment may have been too brief. In the natural IFN-α trial reported by Knobler et al. (11), immune complexes were identified in a number of patients, some of whom developed symptoms suggestive of immune complex disease (35,36). It is likely that the antibodies in the immune complexes were against a contaminating protein related to Sendai virus rather then against IFN.

The effect of IFN-α on both peripheral blood and CSF MNC subsets, identified by cell surface markers, was studied in both relapsing and CP MS patients. Prior to treatment with natural IFN-α, the CD4/CD8 ratio of PBMNCs in RR patients was increased when compared with normal controls (35). Following treatment, the ratio increased again; in some cases, due to an increase in CD4$^+$ cells and in others to a decrease in CD8$^+$ cells. Similar increases in CD4/CD8 ratios were reported with CP MS patients both prior to (41) and following treatment with lymphoblastoid IFN (37). A reduction in CD8$^+$ cells in the peripheral blood was also reported by Kinnunen et al. (21) in six CP MS patients treated with recombinant IFN-α$_{2b}$ but this did not reach significance. In contrast to these studies, Hirsch and Johnson did not find any effect of recombinant IFN-α$_2$ on either CD4 or CD8 cells in the peripheral blood (51). Patients in this study (previously reported by Camenga et al. [15]) received a low dose of IFN compared with other studies, and this likely was an important factor in the lack of change observed. In CSF, Panitch et al. reported a decrease in the CD4/CD8 ratio with IFN treatment, an effect opposite to that observed in blood (35). Similar results with an increase in the percentage of CD8$^+$ cells in the CSF with IFN treatment were reported by Durelli et al. (16). Although these results could be interpreted as indicating a movement of CD8$^+$ cells from the blood to the CSF by some investigators, Durelli (16) failed to identify a significant increase in the absolute count of CD8$^+$ cells in the CSF with treatment, suggesting this interpretation may be simplistic.

The effect of IFN-α on nonspecific suppressor cell function was also studied in both relapsing and CP MS patients. Previously, in vitro studies had shown that IFN-α could induce nonspecific suppressor cell function in MNCs from controls (52–56). Similarly, IFN-α added to MNCs obtained from CP MS patients augmented suppressor function in vitro (57). Hirsch and Johnson reported no improvement in nonspecific suppressor cell function in MS patients receiving recombinant IFN-α_2 although suppressor cell function did decrease during relapses in both IFN and placebo-treated patients (51). Patients in this study received a low dose of IFN and did not show any difference in frequency or severity of relapses (15). A similar lack of effect of lymphoblastoid IFN on nonspecific suppressor function in CP MS was reported by O'Gorman et al. (41); however, suppressor function was not studied beyond the first week of treatment. It is not clear if an effect might have been observed if these studies had continued.

The effect of IFN-α on natural killer (NK) cells was also studied in both relapsing and CP MS patients. Hirsch and Johnson observed in RR MS patients that an 18-hr in vitro culture of PBMCs with 100 U/ml of recombinant IFN-α_2 significantly increased NK cell function where previously it had been abnormally low (58). In relapsing MS patients, natural IFN-α resulted in a significant increase in NK cell functional activity at 48 hr and during the first 7 days after the initiation of therapy in 9 of 12 patients studied (59). Over the subsequent 6 months, NK activity remained at baseline despite continued therapy. Similar results were obtained by Kastrukoff et al. (60) in CP MS patients treated with lymphoblastoid IFN. A similar initial rise in NK cell function was reported by Hirsch and Johnson (61) in patients receiving recombinant IFN-α_2 (15). Unlike the previous two studies, however, NK cell activity decreased significantly at weeks 16, 26, and 34 but increased to prestudy levels when IFN was discontinued. Of interest was an initial increase in NK cell activity in both the placebo and treatment groups reported by both Hirsch and Johnson (61) and Kastrukoff et al. (60). Although the increase was more pronounced in the treatment than the placebo group, the mechanisms mediating this increase have yet to be defined. NK cells were also assessed by phenotypes. In CP MS patients treated with lymphoblastoid IFN, Kastrukoff et al. (60) reported an initial increase in CD16$^+$ cells in the blood, followed by a significant drop at 1 and 3 months. A similar reduction in CD16$^+$ cells at 3 months was reported by Kinnunen et al. (21) in CP MS patients treated with recombinant IFN-α_{2b} CP MS patients treated with lymphoblastoid IFN also developed a significant reduction in CD57$^+$ peripheral blood cells at 3 months (60), but this was not observed by Hirsch and Johnson in relapsing patients treated with recombinant IFN-α_2 (51). In the latter group of patients, the dose of IFN was low and no clinical benefit was observed with treatment. Recent studies in RR MS patients also identified a significant reduction in CD57$^+$ cells throughout the treatment phase with IFN-β-1b, 8 MU s.c. every other day (62).

The effect of IFN-α on IFN synthesis was studied in several trials. In vitro IFN synthesis in relapsing MS patients was normal prior to treatment with natural IFN-α (11). Following treatment, both IFN synthesis and the enhancing effect of IFN on its own synthesis were reduced (63). Durelli et al. (16) studied the effect of high-dose recombinant IFN-α_{2a} on IFN-γ production in RR MS patients. IFN treatment significantly reduced the level of IFN-γ production by lymphocyte cultures.

VII.   SUMMARY OF IFN-α TREATMENT ON THE IMMUNE SYSTEM IN MS PATIENTS

In summary, a limited number of immune evaluations were performed in relation to clinical trials of IFN-α in MS. In many cases, similar effects of IFN-α treatment on the immune system were identified despite differences in the nature of the IFN used, the dosage given, and the course of MS treated. Generally, treatment with IFN resulted in an increase in IgG synthesis both in serum and CSF. Although not entirely clear, it appears that this increase may be related to clinical improvement in some cases. Neutralizing antibodies to IFN along with other types of antibodies such as antithyroid antibodies have not been observed, but the length of treatment with IFN in these studies may have been too brief. This may become a problem as more patients are treated for longer periods of time. Treatment with IFN-α appears to be related to an increase in the CD4/CD8 ratio in the blood and possibly a decrease of the ratio in the CSF. The reason for this is not clear but cannot be explained entirely by the movement of CD8 cells from the blood to the CSF. An effect on nonspecific suppressor cell function was not observed following treatment with IFN-α, but this cannot be entirely excluded as the dosage of IFN was low in one study and only a limited number of observations were available in a second study. Treatment with IFN-α does appear to give rise to an increase in NK cell functional activity between 48 hr and 7 days after treatment is initiated but is not sustained despite continued treatment. Although all these observations must be considered preliminary, they do provide a direction on which to build in future studies.

VIII. CONCLUSION

The purpose of this chapter was to review previous studies with IFN-α in MS and to identify important lessons which might have relevance to future clinical trials. These studies have taught us many lessons both clinically and immunologically and hopefully the review will be of value. Better designed clinical trials in MS in future and the identification of the mechanisms of action of IFN in MS will be the measure of success.

REFERENCES

1. IFNB Multiple Sclerosis Study Group. Interferon beta-1b is effective in relapsing-remitting multiple sclerosis I. Clinical results of a multicenter, randomized, double-blind, placebo-controlled trial. Neurology 1993; 43: 655–661.
2. Paty DW, Li DKB, UBC MS/MRI Study Group, et al. Interferon beta-1b is effective in relapsing-remitting multiple sclerosis. II. MRI analysis results of a multicenter, randomized, double-blind, placebo-controlled trial. Neurology 1993; 43:662–667.
3. Jacobs L. O'Malley J, Freeman A, Ekes R. Intrathecal interferon reduces exacerbations of multiple sclerosis. Science 1981; 214:1026–1028.
4. Jacobs L, Salazar AM, Herndon R, et al. Intrathecally administered natural human fibroblast interferon reduces exacerbations of multiple sclerosis: results of a multicenter, double-blinded study. Arch Neurol 1987; 44:589–595.
5. Isaacs A, Lindenmann J. Virus interference: I. The interferon. Proc R Soc Lond (Biol) 1957; 147:258–267.
6. Lengyel P. Biochemistry of interferons and their actions. Annu Rev Biochem 1982; 51:251–282.
7. Pestka S, Langer JA, Zoon KC, Samuel CE. Interferons and their actions. Annu Rev Biochem 1987; 56:727–777.
8. Baron S, Tyring SK, Fleischmann WR Jr., et al. The interferons: mechanisms of action and clinical applications. JAMA 1991; 266:1375–1383.
9. Cross JC, Roberts RM. Constitutive and trophoblast specific expression of a class of bovine interferon genes. Proc Natl Acad Sci USA 1991; 88: 3817–3821.
10. Stewart HJ, McCann SH, Barker PJ, et al. Interferon sequence homology and receptor binding activity of ovine trophoblast antiluteolytic protein. J Endocrinol 1987; 115:R13–R15.
11. Knobler RL, Panitch HS, Braheny SL et al. Systemic alpha-interferon therapy of multiple sclerosis. Neurology 1984; 34:1273–1279.
12. Cantell K, Hirvonen S. Large-scale production of human leukocyte interferon containing 10^8 units per ml. J Gen Virol 1978; 39:541–543.
13. Panitch HS. Systemic α-interferon in multiple sclerosis. Arch Neurol 1987; 44:61–63.

14. AUSTIMS Research Group. Interferon-α and transfer factor in the treatment of multiple sclerosis: a double-blind, placebo-controlled trial. J Neurol Neurosurg Psychiatry 1989; 52:566–574.

15. Camenga DL, Johnson KP, Alter M, et al. Systemic recombinant α-2 interferon therapy in relapsing multiple sclerosis. Arch Neurol 1986; 43: 1239–1246.

16. Durelli L, Bongioanni MR, Cavallo R et al. Chronic systemic high-dose recombinant interferon α-2a reduces exacerbation rate, MRI signs of disease activity, and lymphocyte interferon gamma production in relapsing-remitting multiple sclerosis. Neurology 1994; 44:406–413.

17. Fog T. Interferon treatment of multiple sclerosis patients. A pilot study. In: Boese A, ed. Search for the Cause of MS and Other Chronic Diseases of the CNS. Weinheimger GER Verlag Chemie, 1980:490–493.

18. Ruutiainen J, Panelius M, Cantell K. Toxic effects of interferon administered intrathecally. Br Med J 1983; 286:940–945.

19. Kastrukoff LF, Oger JJ, Hashimoto SA, et al. Systemic lymphoblastoid interferon therapy in chronic progressive multiple sclerosis. I. Clinical and MRI evaluation. Neurology 1990; 40:479–486.

20. Dayal AS, Jensen MA, Lledo A, Arnason BEW. Interferon-gamma-secreting cells in multiple sclerosis patients treated with interferon beta-1b. Neurology 1995; 45:2173–2177.

21. Kinnunen E, Timonen T, Pirttila T, et al. Effects of recombinant α-2b interferon therapy in patients with progressive MS. Acta Neurol Scand 1993; 87: 457–460.

22. Bever CT, Salazar AM, Neely E et al. Preliminary trial of poly ICLC in chronic progressive multiple sclerosis. Neurology 1986; 36:494–498.

23. Arnason BGW, Reder AT. Interferons and multiple sclerosis. Clin Neuropharmacol 1994; 6:495–547.

24. Basham TY, Merigan TC. Recombinant interferon-γ increases HLA-DR synthesis and expression. J Immunol 1983; 130:1492–1494.

25. Arenzana-Seisdedos F, Lirelizier JL, Fiers W. Interferons as macrophage-activating factors III. Preferential effects of interferon on the interleukin 1 secretory potential of fresh or aged human monocytes. J Immunol 1985; 134: 2444–2448.

26. Gerrard TL, Siegel JP, Dyer DR, Zoon KC. Differential effects of interferon-α and interferon-γ on interleukin 1 secretion by monocytes. J Immunol 1986; 138:2535–2540.

27. Tilg H, Mier JW, Vogel W, et al. Induction of circulating IL-1 receptor antagonist by IFN treatment. J Immunol 1993; 150:4687–4692.

28. Arend WP, Joslin FG, Massoni RJ. Effects of immune complexes on production by human monocytes of interleukin 1 or an interleukin-1 inhibitor. J Immunol 1985; 134:3868–3870.

29. Noronha A, Toscas A, Jensen MA. Interferon β decreases T cell activation and interferon gamma production in multiple sclerosis. J Neuroimmunol 1993; 46:145–154.

30. Brinkman V, Geiger T, Alkan S, Heusser CH. Interferon α increases the frequency of interferon γ producing human CD4$^+$ T cells. J Exp Med 1993; 178:1655–1663.

31. Klimpel GR, Fleischman WR Jr, Klimpel KDA. Gamma interferon and IFN α/β suppress murine myeloid colony formation (CFV-C): magnitude of suppression is dependent upon level of colony stimulating factor (CSF). J Immunol 1982; 129:76–80.

32. Abu-khabar KS, Armstron JA, Ho M. Type I interferons (IFN α and β) suppress cytotoxin (tumor necrosis factor-α and lymphotoxin) production by mitogen-stimulated human peripheral blood mononuclear cells. J Leukocyte Biol 1992; 52:165–172.

33. Maggi E, Del Prete G, Macchia D et al. Profiles of lymphokine activities and helper function for IgE in human T cell clones. Eur J Immunol 1988; 18: 1045–1050.

34. Romagnani S, Del Prete G, Maggi E, et al. Role of interleukins in induction and regulation of human IgE synthesis. Clin Immunol Immunopathol 1989; 50:S13–23.

35. Panitch HS, Francis GS, Hooper CJ, et al. Serial immunological studies in multiple sclerosis patients treated systemically with human alpha interferon. Ann Neurol 1985; 18:434–438.

36. Rice GPA, Woelfel EL, Talbot PJ et al. Immunological complications in multiple sclerosis patients receiving interferon. Ann Neurol 1985; 18: 439–442.

37. Kastrukoff LF, Oger JJ-F, Tourtellotte WW, Sacks SL, Berkowitz J, Paty DW. Systemic lymphoblastoid interferon therapy in chronic progressive multiple sclerosis. II. Immunologic evaluation. Neurology 1991; 41:1936–1941.

38. Goust JM, Hogan EL, Arnaud P. Abnormal regulation of IgG production in multiple sclerosis. Neurology 1982; 32:228–232.

39. Oger J, Antel JP, Kuo HH, Arnason BGW. Influence of azathioprine (Imuran) on immune function in multiple sclerosis. Ann Neurol 1982; 11: 177–183.

40. Tjernlund U, Cesaro P, Tournier E, et al. T-cell subsets in multiple sclerosis: a comparative study between cell surface antigens and function. Clin Immunol Immunopathol 1984; 32:185–189.

41. O'Gorman MRG, Oger J, Kastrukoff LF. Reduction of immunoglobulin G secretion in vitro following long term lymphoblastoid interferon (Wellferon) treatment in multiple sclerosis patients. Clin Exp Immunol 1987; 67:66–75.

42. Choi YS, Lim KH, Sanders FK. Effect of interferon α on pokeweed mitogen-induced differentiation of human peripheral blood B lymphocytes. Cell Immunol 1981; 64:20–25.

43. Parker MS, Mandel AD, Wallace JH, Sonnenfeld G. Modulation of the human in vitro antibody response by human leukocyte interferon preparations. Cell Immunol 1981; 58:464–470.

44. Levinson AI, Dziarksi A, Hooks JJ. Modulation of polyclonal B cell differentiation by human leukocyte alpha interferon. Clin Exp Immunol 1982; 49: 677–684.

45. Ross C, Mansen MB, Schyberg T, Berg K. Autoantibodies to crude human leucocyte interferon (IFN), native human IFN, recombinant human IFN-alpha 2b and human IFN-gamma in healthy blood donors. Clin Exp Immunol 1990; 82:57–62.

46. Öberg K, Alm G, Magnusson A, et al. Treatment of malignant carcinoid tumors with recombinant interferon alpha-2b: development of neutralizing interferon antibodies and possible loss of anti-tumor activity. J Natl Cancer Inst 1989; 81:531–535.

47. Figlin RA, deKernion JB, Mukamel E, et al. Recombinant interferon alpha-2a in metastatic renal cell carcinoma: assessment of antitumor activity and anti-interferon antibody formation. J Clin Oncol 1988; 6:1604–1610.

48. Burman P, Totterman TH, Oberg K, Karlsson FA. Thyroid autoimmunity in patients on long term therapy with leukocyte-derived interferon. J Clin Endocrinol Metab 1986; 110:1086–1090.

49. Fentiman IS, Balkwill FR, Thomas BS, et al. An autoimmune aetiology for hypothyroidism following interferon therapy for breast cancer. Eur J Cancer Clin Oncol 1988; 21:1299–1303.

50. Gisslinger H, Gilly B, Woloszczuk W, et al. Thyroid autoimmunity and hypo-thyroidism during long-term treatment with recombinant interferon-alpha. Clin Exp Immunol 1992; 90:363–367.

51. Hirsch RL, Johnson KP. The effects of long-term administration of recombi-nant alpha-2 interferon on lymphocyte subsets, proliferation, and suppressor cell function in multiple sclerosis. J Interferon Res 1986; 6:171–177.

52. Schnaper HW, Aune TM Pierce CW. Suppressor T cell activation by human leukocyte interferon. J Immunol 1983; 131:2301–2306.

53. Aune TM, Pierce DW. Activation of a suppressor T-cell pathway by inter-feron. Proc Natl Acad Sci USA 1982; 79:3808–3812.

54. Johnson HM, Blalock JE. Interferon immunosuppression: mediation by a suppressor factor. Infect Immun 1980; 29:301–305.

55. Aune TM. Two different pathways of interferon mediated suppression of antibody secretion. Int J Immunopharmacol 1985; 7:65–71.

56. Onsrud M. Enhancement of suppressor cell generation in human mixed lym-phocyte cultures by interferon. Int Arch Allergy Appl Immunol 1982; 67: 315–321.

57. Noronha A, Toscas A, Jensen MA. Contrasting effects of alpha, beta, and gamma interferons on nonspecific suppressor cell functions in multiple scle-rosis. Ann Neurol 1992; 31:103–106.

58. Hirsch RL, Johnson KP. The effect of recombinant alpha$_2$-interferon on de-fective natural killer cell activity in multiple sclerosis. Neurology 1985; 35: 597–600.

59. Rice GPA, Casali P, Merigan TC, Oldstone MBA. Natural killer cell activity in patients with multiple sclerosis given α interferon. Ann Neurol 1983; 14: 333–338.

60. Kastrukoff LF, Morgan NG, Aziz TM, et al. Natural killer (NK) cells in chronic progressive multiple sclerosis patients treated with lymphoblastoid interferon. J Neuroimmunol 1988; 20:15–23.

61. Hirsch RL, Johnson KP. Natural killer cell activity in multiple sclerosis patients treated with recombinant interferon-α_2. Clin Immunol Immunopathol 1985; 37:236–244.

62. Kastrukoff LF, Morgan N, Zecchini D, et al. Multiple sclerosis lesions develop on serial MRIs during a reduction in natural killer (NK) cell functional activity. Neurology 1995; 45(suppl 4):A233.

63. Kamin-Lewis R, Panitch HS, Merigan TC, Johnson KP. Decreased interferon synthesis and responsiveness to interferon by leukocytes from multiple sclerosis patients given natural alpha interferon. J Interferon Res 1984; 4: 423–428.

12

Recombinant Interferon-α in the Treatment of Multiple Sclerosis
Effects on Exacerbation Rate, Magnetic Resonance Imaging of Lesion Activity, and Cytokines

Luca Durelli

University of Turin Medical School, Turin, Italy

I. INTERFERONS ARE CYTOKINES

Interferons (IFNs) were the first cytokines purified and cloned (1). They interact with multisubunit receptors on the cell surface. Cytokines are proteins which carry directives from cell to cell, bind to a specific receptor, and activate a direct signal transduction pathway. The signal transduction pathways activated by IFNs directly activate a recently identified class of enzymes, known as Janus kinases (JAKs) (like the Roman god Janus, they have two faces; i.e., two active sites). Activated JAKs, apparently attached to the intracellular domain of the cytokine receptor, phosphorylate intracellular proteins called signal transducers and activators of transcription (STAT). Phosphorylated STATs form a protein complex that moves to the nucleus and directly binds to the IFN-stimulated response element, a DNA element common to the promoters that control transcription of IFN-inducible genes. Although other cytokines bind different cell receptors, IFNs share JAK or STAT proteins with some cytokines (2). This may explain why IFNs modulate, as well as share, biological effects with other cytokines.

IFNs are divided into two main types based on differences in their structure and other properties. Type I IFNs are IFN-α, IFN-β, IFN-τ, and IFN-ω. The only known type II IFN is IFN-γ. Both IFN types can interfere with viral replication in cells and can modulate immune system functions. Nevertheless, type I IFNs are more effective at bolstering the ability of cells to resist viral infections, and type II IFN is more important to the proper functioning of the immune system.

II. EFFECTS OF IFNs ON IMMUNE FUNCTION

IFNs promote the activity of many components of the immune system, an effect useful for eradicating tumors or infections in cells. They enhance major hystocompatibility complex (MHC) molecule expression and facilitate antigen presentation to lymphocytes. Both types of IFNs induce transcription of MHC class I genes and expression of their products on the cell surface (3). MHC class I molecules present epitopes to $CD8^+$ T cytotoxic lymphocytes, and the cytotoxic response is increased both in vitro and in vivo by all IFN types (4). In contrast, MHC class II gene transcription and expression is mainly induced by IFN-γ (5). MHC class II molecules are involved in antigen presentation to $CD4^+$ T helper lymphocytes, and they are usually expressed at high density on antigen-presenting cells; that is, macrophages and monocytes (6). IFN-γ increases MHC class II molecule expression on antigen-presenting cells (7,8) and also on many other cell types that usually do not express MHC class II molecules; for example, astrocytes and cerebrovascular endothelial cells (9,10).

In plaques of multiple sclerosis (MS), there is abnormal MHC class II molecule expression on astrocytes or endothelial cells (11). Similarly, in autommune diseases, such as thyroiditis or rheumatoid arthritis, target cells (e.g., thyroid or synovial cells) abnormally express MHC class II molecules (12), indicating there is local activation of the immune response and production of IFNs. Both type I and type II IFNs are present in MS demyelinated plaques (13), and IFN-γ mRNA levels are increased in MS lymphocytes of peripheral blood (PB), cerebrospinal fluid (CSF), and brain (14–16). During systemic IFN-γ administration, increased MHC class II molecule expression on PB macrophages is associated with a striking worsening of MS and increased exacerbation rate (8). Similarly, enhancement of the immune response may lead to the appearance or to the worsening of autoimmune diseases. Thyroiditis or rheumatoid arthritis is sometimes reported during type I IFN administration to cancer or hepatitis patients (17,18).

Both IFN-α and IFN-β counteract IFN-γ–induced abnormal MHC class II molecule expression. This effect includes cells where MHC class II molecules are overrepresented in MS, such as astrocytes (19). We have found that chronic IFN-α treatment does not reduce baseline MHC class II molecule expression on monocytes from MS patients (20). Thus, type

I IFNs do not directly inhibit MHC class II molecule synthesis but mainly counteract an IFN-γ–mediated effect. The preferential use of certain intracellular signal transducers (JAK or STAT proteins) by type I rather than type II IFNs (1,2) may well reduce gene transcription sustained by IFN-γ and counteract its effects (see Chapters 1 and 2).

T lymphocytes are another important target of IFN immunomodulatory effects. CD4$^+$ T helper lymphocytes include two different subsets (21) activated by different antigenic stimuli and producing different cytokines. T helper type 1 (Th1) are activated by viral and bacterial antigens. These antigens induce macrophages to secrete interleukin-12 (IL-12) and natural killer (NK) cells to secrete IFN-γ. These two cytokines promote maturation of totipotent progenitor Th0 cells toward Th1 lymphocytes. Th1 cells produce IL-2, IFN-γ, and tumor necrosis factor (TNF), cytokines that sustain Th1 activation. The Th1 lymphocyte activation process is IFN-γ-dependent and can be inhibited by anti–IFN-γ monoclonal antibodies (4). In contrast, the Th2 subset is activated by parasite antigens or allergens, which provoke IL-4 secretion. IL-4 induces the maturation of Th0 toward Th2 lymphocytes, which secrete IL-4, IL-5, IL-6, IL-10, IL-13. The Th1 subset regulates delayed-type hypersensitivity (DTH) reactions and helps IgG2a and suppress IgG1 and IgE antibody production (22). The Th2 subset is involved in allergic and immediate hypersensitivity responses and in IgG1, IgG4, IgA, and IgE antibody production (22).

The two T-lymphocyte subsets are reciprocally inhibitory. IFN-γ/IL-12 directs the development of Th0 lymphocytes toward a Th1 subtype, and IL-4 directs Th0 to a Th2 subtype (23,24). The Th1-derived cytokine IFN-γ inhibits Th2 cell proliferation, whereas the Th2-derived cytokine IL-10 suppresses Th1 cell cytokine production (25–27). The inhibition of Th1 cells by IL-10 occurs via antigen-presenting cells. IL-10 downregulates expression of costimulatory molecules required for the activation of Th1 lymphocytes by macrophages (26). In addition, IL-10 inhibits the production of TNF-α, reactive oxygen intermediates, and nitrogen oxide by macrophages (28,29); thus exerting immunomodulatory effects at two distinct levels of macrophage function. We have found that IFN-α administration in vivo to MS patients inhibits secretion of Th1 cytokines, but this finding was not correlated with changes of IL-10 lymphocyte production (see below).

Th1 lymphocytes specific for myelin basic protein or proteolipid protein induce experimental autoimmune encephalomyelitis (EAE) (30), and Th1 cytokines are probably involved in MS pathogenesis (18–21). IFN-γ induces abnormal MHC class II molecule expression on many cell types, including astrocytes (8–10), cerebrovascular endothelial cells (31), and microglia; secretion of reactive oxygen intermediates and nitrogen oxide from macrophages; and secretion of TNF-α from Th1 lymphocytes (21). Activated macrophage products and TNF-α cause central nervous system tissue damage (32–33). IFN-γ and TNF-α are present in MS demyelinated lesions (13), and lymphocyte IFN-γ and TNF-α mRNA production is increased in active MS (14–16). In contrast, Th2 cytokines may exert a protective effect against inflammation and demyelination. Analysis of several instances of cytokine mRNA expression revealed that only levels of the Th2 cytokine IL-10 correlated with remission of disease activity in EAE (34). Moreover, a Th2 clone which recognizes encephalitogenic proteolipid protein peptides, but does not induce EAE, inhibits the proliferation of an encephalitogenic Th1 clone, probably through an IL-10–mediated effect (35).

The local balance between encephalitogenic and suppressor T-cell clones may be crucial for lesion pathogenesis in demyelinating diseases. IFN effects on Th clone maturation and cytokine secretion probably play a key role in this process. IFN-α/β and IFN-γ exert different biological activities on immune cells (4). Concanavalin A (ConA)–induced or IL-2–induced proliferation of T lymphocytes is dramatically inhibited by IFN-α/β regardless of their phenotype. IFN-γ inhibits IL-2–induced proliferation of Th2 clones only and enhances ConA-induced proliferation of total T cells (36). This differential control of type I and II IFNs on T-cell growth is also reflected at the molecular level. IFN-α/β activates gene transcription for the enzyme 2′,5′-oligoadenylate synthetase in T and B cells, macrophages, and fibroblasts. In contrast, IFN-γ activates this antiviral gene in B cells, macrophages, and fibroblasts but not in T cells stimulated with IL-2. IFN-γ appears to provide signals for functional differentiation of immature T lymphocytes, whereas IFN-α/β regulates the activity of already differentiated T cells.

IFN-γ and IFN-α/β also affect differentiation and function of cytotoxic T lymphocytes (CTLs). Monoclonal antibodies against IFN-γ inhibit the IL-2–dependent growth and maturation of CTL clones (37). Both IL-2 and IFN-γ appear to be required for the majority of precursor CTLs to develop into fully mature CTL clones. IFN-γ enhances the synthesis of IL-2 and of IL-2 cell surface receptors, eventually leading to the functional differentiation of CTL precursors. Human recombinant IFN-α (rIFN-α) induces precursors to differentiate into mature CTL clones and causes rearrangements of the T-cell receptor genes (38). IFN-α/β enhances T-cell cytotoxicity against virus-infected or allogeneic target cells (4), acting at later stages of T-cell differentiation, and increases the production of serine esterase, a putative cytotoxicity-linked protein, with a parallel increase of cytotoxic activity (39).

IFN-α or IFN-β significantly increase nonspecific T suppressor cell function (ConA-induced) of healthy control subjects as well as of MS patients (40). The effect is particularly pronounced in MS patients with active disease. In these patients, whose T suppressor cell function is reduced from normal (41), in vitro treatment with IFN-α or IFN-β brings about a threefold increase of T suppressor cell function, which becomes equivalent to that of controls. In contrast, IFN-γ has no effect on T suppressor cell function of control subjects or on the deficient T suppressor cell function of active MS patients, and it reduces the normal T suppressor cell function of stable MS patients. The reduction of the T lymphocyte suppressor function correlates with disease activity in MS (42), so the correction of this defect by means of IFN-α or IFN-β may well be therapeutic.

All types of IFNs increase natural killer (NK) cell number and function, an important mechanism in host defenses against bacteria, viruses, and tumor growth (43,44). IFNs promote the generation of NK cells from a pre-NK pool and enhance cell killing by inducing the release of potent cytolysins, including TNF and perforins (44). IFN-γ induces TNF-α secretion from NK cells and increases the susceptibility of bacteria-infected fibroblasts to TNF-α–mediated cytolysis by enhancing the expression of cell surface TNF-α receptors (45). In contrast, IFN-α/β are virtually ineffective in potentiating TNF action in several cell lines. NK cell function is reduced in MS patients, and this reduction correlates with disease activity (46–48). The defective NK activity was increased after IFN treatment in a recent trial of natural IFN-α (49), but this immunological effect was not correlated with a significant clinical effect (50) (see Chapter 11). The modulation of NK cell function by type I IFNs in MS patients is probably a secondary immunological effect not directly related to an effect on MS disease activity. Alternatively, the use of higher IFN doses or of recombinant products may be needed to achieve both immunological and clinical effects.

IFN-γ exerts both stimulatory and inhibitory effects on B-cell maturation to Ig secretion. It promotes maturation of Th1 lymphocytes (21), which in turn provide help to B cells for IgG and IgM production. IFN-γ also directly stimulates human B-cell maturation (51). IFN-γ enhances Ig production only in the presence of IL-2. IL-2 acts as a B-cell growth factor, whereas IFN-γ is required for subsequent differentiation.

IFN-γ acts at the earliest IL-2–dependent stages of the B-cell differentiation process, but IFN-α/β regulates the functions of more differentiated B cells. In addition, IFN-γ promotes Ig class switching from IgM to IgG2 and IgG3 and inhibits IgG1 and IgE production induced by IL-4 (52–55) (also see Chapter 7). The effect of IFN-α/β on Ig class switching is partial: in mice, IFN-α/β fails to stimulate IgG2 (56) and inhibits IgG1 and IgE production (57). Long-term IFN-α treatment increases IgG production in serum as well as in the cerebrospinal fluid (CSF) of MS patients (58–60). In contrast, pokeweed mitogen–stimulated IgG production, which is usually higher than normal in MS patients, was inhibited in MS patients treated with natural IFN-α (61). However, no relationship between these laboratory findings and clinical outcome was found.

Table 1 IFN Effects on Immune Functions

	Immunoactivating effects	Immunoinhibiting effects
Type I IFNs (IFN-α and IFN-β)	Increase of MHC class I molecule expression Slight to moderate increase of MHC class II molecule expression on antigen-presenting cells only Increase of activity of differentiated T cytotoxic cells Increase of IgG production	Inhibition of the abnormal IFN-γ–induced MHC class II expression on many cell types (astrocytes included) Inhibition of mitogen-induced T-lymphocyte proliferation Increase of T suppressor cell function (particularly if reduced, as in active MS) Inhibition of mitogen-induced IgG and of IL-4–induced IgG1 and IgE production Reduction of IFN-γ production by T cells
Type II IFN (IFN-γ)	Increase of MHC class I molecule expression Increase of MHC class II molecule expression on APC and other cell types Induction of Th1 lymphocyte differentiation (potentially encephalitogenic lymphocytes) Activation of T cytotoxic and NK lymphocyte maturation and function Activation of B-cell maturation, Ig production, and Ig class switching Enhancement of macrophage function (with release of potentially CNS-damaging products) Enhancement of TNF-α (a potentially demyelinating cytokine) Inhibition of T suppressor lymphocyte maturation and function Inhibition of maturation and function of Th2 lymphocytes (which may counteract encephalitogenic Th1 lymphocyte activity)	

In summary, type I and type II IFNs exert complex effects at different levels of the immune response (Table 1). The effects of the two types of IFNs are different, inasmuch as they bind to different cell surface receptors (1) and activate different sets of genes (62). Nevertheless, the two types of IFNs share some intracellular signal transducers (1,2) and sometimes have common immunological effects. IFN-γ is the main immunoactivating IFN. IFN-γ (1) induces MHC class I and class II molecule expression on cell types that normally express those antigens (3,5,7) as well as on other cell types (such as astrocytes) (9); (2) promotes T helper lymphocyte differentiation toward the Th1 subtype (4,21), which aggravates experimental demyelinating encephalitis (30); (3) enhances TNF-α production and cell susceptibility to TNF-α (21,45,63), a cytokine which is able to damage oligodendrocytes (33); (4) activates CTLs and NK- and B-cell maturation and function (37,43,44,51); (5) inhibits Th2 and Ts maturation and function (27,40); and (6) enhances macrophage function (63).

In contrast, IFN-α and IFN-β often exert lesser immunoactivating effects. IFN-α and IFN-β (1) enhance MHC class I molecule expression on many cell types (3), but have minimal effects on MHC class II molecule expression (5); (2) antagonize IFN-γ–induced MHC class II expression (19); (3) regulate activity of differentiated lymphocytes by increasing suppressor, CTLs, NK cell, and, partially, B-cell function (4,38,39,44,51); and (4) inhibit mitogen-driven T- and B-cell activation (4,36,51). In addition, (5) IFN-α and IFN-β reduce T-lymphocyte IFN-γ production (40,64). Therefore, although IFN-α and IFN-β exert some immunostimulatory effects, they also modulate and inhibit the immune response.

III. DIFFERENTIAL QUALITATIVE AND QUANTITATIVE EFFECTS EXERTED BY IFN-α AND IFN-β

IFN-α and IFN-β share the same cellular receptor complex (1) (see Chapter 1) and have many similar actions. They sometimes exert differential effects for two main reasons—binding the receptor complex with different affinity or binding to separate receptor proteins (65). Type I IFN binding affinity varies according to the cell system tested. In certain mouse cell lines transfected with a human IFN-α/β receptor gene, the sensitivity to one subtype of human IFN-α is a 1000-fold higher than that to human IFN-β (66); on the contrary, cells that respond to IFN-β and not to IFN-α have been identified (67). Furthermore, antibodies capable of neutralizing a particular IFN-α subtype (more than 20 IFN-α subtypes are known) do not always neutralize the other IFN-α subtypes or IFN-β, implying that different type I IFNs may interact with discrete moieties of the same receptor complex (68).

Another difference between IFN-α and IFN-β arises from their bio-availability (also see Chapter 3). IFN-β diffuses poorly from the site of production or injection (68), so that even when injected by the intramuscular route, blood levels are difficult to detect (69). This property probably allows IFN-β to attain the high concentrations required to establish a strong antiviral state in the tissue surrounding infected cells (68). In contrast, IFN-α is highly diffusible. It has complete bioavailability following parenteral injection (70) and easily reaches distant organs. (Pharmacokinetic differences between IFN β-1a and IFN β-1b are still undefined.) In principle, IFN-β should be most effective when used for topical and intralesional administration owing to its localized action; IFN-α, which diffuses better, is more suitable for systemic effects after subcutaneous or intramuscular injection. For this reason, in the first patients in whom IFN-β was proposed as alternative treatment to IFN-α (71–73), IFN-β was administered intravenously. However, many pharmacokinetic and clinical studies have shown that after intramuscular or subcutaneous injection, IFN-β exerts many biological and clinical effects in spite of undetectable blood levels (69,73,74). After intramuscular or subcutaneous IFN-β, the serum contains the products of IFN-inducible genes, such as β_2-microgobulin, 2′, 5′ oligoadenylate synthetase, neopterin (a macrophage-associated protein), and myxovirus (MX) proteins (derived from the Mx gene, which confers resistance to myxoviruses [influenza], and that have been compared to the stress proteins, including heat shock proteins) (75). The recent trial with recombinant IFN β-1b in MS patients (76,77) shows that biological effects of subcutaneous injection can be directly demonstrated in a distant organ. Clinical and magnetic resonance imaging (MRI) signs of disease activity were reduced by therapy.

IV. THERAPEUTIC USE OF IFN-α

Recombinant IFN-α became available worldwide during early 1980s, and clinical trials clearly established its efficacy in many viral and malignant diseases (1). In 1986, rIFN-α became the first IFN to gain U.S. Food and Drug Administration (FDA) approval as therapy for hairy cell leukemia. IFN-α is still considered the treatment of choice for this rare malignancy. Taken in low doses (1–3 million international units) (MIU), IFN-α causes significant regression of the cancer in about 90% of patients, who must then take it indefinitely in order to avoid relapses (1,78). Some patients develop resistance to the antitumor effect of IFN-α, which is attributable to specific neutralizing anti–IFN-α antibodies (79). The administration of other recombinant IFN-α subtypes (79) or of IFN-β (72,73) has been suggested as alternative treatment, and an IFN-β–induced remission in a patient resistant to IFN-α has been reported (80). The results obtained with high-dose IFN-β (6 MIU/m²), even given intravenously to overcome its poor bioavailability, however, are somewhat inferior to those achieved with IFN-α.

IFN-α treatment of patients with chronic myelogenous leukemia is also very promising. High-dose IFN-α (9 MIU) is more effective than conventional chemotherapy, delaying disease progression and prolonging survival (81). IFN-α therapy is able to induce karyotypic negativity in previously Philadelphia chromosome–positive patients, whereas IFN-β has no activity in chronic myelogenous leukemia (82).

Patients with hepatitis also have benefitted from IFN-α. Before IFN-α was licensed in 1991, there was no reliable treatment of chronic hepatitis C (non-α, non-β hepatitis). Now a 6-month course low-dose IFN-α (3 MIU) can eliminate symptoms (83), and prolonged treatment at higher doses (9 MIU) prevents relapses (84). In 1992, IFN-α also became the first approved treatment for chronic hepatitis B.[HB] After a 6-month course of high-dose IFN-α (9 MIU), more than 70% of patients lose serum hepatitis B antigen or virus DNA and seroconvert to anti-HB antibodies (85,86). The serum changes are often stable for prolonged periods. It is of interest that seroconversion and loss of serum virus DNA or antigen is often heralded by a transient exacerbation of the underlying hepatitis (85). The previously described partial proinflammatory actions of IFN-α may explain the transitory exacerbation. Chronic intravenous IFN-β causes seroconversion to anti-HB antibodies, but it is unable to induce the serum clearance of the antigen or virus DNA (72).

V. SIDE EFFECTS ASSOCIATED WITH IFN-α OR IFN-β TREATMENT

Four major types of side effects have been described during IFN-α administration: flu-like, cardiocirculatory, neurological, and hematological (Table 2) (also see Chapters 6 and 16).

A. Flu-Like Syndrome

The flu-like syndrome is dominated by fever, myalgias, headache, and arthralgias (18). A few hours will pass between IFN-α administration and the onset of the febrile reaction, suggesting that IFN may not be pyrogenic itself but rather acts through induction of mediators such as IL-1 or prostaglandin. The flu-like syndrome usually decreases and disappears within

Table 2 Type I IFN Side Effects

Side effect	Rate (%)	Treatment	Adaptation	IFN-α	IFN-β
Flu-like syndrome (fever, myalgias, headache)	60–100	Acetaminophen	Good	+ +	+
Local skin reaction	50–90	Rotating injection site	Poor	–	+ + +
Fatigue	40–60	Amantadine, IFN dose reduction	Poor	+ + +	+ +
Leukopenia or thrombocytopenia	30–50	Usually transitory effect, IFN dose reduction	Good	+	+
Hepatic enzyme elevation	30–50	IFN dose reduction	Good	+	+
Anorexia	30–40	IFN dose reduction	Poor	+ +	+
Depression	10–20	Antidepressants, IFN dose reduction	Poor	+ +	+ +
Mild alopecia, generalized skin rashes	10–20	IFN dose reduction	Good	+	+
Hypotension, tachyrhythmias	1–2	IFN dose reduction	Poor	+	+
Confusion	1–2	IFN dose reduction	Poor	+ +	+
Cognitive disturbances	1–2	IFN dose reduction	Poor	+ +	–
Autoimmune(?) hypothyroidism	1–2	Stopping treatment	Poor	+ +	–
Other autoimmune diseases	Rare	Stopping treatment	Poor	+	+

days provided that IFN-α injections are given at intervals which enhance downregulation of cell surface receptors (<72 hrs), thus promoting tachyphylaxis (87).

With chronic IFN-α administration at high doses, the acute febrile reaction is replaced by persistent fatigue, manifested as tiredness, social withdrawal, or absence of motivation, often associated with anorexia and weight loss. These symptoms could be mediated by other cytokines, such as TNF (68). There is a great range of tolerance, and adaptation may occur at doses lower than 10 MIU. Fatigue is by far the most difficult adverse effect to control. Intermittent schedules, evening administrations, slight dose reduction or transitory discontinuation, and symptomatic drugs for alleviating fatigue will facilitate tolerance (18,87,88).

B. Cardiocirculatory Effects

Cardiocirculatory effects, such as hypotension, tachycardia, or heart arrhythmias are rare (1–2%) they are seen only at doses higher than 10 MIU IFN-α.

C. Neurological Effects

Neurological abnormalities have been described at IFN-α doses higher than 10 MIU (18,87). It causes electroencephographic slowing, lethargy and psychomotor slowing, confusion, and dysfunction in learning and immediate memory recall (89,90). Cognitive tests suggest frontal-subcortical dysfunction (89), although serious methodological questions with this study have been raised (see Chapter 6). Depression occurs in 10% of patients, and is more frequent if the depressive state existed before treatment (18). Mild sensory-motor neuropathy and sensorineural hearing loss also occur during IFN-α or IFN-β therapy (91). Neurological side effects are usually reversible, but they occasionally persist after IFN treatment is stopped (89).

D. Hematological Effects

Leukopenia and thrombocytopenia are rather frequent occurrences during IFN treatment (18,68), but they are somewhat singular, because (1) levels rarely go below 2000 leukocytes or 70,000 platelets per cubic millimeter, even during long term treatment; and (2) the effect is strictly peripheral, since bone marrow cellularity is completely preserved. Reduced blood cell count may be related to redistribution of blood cells from the circulation to other body compartment, and, consequently, the blood count is quickly restored on dose reduction or discontinuation of therapy.

E. Other Effects

Mild alopecia, generalized skin rashes (macular eruptions affecting trunk and extremities), increase of serum hepatic enzymes, and hypothyroidism are also seen during intramuscular IFN-α treatment.

In general, side effect severity is directly related to IFN-α dose, but individual variation is ample. Doses between 1 and 5 MIU are well tolerated even for prolonged periods. Doses between 6 and 10 MIU may be less well tolerated and may require brief treatment interruptions or dose reduction. Doses above 10 MIU usually result in severe toxicity.

Another rare side effect, but relevant to the treatment of a putatively immune-mediated disease such as MS, is the occurrence or the exacerbation of autoimmune diseases. Reversible asymptomatic autoantibodies and also autoimmune thyroiditis, thrombocytopenia, anemia, hepatitis, polyarthropathies, diabetes, or myasthenia gravis sometimes follow IFN-α or IFN-β treatment (17,92–94). The immunoactivating effects of IFN-α and IFN-β may account for the exacerbation of preexisting autoimmune diseases. Possibly for the same reason, worsening of MS symptoms may occur shortly after the first few IFN-α or IFN-β administrations (95,96). In our experience, MS patients may notice a transient increase of preexisting symptoms and signs (sometimes only in the day after IFN-α injection) during the first months of IFN-α treatment.

A thorough search for serum autoimmune antibodies and, in particular, for preexisting hypothyroidism or subclinical hepatic damage is strongly recommended before starting type I IFN therapy.

The flu-like side effects described during IFN-α or IFN-β treatment are qualitatively similar, although the severity seems less and tolerance occurs earlier during IFN-β therapy (see Table 2). The most frequent adverse clinical events reported during chronic IFN-β administration (76,97,98) were fatigue, headache, sense of weakness, depression, local skin erythema, and mild neutropenia. Psychomotor slowing, confusion, and cardiac arrhythmias are rare. Cognitive dysfunction has not been reported during chronic IFN-β administration in these studies (see Chapter 6). However, pain and of local skin reactions at the injection site are observed with IFN-β and not with IFN-α. Most IFN-β side effects, including fatigue but excluding the persistent local skin reaction, rapidly decreased in severity after 3–6 months.

Neutralizing anti-IFN antibodies are found in serum of about 40–50% of patients chronically treated with IFN-α or IFN-β (18,76,97). In cancer or hepatitis patients, relapses are associated with neutralizing antibodies (18,79). In MS the relationships between serum anti-IFN antibody activity and MS exacerbation severity or time between exacerbations are still controversial (also see Chapters 3 and 13).

VI. EFFECTIVENESS OF HIGH-DOSE RECOMBINANT IFN-α_{2a} IN RELAPSING-REMITTING MS

The antagonistic effect of type I IFNs on IFN-γ–induced MHC class II molecule expression on astrocytes (19), their capability to restore the impaired lymphocyte suppressor function in MS (40), and their well-known antiviral activity (1) provided a rationale for their use in MS. The first clinical trials using low doses of either natural or recombinant IFN-α or IFN-β (49,99–102) reported no relevant effects on the course of MS, but a dose-finding study with rIFN-β 1b showed a decreased exacerbation rate with doses of 45 MIU or higher (103). We therefore tested the effect of high-dose rIFN-α-2a in MS because of these prior studies and its wide use in other diseases. We chose a dose of 9 MIU, because lower doses were ineffective in MS treatment (49,99,100,102), yet 9 MIU had acceptable side effects in the treatment of viral or neoplastic diseases (18) and had proven effects on immune function (104) as well. Another consideration was crucial in choosing the dose. Owing to the extremely greater in vivo diffusibility and bioavailability (68,70) of IFN-α compared with IFN-β, we decided that 9 MIU rIFN-α would be comparable or more potent than the 45 MIU rIFN-β dose chosen by the North American Betaseron trial (76) (this decision preceded the subsequent translation of the dosages to a different standard for potency; 45 MIU is now 8 MIU of IFN β-1b).

We studied 20 patients with clinically definite MS of the relapsing-remitting (RR) type (64). All patients had a past history of active disease, with at least two exacerbations in the 2 years preceding entry into the study, and the last exacerbation occurring at least 3 months before entry. All patients regularly visited as outpatients at our institution during the last 3–4 years, and the prestudy exacerbation rate was carefully determined from our clinical files. Patients were stratified by gender and expanded disability status scale (EDSS) (105) score at entry (Table 3).

Table 3 Pretreatment Comparison of the Study Groups of the rIFN-α_{2a} Trial in MS

	IFN-α Group	Placebo group
Number of patients (females)	12(7)	8(4)
Age at disease onset[a]	24.25 ± 1.90(15–36)	30.00 ± 3.75(18–50)
Age at entry[a]	33.00 ± 2.48(18–46)	38.00 ± 3.38(29–57)
Disease duration (years)[a]	8.92 ± 1.47(3–19)	6.37 ± 0.80(3–10)
Exacerbations/year before entry[a]	1.25 ± 0.24(0–2.5)	1.06 ± 0.20(0.5–2.0)
Last exacerbation before entry (days)[a]	142 ± 19.70	153.2 ± 30.54
Disability status scale at entry:		
EDSS[a]	3.42 ± 0.61(1–6)	2.81 ± 0.47(1.5–5.0)
patients at scores 0–2.5:		
number	6	5
EDSS[a]	1.58 ± 0.24(1–2.5)	1.90 ± 0.19(1.5–2.5)
patients at scores 3–6.0:		
number	6	3
EDSS[a]	5.25 ± 0.48(3.5–6.0)	4.33 ± 0.33(4–5)
NRS score[a]	78.42 ± 3.77(59–96)	86.87 ± 2.47(75–96)

[a] Mean ± SEM (and range).
Source: From ref. 64.

Patients were treated with 9 MIU rIFN-α (IFN α-2a, Roferon, Roche S.p.A., Milan, Italy) (12 patients) or placebo (8 patients). IFN-α was injected intramuscularly between 8 and 9 PM on alternate days for 6 months. All patients were also given 1000 mg acetaminophen 2 hr before and 2–8 hr after IFN-α or placebo injection. Patients were regularly examined by blinded physicians who had no knowledge of treatment administered, of treatment duration, or of drug side effects. The follow-up lasted 12 months (6 months of treatment followed by 6 months after stopping treatment). Examinations were repeated every month, and whenever a patient felt that an exacerbation might be occurring. When absolutely necessary, exacerbations were treated with 3 days of 1 g i.v. methylprednisolone therapy tapered over 15 days with oral glucocorticoid.

Disease activity was also monitored with repeat cranial MRI scans (106–109), before treatment, at treatment end, and 6 months after treatment end. A 0.5-tesla (T) superconducting MR imager was used to scan 12 brain slices, 8 mm thick (gap 2 mm), both axially and coronally. External and internal anatomical landmarks were used to duplicate the same imaging plane and patients head position for each study. The MRI criteria for worsening were the occurrence of new lesions or the enlargement of previously seen lesions, or both, on T_2-weighted spin-echo sequences (77). Gadolinium enhancement was not used in this pilot study.

The effects of rIFN-α on cognitive function and on mood depression were monitored with the following neuropsychological tests: Wechsler memory scale, Benton visual retention test, Bender visual motor gestalt test, and Hamilton depression scale.

During rIFN-α treatment (Table 4), two exacerbations occurred in the rIFN-α group versus eight in the placebo group. The exacerbation rate was significantly higher (t-test, $P < .03$) in placebo-treated (1 exacerbation per patient per 6 months) than in rIFN-α–treated (0.17 exacerbations per patient per 6 months) patients. The exacerbation rate significantly decreased in the rIFN-α group from the prestudy exacerbation rate (from 0.75 to 0.17) (t-test, $P < .02$), whereas it was unchanged in the placebo group (Fig. 1). Median time to first exacerbation was almost doubled for the rIFN-α group compared with the placebo group (111 vs 58 days). Exacerbation severity, rated according to the neurological rating scale (NRS) score (110), was milder in the rIFN-α group. No exacerbation in this group required corticosteroid treatment, but three severe exacerbations in the placebo group required hospitalization and high-dose methylprednisolone treatment.

The number of active MRI scans was 1 of 12 in the rIFN-α group and 6 of 8 in the placebo group. The difference is highly significant (Fisher's exact test, $P < .005$). In the rIFN-α group, we found only one active

Table 4 Clinical and MRI Effects of rIFN-α_{2a} Treatment in MS Patients

	rIFN-α group (n = 12)		Placebo group (n = 8)	
	1–6 months	7–12 months[a]	1–6 months	7–12 months
Exacerbations	2[b]	3	8	4
Exacerbation rate	0.17[b]	0.25	1	0.5
Active lesions at MRI	1[b]	14[c]	27	17
Active lesions/patient	0.083[b]	1.17[c]	3.375	2.125
Percentage patients with active lesions at MRI	8.3[b]	50[c]	75	75
Percentage patients with signs of disease activity	16.7[b]	66.7[c]	87.5	75

[a] 1–6 months = 6-month treatment period; 7–12 months = 6-month follow-up after treatment.
[b] Significantly different from placebo or [c] from treatment period (means were compared using Student's paired t-test and two sample t-test for parametric data, or Wilcoxon's signed rank test and Rank sum test for nonparametric data. Discrete data were compared using a two-tailed Fisher's exact test).

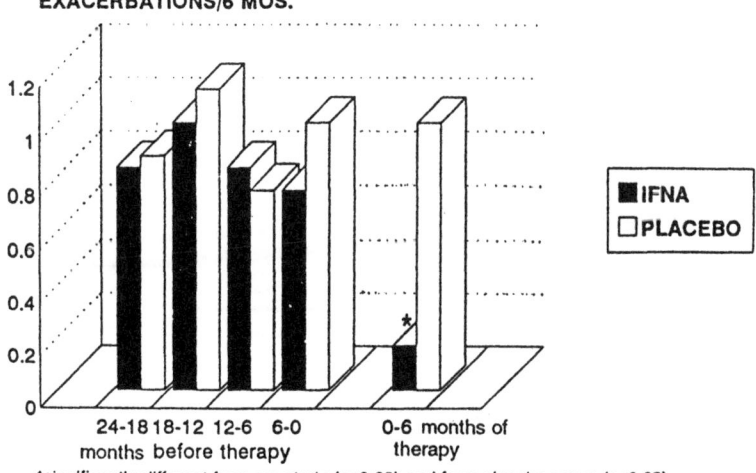

EXACERBATIONS/6 MOS.

■ IFNA
☐ PLACEBO

24-18 18-12 12-6 6-0 months before therapy   0-6 months of therapy

*significantly different from pre-study (p<0.03) and from placebo group (p<0.03)

Figure 1 Exacerbation rate (calculated on a 6-month base) in the 2 years before and during treatment for patients receiving high-dose systemic recombinant IFN-α_{2a} (IFNA) or placebo. *Significantly different from prestudy ($P < .03$) and from placebo group ($P < .03$). (From ref. 64.)

lesion out of the 12 patients studied, whereas in the placebo group, we found 27 active lesions. The mean number of active lesions per patient was 0.08 ± 0.08 in the rIFN-α and 3.37 ± 1.03 in the placebo group (t-test, $P < .01$). Based on both clinical and MRI data, signs of disease activity were observed in 2 of 12 patients of the rIFN-α group and in 7 of 8 patients of the placebo group (Fisher's exact test, $P < .005$).

At the end of the 6-month treatment period, the mean EDSS and NRS scores did not show any significant change from baseline in both groups, indicating that rIFN-α treatment did not lead to overall improvement or worsening of neurological status. The neuropsychological tests did not show any significant change from baseline in either study group. The Hamilton depression scale indicated one case of depression among rIFN-α–treated patients.

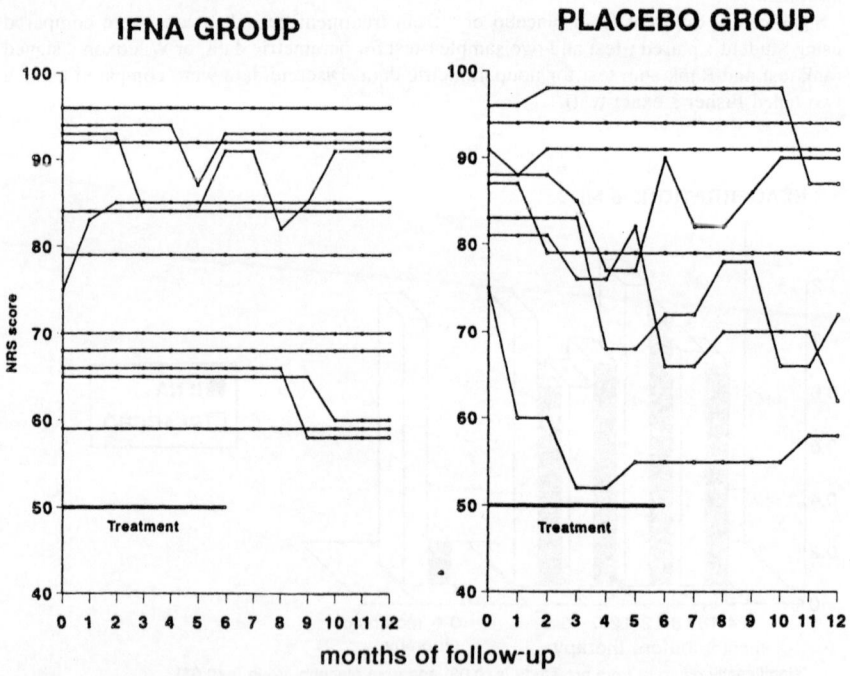

Figure 2 Serial NRS scores at the monthly clinical evaluation during a 6-month period of treatment (solid horizontal bars), randomized between high-dose systemic recombinant IFN-α_{2a} (IFNA) or placebo. Follow-up continued for 6 months after treatment was discontinued.

During the 6 months after stopping treatment (Fig. 2; see Table 4), three exacerbations were observed in the previously rIFN-α–treated group versus four in the placebo group. Exacerbation severity and median time to first exacerbation were similar in both groups. At the final MRI scan, 14 active lesions could be detected in the previously rIFN-α–treated group versus 17 in the placebo-treated group. The proportion of patients with active lesions at MRI was 6 of 12 in the previously rIFN-α–treated group and 6 of 8 in the other. By combining clinical and MRI data, the proportion of patients with either clinical or MRI signs of disease activity was 7 of 12 in the previously rIFN-α–treated group versus 6 of 8 in the other. The Hamilton depression scale score returned to baseline values in the previously rIFN-α–treated group, and the results of the other neuropsychological tests did not show any significant change in both study groups. Thus, 6 months after stopping rIFN-α, there were no more significant differences between the two groups, and in many cases, the figures of the previously rIFN-α–treated group were significantly different from the treatment period (see Table 4).

VII. REDUCTION OF LYMPHOCYTE PRODUCTION OF PROINFLAMMATORY CYTOKINES IN VIVO IN CHRONIC rIFN-α_{2a} TREATMENT

The in vivo immunological effects of chronic rIFN-α treatment in MS patients (Tables 5 and 6) were assessed by studying cytokine production by peripheral blood (PB) lymphocyte cultures, MHC class II molecule expression by cultured PB monocytes, cell surface differentiation antigen expression by PB and CSF lymphocytes, and the serum level of β_2-microglobulin, a class I MHC–associated protein which is elevated by IFNs (111).

Before treatment, at the treatment end, and 6 months after treatment end, 30 ml of PB was drawn in heparinized tubes by venipuncture and diluted with an equal volume of phosphate-buffered saline (PBS). Mononuclear cells (MCs) were separated by Lymphoprep density gradient centrifugation. Before and after treatment, 15 ml of CSF was slowly drawn with a 22-gauge spinal needle, divided in Eppendorf tubes, and centrifugated at 1000 rpm for 3 min. CSF was removed and MCs washed and resuspended in PBS.

Lymphocyte differentiation antigens of PB and CSF MC suspensions were analyzed with a direct immunofluorescence technique using fluorescein isothiocyanate–conjugated or phycoerythrin-conjugated monoclonal antibodies. Particular attention was given to the $CD8^+$ $CD11b^+$ popula-

Table 5 Immunological Effects of rIFN-α Treatment in MS Patients

	rIFN-α Group (n = 12)			Placebo Group (n = 8)		
	baseline	6 months[a]	12 months[a]	baseline	6 months[a]	12 months[a]
Serum β_2 Microglobulin (ng/ml)	1,091 ± 43	1,791 ± 168[b,c]	1,098 ± 50[d]	1,200 ± 85	1,086 ± 39	1,053 ± 25
Lymphocyte IFN-γ Production (U/ml)	19.1 ± 7.1	3.03 ± 0.7[b,c]	12.4 ± 2.2[d]	21.7 ± 9.7	15.4 ± 3.6	12.2 ± 2.1
Lymphocyte TNF-α Production (pg/ml)	18.1 ± 5.3	5.8 ± 0.9[b,c]	18.9 ± 6.3	21.0 ± 7.7	20.6 ± 5.7	28.2 ± 8.4
Lymphocyte TGF-β Production (pg/ml)	16.9 ± 1.7	17.6 ± 2.1	16.6 ± 0.9	16.6 ± 1.8	16.1 ± 1.8	17.8 ± 1.7
Lymphocyte IL-10 Production (pg/ml)	131.5 ± 12	219.1 ± 79	131.7 ± 15	132.9 ± 27	259.5 ± 82	141.0 ± 23
Macrophage HLA-DR antigen expression (mean fluorescence intensity)						
with IFN-γ 500 U/ml	959 ± 251	807 ± 103	944 ± 116	1,169 ± 220	1,134 ± 328	977 ± 165
without IFN-γ	440 ± 89	418 ± 54	450 ± 79	488 ± 101	549 ± 231	588 ± 101

[a] 6 months = end of the 6-month treatment period; 12 months = end of the 6-month follow-up after treatment period.
Significantly different [b] from baseline ($P < .04$), [c] from placebo ($P < .04$), or [d] from treatment period ($P < .05$). Means were compared using Student's paired t-test and two-sample t-test for parametric data, or Wilcoxon's signed rank test and rank sum test for nonparametric data.

Table 6 Effects of rIFN-α Treatment on Lymphocyte Surface Antigen Expression in MS Patients

		rIFN-α group (n = 12)			Placebo group (n = 8)		
		baseline	6 months[a]	12 months[a]	baseline	6 months[a]	12 months[a]
CSF							
lymphocytes/mm³		2.8 = 0.9 (11)	1.6 ± 0.3 (11)	ND	5.1 ± 1.1	5.3 ± 1.8 (7)	ND
CD4+	%	36.5 ± 8.9 (6)	24.6 ± 3.6 (7)		30.2 ± 6.7 (3)	37.4 ± 10.6 (4)	
	cells/mm³	0.4 ± 0.1 (6)	0.2 ± 0.1[b] (7)		0.6 ± 0.3 (3)	0.9 ± 0.3 (4)	
CD8+	%	23.3 ± 2.6 (7)	36.8 ± 2.9[b] (8)		15.7 ± 2.79[b] (6)	22.7 ± 5.9 (4)	
	cells/mm³	0.8 ± 0.3 (7)	0.6 ± 0.1 (8)		0.5 ± 0.1 (6)	0.7 ± 0.2 (4)	
CD8+CD11b+	%	2.4 ± 0.7 (7)	6.9 ± 1.3[c] (8)		3.9 ± 0.9 (6)	4.3 ± 1.5 (4)	
	cells/mm³	0.1 ± 0.02 (7)	0.1 ± 0.03 (8)		0.2 ± 0.04 (6)	0.1 ± 0.02 (4)	
CD3−CD16/56+	%	6.0 ± 1.1 (8)	16.7 ± 2.7 (7)		14.5 ± 4.2 (7)	20.1 ± 2.8 (4)	
	cells/mm³	0.21 ± 0.10 (8)	0.23 ± 0.08[b] (7)		0.56 ± 0.22 (7)	0.29 ± 1.28 (4)	
PB							
lymphocytes/mm³		2,165 ± 147	1,646 ± 195[d]	1,892 ± 126.7	1,958 ± 77	1,840 ± 107	1,977 ± 76.1
CD4+	%	50.2 ± 2.7	52.7 ± 2.9[b]	51.4 ± 2.4	49.9 ± 2.5	45.6 ± 5.0	50.3 ± 1.8
	cells/mm³	1,091 ± 101	883 ± 109	968 ± 73.6	972 ± 52	857 ± 113	993 ± 47.8
CD8+	%	17.9 ± 1.4	17.1 ± 1.6	18.2 ± 2.3	16.7 ± 2.4	19.3 ± 1.3	17.8 ± 1.4
	cells/mm³	438 ± 53	307 ± 59	348 ± 50.7	367 ± 53	279 ± 48	350 ± 29
CD8+CD11b+	%	4.05 ± 0.7	4.41 ± 0.8	4.15 ± 0.6	6.38 ± 1.9	3.94 ± 1.58	4.27 ± 1.2
	cells/mm³	85 ± 13	74 ± 15	76 ± 12	142 ± 40	196 ± 116	88 ± 27
CD3−CD16/56+	%	9.7 ± 1.6	14.8 ± 1.5	13.2 ± 2	14.7 ± 2.9	12.4 ± 2.3	14.4 ± 2.6
	cells/mm³	251 ± 38	243 ± 38	222 ± 31	292 ± 61	227 ± 43	285 ± 54

ND, Lumbar punctures were not repeated 6 months after stopping treatment. The number of patients studied is given in parentheses if less than the total number of patients in the trial.

[a] 6 months = end of the 6-month treatment period; 12 months = end of the 6-month follow-up after treatment period.

Significantly different from baseline values ([b] $P < .03$, [c] $P < .04$, [d] $P < .02$); [e] significantly different from IFN-α group values ($p < .01$). Means were compared with Student's paired t test and two-sample t test for parametric data or Wilcoxon's signed-rank test and rank-sum test for nonparametric data.

tion. The cytofluorometer window was set to study cells with CD8 high-
and CD11b low-fluorescent staining intensity (CD8^{high} CD11b^{low}), a CD8$^+$
subset with suppressor-effector function (112).

The remaining PBMCs were washed three times with PBS and resuspended at a final concentration of 2×10^6 cells/ml in complete medium
and 5% heat inactivated fetal bovine serum (FBS). To avoid nonspecific
effects due to lot-to-lot variations in the FBS, the same media preparation
was stored at $-20°C$ and used throughout the study. Macrophages were
removed by plastic adherence after incubation for 45 min in sterile flasks.
The adherent cells were cultured for 24 hr in complete medium with or
without 500 U/ml IFN-γ, collected after incubation at 4°C with EDTA,
and labeled for CD14 and HLA-DR antigen expression. The nonadherent
cells were washed twice in PBS, resuspended at a final concentration of
1.5×10^6 cells/ml in complete medium with 10% FCS, and cultured for
3 days in triplicate without mitogens. Phenotypical analysis demonstrated
that cultured cells were mainly lymphocytes, namely, 65% CD3$^+$ (T lymphocytes), 15% CD3$^-$CD16/56$^+$ (NK lymphocytes), and only 3% CD14$^+$
(macrophages), without significant differences before and after treatment.
Spontaneous cytokine production by lymphocyte cultures was determined
in 72-hr culture supernatants: IFN-γ by radioimmunoassay, and TNF-α,
transforming growth factor-β (TGF-β), IL-4, and IL-10 by commercially
available ELISA kits.

The β_2-microglobulin serum level was monitored using a commercially
available microparticle enzyme immunoassay kit.

Baseline cytokine production by PBMC cultures was similar in both
study groups. After 6 months of IFN-α treatment, production of IFN-γ
and TNF-α was decreased from baseline (t-test, $P < .04$), whereas it was
unchanged in controls. IFN-γ and TNF-α production in the treated group
was significantly lower than that of placebo group (t-test, $P < .04$). TGF-
β production was slightly (but not significantly) increased, IL-10 was unchanged, and IL-4 was undetectable in the culture supernatants both before and after therapy. PB monocyte HLA-DR antigen expression of both
unstimulated and IFN-γ–stimulated cultures did not change from baseline
or between groups.

Baseline PB and CSF lymphocyte counts and phenotypes were similar
in both study groups (see Table 6). After rIFN-α treatment, PBMC and
CSF CD4$^+$ T-cell counts were significantly decreased, and the percentage
of CSF CD8$^+$ T cells, CD8^{high}CD11b^{low} T cells (the suppressor-effector
subset), and CD3$^-$CD16$^+$CD56$^+$ cells (NK lymphocytes) significantly
increased from baseline. In the placebo group's CSF, these subsets did
not significantly change from baseline. In both study groups, percentage

and absolute counts of PB CD4$^+$, CD8$^+$, and CD8^{high}CD11b^{low} T cells were constant.

At the end of treatment period, β_2-microglobulin serum level was significantly increased from baseline in rIFN-α–treated patients, whereas it remained unchanged in placebos.

VIII. INHIBITION OF DISEASE ACTIVITY AND OTHER BIOLOGICAL EFFECTS OF rIFN-α-2a IN MS PATIENTS CEASE AFTER TREATMENT STOPS

A decrease of both clinical and MRI signs of disease activity was associated with decreased production of the proinflammatory cytokines IFN-γ and TNF-α during high-dose rIFN-α treatment. After stopping treatment, many signs of disease activity resumed. The reappearance of clinical or laboratory signs of disease activity after stopping IFN-α treatment has been well documented in other diseases (such as chronic hepatitis or lymphoproliferative diseases), where the efficacy of IFN-α treatment is well established (78,83). During the 6 months after stopping treatment, the exacerbation rate of previously rIFN-α-2a–treated patients showed a slight increase, from 0.17 to 0.25 exacerbations per 6 months, becoming similar to that of controls; that is, 0.50 exacerbations per 6 months. The exacerbation rate randomly fluctuates over the course of RR MS, with a usual trend for a slight progressive decrease in the attack rate with time (113). In addition, MRI signs of disease activity, which were greatly reduced during rIFN-α treatment, remarkably and significantly increased after stopping treatment, becoming equivalent to the activity of controls. Longitudinal studies with MRI show that changes of disease activity in RR MS may be detected by MRI even in the absence of changes of exacerbation rate (114,115). The abrupt increase of the active lesion number strongly suggests that disease activity, reduced during rIFN-α administration, resumed after stopping treatment.

Many other biological effects disappeared after stopping rIFN-α treatment. The increase of serum β_2-microglobulin and the PB lymphopenia (two well-known effects of IFN-α treatment) (18,111), and the changes of PB lymphocyte phenotypes and of lymphokine production returned toward pretreatment values. In conclusion, we observed many sudden biological changes, simultaneously occurring during rIFN-α administration and disappearing after stopping the drug, indicating that high-dose rIFN-α affected immune function and disease activity in RR MS. Since the reduction of signs of disease activity was temporary and restricted to the period of rIFN-α administration, chronic rIFN-α treatment seems needed to maintain therapeutic effects in MS, as has been demonstrated in many other diseases where IFN-α efficacy is widely accepted (1,78,84).

IX. POSITIVE THERAPEUTIC EFFECT OF rIFN-α IN MS IS ASSOCIATED WITH MODULATION OF CYTOKINE PRODUCTION RATHER THAN WITH DOWNREGULATION OF THE ANTIGEN PRESENTATION PROCESS

Type I IFN antiviral and immunomodulatory actions may counteract the inflammatory mechanisms and the immune activation underlying disease activity in MS (30,116). IFN-β or IFN-α may decrease Th1 lymphocyte production of proinflammatory cytokines (64) (also see Chapter 7). Cytokine production is enhanced during viral infections (117) and may trigger MS exacerbations (118–120). IFN-γ and TNF-α are found in MS-active plaques (13) and enhance immune responses (8–10,30), lysis of oligodendrocytes (33), and MS disease activity (8,121). In contrast type I IFNs downregulate IFN-γ–induced HLA-DR expression (19) and increase the reduced suppressor activity of MS lymphocytes (40).

We show, for the first time, that chronic rIFN-α treatment in RR MS is associated both with reduced clinical and MRI signs of disease activity as well as with the reduced production of two proinflammatory cytokines IFN-γ and TNF-α. rIFN-α treatment is not associated with changes of monocyte MHC class II molecule expression. These data suggest that the beneficial in vivo effect of rIFN-α in MS is probably mediated by downregulation of lymphocyte proinflammatory cytokine synthesis rather than by inhibition of class II–regulated antigen presentation. Systemic rIFN-β treatment increases lymphocyte suppressor activity and could decrease cytokine production (122). We have also now demonstrated the increased availability of CSF $CD8^{high}CD11^{low}$ T cells and of $CD3^-CD16^+CD56^+$ NK cells; both subsets contain suppressor-effector cells (123). The increased number of suppressor-effector cells may reduce disease activity in MS.

X. IS rIFN-α TREATMENT OF RR MS MORE EFFECTIVE THAN rIFN-β?

Three controlled trials of high-dose chronic systemic type I rIFNs in MS have been finished so far, (64,76,124). In all trials, a significant reduction of clinical and MRI signs of disease activity has been documented (Table 7). The North American Betaseron trial of 372 patients (76,77) demonstrated that subcutaneous 8 MIU rIFN β-1b on alternate days brought

Table 7 Comparison of Clinical and MRI Signs of Disease Activity After Treatment Reported in the Three Trials with Type I IFNs in MS Described in the Text (64,76,77,124)

	rIFN β-1b		rIFN β-1a		rIFN α_{2a}	
	IFN	placebo	IFN	placebo	IFN	placebo
Weekly dose	28 MIU s.c.	—	6 MIU i.m.	—	31.5 MIU i.m.	—
Exacerbation rate (mean/6 months)	0.42	0.63	0.31	0.45	0.17	1.00
Active lesion rate at MRI (mean/6 months)	1.0	2.4	0.4	0.8	0.08	3.37

about a 34% reduction of exacerbation rate and a 59% reduction of active MRI lesion number in comparison with controls. These data have been recently confirmed by the study of Jacobs et al. (124), who observed, in 301 patients treated with intramuscular 6 MIU rIFN β-1a weekly, a 31% reduction of exacerbation rate, a 40% decrease of 1- and 2-year progression rates, and a 52% reduction of active MRI lesion number. Finally, we have shown that intramuscular 9 MIU rIFN-α_{2a} on alternate days also reduced both clinical and MRI signs of disease activity in 20 RR MS patients (64). In rIFN-α–treated patients, the exacerbation rate was reduced by 77% compared with the rate before the study and by 83% compared with the rate in placebo-treated controls. The number of active MRI lesions was reduced by 97% compared with controls. In addition, proinflammatory lymphokine production was reduced by 84% compared with baseline and by 80% compared with controls. The efficacy of high-dose chronic IFN-α treatment in reducing clinical signs of disease activity in RR MS has been recently supported by Sheremata et al. (125), who reported an 82% reduction of exacerbation rate in nine patients, after 0.5–1.0 year of 20 MIU/week natural IFN-α.

The two small studies with chronic high-dose IFN-α in MS so far published (64,125) have, therefore, confirmed the 77–96% reduction of clinical or MRI signs of disease activity in comparison with baseline or placebo. On the other hand, the large trials with high-dose rIFN-β (76,77,124) showed a 31–59% reduction of clinical and MRI signs of disease activity; a somewhat worse result than with IFN-α. IFN-α is the IFN most widely used in therapy and is registered for many more diseases than IFN-β (1). In some viral or lymphoproliferative diseases, where IFN-β has been used as an alternative for patients who developed resistance to IFN-α, therapeutic results have been worse (72,73,79,80). In chronic myelogenous leukemia, IFN-β is ineffective, but IFN-α is antileukemic (82). The greater bioavailability and in vivo diffusion from the injection site (68), and some differences in affinity for the cell surface human type I IFN receptor (66; and see Chapter 1) of IFN-α in comparison with IFN-β may explain the better results obtained with IFN-α in many clinical applications.

XI. SIDE EFFECTS OF HIGH-DOSE rIFN-α TREATMENT IN MS

The major drawbacks for the use of chronic high-dose rIFN-α in MS certainly arise from side effects. We observed all the common side effects of IFN-α therapy (18) (Table 8). A flu-like syndrome (fever, headache, arthralgias, and myalgias) occurred in more than 60% of patients but progressively disappeared 1–3 months after starting treatment. Mild labora-

Table 8 Frequency of Side Effects During 6 Months of High-Dose rIFN-α_{2a} Treatment in RR MS

Side effect	IFN-α group	Placebo group
Fever	8/12	1/8
Fatigue	6/12	2/8
Arthralgias/myalgias	1/12	0/8
Headache	2/12	1/8
Anorexia/nausea/vomiting/weight loss	0/12	0/8
Hair loss	3/12	0/8
Depression	1/12	0/8
Infections		
Urinary tract infections	1/12	1/8
Upper respiratory tract infections	1/12	0/8
Severe infections or septicemias	0/12	0/8
Lymphoadenopathies	0/12	0/8
Mild neutropenia (cell number <2000)	6/12	0/8
Severe neutropenia (cell number <1000)	0/12	0/8
Mild hepatic enzyme elevation (2 × normal)	4/12	0/8
Severe hepatic enzyme elevation (3 × normal)	2/12	0/8
Thrombocytopenia	0/12	0/8
Generalized skin rashes	1/12	0/8

Source: From ref. 64.

tory abnormalities also occurred frequently: mild neutropenia (cell number between 1000 and 2000/mm^3) (50%), and mild (two times normal) or moderate (three times normal) hepatic enzyme elevation (50%). Hair loss (25%) and generalized skin rashes (9%) were rarer.

The major problems were fatigue (50%) and depression (9%). These symptoms usually started after 1–3 months of treatment, and once present did not disappear during treatment. Since fatigue is a symptom of MS and depression is a common complaint of patients with MS, a drug which can increase both symptoms must be used with caution. In two patients, IFN-α–induced fatigue was sufficiently debilitating to affect employment and to discourage them from staying on treatment for a longer period. Fatigue was particularly severe in patients already suffering from this symptom before starting rIFN-α.

Selection of patients without preexisting fatigue, and the use of symptomatic drugs or the reduction of rIFN-α dose at the occurrence of fatigue, must be considered in future rIFN-α trials. A more prolonged interval between drug administrations, such as the weekly dose recently used in the rIFN β-1a trial (124,126), would be counterproductive with rIFN-α. Tachyphylaxis to fever only develops if repeated IFN-α injections are given at intervals of <72 hr (87).

From the long-term trials with IFN-α in chronic hepatitis patients (18), and from our increasing experience with MS patients treated with rIFN-α for more than 6 months, it appears that adaptation to chronic side effects occurs to some extent in most patients. Side effects decrease in frequency after a few months of treatment and fatigue is only rarely debilitating. The side effects of chronic rIFN-β (76,97) in MS are qualitatively similar to those described with rIFN-α, and although rIFN-β seemed more tolerated by patients according to the original report of the Betaseron trial (76), a recent report (98) described a high dropout rate during long-term rIFN β-1b treatment in MS patients. Dropouts were mainly caused by fatigue and depression. Dropouts were more frequent in patients affected with relapsing-progressive or secondary-progressive MS; patients who usually suffer from fatigue before starting IFN treatment.

Type I IFN side effects certainly depend on dose, treatment duration, and patient body size, and the weekly doses used in the above-mentioned trials are extremely variable (see Table 7). A multicenter trial comparing high (9 MIU) and intermediate (4.5 MIU) intramuscular rIFN-α$_{2a}$ doses in RR MS is underway in Europe (R. Nilsen, personal communication, November 1995). A more prolonged follow-up with chronic rIFN-α$_{2a}$ treatment in MS is certainly needed, and direct comparisons of IFN-α and IFN-β treatment in MS are warranted for the exact definition of doses, schedules, and indications of the two drugs. The possibility that type I

IFN treatment might induce or exacerbate autoimmune disease in the dysimmune MS patient must be emphasized. Careful monitoring of serum autoantibodies and of signs of thyroid or liver damage must precede and accompany long-term type I IFN therapy.

REFERENCES

1. Johnson HM, Bazer FW, Szente BE, Jarpe MA. How interferons fight disease. Sci Am 1994; 270(5):68–75.
2. Darnell JE Jr, Kerr IM, Stark GR. Jak-STAT pathways and transcriptional activation in response to IFNs and other extracellular signaling proteins. Science 1994; 264:1415–1421.
3. Tanaka K, Yoshioka T, Bieberich C, Jay G. Role of the major histocompatibility complex class I antigens in tumor growth and metastasis. Ann Rev Immunol 1988; 6:359–380.
4. Landolfo S, Cofano F, Gariglio M, Gribaudo G, Lembo D, Gaboli M, Cavallo R. IFN regulation of T cell function. In: Baron S, Coppenhaver DH, Dianzani F, Fleischmann Jr. WR, Hughes Jr. TK, Klimpel GR, Niesel DW, Stanton GJ, Tyring SK, eds. Interferon: Principles and Medical Applications. Galveston, TX: University of Texas Medical Branch, Department of Microbiology, 1992:353–360.
5. DeMaeyer EM. Modulation of the expression of the major histocompatibility antigens. In: DeMaeyer EM, DeMaeyer-Guignard J, eds. Interferons and Other Regulatory Cytokines. New York: Wiley, 1988:174–193.
6. Unanue ER. Macrophages, antigen presenting cells, and the phenomena of antigen handling and presentation. In: Paul E, ed. Fundamental Immunology. New York: Raven Press, 1989:95–115.
7. Sztein MB, Steeg PS, Johnson HM, Oppenhezim J. Regulation of human peripheral blood monocyte DR antigen expression by lymphokines and recombinant interferons. J Clin Invest 1982; 73:556–563.
8. Panitch HS, Hirsch RL, Schindler J, Johnson KP. Treatment of multiple sclerosis with gamma interferon: exacerbations associated with activation of the immune system. Neurology 1987; 37:1097–1102.
9. Fierz W, Endler B, Reske K, Wekerle H, Fontana A. Astrocytes as antigen-presenting cells. I. Induction of Ia antigen expression on astrocytes by T cells via immune interferon and its effect on antigen presentation. J Immunol 1985; 134:3785–3793.
10. Pober JS, Gimbrone MA Jr, Cotran RS, Reiss CS, Burakoff SJ, Fierz W, Ault KA. Ia expression by vascular endothelium is inducible by activated T cells and by human γ-interferon. J Exp Med 1983; 157:1339–1353.
11. Traugott U, Scheinberg LC, Raine CS. On the presence of Ia-positive endothelial cells and astrocytes in multiple sclerosis lesions and its relevance to antigen presentation. J Neuroimmunol 1988; 8:1–14.
12. Schwartz RS, Datta SK. Autoimmunity and autoimmune diseases. In: Paul E, ed. Fundamental Immunology. New York: Raven Press, 1989:819–866.

13. Traugott U, Lebon P. Multiple sclerosis: involvement of interferons in lesion pathogenesis. Ann Neurol 1988; 24:243–251.
14. Woodroofe MN, Cuzner ML. Cytokine mRNA expression in inflammatory multiple sclerosis lesions: detection by nonradioactive in situ hybridization. Cytokine 1993; 5:583–588.
15. Link J, Soderstrom M, Olsson T, Hojeberg B, Ljungdahl A, Link H. Increased transforming growth factor-β, interleukin-4, and interferon-γ in multiple sclerosis. Ann Neurol 1994; 36:379–386.
16. Rieckmann P, Albrecht M, Kitze B, Weber T, Tumani H, Broocks A, Luer W, Poser S. Cytokine mRNA levels in mononuclear blood cells from patients with multiple sclerosis. Neurology 1994; 44:1523–1526.
17. Conlon KC, Urba WJ, Smith JW II, Steis RG, Longo DL, Clark JW. Exacerbation of symptoms of autoimmune disease in patients receiving α-interferon therapy. Cancer 1990; 65:2237–2242.
18. Quesada JR. Toxicity and side effects of interferons. In: Baron S, Coppenhaver DH, Dianzani F, Fleischmann Jr. WR, Hughes Jr. TK, Klimpel GR, Niesel DW, Stanton GJ, Tyring SK, eds. Interferon: Principles and Medical Applications. Galveston, TX: University of Texas Medical Branch, Department of Microbiology, 1992:427–432.
19. Barna BP, Chou SM, Jacobs B, Yen-Lieberman B, Ransohoff RM. Interferon-β impairs induction of HLA-DR antigen expression in cultured adult human astrocytes. J Neuroimmunol 1989; 23:45–53.
20. Bongioanni MR, Durelli L, Ferrero B, Imperiale D, Ogpero A, Verdun E, Aimo G, Pagni R, Geuna M, Bergamasco B. Systemic high-dose recombinant-alpha-2a-interferon therapy modulates lymphokine production in multiple sclerosis. J Neurol Sci (in press).
21. Romagnani S. Induction of T_H1 and T_H2 response: a key role for the 'natural' immune response? Immunol Today 1992; 13:379–381.
22. Romagnani S. Lymphokine production by human T cells in disease states. Ann Rev Immunol 1994; 12:227–258.
23. Maggi E, Parronchi P, Manetti R, Simonelli C, Piccinni MP, Rugiu FS, De Carli M, Ricci M, Romagnani S. Reciprocal regulatory effect of IFN-γ and IL-4 on the in Th1 and Th2 clones. J Immunol 1992; 148:2142–2147.
24. Hsieh CS, Macatonia SE, Tripp CS, Wolf SF, O'Garra A, Murphy KM. Development of T_H1 CD4$^+$ T cells through IL-12 produced by Listeria-induced macrophages. Science 1993; 260:547–549.
25. Gajewski TF, Schell RS, Nau G, Fitch FW. Regulation of T-cell activation: differences among T-cell subsets. Immunol Rev 1989; 111:79–110.
26. Fiorentino DF, Zlotnik A, Vieira P, Mosmann TR, Howard M, Moore KW, O'Garra A. IL-10 acts on the antigen-presenting cells to inhibit cytokine production by Th1 cells. J Immunol 1991; 146:3444–3451.
27. Mosmann TR. Cytokine secretion patterns and cross-regulation of T cell subsets. Immunol Res 1991; 10:183–188.
28. Bogdan C, Vodovotz Y, Nathan C. Macrophage deactivation by Interleukin 10. J Exp Med 1991; 174:1549–1555.
29. Oswald IP, Wynn TA, Sher A, James SL. Interleukin 10 inhibits macro-

phage microbicidal activity by blocking the endogenous production of tumor necrosis factor required as a costimulatory factor for interferon gamma-induced activation. Proc Natl Acad Sci USA 1992; 89:8676–8680.

30. Olsson T. Role of cytokines in multiple sclerosis and experimental autoimmune encephalomyelitis. Eur J Neurol 1994; 1:7–19.

31. McCarron RM, Wang L, Racke MK, et al. Cytokine-regulated adhesion between encephalitogenic T lymphocytes and cerebrovascular endothelial cells. J Neuroimmunol 1993; 43:23–30.

32. Ruddle N, Bergman CM, McGrath KM, Lingenheld EG, Grunnet ML, Padula SJ, Clark RB. An antibody to lymphotoxin and tumor necrosis factor prevents transfer of experimental allergic encephalomyelitis. J Exp Med 1990; 172:1193–1200.

33. Selmaj KW, Raine CS. Tumor necrosis factor mediates myelin and oligodendrocyte damage in vitro. Ann Neurol 1988; 23:339–346.

34. Kennedy MK, Torrance DS, Picha KS, Mohler KM. Analysis of cytokine mRNA expression in the central nervous system of mice with experimental autoimmune encephalomyelitis reveals that IL-10 mRNA expression correlates with recovery. J Immunol 1992; 149:2496–2505.

35. Van der Veen RC, Stohlman SA. Encephalitogenic Th1 cells are inhibited by Th2 cells with related peptide specificity: relative roles of interleukin (IL)-4 and IL-10. J Neuroimmunol 1993; 48:213–220.

36. Klimpel GR, Infante AJ, Patterson J, Hess CB, Asuncion M. Virus induced interferon-α/β (IFN-α/β) production by T cells and by Th1 and Th2 helper T cell clones: a study of the immunoregulatory actions of IFN-γ versus IFN-α/β on functions of different T cell populations. Cell Immunol 1990; 128:603–607.

37. Simon MM, Landolfo S, Diamanstein T, Hochgeschwender U. Antigen- and lectin-sensitized murine cytolitic T lymphocyte precursors require both interleukin 2 and endogenously produced interferon-γ for their growth and differentiation into effector cells. Curr Top Microbiol Immunol 1986; 126:173–180.

38. Chen LK, Mathieu-Mahul D, Back FH, Dausset J, Bensussan A, Sasportes M. Recombinant interferon-α can induce rearrangement of T-cell antigen receptor α-chain genes and maturation to cytotoxicity in T-lymphocyte clones in vitro. Proc Natl Acad Sci USA 1986; 54:4887–4892.

39. Wagner L, Goldstone AH, Worman CP. Demonstration of the increase of serine esterase-positive T cells in hairy-cell leukemia patients undergoing α-interferon therapy. Leukemia 1989; 3:373–379.

40. Noronha A, Toscas A, Jensen MA. Contrasting effects of alpha-, beta-, and gamma-interferons on nonspecific suppression function in multiple sclerosis. Ann Neurol 1992; 31:103–106.

41. Antel J, Arnason BGW, Medof ME. Suppressor cell function in multiple sclerosis—correlation with clinical disease activity. Ann Neurol 1979; 5:338–342.

42. Oger J, Kastrukoff LF, Li DKB, Paty DW. Multiple sclerosis: in relapsing

patients, immune functions vary with disease activity as assessed by MRI. Neurology 1988; 38:1739–1744.

43. Niesel DW, Klimpel GR. Interferon as a mediator of host defense against bacteria. In: Baron S, Coppenhaver DH, Dianzani F, Fleischmann Jr. WR, Hughes Jr. TK, Klimpel GR, Niesel DW, Stanton GJ, Tyring SK, eds. Interferon: Principles and Medical Applications. Galveston, TX: University of Texas Medical Branch, Department of Microbiology, 1992:311–328.

44. Fleischmann WR Jr, Fleischmann CM. Mechanisms of interferons' antitumor actions. In: Baron S, Coppenhaver DH, Dianzani F, Fleischmann Jr. WR, Hughes Jr. TK, Klimpel GR, Niesel DW, Stanton GJ, Tyring SK, eds. Interferon: Principles and Medical Applications. Galveston, TX: University of Texas Medical Branch, Department of Microbiology, 1992:299–309.

45. Tsujimoto M, Yip YK, Vilcek J. Interferon-γ enhances expression of cellular receptors for tumor necrosis factor. J Immunol 1986; 136:1441–1447.

46. Neighbor PA, Grayzel AI, Miller AE. Endogenous and interferon-α natural killer activity of human peripheral blood mononuclear cells in vitro: study of patients with multiple sclerosis, systemic lupus erythematosus, or reumathoid arthritis. Clin Exp Immunol 1982; 49:11–21.

47. Oger J, Kastrukoff L, O'Gorman M, Paty DW. Progressive multiple sclerosis: abnormal immune functions in vitro and aberrant correlation with enumeration of lymphocyte subpopulations. J Neuroimmunol 1986; 12: 37–48.

48. Vranes Z, Poljakovic Z, Marusic M. Natural killer cell number and activity in multiple sclerosis. J Neurol Sci 1989; 94:115–123.

49. Kastrukoff LF, Oger JJ, Hashimoto SA, Sacks SL, Li DK, Palmer MR, Koopmans RA, Petkau AJ, Berkovitz J, Paty DW. Systemic lymphoblastoid interferon therapy in chronic progressive multiple sclerosis. I. Clinical and MRI evaluation. Neurology 1990; 40:479–486.

50. Kastrukoff LF, Morgan NG, Aziz TM, Zecchini D, Berkovitz J, Paty DW. Natural killer (NK) cells in chronic progressive multiple sclerosis treated with lymphoblastoid interferon. J Neuroimmunol 1988; 20:15–23.

51. Snapper CM. The regulation of B cell function by interferon-γ. In: Baron S, Coppenhaver DH, Dianzani F, Fleischmann Jr. WR, Hughes Jr. TK, Klimpel GR, Niesel DW, Stanton GJ, Tyring SK, eds. Interferon: Principles and Medical Applications. Galveston, TX: University of Texas Medical Branch, Department of Microbiology, 1992:373–385.

52. Snapper CM, McIntyre T, Mandler R, Pecanha LMT, Finkelman FD, Lees A, Mond JJ. Induction of IgG3 secretion by interferon-γ: a model for T cell independent type 2 antigens. J Exp Med 1992; 175:1367–1371.

53. Snapper CM, Paul WE. Interferon-γ and B cell stimulatory factor-1 reciprocally regulate Ig isotype production. Science 1987; 236:944–946.

54. Coffmann RL, Carty J. A T cell activity that enhances polyclonal IgE production and its inhibition by interferon-γ. J Immunol 1986; 136:949–953.

55. Finkelman FD, Katona IM, Mosmann T, Coffmann RL. IFN-γ regulates the isotypes of Ig secreted during in vivo humoral immune responses. J Immunol 1988; 140:1022–1025.

56. Snapper CM, Peschel C, Paul WE. IFN γ stimulates IgG2a secretion by murine B cells stimulated with bacterial lipopolysaccharide. J Immunol 1988; 140:2121–2125.

57. Finkelman FD, Svetic A, Gresser I, Snapper C, Holmes J, Trotta PP, Katona I, Gause WC. Regulation by interferon-α of immunoglobulin isotype selection and lymphokine production in mice. J Exp Med 1991; 174: 1179–1184.

58. Panitch HS, Francis GS, Hooper CJ, Merigan TC, Johnson KP. Serial immunological studies in multiple sclerosis patients treated systemically with α-interferon. Ann Neurol 1985; 18:434–438.

59. Rice GPA, Woelfel EL, Talbot PI, Braheny SL, Sipe JC. Immunological complications in multiple sclerosis patients receiving interferon. Ann Neurol 1985; 18:439–442.

60. Kastrukoff LF, Oger JJ, Tourtellotte WW, Sacks SL, Berkowitz J, Paty DW. Systemic lymphoblastoid interferon therapy in chronic progressive multiple sclerosis. II. Immunological evaluation. Neurology 1991; 41: 1936–1941.

61. O'Gorman MR, Oger J, Kastrukoff LF. Reduction of immunoglobulin G secretion in vitro following long term lymphoblastoid interferon (Wellferon) treatment in multiple sclerosis patients. Clin Exp Immunol 1987; 67:66–75.

62. Gupta SL. Regulation of interferon inducible genes. In: Baron S, Coppenhaver DH, Dianzani F, Fleischmann Jr. WR, Hughes Jr. TK, Klimpel GR, Niesel DW, Stanton GJ, Tyring SK, eds. Interferon: Principles and Medical Applications. Galveston, TX: University of Texas Medical Branch, Department of Microbiology, 1992:193–211.

63. Adams DO. Regulation of macrophage function by interferon-γ. In: Baron S, Coppenhaver DH, Dianzani F, Fleischmann Jr. WR, Hughes Jr. TK, Klimpel GR, Niesel DW, Stanton GJ, Tyring SK, eds. Interferon: Principles and Medical Applications. Galveston, TX: University of Texas Medical Branch, Department of Microbiology, 1992:341–351.

64. Durelli L, Bongioanni MR, Cavallo R, Ferrero B, Ferri R, Ferrio MF, Bradac GB, Riva A, Vai S, Geuna M, Bergamini L, Bergamasco B. Chronic systemic high-dose recombinant interferon-α_{2a} reduces exacerbation rate, MRI signs of disease activity, and lymphocyte interferon-γ production in relapsing-remitting multiple sclerosis. Neurology 1994; 44:406–413.

65. Novick D, Cohen B, Rubinstein M. The human interferon alpha/beta receptor: characterization and molecular cloning. Cell 1994; 77:391–400.

66. Uzé G, Lutfalla G, Gresser I. Genetic transfer of a functional human interferon-α receptor into mouse cells: cloning and expression of its cDNA. Cell 1990; 60:225–234.

67. Borden EC, Hogan TF, Voelkel JC. Comparative antiproliferative activity in vitro of natural interferons α and β for diploid and transformed human cells. Cancer Res 1982; 42:4948–4953.

68. Dianzani F. Interferon treatments: how to use an endogenous system as a therapeutic agent. J Interferon Res 1992; May, special issue: 109–118.

69. Goldstein D, Sielaff KM, Storer BE, Brown RR, Datta PL, Witt PL, Teitelbaum AP, Smalley RV, Borden EC. Human biologic response modification by interferon in the absence of measurable serum concentrations: a comparative trial of subcutaneous and intravenous interferon-β serine. J Natl Cancer Inst 1989; 81:1061–1068.

70. Ahstrom L, Dohlwitz A, Strander H, Carlstrom G, Cantell K. Interferon in acute leukemia in children. Lancet 1974; 1:166–167.

71. Glapsy JA, Marcus SG, Ambersley J, Golde DW. Recombinant beta-serine-interferon in hairy cell leukemia compared prospectively with results with recombinant alpha-interferon. Cancer 1989; 164:409–413.

72. Kagawa T, Morizane T, Saito H, Tsunematsu S, Tada S, Kumagai N, Tsuchimoto K, Sugiura H, Mukai M, Tsuchiya M. A pilot study of long-term weekly interferon-β administration for chronic hepatitis B. Amer J Gastroenterol 1993; 88:212–216.

73. Liberati AM, Fizzotti M, Di Clemente F, Senatore M, Berruto P, Falini B, Martelli MF, Grignani F. Response to intermediate and standard doses of IFN-β in hairy cell leukemia. Leukemia Res 1990; 14:779–784.

74. Liberati AM, Horisberger MA, Palmisano L, Astolfi S, Nastari A, Mechati S, Villa A, Mancini S, Arzano S, Grignani F. Double-blind randomized phase I study on the clinical tolerance and biological effects of natural and recombinant interferon-β. J Interferon Res 1992; 12:329–336.

75. Horisberger MA. Mx protein: function and mechanism of action. In: Baron S, Coppenhaver DH, Dianzani F, Fleischmann Jr. WR, Hughes Jr. TK, Klimpel GR, Niesel DW, Stanton GJ, Tyring SK, eds. Interferon: Principles and Medical Applications. Galveston, TX: University of Texas Medical Branch, Department of Microbiology, 1992:215–224.

76. The IFN-β Multiple Sclerosis Study Group. Interferon β-1b is effective in relapsing-remitting multiple sclerosis. I. Clinical results of a multicenter, randomized, double-blind, placebo-controlled trial. Neurology 1993; 43: 655–661.

77. Paty DW, Li DKB, the UBC MS/MRI Study Group, and the IFN-β Multiple Sclerosis Study Group. Interferon β-1b is effective in relapsing-remitting multiple sclerosis. II. MRI analysis results of a multicenter, randomized, double-blind, placebo-controlled trial. Neurology 1993; 43:662–667.

78. Platanias LC, Golomb HM. Clinical use of interferons: hairy cell, chronic myelogenous and other leukemias. In: Baron S, Coppenhaver DH, Dianzani F, Fleischmann Jr. WR, Hughes Jr. TK, Klimpel GR, Niesel DW, Stanton GJ, Tyring SK, eds. Interferon: Principles and Medical Applications. Galveston, TX: University of Texas Medical Branch, Department of Microbiology, 1992:487–499.

79. Steis RG, Smith II JW, Urba WJ, Clark JW, Itri LM, Evans LM, Schoenberger C, Longo DL. Resistance to recombinant interferon-α-2a in hairy-cell leukemia associated with neutralizing anti-interferon antibodies. N Engl J Med 1988; 318:1409–1413.

80. Michalevicz R, Aderka D, Frisch B, Revel M. Interferon-β induced remis-

sion in a hairy cell leukemia patient resistant to interferon-α. Leukemia Res 1988; 12:845–851.

81. The Italian Cooperative Study Group on Chronic Myelogenous Leukemia. Interferon α-2a as compared with conventional chemotherapy for the treatment of chronic myeloid leukemia. N Engl J Med 1994; 330:820–825.

82. Aulitzky WE, Peschel C, Depres D, Aman J, Trautman T, Tilg H, Rudolf G, Huttmann H, Obermeier J, Herold M, Huber C. Divergent in vivo and in vitro antileukemic activity of recombinant interferon β in patients with chronic-phase chronic myelogenous leukemia. Ann Hematol 1993; 67: 205–211.

83. Saracco G, Rosina F, Abate ML, Chiandussi L, Gallo V, Cerutti E, Di Napoli A, Solinas A, Deplano A, Tocco A, Cossu P, Chien D, Quo G, Polito A, Weiner AJ, Houghton M, Verme G, Bonino F, Rizzetto M. Long-term follow-up of patients with chronic hepatitis C treated with different doses of interferon-α-2b. Hepatology 1993; 18:1300–1305.

84. Hoofnagle JH. Interferon therapy of viral hepatitis. In: Baron S, Coppenhaver DH, Dianzani F, Fleischmann Jr. WR, Hughes Jr. TK, Klimpel GR, Niesel DW, Stanton GJ, Tyring SK, eds. Interferon: Principles and Medical Applications. Galveston, TX University of Texas Medical Branch, Department of Microbiology, 1992:433–462.

85. Saracco G, Mazzella G, Rosina F, Cancellieri C, Lattore V, Raise E, Rocca G, Giorda L, Verme G, Gasbarrini G, Barbara L, Bonino F, Rizzetto M, Roda E. A controlled trial of human lymphoblastoid interferon in chronic hepatitis B in Italy. Hepatology 1989; 10:336–341.

86. Fattovich G, Farci P, Rugge M, Brollo L, Mandas A, Pontisso P, Giustina G, Lai ME, Belussi F, Busatto G, Balestrieri A, Ruol A, Alberti A. A randomized controlled trial of lymphoblastoid interferon-α in patients with chronic hepatitis B lacking HBeAg. Hepatology 1992; 15:584–589.

87. Gauci L. Management of cancer patients receiving interferon-α-2a. Int J Cancer 1987; 40(suppl 1):21–30.

88. Mitchell G. Update on multiple sclerosis therapy. Med Clin North Am 1993; 77:231–249.

89. Meyers CA, Scheibel RS, Forman AD. Persistent neurotoxicity of systemically administered interferon-α. Neurology 1991; 41:672–676.

90. Iivanainen M, Laaksonen R, Niemi ML, Farkkila M, Bergstrom L, Mattson K, Niranen A, Cantell K. Memory and psychomotor impairment following high-dose interferon treatment in amyotrophic lateral sclerosis. Acta Neurol Scand 1985; 72:475–480.

91. Kanda Y, Shigeno K, Kinoshita N, Nakao K, Yamo M, Matsuo H. Sudden hearing loss associated with interferon. Lancet 1994; 343:1134–1135.

92. Papo T, Marcellin P, Bernuau J, Durand F, Poynard T, Benhamou JP. Autoimmune chronic hepatitis exacerbated by α-interferon. Ann Intern Med 1992; 116:51–53.

93. Waguri M, Hanafusa T, Itoh N, Inagawa A, Miyagawa J, Kawata S, Kono N, Kuwajoima M, Matsuzawa Y. Occurrence of IDDM during interferon therapy for chronic viral hepatitis. Diabetes Res Clin Pract 1994; 23:33–36.

94. Batocchi AP, Evoli A, Servidei S, Palmisani MT, Apollo F, Tonali P. Myasthenia gravis during interferon alfa therapy. Neurology 1995; 455:382–383.
95. Huber M, Bamborschke S, Assheuer J, Heiss WD. Intravenous natural interferon treatment of chronic exacerbating-remitting multiple sclerosis: clinical response and MRI/CSF findings. J Neurol 1988; 235:171–173.
96. Kinnunen E, Timonen T, Pirttila T, Kalliomaki P, Ketonen L, Matikainen E, Sepponen R, Juntunen J. Effects of recombinant α-2b interferon therapy in patients with progressive MS. Acta Neurol Scand 1993; 87:457–460.
97. Knobler RL, Greenstein JI, Johnson KP, Lublin FD, Panitch HS, Conway K, Grant-Gorsen SV, Muldoon J, Marcus SG, Wallenberg JC, Williams GJ, Yoshizawa CN. Systemic recombinant human interferon-β treatment of relapsing-remitting multiple sclerosis: pilot study analysis and six-year follow-up. J Interferon Res 1993; 13:333–340.
98. Neilly LK, Goodin DS, Goodkin DE, Mohr D, Hauser SL. Side-effect profile of interferon beta-1b in MS: results of an open label trial. Neurology 1996; 46:552–554.
99. AUSTIMS Research Group. Interferon-α and transfer factor in the treatment of multiple sclerosis: a double-blind, placebo-controlled trial. J Neurol Neurosurg Psychiatry 1989; 52:566–574.
100. Camenga DL, Johnson KP, Alter M, Engelhardt D, Fishman PS, Greenstein JI, Haley AS, Hirsch RL, Kleiner JE, Kofie WY, Koski CL, Margulies SL, Panitch HS, Valero R. Systemic recombinant α2 interferon therapy in relapsing multiple sclerosis. Arch Neurol 1986; 43:1239–1246.
101. Jacobs L, Salazar AM, Herndon R, Reese PA, Freeman A, Josefowicz R, Cuetter A, Husain F, Smith WA, Ekes R, O'Malley JA. Multicentre double blind-study of effect of intratechally administered natural human fibroblast interferon on exacerbations of multiple sclerosis. Lancet 1986; 2:1411–1413.
102. Knobler RL, Panitch HS, Braheny SL, Sipe JC, Rice GPA, Huddlestone JR, Francis GS, Hooper CJ, Kamin-Lewis RM, Johnson KP, Oldstone MBA, Merigan TC. Systemic α-interferon therapy of multiple sclerosis. Neurology 1984; 34:1273–1279.
103. Greenstein JI, Knobler RL, Johnson KP, Marcus SG, Panitch HS, Lublin FD, Hassett RM, Wilson JR, Russick AM, Haley AS, Grant SV. A phase I clinical trial of human recombinant β-interferon in relapsing-remitting multiple sclerosis. J Neuroimmunol 1987; 16(suppl 1):66.
104. Krown SE. Clinical trials of interferons in human malignancy. In: Pfeffer LM, ed. Mechanisms of Interferon Actions. Vol. II. Boca Raton, FL: CRC Press, 1987:144–178.
105. Kurtzke JF. Rating neurologic impairment in multiple sclerosis: an expanded disability status scale (EDSS). Neurology 1983; 33:1444–1452.
106. Koopmans RA, Li DKB, Oger JJF, Mayo J, Paty DW. The lesion of multiple sclerosis: imaging of acute and chronic stages. Neurology 1989; 39:959–963.
107. Miller DH, Barkhof F, Berry I, Kappos L, Scotti G, Thompson AJ. Magnetic resonance imaging in monitoring the treatment of multiple sclerosis: concerted action guidelines. J Neurol Neurosurg Psychiatry 1991; 54:683–688.

108. McFarland HF, Frank JA, Albert PS, Smith ME, Martin R, Harris JO, Patronas N, Maloni H, McFarlin DE. Using gadolinium-enhanced magnetic resonance imaging lesions to monitor disease activity in multiple sclerosis. Ann Neurol 1992; 32:758–766.

109. Nauta JJP, Barkhof F, Thompson AJ, Miller DH. Magnetic resonance imaging in monitoring the treatment of multiple sclerosis patients: statistical power of parallel-groups and crossover designs. J Neurol Sci 1994; 122: 6–14.

110. Sipe JC, Knobler RL, Braheny SL, Rice GPA, Panitch HS, Oldstone MBA. A neurologic rating scale (NRS) for use in multiple sclerosis. Neurology 1984; 34:1368–1372.

111. Borden E, Paulnock D, Spear G, Byrne G, Merrit J, Brown R. Biological response modification in man: measurement of interferon-induced proteins. In: Baron S, Dianzani F, Stanton GJ, Fleischmann WR Jr, eds. The Interferon System: A Current Review. Austin, TX: University of Texas Press, 1986:1–7.

112. Durelli L, Poccardi G, Cavallo R. CD8^{+high} CD11b^{+low} T cells (T suppressor-effectors) in multiple sclerosis cerebrospinal fluid are increased during high dose corticosteroid treatment. J Neuroimmunol 1991; 31:221–228.

113. Weinshenker BG, Bass B, Rice GPA, Noseworthy J, Carriere W, Baskerville J, Ebers GC. The natural history of multiple sclerosis: a geographically based study. 2. Predictive value of the early clinical course. Brain 1989; 112:1419–1428.

114. Willoughby EW, Grochowski E, Li DKB, Oger J, Kastrukoff LF, Paty DW. Serial magnetic resonance scanning in multiple sclerosis: a second prospective study in relapsing patients. Ann Neurol 1989; 25:43–49.

115. Harris JO, Frank JA, Patronas N, McFarlin DE, McFarland HF. Serial gadolinium-enhanced magnetic resonance imaging scans in patients with early, relapsing-remitting multiple sclerosis: implications for clinical trials and natural history. Ann Neurol 1991; 29:548–555.

116. Panitch HS. Interferons in multiple sclerosis. A review of the evidence. Drugs 1992; 44:946–962.

117. Baron S, Coppenhaver DH, Dianzani F, Fleischmann Jr. WR, Hughes Jr. TK, Klimpel GR, Niesel DW, Stanton GJ, Tyring SK. Introduction to the interferon system. In: Baron S, Coppenhaver DH, Dianzani F, Fleischmann Jr. WR, Hughes Jr. TK, Klimpel GR, Niesel DW, Stanton GJ, Tyring SK, eds. Interferon: Principles and Medical Applications. Galveston, TX: University of Texas Medical Branch, Department of Microbiology, 1992:1–15.

118. Sibley WA, Bamford CR, Clark K. Clinical viral infections and multiple sclerosis. Lancet 1985; 1:1313–1315.

119. Panitch HS, Bever CT, Katz E, Johnson KP. Upper respiratory tract infections trigger attacks of multiple sclerosis in patients treated with interferon (abstr). J Neuroimmunol 1991; 35(suppl 1):125.

120. Panitch HS. Influence of infection on exacerbations of multiple sclerosis. Ann Neurol 1994; 36(suppl 1):S25–S28.

121. Compston A. Future prospects for the management of multiple sclerosis. Ann Neurol 1994; 36(suppl 1):S146–S150.
122. Noronha A, Toscas A, Jensen MA. IFN-β down-regulates IFN-γ production by activated T cells in MS (abstr). Neurology 1991; 41(suppl 1):219.
123. Katz P, Whalen G, Mitchell RS, Cupps TR, Evans M. Modulation of suppression of mitogen-induced T cell-dependent B cell responses by natural killer cells. Clin Immunol Immunopathol 1990; 55:148–155.
124. Jacobs LD, Cookfair DL, Rudick RA, Herndon RM, Richert JR, Salazar AM, Fischer JS, Goodkin DE, Grauger CV, Simon JH, Alan JJ, Bartoszak DM, Bourdette DN, Braiman J, Brownscheidle CM, Coats ME, Cohan SL, Dougherty DS, Kinkel RP, Mass MK, Munschauer FE, Priore RL, Pullicino PL, Scherokman BJ, Weinstock-Guttman B, Whitham RH and The Multiple Sclerosis Collaborative Research Group (MSCRG). Intramuscular interferon beta-1a for disease progression in relapsing multiple sclerosis. Ann Neurol 1996; 39:285–294.
125. Sheremata WA, Squillacote D, Sazant A. Stabilization of relapsing-remitting and progressive multiple sclerosis with natural interferon-α: a preliminary trial (abstr). Ann Neurol 1994; 36:327.
126. Jacobs L, Munschaner F. Treatment of multiple sclerosis with interferons. In: Rudick R, Goodkin D, eds. Treatment of Multiple Sclerosis. London: Springer-Verlag, 1992:233–250.

13

Interferon β-1a Treatment of Multiple Sclerosis

Robert M. Herndon

Jackson Veterans Administration Medical Center, Jackson, Mississippi

I. INTRODUCTION

The Multiple Sclerosis Collaborative Research Group (MSCRG) was formed initially by Lawrence Jacobs, M.D., Andres Salazar, M.D. and Robert Herndon, M.D. in the early 1980s shortly after β interferons (IFNs) became available in sufficient quantities for testing. Dr. Jacobs did a preliminary trial with intrathecal natural IFN-β (1,2) based on evidence that IFNs do not cross the blood-brain barrier in appreciable concentrations (3) later confirmed (4) and the assumption that they would have to get into the central nervous system to have an effect. This initial pilot trial was followed by a modified double-blind study using 1×10^6 international units, (IU) of natural human IFN-β dissolved in 9 ml of Elliot's B solution and 1 ml sterile water injected intrathecally once weekly for 4 weeks and then monthly for 5 additional months. Control multiple sclerosis (MS) patients had an initial and final lumbar puncture (LP) to collect cerebrospinal fluid with sham LPs at other times. That is, they were prepped and anesthetized in the normal manner, the needle was inserted but did not penetrate the dura, and 5 ml of sterile water was injected before withdrawing the needle (5).

The data revealed a decrease in attack rate from 1.79 to 0.76 per year in treated MS patients versus a drop from 1.98 to 1.48 per year in the placebo group over a period of 2 years following initiation of treatment.

This was statistically significant at the 0.001 level. Thus, the effect of intrathecal administration appeared to continue after completion of treatment. However, in addition to the disadvantage represented by a cumbersome method of administration, intrathecal IFN, like peripherally administered IFNs, caused flu-like muscle aches and pains. In addition, a chemical meningitis with elevated cerebrospinal (CSF) cell counts which ranged from 12 to 560/mm^3 and elevated protein, mean 59 mg/dl, range 24–160 mg/dl, were seen in the first 4 weeks of treatment with lesser elevations seen when treatments were a month apart. Whether the pleocytosis resulted from the IFN per se or from contaminants in the lyophilized preparation is not clear; although given the limited purity of the preparation, contaminants may well have been responsible for the reaction (see Chapter 11). Post–lumbar puncture headaches were occasionally seen but were rarely a problem, and few patients experienced meningismus despite the CSF pleocytosis (6).

The decision to investigate the efficacy of intramuscular recombinant IFN β-1a by the MSCRG was a direct outgrowth of the study of natural IFN-β administered intrathecally. Experience from the intrathecal study strongly influenced the design of the subsequent intramuscular study. In particular, the trend toward a slower rate of progression on the Kurtzke scores suggested that progression on the Kurtzke scale could be used as a primary endpoint. By the time of the subsequent study application, studies had shown that IFN effects could be detected in the CSF even if the IFN itself did not cross the blood-brain barrier in measurable quantities (7,8) (see chapter by Witt). As a result, the investigators believed that peripheral administration might be effective and if so, it would be much more acceptable to patients. The initial proposal to the National Institutes of Health (NIH) for the subsequent study included an intrathecal arm which was felt to be indicated given the previous positive result. However, this arm was dropped on the recommendation of the NIH review committee, to the relief of the investigators who felt the intrathecal arm would complicate the study and make recruitment more difficult.

II. INTRAMUSCULAR IFN β-1a TRIAL

A. Dose and Dosing Schedule

Natural sequence glycosylated recombinant IFN β-1a (Avonex, Biogen), produced in Chinese hamster ovary cells, lyophilized and stabilized in human albumin was used for the study, with placebo patients receiving lyophilized human albumin. The dose of 6 × 10^6 IU was arrived at from a preliminary trial indicating that this was the highest dose in which the side effects could be consistently suppressed by acetaminophen (9). It was felt that higher doses would carry too high a risk of unmasking due to side effects. The once a week dosing schedule was also based on the preliminary trial which demonstrated that β_2-microglobulin in the CSF remained elevated for a week following intramuscular injection of 6 × 10^6 IU of IFN β-1a (9). Acetaminophen was used just before and 3–4 hrs after each dose to minimize side effects.

B. Trial Design

The trial was designed as a double-blind placebo-controlled study using separate treating and examining physicians to avoid any possibility that laboratory abnormalities or side effects of the medication would compromise the blind. Examining physicians were not allowed to discuss symptoms, side effects, or examination results with the patients. Examinations were done every 6 months. Interval examinations were also performed when the treating physician or patient reported new symptoms suggestive of an exacerbation.

C. Clinical Evaluation

Time to disease progression on the Kurtzke extended disability status scale (EDSS) was used as the endpoint. This was viewed by the investigators as a more stringent but also more reliable endpoint than attack frequency. It was felt to be more reliable because the patients' subjective judgment is needed to identify many of the new attacks. Additionally, some patients, particularly those who live at a distance, may not report attacks, because it is inconvenient for them to come in for examination. Once a new attack is suspected, arrangements for examination alert the examining physician to the fact that the patient thinks an attack is occurring. Thus, if there is any risk that the patient is not blind to treatment, it could alter the result. Although such an interval attack could presumably influence the examining physician's subsequent examination, this was felt to be a low risk. We did elect to use exacerbation frequency as a secondary endpoint to allow comparison of this study with other recent studies (10,11).

The investigators had extensive discussions regarding use of disability as the primary endpoint. It was felt to carry considerable risk of failure, since no drug had ever been found to be effective using disability as a standard in a double-blind setting. On the other hand, slowing of the rate of progression of disability has far more important implications than a reduction in attack rate. Following a preliminary training session, it was determined that the examining physicians could reliably detect a one point change on the Kurtzke EDSS in the range from 1.0 to 4.5 (12). It was also the opinion of the investigators that the EDSS, which despite its flaws is widely regarded as the standard for MS trials, would provide a more meaningful measure of the effect of the drug on the course of the disease than would the number of new attacks. The primary outcome was thus chosen as time to treatment failure defined as a one-point increase in EDSS score found on two successive examinations 6 months apart; that is, "sustained" progression. Basically, if the score was more than one point worse than baseline at two successive examinations 6 months apart, the subject was considered a treatment failure. For example, if entry score was 2, the score following an attack was 5, and 6 months later was 2, it was not a treatment failure; if the 6-month score was 3 or higher, it was considered treatment failure. Similarly, scores of 2, 5, 4 were counted as sustained progression at an EDSS of 4. The 6-month time interval was chosen to eliminate the possibility that the change was temporary worsening due to a recent attack. The number of new attacks, magnetic resonance imaging (MRI) plaque load, number and volume of enhancing lesions on MRI, timed gait, nine-hole peg test, and neuropsychological testing were planned secondary outcome measures. MRI with and without contrast was done annually using a standardized protocol. Examinations by the examining physicians were done every 6 months on study and additional examinations were done whenever the patient reported worsening or was suspected of having an exacerbation of MS on a scheduled telephone interview. An on-study exacerbation was defined as the development of new or worsening of preexisting neurological symptoms, lasting more than 48 hrs, in a patient who had been stable or improving for the past 30 days. On-study exacerbation required objective change on neurological examination, defined as a change of 0.5 points on the EDSS or a worsening by 1 point on the pyramidal, cerebellar, brainstem, or visual functional status scale.

Patients selected for this study were between the ages of 18 and 55 years with definite relapsing-remitting MS of greater than 1 year of duration, with at least two attacks in the last 3 years. Exacerbations had to be documented in the medical record to be accepted for study entry purposes. The patients had to have an EDSS of 1.0–3.5 inclusive and to be at least 2 months from their last exacerbation. Exclusion criteria included prior use of IFNs, prior use of immunosuppressant drugs other than steroids, and any disease requiring specific continuing treatment or compromising organ function. Patients of both sexes had to be using an acceptable form of birth control to prevent pregnancy.

D. Statistical Assumptions

Sample size was calculated for survival analysis with time to sustained worsening by one point on the EDSS as the primary outcome using an intent to treat methodology. It was assumed the 50% of the placebo patients would progress in 2 years, whereas only 33% of the treated patients would progress (12,13). It was planned to have a statistical power of 80% to detect the group difference at the 0.05 level of significance. Sample size estimates were conservative in that they allowed for a 25% treatment discontinuation in the treatment arm and that these patients would behave similarly to the placebo group. It also assumed that 10% of patients would be lost to follow-up.

When the statistician reported that only 5% of patients had stopped treatment and only 1% were lost to follow-up, and as a result, the study had reached the calculated statistical power, discussion ensued regarding whether or not to continue the study as planned or to terminate early. Some investigators argued that we should continue the study to gain any additional power we could. Others argued that if we could not show an effect with the power assumptions we had calculated initially, the amount of benefit would not be enough to be worthwhile. The latter argument carried the day, and the study was terminated early. A total of 301 patients had been randomized between the treatment and placebo arms at the four clinical sites: Buffalo, NY, Cleveland, OH, Portland, OR, and Washington, DC.

E. On-Study Therapy of Attacks

Treatment of on-study attacks was permitted. Initially, this was limited to adrenocorticotropin (ACTH); however, early in the study, it became apparent that in the general neurological community, the standard treatments with ACTH or oral prednisone had been superseded by intravenous (i.v.) methylprednisolone, so a standard methylprednisolone protocol was established which could be used to treat on-study attacks. The protocol was approved by the institutional review boards of each of the participating institutions. The study was monitored by an NIH safety monitoring committee.

F. Results

Time to sustained progression, the primary outcome, was significantly longer in treated than in control patients. The change in EDSS over 2 years was +0.247 in treated patients and +0.736 in placebo recipients (*P*

= .02). Projected median time to progression was increased by 74% with a decrease in estimated progression rate at 1 and 2 years of 40% (14).

Annual exacerbation rate among patients who were on study for 2 or more years was 0.90 in placebo patients and 0.61 in IFN β-1a recipients, a 32% reduction (P = .002). The number of exacerbation-free patients in the treated group was reduced, but this did not reach statistical significance (P = .099). Median time to first exacerbation was longer in treated than in placebo patients, but the difference did not reach statistical significance (P = .34). More than twice as many placebo patients as treated patients had three or more exacerbations. Subsequent analyses using a two point change on the Kurtzke scale, time to Kurtzke 4, and time to Kurtzke 6, all showed a statistically significant difference at a better than 0.05 level for each of these measures.

G. MRI

Standard T_1- and T_2-weighted MRI scans and gadolinium-enhanced scans were obtained at baseline, 1 year, and 2 years using a standardized positioning and imaging technique (14). No difference between treated and placebo groups was seen in the accumulation of T_2-weighted high signal areas over the course of the study. On the other hand, there were significant reductions in the volume (P = .02) and number (P = .02) of gadolinium-enhancing lesions at year 1, and these differences were maintained at year 2 (14).

H. Adverse Events

Flu-like muscle aches and pains, chills, fever, and asthenia were reported more frequently in recipients than in controls (P < .08). Such symptoms were generally mild, and the median number of days on which they occurred was 7. Mild anemia was seen in 8% of treated and 3% of placebo patients. This was never severe enough to warrant transfusion, reduction in dosage, or discontinuation of study drug. Injection site reactions and menstrual disorders were seen in equal number in both arms of the study. There was no evidence of leukopenia, liver enzyme elevation, or thrombocytopenia in treated patients.

Serum anti-IFN activity occurred in 14% of treated patients at 52 weeks and 23% at 104 weeks. Such activity was seen at some time in 4% of placebo patients but was not found on repeat testing.

There was one death in the study which occurred in a patient on drug. The patient had an underlying cardiac condition, and death was attributed to cardiac arrhythmia induced by small pulmonary emboli which were found at autopsy. This was thought to be unrelated to the treatment.

There was no increase in depression in either group on the Beck depression scale. Depression occurred in 12% of placebo patients and 11% of treated patients.

III. DISCUSSION

Results of the IFN β-1a and the IFN β-1b (Betaseron) trials are quite comparable despite major differences in dose,* dosing frequency, and route of administration. It appears that the alternate-day 8.3×10^6 IU subcutaneous dose of IFN β-1a results in a fairly constant, low blood level of IFN, whereas the weekly intramuscular IFN β-1a provides a bolus. There is evidence that blood levels are higher, although transient, with IFN β-1a (15,16). Although this presumably could be due to the intramuscular versus subcutaneous injection, it seems more likely that water solubility is enhanced by the glycosylation of IFN β-1a, leading to more rapid absorption.

There are several reasons why the less frequent dosing with IFN β-1a might be as effective as every other day doses. First, the changes induced by a fairly constant low level of IFN may be subject to tachyphylaxis, with a reduced response compared with the intermittent dosage. Alternatively, the antiviral effect of the drug or the maximal immunological effect may depend as much or more on maximum blood or tissue level as it does on total dose.

The recent work by Challoner et al. (17) implicating herpesvirus type 6 in MS is particularly interesting in this regard. Although this work has generally been downplayed as just another viral candidate, the author believes this is an extremely important discovery highly relevant to the use of IFNs in MS. First, most, if not all, human herpes viruses are latent in nervous tissue and when latent, cannot be structurally identified, so they would not be likely to be found on electron microscopy. Second, herpes viruses, like MS, are activated by other viral infections. Third, a number of herpes viruses cause demyelination. Fourth, herpes viruses are transported within axons and spread, in part, by axonal transport often causing patchy involvement of the nervous system. Finally, as with most other childhood exanthems, including measles, mumps, and chickenpox,

---

* Dosage of interferon β-1a (30 mcg or 6×10^6 IU) and β-1b (300 mcg and 8.3×10^6 IU) cannot be directly compared. IFN β-1a is tested against a natural human IFN reference standard and IFN β-1b against a recombinant standard. The units may not be equivalent. The author has been unable to locate or obtain a direct comparison between these two. Additionally, units are measured in tissue culture based on the ability of the compound to induce viral resistance in tissue cultures, which may not correlate with in vivo biological effects in MS where there may be additional differences between the effects of the drugs.

MS would represent an infrequent chronic central nervous system viral sequel to the primary illness.

The occurrence of anti-IFN activity in the serum of patients using the two different preparations was quite different. Patients receiving Betaseron appear to be much more likely to have anti-IFN activity than recipients of IFN β-1a. To our knowledge, however, there has not been a direct comparison of anti-IFN activity in these two groups using the same test. Whether the anti-IFN activity results wholley or in part from antibody formation, or if other factors are involved, has also not been established. IFN β-1b, which has an amino acid substitution and is not glycosylated, would be expected to be more antigenic than IFN β-1a, and this could account for some of the difference in clinical effectiveness (18).

IV. FUTURE STUDIES

There is, at present, no reason to believe that we have found or are anywhere near optimal dosing with IFNs in MS. Dose selection for IFN β-1b was based on pilot trials which included a dose twice that used in the phase III trial. Apparently, the higher dose was poorly tolerated and would have been very difficult to mask. A decision was made not to use the higher dose in the controlled trial. In the case of IFN β-1a, the dose was the highest the investigators thought they could give in a double-blind trial without a significant risk of breaking the blind, at least for the patients and treating physicians.

Side effects and laboratory abnormalities have rarely been limiting in these patients, and both higher doses and more frequent dosing could be tried. It took more than 30 years after the introduction of steroids before the current high-dose regimens were tested and accepted. We need to begin to look at the effects of different doses and dosing intervals if we are to optimize therapy. In addition, we need to look at the possibility of combined therapies with COP-1. If the work of Challoner et al. (17) holds up, combinations with antiviral agents such as ganciclovir known to be effective against herpes virus type VI with IFNs are possible. We also need to understand in much more detail the effect of steroids used in conjunction with IFNs.

REFERENCES

1. Jacobs L, O'Malley J, Freeman A, Ekes R. Intrathecal interferon reduces exacerbations of multiple sclerosis. Science 1981; 214:1026–1028.
2. Jacobs L, O'Malley J, Freeman A, Ekes R. Intrathecal interferon in multiple sclerosis. Arch Neurol 1982; 39:609–615.
3. Emodi G, Just M, Hernandez R, et al. Circulating interferon in man after administration of exogenous human leukocyte interferon. J Natl Cancer Inst 1975; 54:1045–1049.

4. Smith RA, Norris F, Palmer D, et al. Distribution of alpha interferon in serum and cerebrospinal fluid after systemic administration. Clin Pharmacol Ther 1985; 37:85–88.

5. Jacobs L, Herndon R, Freeman, A, et al. Multicentre double-blind study of effect of intrathecally administered natural human fibroblast interferon on exacerbation of multiple sclerosis. Lancet 1986; 2:1411–1413.

6. Jacobs L, Salazar A, Herndon R, et al. Intrathecally administered natural human fibroblast interferon reduces exacerbations of multiple sclerosis: results of a multicenter double-blind study. Arch Neurol 1987; 44:589–595.

7. Flenniken A, Galabru J, Rutherford M, et al. Expression of interferon-induced genes in different tissues of mice. J Virol 1988; 62:3077–3083.

8. Wong GH, Bartlett PH, Clark LI, et al. Inducible expression of H-2 and Ia antigens on brain cells, Nature 1984; 310:688–691.

9. Jacobs L, Munschauer FE. Treatment of multiple sclerosis with interferons. In: Rudick RA, Goodkin DE, eds. Treatment of Multiple sclerosis: Trial Design, Results and Future Perspectives. London: Springer-Verlag 1992: 223–250.

10. The IFNB Multiple Sclerosis Study Group. Interferon beta-1b is effective in relapsing-remitting multiple sclerosis. I. Clinical results of a multicenter, randomized, double-blind placebo-controlled trial. Neurology 1993; 43: 655–661.

11. Bornstein M, Miller A, Slagle S, et al. A pilot trial of COP-1 in exacerbating-remitting multiple sclerosis. N Engl J Med 1987; 317:408–414.

12. Goodkin DE, Cookfair D, Wende K, et al. Inter- and intrarater scoring agreement using grade 1.0 to 3.5 on the Kurtzke expanded disability status scale. Neurology 1992; 42:859–863.

13. Jacobs L, Cookfair D, Rudick R, et al. A Phase III Trial of Intramuscular Recombinant Interferon Beta for Exacerbating-Remitting Multiple Sclerosis: Design and Conduct of Study; Baseline Characteristics of Patients. Multiple Sclerosis 1995; 1:118–135.

14. Jacobs LD, Cookfair DL, Rudick RA, et al. Intramuscular interferon beta-1a for disease progression in relapsing multiple sclerosis. Ann Neurol 1996; 39:285–294.

15. Gomi K, Morimoto M, Inoue A, et al. Pharmacokinetics of human recombinant interferon-β in monkeys and rabbits. Gann 1984; 75:292–300.

16. Alam J, Biogen Corp. Personal communication.

17. Challoner PB, Smith KT, Parker JD et al. Plaque-associated expression of human herpesvirus 6 in multiple sclerosis. Proc Natl Acad Sci 1995; 92: 7440–7444.

18. The IFNB Multiple Sclerosis Study Group and the University of British Columbia MS/MRI Analysis Group. Interferon beta 1b in the Treatment of Multiple Sclerosis. Final Outcome of the Randomized Trial. Neurology 1995; 45:1277–1285.

19. Sediq SA, Revesz KJ, Lassman AB, Miller JR. Antibodies to interferon β in patients with multiple sclerosis: detection and clinical effects. Neurology 1996; 42:A136.

14

Interferon β-1b (Betaseron) Treatment of Multiple Sclerosis

Robert L. Knobler

Jefferson Medical College, Philadelphia, Pennsylvania

I. OVERVIEW: WHAT IS MULTIPLE SCLEROSIS?

Multiple sclerosis (MS) is characterized by patchy areas of demyelination within the central nervous system (CNS), which includes the brain, spinal cord, and optic nerves but excludes the peripheral nervous system (1). The demyelinated lesions, typically located around postcapillary venules of the myelin-rich CNS white matter, are characterized by perivascular cuffing of inflammatory cells which then infiltrate into the surrounding tissue (Fig. 1).

In the brain, the areas surrounding the ventricles are most commonly affected in MS. (Fig. 2). A predeliction for periventricular and related sites may be a reflection of the slower rate of blood flow which occurs in these territories. Adhesion is a prerequisite of the penetration and passage of activated inflammatory cells through the lining of the blood vessel wall (transendothelial migration). Adhesion is facilitated by slow blood flow (sludging), and the presence of specific adhesion molecules, which have corresponding counterpart molecules on the invading inflammatory cells (Fig. 3).

Experimental models of MS, such as experimental allergic encephalomyelitis (EAE), have been used to demonstrate that this step of inflammatory cell adhesion and then penetration can be blocked by specific antibodies to the relevant adhesion molecules (2), demonstrating that adhesion

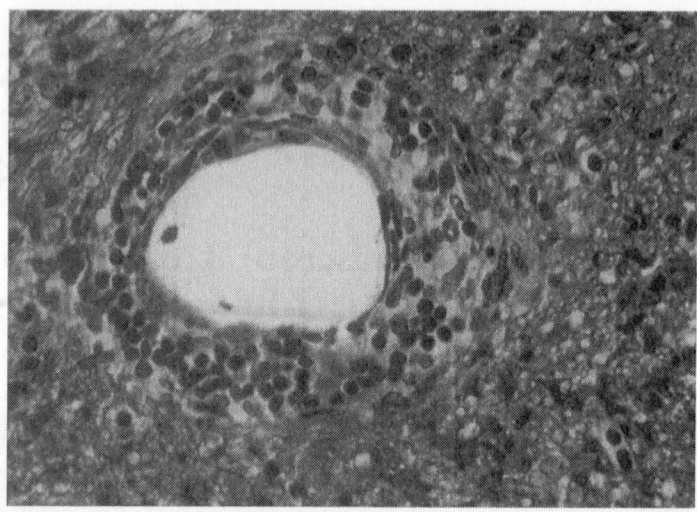

Figure 1 Perivascular infiltrate forming a cuff, surrounding a postcapillary ven-ule, located at the border of an active MS lesion in the cerebral white matter. Hypertrophic, sometimes multinucleated astrocytes are also present in the area surrounding the perivascular cuff. Magnification × 140. (Adapted from Traugott U. In: Cook SD, ed. Handbook of Multiple Sclerosis. New York: Marcel Dekker, 1990:107.)

is an essential step in the development of an inflammatory demyelinating lesion. This is an important focus of current research directed at prevent-ing the entry of these inflammatory cells into the CNS compartment in MS.

Demyelination and edema occur in MS lesions after the entry of inflam-matory cells. This usually leaves the structure of the demyelinated nerve fiber (axon) intact, with the potential for recovery by remyelination. How-ever, axonal loss, with the consequence of permanent atrophic changes in the tissue over time (3), may occur as a result of particularly severe lesions or repeated inflammatory assaults.

II. ELECTROPHYSIOLOGY

In classic demyelination, conduction of the nerve impulse is most com-monly disrupted by at least two mechanisms (4). One is from the loss of myelin (Fig. 4A,B), whereas the other is from the impact of local edema (Fig. 5) (see also direct effects of cytokines in chapters by Dafney and

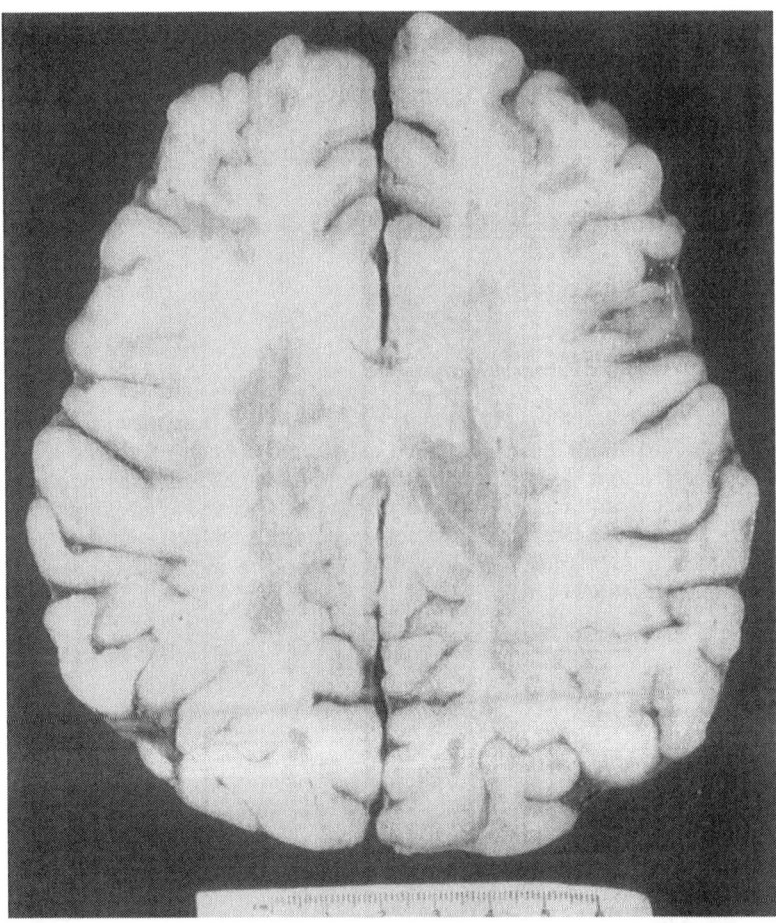

Figure 2 Brain slice demonstrating periventricular plaques (MS lesions). The plaques are characterized as darker areas of the cerebral white matter near the ventricles and can be identified by the absence of myelin staining when the normal myelin of the surrounding white matter has been highlighted to appear as black through the use of a special myelin stain. (Adapted from Prineas JW. In: Cook SD, ed. Handbook of Multiple Sclerosis. New York: Marcel Dekker, 1990:188.)

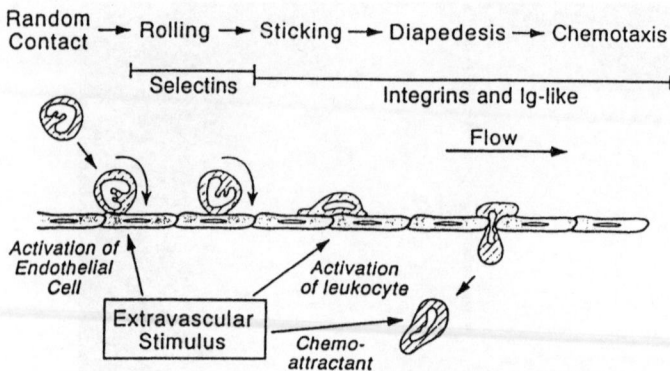

Figure 3 Adhesive interactions during leukocyte emigration from the circulation into the surrounding tissue are represented as random contact → rolling with endothelial cell activation → sticking (firm adhesion) → diapedesis (transendothelial migration) → chemotaxis (subendothelial migration). (Derived as an adaptation of Lasky LA. Selectins: Interpreters of cell-specific carbohydrate information during inflammation. In: Carlos TM, Harlan JM. Leukocyte-endothelial adhesion molecules. Blood 1994; 84(7):2068–2101.)

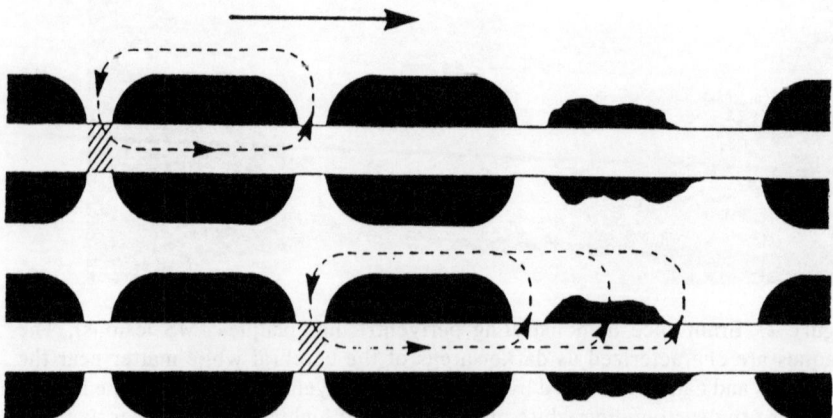

Figure 4 Conduction in a normal portion (top) and a demyelinated portion (bottom) of an axon. In the normal myelinated regions (top), high-resistance myelin serves as an insulator so that the action potential is shunted from one node of Ranvier to the next, to facilitate saltatory conduction. This permits rapid, energy-efficient, repetitive conduction. In contrast, in the demyelinated region (bottom), the action potential is diffused over a larger area, reducing conduction velocity, energy efficiency, and the capacity for reptitive conduction. Under severe circumstances, conduction may be completely blocked. Demyelinated fibers are extremely sensitive to elevated temperatures, which further reduce their efficiency, worsening symptoms. (From Waxman SG. In: Cook SD, ed. Handbook of Multiple Sclerosis. New York: Marcel Dekker, 1990:230.)

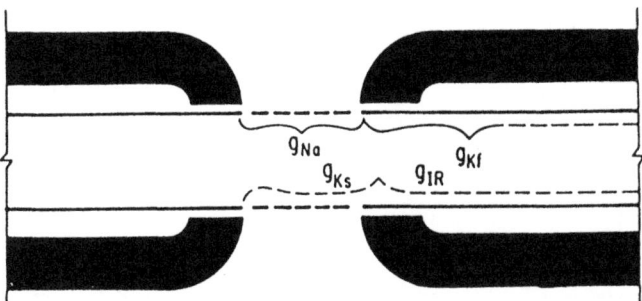

Figure 5 Distribution of ion channels at the node of Ranvier (g_{Na} = sodium channels, clustered at the node of Ranvier; g_{Kf} = fast potassium channels, responsible for repolarization of the action potential, are present in the internodal axonal membrane; g_{Ks} = slow potassium channels; g_{IR} = inward rectifier channels). Following demyelination, which is usually initiated in the paranodal region, there is a change in the distribution of ion channels. There is a lower density of sodium channels, and a higher density of fast potassium channels, both of which negatively impact upon conduction. Clinically, this is worsened by edema. Agents such as 4-aminopyridine improve conduction by blocking these potassium channels. Steroid use in clinical practice also has an immediate benefit through the reduction of edema with a resulting positive impact on impulse conduction, as well as an additional long-term impact associated through reduction of the cellular inflammatory response, thus reducing their sequelae as well. (From Waxman SG. In: Cook SD, ed. Handbook of Multiple Sclerosis. New York: Marcel Dekker, 1990:229.)

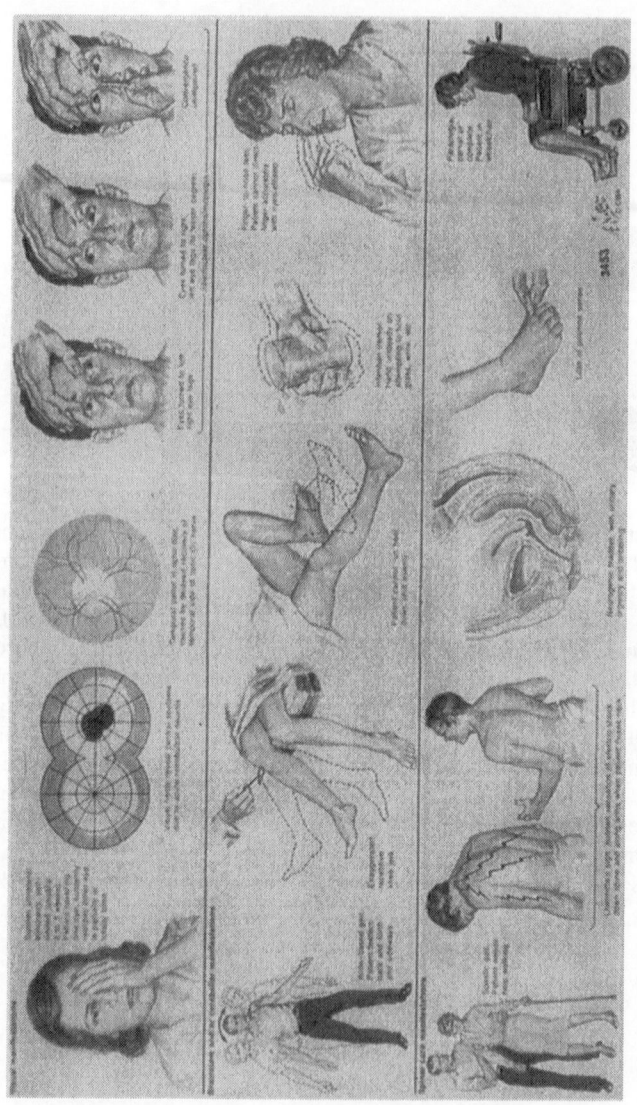

Figure 6 Clinical manifestations of MS, focusing on visual manifestations affecting either visual acuity or control of eye movements, brainstem, cerebellar, and spinal cord manifestations. (From Netter FH, Kott HS, Jones HR Jr, eds. Multiple sclerosis: Clinical manifestations. Section IX: Demyelinating Disorders of Central Nervous System. The CIBA Collection of Medical Illustrations, Volume I, Nervous System, Part II, Neurologic and Neuromuscular Disorders. West Caldwell, NJ: CIBA, 1986: 174–175.)

Table 1 Clinical Evoked Potentials

Visual evoked potential (VEP)	Motor evoked potential (MEP)
Brainstem auditory evoked potential (BAEP)	Central motor conduction time
Somatosensory evoked potential (SSEP)	Upper extremity
Upper extremity	Lower extremity
Lower extremity	

Source: Nuwer MR. Evoked potentials. In: Cook SD, ed. Handbook of Multiple Sclerosis. New York: Marcel Dekker, 1990:271–290.

Pliskin. In any case, altered nerve conduction leads to symptoms which reflect the location of these demyelinating and edematous lesions (Fig. 6). Clinical evoked potential tests are used to quantitatively measure these abnormalities (Table 1).

III. EXACERBATION OF SYMPTOMS

The onset of symptoms in MS can be quite sudden. This is commonly referred to as an acute attack (exacerbation/relapse/flare). Initially, symptoms are more due to the rapid onset of edema than to demyelination. In other cases, lesion development may be slower, suggesting there is less immediate edema and that inflammation gradually produces demyelination and gliosis. Under these circumstances, the recognition of progressive clinical worsening only occurs with the passage of time.

IV. BLOOD-BRAIN BARRIER DISRUPTION

The blood-brain barrier (BBB) is a unique restriction to the passage of cells and other substances into the CNS (Fig. 7). The BBB gets disrupted as new lesions form (5). Our current perceptions assume that this step must occur in order for inflammatory cells to enter the CNS and for a lesion to develop. However, disruption of the BBB may be the consequence of inflammation rather than a prerequisite for its occurrence (6). In both laboratory models of MS and the human disease, lesions preferentially occur at sites in which the BBB is present. They are not localized to those regions of the brain in which cells can freely enter the CNS because the BBB is not naturally present. This strongly suggests that the entry of inflammatory cells into the brain is highly selective, locally regulated, and can occur independently of the breakdown of the BBB (Fig. 8).

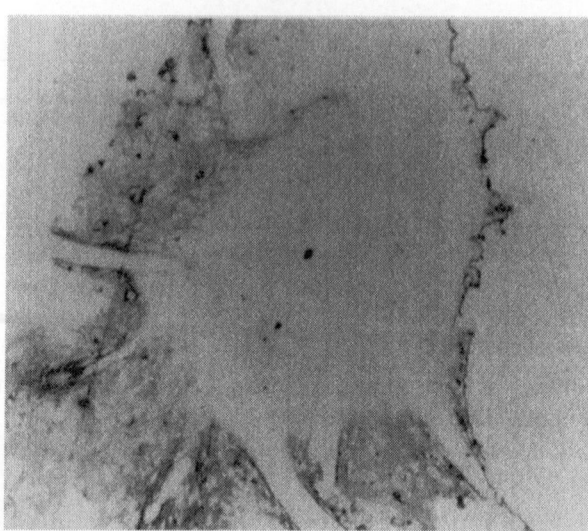

Figure 7 Normal exclusion of molecules by function of the blood-brain barrier. Horseradish peroxidase is excluded from the tissue because of the integrity of the blood-brain barrier. (From Knobler RL, Marini JC, Goldowitz D, Lublin FD. Distribution of the blood-brain barrier in heterotopic brain transplants and its relationship to the lesions of EAE. J Neuropathol Exp Neurol 1992; 51:36–39.)

$\longrightarrow$

Figure 9 Use of gadolinium as a contrast agent in T1-weighted (short relaxation time; TR, 600 msec; TE, 20 msec), axial images, which typically show new lesions as having low signal intensity. Use of the high signal contrast agent gadolinium, which passes through the damaged blood-brain barrier (BBB), serves as the earliest detectable indicator of tissue damage in early MS lesions. Typically, these lesions have no associated mass effect. In the unenhanced T1-weighted image (left), the lesion is demonstrated as a low signal intensity focus (arrow). This lesion enhances (right), appearing as a high signal area (double arrows), after the administration of gadolinium. Of significant interest, there is loss of gadolinium enhancement following treatment of patients with Betaseron (IFN beta-1b), as well as following treatment with steroids, suggesting such therapy improves the integrity of the BBB (Stone LA, Frank JA, Alberts PS, et al. The effect of interferon-β on blood-brain barrier disruption demonstrated by contrast-enhanced magnetic resonance imagery in relapsing-remitting multiple sclerosis. Ann Neurol 1995; 37:611–619). (From Yetkin FZ, Haughton VM. Common and uncommon manifestations of MS on MRI. MRI Decisions 1992; (Nov/Dec):13–18.)

Activated Lymphocyte ->

Random Contact of Cerebrovascular Endothelium ->

Lymphocyte Rolling Along the Cerebrovascular Endothelium ->

Cerebrovascular Endothelial Cell Activation ->

Lymphocyte Sticking (Firm Adhesion) ->

Lymphocyte Transendothelial Migration ->

Subendothelial Migration ->

Local Lesion Chemotaxis Signals ->

BBB Breakdown ->

Recruitment of Additional Cells

Figure 8 Postulated sequence of events at the blood-brain barrier (BBB), based on various sources of data, indicates multiple steps involved in the initial entry of immune-mediated inflammatory cells into the central nervous system compartment. In this model, available data suggest that the initial entry of activated inflammatory cells selectively occurs at BBB sites and precedes BBB breakdown. After BBB breakdown, there is enhanced recruitment and entry of a greater variety of additional inflammatory cells due to local chemoattractants. (Adapted from Knobler RL, Marini JC, Goldowitz D, Lublin FD. Distribution of the blood-brain barrier in heterotopic brain transplants and its relationship to the lesions of EAE. J Neuropathol Exp Neurol 1992; 51:36–39.)

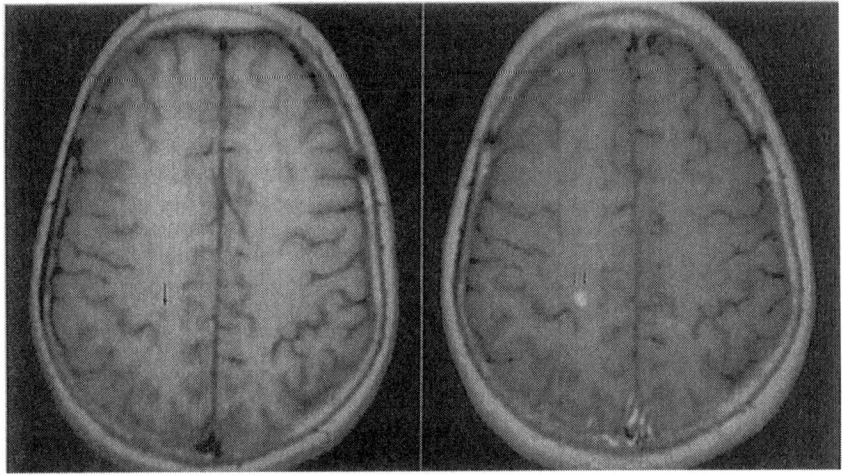

Figure 9

BBB breakdown, however, does occur as a lesion progresses, allowing more cell entry into the brain. This is used clinically as a marker of an active MS lesion, that is, "lesion activity." Intravenous injection of salts of the heavy metal gadolinium have successfully been used to mark those brain areas in which the BBB is disrupted (7). BBB breakdown allows gadolinium to leak into the brain, and this is visualized by using T_1-weighted magnetic resonance imaging (MRI). These gadolinium-enhancing lesions are scored as active lesion sites or lesion activity, and they serve as one measure of disease activity (Fig. 9).

V. SERIAL MRI—CHANGING CONCEPT OF MS

The use of serial MRI studies, at 2- to 6-week intervals (8–10) has demonstrated that new lesions can appear at the same time that old lesions disappear and presumably are resolving (Fig. 10A,B). Recognition of the simultaneous appearance and occurrence of these two opposing processes, new lesion development and lesion resolution, has necessitated a dramatic departure from the previously held notions defining an MS exacerbation.

In the past, it was believed that lesions developed only during the time of an exacerbation, and that this was a systemically regulated event reflecting an all out attack on the CNS. A clinical state of remission was believed to be associated with lesion resolution. However, based on serial brain MRI studies, it is now recognized that at any given point in time a new lesion can be forming while another is resolving, and this may or may not be associated with the appearance or resolution of clinical symptoms.

Thus, lesion formation is not confined to the time of a clinical exacerbation, and remission is not confined to the time of lesion resolution. Instead, the picture is broadened to include some lesions which become clinically relevant and others which may remain subclinical. This suggests that local vascular and tissue factors, which may be influenced by systemic events, control the tempo of this disease. This further focuses attention on events at the local BBB regulating lesion development and resolution. If there is no transendothelial migration of mononuclear cells across the BBB, there will be no new lesion activity.

Although activated inflammatory cells may be found with increased frequency in the circulation of patients with MS during the time of an acute viral infection, it is the local milieu at any given postcapillary venule that determines whether a new lesion will form, whether edema will resolve, and whether gliosis rather than remyelination will prevail. Because these inflammatory events are ongoing, as demonstrated by the serial MRI studies, it is quite likely that the most effective approach to the treatment

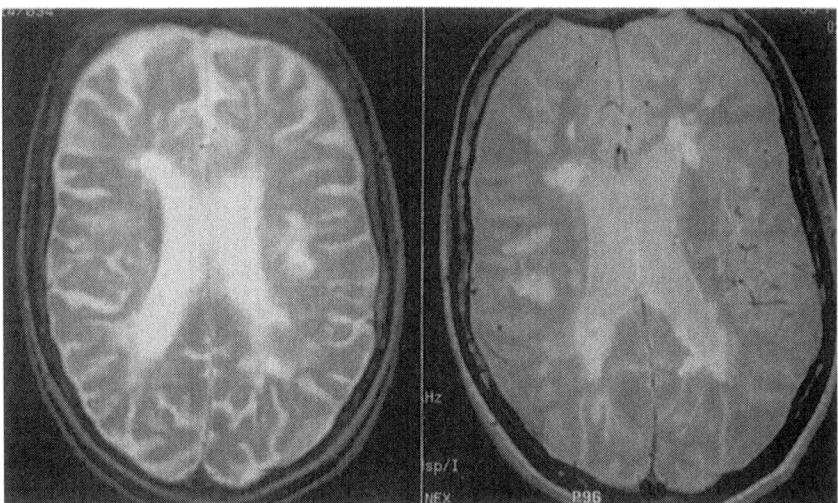

Figure 10 Magnetic resonance images of the same patient are provided at two different time points, 3 months apart, to illustrate the changing appearance of MS lesions in the brain of a patient with relapsing-remitting MS. These images demonstrate that new lesions appear in some areas, while older lesions are resolving, and indicate that the local environment has a significant influence on lesion formation and resolution. The scan on the left was obtained with a long relaxation time (TR: 2216.7 msec; TE: 90 msec). The scan on the right was obtained 3 months later (TR: 4000 msec; TE: 18 Ef—fast spin echo). (Adapted from Frank JA, Stone LA, Smith ME, et al. Serial contrast-enhanced magnetic resonance imaging in patients with early relapsing-remitting multiple sclerosis: Implications for treatment trials. Ann Neurol 1994; 36(Suppl):S86–S90.)

of MS will be one which is preemptive and impacts on these processes in an ongoing fashion rather than past strategies that have focused primarily on treatment after the occurrence of a clinical attack.

VI. LESION BURDEN: A SURROGATE MARKER FOR MS

Lesion activity on the cerebral MRI seems to be a good indicator of future clinical course rather than a direct correlate of neurological disability. Neuropsychological deficits are an exception and do correlate with lesion burden (11–13). Specifically, the more lesion activity detected on cerebral MRI, the more likely is greater future neurological disability. This is based on the notion that MRI "lesion activity" is predictive of future "lesion burden" (Fig. 11) and "clinical disability" (Fig. 12). In this way, the MRI is useful as a "surrogate" marker of disease activity rather than as a precise measure of how a patient is clinically affected at a specific point in time.

Although MRI lesion activity may be in a constant state of flux, new clinical symptoms only become apparent when either a critical CNS volume or specific neuroanatomical pathway is affected by demyelination or edema. It must be emphasized that some lesions observed on the MRI are clinically silent (Fig. 13). Moreover, the correlation between the Kurtzke

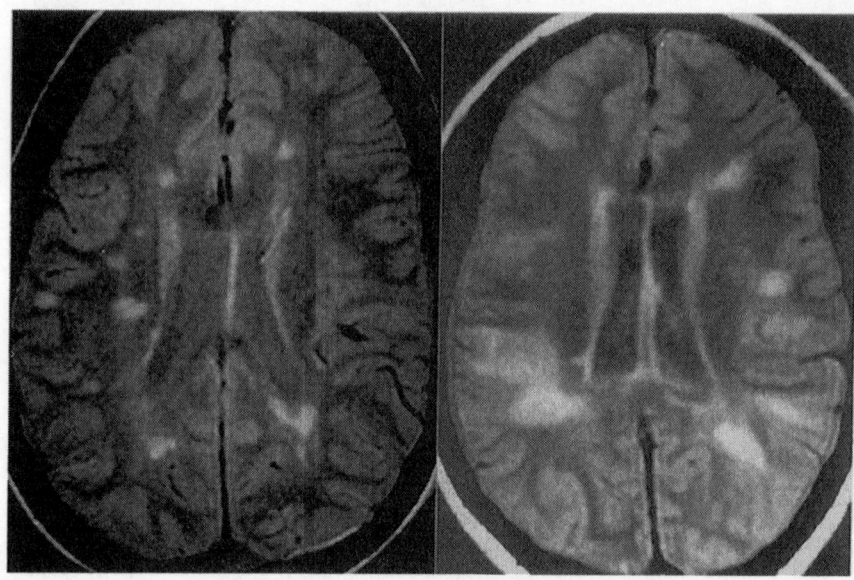

Figure 11 Lesion burden refers to the accumulated lesion load as calculated by either the tracing of lesions and the addition of their accumulated areas, or through the use of newer computer-assisted methods which are dependent upon the application of sophisticated algorhythms. The two different images provided demonstrate the inherent difficulty in manually defining the MS lesion load from the surrounding tissue. (From Paty DW, Li DKB, The IFNB Multiple Sclerosis Study Group. Interferon beta 1b is effective in relapsing-remitting multiple sclerosis: MRI results of a multicenter randomized double blind, placebo controlled trial. Neurology 1993; 43:662–667; Gonzalez CF, Vinitski S, Lublin FD, et al. Tissue segmentation and volumetric measurements as a marker of disease activity in MS (abstract). Neurology 1995; 45(Suppl):4251.)

Lesion Activity (new or enlarging lesions) ->

Lesion Burden (accumulated lesion load)->

Clinical Disability (neurological impairment)

Figure 12 Lesion activity—the new appearance or enlargement of either a T2-weighted lesion or a gadolinium-enhanced T1-weighted lesion on the cerebral MRI. The best clinical correlate of cerebral MRI lesions is a change in either mood (i.e., depression, euphoria, mixed mood state) or cognitive function. Lesion burden indicates the accumulated lesion load on a T2-weighted cerebral MRI. Clinical disability addresses a variety of issues, such as the clinical impairment of the patient. Efforts are often directed toward correlating the Kurtzke Expanded Disability Status Score (EDSS), with the MRI lesion burden. However, it must be kept in mind that the EDSS is typically more affected by the brainstem and spinal cord lesions of MS than by the cerebral lesions being measured in such a paradigm. (Adapted from Swirsky-Sacchetti T, Mitchell DR, Seward J, et al. Neuropsychological and structural brain lesions in multiple sclerosis: A regional analysis. Neurology 1992; 42:1291–1295.)

expanded disability status score (EDSS), a 10-step scale divided by half-step intervals (14), and MRI findings is only $r = 0.3$, which, although highly significant, indicates that a big piece of the picture is being missed. It is this gap between a given MRI observation and the actual clinical state of the patient that remains a bit difficult to predict with accuracy at present, but the concept that increased lesion activity will lead to increased lesion burden and increased clinical disability over time is quite accurate.

Therefore, MRI is clearly an important adjunct to the clinical examination of patients with MS. Through the use of MRI segmentation analysis, which allows computer-aided visual separation of different tissue components, it is now feasible further to differentiate tissue components. MRI segmentation analysis can identify the total MS lesion burden as an objectively measured endpoint (15) even more accurately than by previous manual lesion tracing techniques (16). For example, gliosis can now be visually separated from demyelination/edema (Fig. 14). In this way, MRI can be used as a screening tool in future MS therapeutic clinical trials to differentiate patients with demyelination/edema, who are more likely to be responsive to treatments, from those with significant fixed lesions and gliosis, who are less likely to be responsive to treatments.

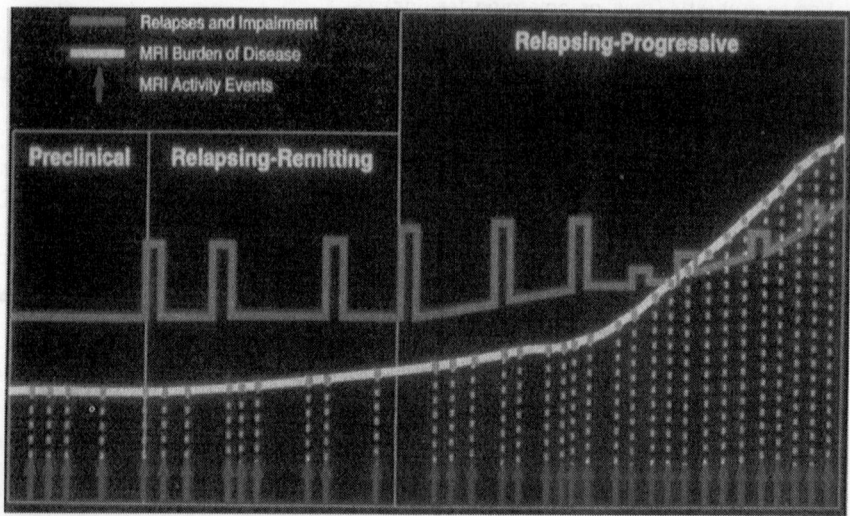

Figure 13 Overview of current thinking regarding the natural history of MS. It is now appreciated that there are many subclinical events initially; although detected as new lesion activity when performing frequent cerebral MRI examinations, these lesions are not associated with detectable clinical symptoms. MRI lesion activity is indicated in the bottom row of arrows. The continuous line, immediately above the arrows, represents the accumulated cerebral lesion burden, which increases over time in studies of the natural history of MS. The interrupted top line represents changes in clinical course and degree of neurological impairment over time. No clinical activity is noted during the asymptomatic preclinical stage of the disease, although MRI cerebral lesion activity is evident. There are periods of worsening (exacerbations or relapses), followed by improvement (remissions), sometimes back to baseline, during the relapsing-remitting phase of MS. Over time, with accumulated lesion burden, there is increased clinical impairment, during the secondary progressive phase (also previously called the chronic progressive or the relapsing-progressive phase). The correlation between the cerebral MRI and neurological impairment is best evident when using cognitive impairment as the measure of clinical deficit. (Derived from Paty DW, adapted from Wolinsky JS.)

VII. CLINICAL DISABILITY IN MS

Clinical disability in MS is scored, at present, through the use of several scales (17). Unfortunately, none of these scales is ideal. All of the scales have been devised to display data generated from clinical trials to evaluate the impact of different therapies on neurological disability (Table 2), and

Table 2   Clinical Scales

Kurtzke Expanded Disability Status Scale (EDSS)
Scripps Neurological Rating Scale (NRS)
The Troiano Scale
The Upper Limb Scale
The Ambulation Index (AI)
The Quantitative Examination of Neurologic Function (QENF)

Source: Whitaker JN, McFarland HF, Rudge P, Reingold SC. Outcomes assessment in multiple sclerosis clinical trials: A critical analysis. Mult Scler 1991; 1:37–47. Goodkin DE, Hertsgaard D, Seminary J. Upper extremity function in multiple sclerosis: Improving assessment sensitivity with box-and-block and nine-hole peg tests. Arch Phys Med Rehabil 1988; 69:850–854. Hauser SL, Dawson DM, Lehrich JR, et al. Intensive immunosuppression in progressive multiple sclerosis. N Engl J Med 1983; 308:173–180.

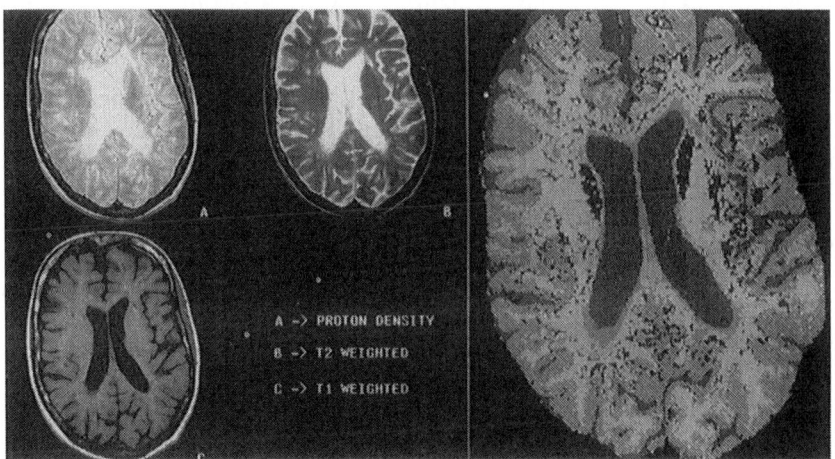

Figure 14   Tissue segmentation image of MS lesions is presented and the MR images from which it was derived. (Left) (A) proton density, (B) T2-weighted, and (C) T1-weighted images, respectively, from which the segmentation analysis (tissue separation), was performed. In this way, different tissue components were defined, and colors were assigned to illustrate these findings. In the original, the cerebrospinal fluid is blue, the cerebral cortex is gray, the normal white matter is yellow, the deep gray matter is green, and the MS lesions are illustrated in red and pink; the red areas correspond to gliotic lesions, with less potential for remyelination; the pink areas correspond to demyelination and edema, areas with greater potential for remyelination. Such analysis can be used to measure lesion volume over time as well, so that it has applicability in the conduct of future therapeutic clinical trials. (Adapted from Gonzalez CF, Vinitski S, Lublin FD, et al. Tissue segmentation and volumetric measurements as a marker of disease activity in MS (abstract). Neurology 1995; 45(Suppl):4251.)

there is a correlation between increased lesion burden and worsened clinical disability status. The EDSS, a nonlinear scale, has been most widely used, but it was designed to reflect whether a patient is better, the same, or worse after treatment. Unfortunately, it has not been used that way. Instead, it has been abused when treatments are evaluated as producing a "one point improvement" on the EDSS, since this does not have the same impact on the patient at the low end of the scale as it would if that improvement had occurred for patients classified in the middle and higher ends of the scale, and is, therefore, misleading as used.

At this time, I personally favor the Scripps neurological rating scale (NRS) (18), since it is a direct numerical representation of the overall clinical findings obtained during the neurological examination and is weighted to reflect the impact of such changes on the patient. The NRS too is not perfect, since the "weightings" were arbitrarily chosen, but changes in this score with treatment are a closer approximation to the true status of the patient. The Scripps score fluctuates most when there are changes in the neurological examination that have a dramatic impact on the overall function of the patient. The NRS has been used in at least four clinical trials to date (19–22), and all investigations have agreed on its usefullness in assessing severity of neurological deficits.

VIII. CLINICAL COURSE OF MS

Quite typically, the MS lesion process of inflammation, edema, and demyelination is self-limited, and symptoms associated with a given lesion will begin to resolve over a 4- to 6-week period after onset. This corresponds to the phase of remission, a time at which edema has resolved and remyelination, if any, has begun. Differences in clinical course between relapsing-remitting (RR), secondary progressive (SP), and primary progressive (PP) forms of MS can be appreciated clinically and with the MRI.

In RR MS, there is relatively little residual glial scarring (gliosis) or axonal loss (Fig. 15). In contrast, in the SP form of MS, there is progressive gliosis and axonal loss, as detected by an increased degree of white matter atrophy on the cerebral or spinal MRI (Fig. 16). The SP and PP courses of MS have usually been grouped as forms of relapsing progressive and chronic progressive MS, but there has been an effort at redefining these descriptors more accurately to reflect differences in their natural history and potentially their responses in clinical trials. In PP MS, lesions and their sequelae are usually localized to the spinal cord. The sequelae include slow expansion of foci of spinal cord demyelination and edema, progressing to gliosis and atrophy, without evident remission.

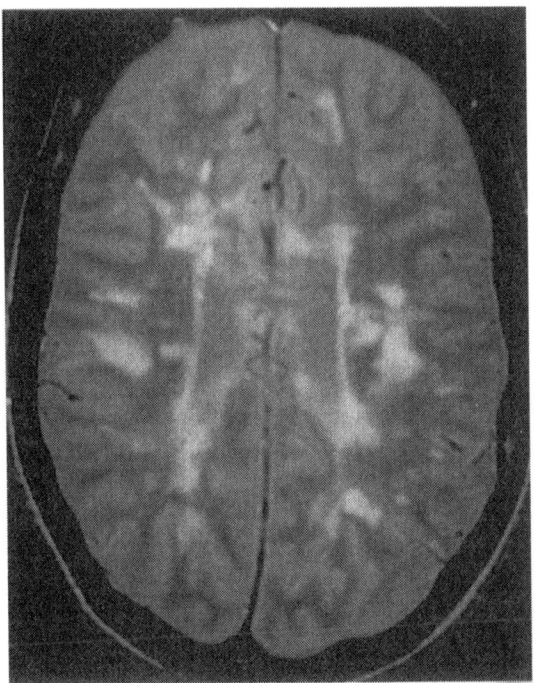

Figure 15 MRI characteristics of relapsing-remitting MS. Proton density cerebral MR image (long relaxation time; TR, 2500 msec; TE, 30 msec), of a patient with relapsing-remitting MS. Many oblong, periventricular, and subcortical high signal intensity lesions are present. These are referred to as "Dawson's fingers." When three or more such lesions are present, the likelihood of MS in the differential diagnosis of the image is high. These high signal lesions are scattered throughout the cerebral white matter and have a "fluffy" character most often associated with a relapsing-remitting course of MS. Such lesions will typically appear and disappear independently over time. (Adapted from Horowitz AL, Kaplan RD, Grewe G, et al. The ovoid lesion: A new MR observation in patients with multiple sclerosis. AJNR 1983; 10:303–305.)

Patients with abundant gliotic and/or atrophic areas would be expected to be less likely to respond to current therapeutic intervention strategies. Therefore, alternative therapeutic approaches must be sought and applied for this population. In contrast, patients with primarily demyelination and edema are most likely to respond to a variety of forms of therapeutic

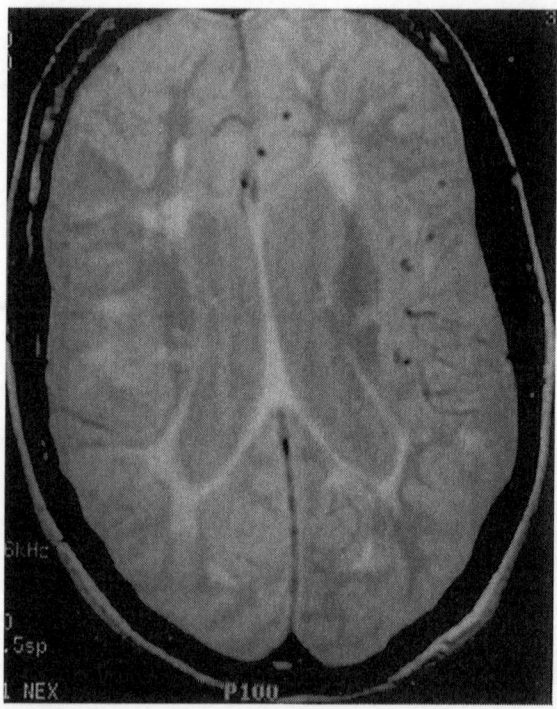

Figure 16 MRI signal characteristics of secondary-progressive MS. Proton density cerebral MR image (long relaxation time; TR, 2433 msec; TE, 30 msec), of the same patient shown in Figure 15, but 3 years later, now manifesting features of secondary-progressive MS. Dawson's fingers are no longer the most obvious feature on the scan, although many periventricular and subcortical high signal intensity lesions are present. There has been a change in the the appearance of the lesions and the size of the ventricles, which also corresponds to a change in the neuropsychological status of this patient. The lesions are primarily confluent and "smoothed," in appearance, more characteristic of gliosis associated with the secondary-progressive course of MS. Cerebral atrophy is also identified in this scan, and associated hydrocephalus ex vacuo is noted, which in part represents both the more compacted structure of gliotic tissue, as well as axonal loss. The patient had greater cognitive difficulties at this time, which correlate with the appearance of this scan. (Adapted from Rao SM, Leo GJ, Haughton VM, et al. Correlation of magnetic resonance imaging with neuropsychological testing in multiple sclerosis. Neurology 1989; 39:161–166; Swirsky-Sacchetti T, Mitchell DR, Seward J, et al. Neuropsychological and structural brain lesions in multiple sclerosis: A regional analysis. Neurology 1992; 42:1291–1295.)

intervention. The earlier any therapy which can limit the development of new lesions from forming can be applied, the greater the likelihood this will prevent further progression of this disease.

IX. ETIOLOGY OF MS

The cause of MS remains unknown at the present time, although current thinking implicates a genetic predisposition, sensitivity to an environmental trigger, such as a coincidental viral infection, and an elicited immune response resulting in CNS demyelination. The nature of the genetic predisposition for MS presently remains unknown, but is likely multigenic. MS is not considered an inherited disease, although there are hereditary diseases with abnormalities of myelin, such as adrenoleukodystrophy and Leber's hereditary optic atrophy (23–25). Concordance of MS in identical twins is at most 30% (26–28), which is similar to another multigenic autoimmune disease, diabetes mellitus (29). Lack of 100% concordance in identical twins supports the importance of environmental factors in the pathogenesis of MS, but it does not exclude the possible contribution of mitochondrial DNA, which can be distributed to identical twins in some disequilibrium (30).

An intriguing hypothesis on the etiology of MS suggests the possibility that the genetic predisposition to MS reflects a heightened immune response, providing increased antibody production and an enhanced capacity of immune cells to infiltrate the CNS (Fig. 17). This may have afforded

Hypothesis - "MS Affords Survival Value"
    Increased antibody protection and
    Enhanced capacity of cells to infiltrate into the CNS
    A "naïve" host, without such abilities would not likely survive
        neuronal infection with a neuropathic agent

A consequence of heightened "immune reactivity" is
    varying degrees of rapid and abundant release of
    inflammatory cytokines (i.e, TNF), complement,
    proteolytic enzymes, hydrogen peroxide, nitric oxide
    in myelinated pathways, and inflammatory demyelination

Myelinated pathways may selectively be affected not because of
    antigen specificity, but because of slower flow (rheology),
    allowing adhesion and entry of inflammatory cells
    Antigen reactivity may then occur in individuals
        with heightened immune reactivity
        in response to myelin breakdown

Figure 17 Hypothesis of pathogenesis of MS.

survival value in populations possessing such a trait when they encountered viruses or other pathogens having the capacity to infect and perhaps kill cells of the CNS. In a "naive" host, encounter with such a pathogen would have been expected to lead to death, particularly by loss of neurons. However, possession of the "survival trait" would have led to the generation of a rigorous immune response within the CNS, permitting survival of neuronal cells, and thus the host. Demyelination could have occurred as a direct effect of the pathogen or as a consequence of this vigorous inflammatory response. A variety of "environmental triggers," including viruses (31) and seasonal allergens (32), could serve to "activate" the immune system, thus leading to the entry of inflammatory cells into the CNS compartment, initiating this process.

X. TARGET ANTIGEN

A specific antigenic target to which the immune system responds in MS has not yet been found despite repeated efforts. MS plaques could represent a response within the CNS to a latent or persistent infectious agent, which has been a focal point of much of the research over the past 40 years (33); expression of a sequestered developmental form of myelin antigen (exon 2) during remyelination (34); or alternatively, a response characterized as "molecular mimicry" (35). In the latter, the immune system targets a pathogen which has a shared amino acid sequence or configuration which is also present within the CNS white matter, such as myelin basic protein (MBP), proteolipid protein (PLP), or some other component of myelin (36). Heat shock proteins crossreacting with MBP (37), and bacterial molecules acting as superantigens (38; see also Chapter 17) have also been suggested as possible mechanisms of immune reactivity, but it is also possible that there may be no specific antigen in MS, and that the disease represents a disorder of cell trafficking.

Identification of the antigenic target in MS would be important in developing a specific immunotherapy for this disease by blocking reactivity to this molecule. Nevertheless, activation of the immune system by any target may be sufficient to allow immune cells to enter into the CNS of people with MS (39). The occurrence of the inflammatory process locally within the CNS can lead to "bystander" demyelination (40). This is currently believed to occur through the local release of cytokines, such as tumor necrosis factor (TNF) (41), which has experimentally been observed to cause demyelination at pathological doses (42) and to disrupt the function of the myelin-forming oligodendrocytes at more physiological doses (43).

Demyelination could also be the consequence of an immune-mediated attack directed at antigenic determinants of the astrocyte (44), a supporting glial cell, which is in immediate proximity to oligodendrocytes. If the astrocyte is indeed the target of immune attack in MS, then efforts directed at the identification of antigenic determinants in the oligodendrocyte or its myelin sheath in MS for the purpose of treatment (i.e., oral tolerization to myelin) might not alter the response to this target of immune attack. The role of the astrocyte in MS, is an important developing area of study.

XI. MS THERAPY

A. Adrenocorticotropin/Steroids

Recognition that MS lesions are caused by the action of the immune system has focused attention on the need to block the entry of inflammatory cells into the CNS. This can be accomplished in a variety of ways.

When the antigen is known, the afferent limb of the immune system can be blocked through desensitization to that antigen (tolerization). This is the theoretical basis for the therapeutic protocol of oral tolerization to myelin. Unfortunately, the antigen(s) of MS is unknown, although novel potential candidate molecules, such as heat shock proteins described above (37), and the mechanisms regulating their expression, are continually being sought. Therefore, this approach remains under active investigation.

Alternatively, adhesion molecules (see Fig. 3), important in mononuclear cell trafficking into the CNS, can be blocked through the use of specific monoclonal antibodies in animal models of MS (2). This strategy will likely require repetitive pulses of treatment to suppress new lesion formation in humans, since the MRI data shows that lesion activity is ongoing. Studies to determine the effectiveness of such an approach in humans await the availability of the specific monoclonal antibodies for human use.

Treatment of the inflammatory lesion with intravenous (i.v.) adrenocorticotropin (ACTH) or corticosteroids has been the mainstay for addressing the immediate consequences of tissue disruption and edema during acute exacerbations in both RR and SP MS. A variety of toxic immunosuppressive agents (Table 3) has been evaluated for use in MS patients when they no longer respond to the use of ACTH or corticosteroids. The most aggressive approach involves the suppression of either the effector arm alone or the immune system globally. In general, this strategy is less desirable because of the generally toxic properties of the drugs needed to achieve this goal, and the need for an intact immune system for immune surveillance against malignancies and to prevent opportunistic infections with viruses or fungi (e.g., PML, herpes simplex virus 1, candidiasis).

Table 3 Toxic Immunosuppressive Agents

Azathioprine (Imuran)	Cyclosporine (Sandimmune)
Cladribine (Leustatin)	Methotrexate
Cyclophosphamide (Cytoxan)	Mitoxantrone (Novantrone)

Source: Ellison GW. Experimental therapies for multiple sclerosis: Historical perspective. In: Rudick RA, Goodkin DE, eds. Treatment of Multiple Sclerosis: Trial Design, Results and Future Perspectives. Heidelberg, Germany: Springer-Verlag, 1992:1–15. Sipe JC, Romine JS, Koziol JA, et al. Cladribine in treatment of chronic progressive multiple sclerosis. Lancet 1994; 344:9–13.

The clinically used protocols for treatment with ACTH/steroids (Table 4) have been developed through trial and error, with only ACTH having undergone the rigors of a therapeutic clinical trial (45). In recent years, the relative merits of i.v. over oral therapy with corticosteroids has been described through anecdotal reports. Intravenous methylprednisolone is generally accepted, although not proven, as the standard form of therapy for an acute exacerbation of MS (46).

The value of i.v. over oral steroid treatment protocols have been supported by a direct comparison of the effectiveness of these agents in an optic neuritis treatment trial (47). However, the observed superiority of i.v. dosing may be more of a reflection of the 10-fold higher i.v. dose of drug as compared with the oral dose administered in that trial than of a true route-based difference in effectiveness of methylprednisolone. Further exploration of the effectiveness of orally delivering higher doses of methylprednisolone is needed.

The use of IV ACTH or methylprednisolone hastens the resolution of symptoms, especially when administered soon after their onset. These drugs do not work by promoting immediate remyelination but instead rapidly resolve tissue edema, which itself can lead to altered nerve conduction and symptoms (4). This mechanism of effectiveness of the steroids has been corroborated through the use of MRI studies (48).

ACTH and corticosteroids likely impact disability in MS through both immunosuppressive mechanisms, reducing inflammation, and through improved conduction of nerve impulses. Since these are anti-inflammatory molecules, they also lead to a decreased secretion of cytokines such as TNF, which are cytotoxic to oligodendrocytes, and interleukin-1 (IL-1) and other molecules which have been implicated as a causes of fatigue. Patients often "feel better" after a course of steroids, but this is usually transient.

Table 4 ACTH and Steroid Protocols for Treatment of MS

ACTH
　100 units intravenously in 250 cc D5W
　Infuse over 6 hr for each of 10 days

Prednisone (10 mg tablets orally), 110 tablets
　80 mg daily for three days = 24 pills
　70 mg daily for three days = 21 pills
　60 mg daily for three days = 18 pills
　50 mg daily for three days = 15 pills
　40 mg daily for three days = 12 pills
　30 mg daily for three days = 9 pills
　20 mg daily for three days = 6 pills
　10 mg daily for three days = 3 pills
　Break the remaining two pills in half, using one half per day until done

Methylprednisolone—five options
　1 g intravenously in 250 cc D5W
　5 g infuse over 6 hr for each of 3–10 days, as needed
　5 g intravenously over a 24-hr period, divided as 1.25 g every 6 hr for a 6-hr
　　infusion each time
　Medrol 4 mg orally, 100 tablets
　　4 tablets three times a day for 3 days
　　3 tablets three times a day for 3 days
　　2 tablets three times a day for 3 days
　　1 tablet three times a day for 3 days
　　1 tablet daily until done
　Medrol 32 mg orally
　　10 tablets, four times daily, for each of 3 days, in lieu of intravenous methyl-
　　　prednisolone
　　This course is then followed by the oral 4 mg course

In all cases:
Consider the use of an oral prednisone taper, if prednisone has not been used
Consider the use of a single day of 100 units of intravenous ACTH following high-
　dose steroids
Watch serum potassium, glucose, and blood pressure
Provide H_2 antagonists for GI prophylaxis
Ativan for agitation
Consider evaluation of urinalysis to check for asymptomatic infections
Begin physical therapy when appropriate

Source: Personal experience. Myers LW. Treatment of multiple sclerosis with ACTH and corticosteroids. In: Rudick RA, Goodkin DE, eds. Treatment of Multiple Sclerosis: Trial Design, Results and Future Perspectives. Heidelberg, Germany: Springer-Verlag, 1992: 135–156.

ACTH and corticosteroids were not believed to alter the natural history of the disease until recently, since they are most effective on those lesions present at the time of treatment. However, there was less progression from optic neuritis to MS in i.v. methylprednisolone–treated patients in the optic neuritis treatment trial (49). This suggests a change in the natural history of the disease as an effect of such treatment.

The duration of steroid use should be somewhat limited because of associated side effects which can, and often do, affect a number of organ systems (Table 5). This precludes their continual use and limits their value to the treatment of acute exacerbations. Short-term therapy is recognized as a problem in treatment because of the demonstration of ongoing lesion activity in serial MRI studies of untreated MS patients, and thus the likely need for ongoing therapy. The need for ongoing treatment may underly the anecdotally reported success of 3-day pulses of i.v. methylpredniso-lone, given at a frequency of 1-, 2-, or 3-month intervals, depending on the needs of the patient.

Some individuals appear to lose their ability to respond to ACTH and corticosteroids over time. This may reflect the greater degree of gliosis around demyelinated axons in addition to freshly demyelinated axons. Such individuals appear immediately to get worse at the time of administration of steroids, but then their symptoms improve over a course of several weeks, and they do well until the next bout of demyelination. A similar clinical decline often occurs in myasthenics (50), suggesting that this steroid sensitivity is a membrane property of the axons in the gliotic milieu (Fig. 18) rather than a true failure to respond to the steroids. This

Table 5 Steroid Side Effects

Mood alteration	GI irritation, ulceration
Insomnia	Myopathy
Restlessness, agitation	Neuropathy
Fluid retention and edema	Skin thinning
Hypertension	Osteoporosis
Potassium loss	Aseptic necrosis of bone
Hair loss on the scalp, hirsutism	Cataract formation
Acne	Fatal anaphylaxis
Menstrual irregularities	Cardiovascular collapse
Moon facies, buffalo hump	Facial flushing

Source: Myers LW. Treatment of multiple sclerosis with ACTH and corticosteroids. In: Rudick RA, Goodkin DE, eds. Treatment of Multiple Sclerosis: Trial Design, Results and Future Perspectives. Heidelberg, Germany: Springer-Verlag, 1992:135–156.

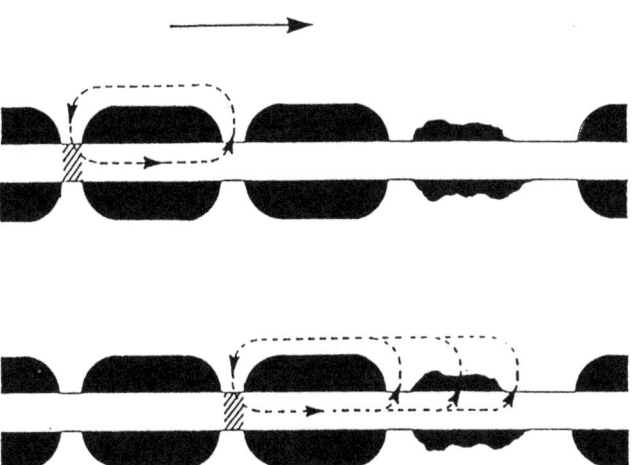

Figure 18 Steroid response on nongliotic versus gliotic axons. Conduction in the normal "nongliotic" myelinated portion (top) and the "gliotic" demyelinated portion (bottom) of an axon is schematically represented, as in Figure 4. In the "nongliotic" axon, steroid treatment leads to a quick return of rapid, energy-efficient impulse conduction. In contrast, in a "gliotic" region (bottom) the action potential is diffused over a larger area, and conduction may be completely blocked. Steroid treatment may have less immediate impact on axonal conduction in such a region, but can produce delayed benefit by reduction of inflammatory cells and their mediators in the vicinity of the demyelinated axon. (From Waxman SG. In: Cook SD, ed. Handbook of Multiple Sclerosis. New York: Marcel Dekker, 1990: 230.)

clinical scenario calls for the application of treatment which will limit the occurrence of new lesions, an issue that has not yet been fully studied in this particular patient population.

B. MS Symptomatic Treatments

Symptomatic treatments are not meant to alter the natural history of MS but to reduce the severity of symptoms which may result from the decreased nerve impulse conduction characteristic of MS or effects of inflammatory cytokines released into the CNS. Such symptoms include urinary urgency and frequency, spasticity, spasms, and fatigue (Table 6). Issues surrounding treatment of symptoms are not trivial. For example, fatigue is often the most common complaint of MS patients, because it limits their quality of life. It reflects impaired nerve impulse conduction (see Fig. 4B) and the effects of cytokines.

Table 6   Symptomatic Treatments

Fatigue	Pain
Amantidine (Symmetrel)	Antispasticity agents as above
Pemoline (Cylert)	Clonazepam (Klonopin) for muscle spasm
Methylphenidate (Ritalin)	Amitriptyline (Elavil)
Fluoxetine (Prozac)	Gabapentin (Neurontin)
Spasticity	Bladder dysfunction
Baclofen (Lioresal)	Failure to store
Diazepam (Valium)	Amitriptyline (Elavil)
Tizanidine (Zanaflex)	Oxybutinin (Ditropan)
Depression	Failure to empty
Amitriptyline (Elavil)	Intermittent catheterization
Fluoxetine (Prozac)	
Sertraline (Zoloft)	

Source: Lechtenberg R. Multiple Sclerosis Fact Book, 2nd ed. Philadelphia: FA Davis, 1988.

Urinary tract infections (UTIs), for example, present a unique set of problems to the patient with MS (51). Such infections are often asymptomatic and go undetected for prolonged periods of time. Patients frequently have limited bladder sensation and also do not immediately recognize a UTI problem when experiencing symptoms of urinary urgency and frequency—they may be accustomed to these symptoms, because these are characteristic of MS. Furthermore, patients with a UTI frequently may experience increased spasticity and more profound signs and symptoms, because a fever further reduces the ability of demyelinated fibers to conduct nerve impulses. In addition, the release of inflammatory mediators and activation of immune cells during a UTI may play a role in triggering a clinical exacerbation. For these reasons, management of urinary tract problems plays an essential role in the symptomatic management of the patient with MS.

Table 7   Pleiotropic Properties of IFNs

Antiviral effects
Antiproliferative effects
Immunomodulatory effects

Source: Baron S, Tyring SK, Fleishmann R, et al. The interferons: Mechanisms of action and clinical applications. JAMA 1991; 266:1375–1383.

In contrast to symptomatic treatments, the recent introduction of therapy with interferon β-1b (Betaseron) has reduced the frequency and severity of relapses (21,52), as well as dramatically altering the detectable accumulating lesion burden, using the cerebral MRI as a surrogate marker of this aspect of the disease (16,52). The remainder of this chapter addresses the use of Betaseron therapy in MS.

XII. OVERVIEW: WHAT ARE THE INTERFERONS?

Interferons (IFNs) were first described by Isaacs and Lindenmann in 1957 (53). This term was suggested to describe a biological activity noted in tissue culture when it was realized that during viral infection a soluble substance was released into the surrounding milieu. This tissue culture fluid could be harvested and later used to treat and "protect" other cells. This protective treatment of cells "interfered" with the capacity of the newly treated cells to be infected by virus. It soon became apparent that there were additional biological effects of this substance, such as antiproliferative and immunomodulatory properties (Table 7).

Three different types of IFNs were initially recognized (Table 8), and these were named based on their primary cells of origin. This led to names such as leukocyte, fibroblast, and immune IFNs (54). Both leukocyte and fibroblast IFN shared many properties and characteristics, and they became known as type I IFNs (acid stable), and the distinct form of immune IFN was then recognized as type II IFN (acid labile). The two type I IFNs were later renamed as α and β IFNs, respectively, whereas type II IFN was renamed γ. In recent years, other types of IFNs have been recognized, including IFN-τ (55), and IFN-ω (56). Their properties are still being characterized, and IFN-τ shows promise experimentally in the treatment of EAE (57) (see Chapter 17).

Table 8 Types of IFN

Type I IFNs	Type I IFNs (cont.)
Alpha	Omega
Beta	Type II IFNs
Tau	Gamma

Source: Charlier M, L'Haridon RL, Boisnard M, et al. Cloning and structural analysis of four genes encoding interferon-omega in rabbit. J IFN Res 1993; 13:313–322. Arnason BGW, Reder AT. Interferons and multiple sclerosis. Clin Neuropharm 1994; 17(6):495–547.

Table 9 FDA Approved IFNs—1996

Interferon	Trade name	Disease
IFN-γ-1b	Actimmune	Chronic granulomatous disease[a]
IFN-α-n3	Alferon	Genital warts
rIFN-α-2b[b]	Intron A	Hairy-cell leukemia, genital warts, AIDS-related Kaposi's sarcoma, hepatitis B, hepatitis C
rIFN-α-2a[b]	Roferon	Hairy-cell leukemia, AIDS-related Kaposi's sarcoma
rIFN-β-1a	Avonex	Relapsing-remitting multiple sclerosis
rIFN-β-1b	Betaseron	Relapsing-remitting multiple sclerosis

[a] This disease is characterized by life-threatening bacterial and fungal infections.
[b] IFN-α-2a and IFN-α-2b are now known as IFN-ω.
r = recombinant.
Source: Physician's Desk Reference, 1996; Package insert, Avonex.

The antiproliferative properties of the IFNs, initially explored with the use of crude natural preparations, led to the hope of developing a novel, anticancer therapy with activity against a large number of tumors. This served as the major force behind the cloning and development of recombinant forms of IFNs in the late 1970s and early 1980s. However, with the exception of antileukemic therapy, which is the primary Food and Drug Administration (FDA), anticancer indication currently approved (Table 9) the clinical application of IFN monotherapy in malignant diseases never quite blossomed. Nevertheless, increased experience in the clinical use of the IFNs was obtained during clinical trials in cancer and viral diseases.

XIII. IFN THERAPY OF MS

A. Origins

The rationale for exploration of the IFNs as a therapeutic modality for the treatment of multiple sclerosis was developed in a parallel fashion in three locations (Table 10). The antiviral, antiproliferative, and immunomodulatory properties of the IFNs all provided bases for their use in MS.

Fog and colleagues (58) used the Cantell preparation of natural IFN-α (59) made from human leukocytes collected by the national Finnish Red Cross blood donor program. These cells were stimulated with killed Sendai virus. This technique of IFN preparation was used in the 1970s in the earliest trials suggesting the usefulness of IFN-α as an anticancer drug

(60,61), which was before recognition of the potentional blood-borne risk of acquired immunodeficiency syndrome (AIDS) inherent in the method.

In those days, international units (IU) of IFN activity were not measured by the content of IFN protein as is done at present, but through a biological assay which measured the capacity of the preparation to inhibit the replication of a standard quantity of test virus. This was known as the "virus-neutralizing activity." Using a titer of 1×10^6 IU subcutaneously (s.c.), on a daily basis, Fog et al. attempted to treat acute exacerbations of RR MS in an open-label study. The outcome was disheartening because of a lack of efficacy and severe side effects, reflecting the temperature sensitivity of MS patients and significant febrile reactions to the IFN preparations used at that time. These side effects were mostly related to contaminants in that "natural" preparation, an issue that only later became better understood.

About the same time, laboratory studies showed a defect in natural killer (NK) cell activity in RR MS (62), (which later became a hotly disputed topic for much of the early 1980s). In response, the same Cantell preparation was used in a study initiated through the U.S. National Multiple Sclerosis Society (19). This was an effort to correct such an NK defect, based on the immunomodulatory ability of IFNs to upregulate NK activity (63).

The Cantell preparation was used in a two-center, 24-patient California study at Scripps Clinic and Research Foundation in La Jolla, and the University of California, San Francisco, in an effort to limit the occurrence

---

Table 10 IFN Studies in MS—Initial Three

Natural IFN alpha
   Subcutaneously, to treat exacerbations
   Subcutaneously, to limit exacerbations
Natural IFN beta
   Intrathecally, to limit exacerbations

Source: Fog T. Interferon treatment of multiple sclerosis patients: A pilot study. In: Boese A, ed. Search for the Cause of Multiple Sclerosis and Other Chronic Diseases of the Nervous System. Weinheim: Verlag Chemie, 1980:491–493. Knobler RL, Panitch HS, Braheny SL, et al. Systemic alpha-interferon therapy of multiple sclerosis. Neurology 1984; 34:1273–1279. Jacobs L, O'Malley J, Freeman A, Ekes R. Intrathecal interferon in multiple sclerosis. Science 1981; 214:1026–1028.

of exacerbations in RR MS (19). Reduction in exacerbation frequency was selected as a clinical outcome measure at that time, because exacerbation frequency was the best and most obvious marker of MS clinical disease activity available (64). There had not yet been either detailed clinical or MRI-based natural history studies of MS to draw attention to the role of accumulated lesion burden and progression of disability.

This study was performed in a double-blind placebo-controlled fashion and included a crossover design requiring 2 years on study protocol. This involved 6 months of treatment with daily dosing of either 5×10^6 IU of natural IFN-α or placebo injected s.c. followed by a 6-month washout period. The crossover design (Fig. 19) was needed because of the limited, and costly, supplies of natural IFN-α available for testing at that time (approximately \$24,000/6 months of daily s.c. treatment). This was a trial with a highly anticipated outcome, and the subject of a poignant article in the lay literature (65). It also underscored the willingness of many affected by MS to meet almost any price for a "cure."

Unfortunately, most patients showed little response to treatment, although they subjectively reported feeling better after the IFN treatment arm had been concluded. Two patients of the 24 showed a dramatic curtailment of clinical exacerbations during the IFN phase of the treatment; however, there was no statistically significant impact of treatment despite positive response trends.

The study was considered nondefinitive, because, in large part, it had been vastly underpowered statistically owing to the costs involved. A minimum of 60 patients per study arm would have been required to show a statistically significant difference in exacerbation frequency. MRI was not available as a clinical tool at that time, and evaluation of clinical effi-

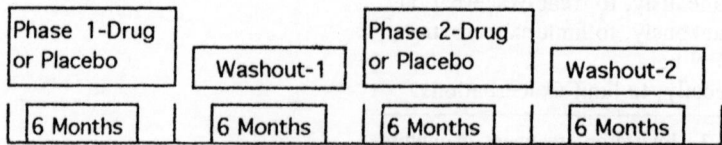

Figure 19 Crossover design utilized in the natural IFN alpha study performed in California in the early 1980s. Patients with two or more exacerbations in the 2 years prior to study entry were randomized to receive either drug or placebo daily for the first 6 months and then underwent a 6-month washout period. This was then followed by treatment with either drug or placebo for the next 6 months and then a second 6-month washout period. (From Knobler RL, Panitch HS, Braheny SL, et al. Systemic alpha-interferon therapy of multiple sclerosis. Neurology 1984; 34:1273–1279.)

cacy in this preliminary study was determined solely by the frequency and severity of exacerbations in these 24 RR MS patients.

A third study on RR MS was conducted in Buffalo (66), NY, utilizing natural IFN-β administered directly into the spinal fluid (intrathecally) by lumbar puncture (LP). The rationale for this approach was based on the hypothesis that there was a viral cause of MS, and the desire to exploit the antiviral properties of IFNs. The intrathecal administration had the specific aim of providing the IFN-β closer to the target CNS, since blood levels from s.c. administration are very low and distribution across the blood-brain barrier was known to be limited (see Chapter 3).

This study compared 10 IFN-β–treated patients to 10 control MS patients, and showed a statistically significant reduction in the number of exacerbations and disease severity in treated patients. However, this study was heavily criticized, because the control group was not subjected to the same number of LPs over the course of treatment, and therefore it was considered a biased study.

Important information was learned from each of these three pioneering studies of IFNs in RR MS. First, continuous treatment of RR MS patients rather than IFN treatment of acute exacerbations alone would be the preferred method of treatment because of the lack of efficacy for an acute exacerbation. Second, side effects were a property of the natural IFNs used in these initial studies. The natural IFNs were less desirable than the more highly purified recombinant products that were becoming available, since the natural IFNs, especially IFN-α, retained components of the viral proteins used in their preparation. This presented a particular problem for patients with MS because of their heightened capacity to produce antibodies, which led to the generation and deposition of immune complexes following repeated injections in the natural IFN-α trial (67,68) (see Chapter 11). Third, the s.c. route of IFN administration provided improved access, preferable to other alternatives, such as LP or an indwelling catheter into the spinal fluid or a vein.

B. Second Wave of Clinical Studies

During the course of cloning and development of recombinant IFNs, it was recognized that there were numerous subtypes of IFN-α, whereas there were only single forms of IFN-β and IFN-γ. There were multiple forms of IFN-α to choose from (61,68), and a clinical trial with one of the available cloned forms of IFN-α was performed using lower doses of this agent in an effort to reduce side effects (69). This was done with the hope of making the injections more tolerable and to improve efforts at maintaining a double-blind clinical trial protocol. However, lower doses were not as therapeutically effective, which highlighted the need to consider a dose-dependent trial to achieve better efficacy. This was corroborated in other trials using different forms of type I IFNs (Tables 11 and 12).

A clinical trial of recombinant IFN-α was performed based on its antiviral and NK-enhancing effects. However, it demonstrated increased exacerbations, as would be expected from other preclinical laboratory studies and observations of the role played by IFN-α in other autoimmune diseases (70,71). Of note, the worsening that occurred was confined to portions of the nervous system that were previously symptomatic. This suggested a possible mechanism of worsening, in which the upregulation of major histocompatibility (MHC) class II antigens, a known response to IFN-α, was preferentially occurring at the old lesion sites. This would then trigger recurrence of symptoms. The observed clinical worsening of MS on administration of IFN-α became viewed as positive evidence that IFN-α, and increased MHC class II expression, played a role in the pathogenesis of MS. This supported the notion that MS was appropriately classified as an immune-mediated disease.

C. Laboratory Evidence

Laboratory studies of MS tissues and models of MS further support a role for the IFNs during different stages of lesion development and resolution. Through immunohistochemistry, it has been demonstrated that IFN-β and

Table 11 IFN Alpha Trials

Knobler RL, Panitch HS, Braheny SL, et al. Systemic alpha-interferon therapy of multiple sclerosis. Neurology 1984; 34:1273–1279.

AUTIMS Research Group. Interferon-alpha and transfer factor in the treatment of multiple sclerosis: A double-blind, placebo-controlled trial. J Neurol, Neurosurg Psychiatry 1989; 52:566–574.

Kastrukoff LF, Oger JJ, Hashimoto SA, et al. Systemic lymphoblastoid interferon therapy in chronic progressive multiple sclerosis. I. Clinical and MRI evaluation. Neurology 1990; 40:479–486.

Camenga DL, Johnson KP, Alter M, et al. Systemic recombinant alpha 2 interferon therapy in relapsing remitting multiple sclerosis. Arch Neurol 1986; 43: 1239–1246.

Source: Panitch HS. Interferons in multiple sclerosis: A review of the evidence. Drugs 1992; 44(3):946–962. Durelli L. Effects of interferon alpha on cytokines and immune function in MS. In: Reder AT, ed. Interferon Therapy of Multiple Sclerosis. New York: Marcel Dekker, 1996, Chapter 12.

Table 12 IFN Beta Trials

Jacobs L, O'Malley J, Freeman A, Ekes R. Intrathecal interferon in multiple sclerosis. Science 1981; 214:1026–1028.

Jacobs L, Salazar AM, Herndon R, et al. Intrathecally administered natural human fibroblast interferon reduces exacerbations of multiple sclerosis: Results of a multicenter, double-blinded study. Arch Neurol 1987; 44:589–595.

Knobler RL, Greenstein JI, Johnson KP, et al. A pilot trial of recombinant human beta interferon in the treatment of relapsing-remitting multiple sclerosis. In: Gonsette RE, Delmotte P, eds. Recent Advances in Multiple Sclerosis Therapy. Amsterdam: Elsevier, 1989:121–124.

Knobler RL, Greenstein JI, Johnson KP, et al. Systemic recombinant human interferon-β treatment of relapsing-remitting multiple sclerosis: Pilot study analysis and six-year follow up. J IFN Res 1993; 13:333–340.

The IFNB Multiple Sclerosis Study Group. Interferon beta 1B is effective in relapsing remitting multiple sclerosis: Clinical results of A multicenter randomized double blind, placebo controlled trial. Neurology 1993; 43:655–661.

The IFNB Multiple Sclerosis Study Group and the University of British Columbia MS/MRI Analysis Group. Interferon beta-1b in the treatment of multiple sclerosis: Final outcome of the randomized controlled trial. Neurology 1995; 45(7): 1277–1285.

Jacobs LD, Cookfair DL, Rudick RA, et al. Intramuscular interferon beta-1a for disease progression in relapsing multiple sclerosis. Ann Neurol 1996; 39: 285–294.

IFN-α are localized in the perivascular lesion (72). The presence of IFN-β correlates with resolution of the lesion, whereas IFN-γ is associated with increased expression of MHC class II antigens on astrocytes and endothelial cells, which is consistent with lesion development. These associations corroborate our present concept of autoimmune disease; that is, there is enhanced expression of MHC class II molecules in the region of acute inflammation.

A critical perspective is needed, however, since experiments using antibodies to IFN-γ in mouse EAE, which presumably would block the enhanced expression of MHC class II antigens and consequent inflammation that is expected following IFN-γ administration, do not produce the anticipated result. Instead, antibodies to IFN-γ lead to more severe inflammation and disease in EAE than what is ordinarily observed, presumably by blocking a "suppressor cell"–generating step (73) (see Chapter 9). Further work is needed in order to clarify the role of IFN molecules at different times during the pathogenesis of this disease and its resolution.

D. The Betaseron Era

A potential therapeutic role for IFN-β in the treatment of MS deserved further attention. Early clinical studies with intrathecal IFN-β demonstrated a reduction in the frequency of exacerbations (66,74,75). Potential mechanisms of action of IFN-β proposed included both antiviral and immunomodulatory properties (Fig. 20). Antiviral activity of IFN-β might limit coincidental viral infections which trigger exacerbations (31). Alternatively, immunomodulatory effects of IFN-β had been observed: It downregulated the expression of MHC class II molecules (76) and depressed IFN-γ synthesis (77), which could in turn constrain antigen presentation and passage of activated cells of the immune system into the CNS (39). In addition IFN-β enhanced suppressor cell function, which is subnormal in MS (78,79). However, three new questions arose regarding the potential use of IFN-β in the treatment of MS.

1. Would s.c. administration of IFN-β be adequate to produce a biological effect in MS? Serum levels were only transiently detectable following s.c. administration of IFN-β, and the molecule did not readily cross the BBB (80) (see Chapter 3). It was widely assumed that IFN-β had to be administered directly into the spinal fluid to exert a biological effect on the CNS (66). However, the s.c. route would be preferable because of greater ease of administration and acceptability for repeated dosings over extended periods. Moreover, the s.c. route of IFN-β administration did produce dose-dependent biological effects in therapeutic clinical trials performed in patients with malignant diseases (81). Thus, there was precedent to test this route in an MS IFN-β pilot study.

Immune system modulation

    Limiting Type II (gamma) Interferon Production
        IFN gamma worsens MS
        IFN gamma promotes antigen presentation
        IFN gamma promotes MHC class II expression
        IFN gamma activates macrophages
        IFN gamma promotes TNF and Lymphotoxin release

    Limiting T-cell proliferation

Promoting suppressor cell function
    Enhancing TGF-beta release
    Reducing IFN-gamma production

Figure 20 Proposed mechanism of IFN beta (type I IFN) action in MS. (From Arnason BGW. Interferon beta in multiple sclerosis. Neurology 1993; 43:641–643.)

2. Would IFN-β side effects be harmful to patients with MS? Specifically, IFN-β therapy increased MHC class II antigen expression on monocytes derived from patients with malignant disease (82). Enhanced MHC class II expression is also a prominent effect of exposure to IFN-γ (83). In laboratory studies, it had been learned that IFN-β could lead to the release of IFN-γ (84), or at very low dosages, it could act synergistically with IFN-γ to enhance MHC class II expression (76). As stated above, treatment of MS patients with IFN-γ led to clinical worsening and reemergence of prior neurological symptoms, possibly through upregulating MHC class II expression at old lesion sites (70,71). Would treatment of MS patients with IFN-β lead to the reemergence of previous MS symptoms or perhaps even new clinical exacerbations of the disease?

3. Prior clinical studies with IFN beta had established that its side effects were dose dependent (81), whereas prior studies with other IFNs suggested the conflicting need to maximize the dose for efficacy. To maintain masking in a double-blind therapeutic clinical trial of IFN-β in MS, it was essential to identify the maximal dose range for efficacy without excessive side effects while retaining biological effectiveness. A corollary issue related to whether antibodies would be generated which could alter the biological action of the molecule (67).

1. Betaseron Pilot Study

a. Design　To address issues of the s.c. route of administration, clinical safety for patients with MS, and the relationship between dose and side effects, a 2-year pilot study of Betaseron in MS was enacted. This period was selected as the minimum time needed to discover the patterns of responses in a small sample of patients with RR MS. Based on prior clinical experience, a s.c. dosing schedule of three times per week was chosen in an effort to increase compliance over the use of a daily dosing protocol.

The safety of Betaseron administration in MS was evaluated by looking for changes in neurological symptoms and signs, as well as in the general physical examination, to determine whether there were positive or negative changes in clinical status. In this pilot study, MRI data were used only as a screening tool to confirm the diagnosis of MS rather than being used as a surrogate marker for following the course of the disease. The clinical and laboratory side effect profile was carefully documented, with every effort being made to maintain double blinding, to determine whether there were any substantial differences in side effects observed at the different doses administered (85).

Thirty patients of both sexes with clinically definite RR MS (86) and between the ages of 18 and 50 were randomized into five groups of six patients each. Patients were enrolled between June and October, 1986, after signing an informed consent. Women of childbearing potential agreed to use contraceptive methods during the period of the study; they were made aware of the unknown potential risk of IFN therapy to the developing fetus.

Five dosage groups received either placebo or 0.8, 4.0, 8.0, or 16.0 million units (MU) of Betaseron (1993 WHO Standard; 80). Because of the formulations available, Betaseron doses were delivered in one of two possible volumes—0.5 and 1.0 ml per injection. After blinding was broken, it was learned that patients treated with 0.5 ml per injection received either 0.8, 4.0, or 16.0 MU, whereas those given 1.0 ml per injection received either placebo or the 8.0-MU dosage. There were two patients on each of the five possible dosages at each of three university centers (Temple University Hospital and Thomas Jefferson University Hospital, Philadelphia, PA; University Hospital, Baltimore, MD).

Patients and investigators had no prior knowledge of the relationship between the injection volume delivered and the dosage group to which they were assigned. Patients were taught self-injection or had a significant other available who was taught how to inject IFN. The supplies of Betaseron and placebo were identical in appearance. Composition of the placebo was identical to the Betaseron diluent and contained 15 mg USP (U.S. Pharmacopeia) human serum albumin and 15 mg dextrose per vial.

The Betaseron dose range selected for this study was determined by a number of factors. These included the concentrations available in different production formulations of the drug (a regulatory issue) and knowledge regarding the dose dependency for biological effectiveness and associated side effects (81). Selection of a dose out of the range of those for which approval for testing already existed would have required reapplication to the FDA, which would have delayed the onset of this clinical trial.

After 24 weeks, all patients initially randomized to any of the Betaseron doses were switched to the 8-MU dose, if tolerated, while the others continued to take the placebo. This meant a change in volume delivered, and this had been accomodated in the study by informing patients that they would start on 0.5 ml and then later be switched to 1.0 ml at some point in the protocol. The study was continued in a blinded fashion for a period of 3 years rather than the initial 2-year period planned to allow the continued collection of safety data, and after which all patients remaining as protocol participants were afforded the opportunity to voluntarily receive open-label drug at a dose of 8.0 MU in a volume of 1.0 ml three times weekly.

Entry criteria included patients with a clinically definite diagnosis of RR MS for not less than 1 year and not more than 15 years and who had experienced at least two clearly defined exacerbations in the 2 years prior to entry into the study. Study patients included had a wide range of Kurtzke EDSS scores (14); in the range of 0–5.5 (ambulatory without assistance). The patients were required to be clinically in remission and to be free of steroid for the month prior to the time of entry into the study. Exacerbations were defined as a new symptom or worsening of an old symptom attributable to MS of at least 24 hr in duration, in the absence of a fever, which followed a period of clinical stability or improvement of at least 30 days' duration.

To secure double-blinding, one neurologist at each center performed the neurological examination for each patient and verified clinical exacerbations. A second neurologist independently evaluated the battery of clinical laboratory tests of hematological, renal, and hepatic functions performed at regular 3-month intervals to identify adverse reactions. At each patient visit, a nurse coordinator collected patient diaries of daily events and documented adverse events noted in these records.

Patients were evaluated biweekly for 6 weeks, every 6 weeks over the next 18 weeks, and then every 3 months for the remainder of the 3-year double-blind study period. Exacerbations were recorded when objective changes in neurological states accompanied clinical symptoms, as verified by the evaluating neurologist. These relapses were treated with either intravenous ACTH, methylprednisolone, or a course of oral prednisone. Although such treatment was acceptable during the course of the study, it was limited to a period no longer than 28 days, and administration of the protocol drug was continued throughout this period. ACTH or steroid use was not allowed during the initiation of protocol drug administration. This paradigm would be carried through the pivotal study as well, and this resulted in missing the observation that steroid administration during the onset of Betaseron treatment greatly reduced side effects observed.[86a]

Kurtzke EDSS and Scripps NRS scores were used to quantitate neurological disability and exacerbation severity, respectively. Withdrawal criteria included the following: steady progression of disability (greater than one-point increase on the EDSS) for a period of 6 months; treatment with more than three courses of ACTH or steroids in a 1-year period; failure to continue scheduled use of study medication for more than 2 consecutive weeks; and persistence or recurrence of moderate or severe drug toxicity after withdrawal and rechallenge with half-strength dosage.

Neutralizing antibodies to Betaseron were assayed by the reduction of IFN activity in a bioassay using an endpoint of cytopathic effect (87). Neutralizing titers were expressed relative to an NIH standard, with the limit of detection at 20 neutralizing units per milliliter.

As an indicator of the biological effects of Betaseron in this patient

Table 13 Exacerbation Rate over the First 24 Weeks of Treatment with Different Doses of Betaseron in the Initial Pilot Study, Undertaken in 1986

Treatment	Number of patients	Number with exacerbation	Number of exacerbation (mean duration)	Years use	Annualized rate[a]
Placebo	7	4/7 (57%)	5 (32 days)	2.8	1.8 (0.7–3.7)
0.8 mU	6	2/6 (33%)	2 (35 days)	2.5	0.8 (0.1–2.5)
4 mU	6	4/6 (67%)	6 (18 days)	2.8	2.2 (0.9–4.3)
8 mU	6	2/6 (33%)	2 (20 days)	2.3	0.9 (0.2–2.7)
16 mU	6	0	0	2.5	0.0 (0.0–1.2)

[a] 95% confidence interval.

Although the exacerbation rate was the lowest (zero), with 16 mU, patients started on this dose did not tolerate the drug because of side effects. However, side effects were minimal at lower doses of Betaseron, suggesting the eventual protocol of slow-dose escalation to reach the maximally effective dose currently in use in the secondary progressive trial of Betaseron in MS.

Source: Knobler RL, Greenstein JI, Johnson KP, et al. Systemic recombinant human interferon-β treatment of relapsing-remitting multiple sclerosis: Pilot study analysis and six-year follow up. J IFN Res 1993; 13:333–340.

population, serum neopterin levels were performed (88) using a commercially available radioimmunoassay kit (Neopterin-RIA, Henning Berlin GMBH, distributed by DRG International, Inc., Mountainside, NJ). Serum neopterin concentrations were extrapolated from a neopterin concentration standard curve. Each sample was assayed in duplicate. The sensitivity of the assay was 0.9 pmol/ml. Serum samples were collected prior to the first injection and then within 14 days of the 6th week on study.

    b. Outcome Analysis at 6 months (24 weeks) suggested a dose-related therapeutic trend for reduction of the exacerbation rate and the fraction of patients free of exacerbations. The fewest exacerbations were seen in patients treated with the higher doses of Betaseron (Table 13). Too few patients were studied for too short a period of time in this pilot study for this result to achieve statistical significance (20,85), but $P = .10$ in a test for a therapeutic trend. Adverse effects, including fever, fatigue, and injection site reactions, were present in all treated groups, but they were most prominent in the those initially dosed at 16 MU. This contributed to patient intolerance of the highest dose of Betaseron, but the problem was effectively resolved with dose reduction.

    At 6 months, all patients receiving Betaseron had their dose adjusted, so that they then received 8 MU three times per week unless previously dose reduced to an even lower level. Patients already on placebo continued to receive three injections of human serum albumin per week. Blinding was effectively maintained between the 8-MU versus placebo groups, indicating tolerance to side effects.

Over the first 3 years of the study period, there tended to be longer times to the first exacerbation for patients on Betaseron as compared with those on placebo and a greater proportion of exacerbation-free patients (85,89). There were no significant differences in severity of attacks, attack incidence rates, or changes from baseline in EDSS or NRS scores.

c. Side Effects The most frequently occurring adverse clinical events were fatigue (termed "myasthenia," although different from myasthenia gravis), headache, sense of weakness (labeled as "asthenia"), and skin reactions at the injection sites (Table 14). These were dose related and most pronounced in the group initiated at 16 MU three times per week. However, side effects were found in all Betaseron-treatment groups, as well as in the placebo patients, thus allowing preservation of blinding.

There was only one life-threatening adverse event which occurred during the course of the entire pilot study. This suicide attempt was judged by the specific investigator as not drug related.

Dose reductions occurred for six patients because of adverse dose-related events, and two patients were withdrawn because of adverse events. Withdrawal rates were comparable in the different treatment groups. Twelve patients withdrew from the study during treatment, three were from the placebo group and nine were from the Betaseron groups.

The most notable laboratory abnormality was lymphopenia (<1000/mm^3) in eight Betaseron and three placebo patients. Side effects tended to abate after several months of treatment. There was no apparent increase of exacerbations in patients treated with Betaseron as compared with placebo-treated patients. No late sequelae have been observed after 9 years of continuous dosing.

Table 14 IFN Beta-1b Side Effects

Injection site reactions	85%	Neutropenia	18%
Flulike symptom complex	76%	Menstrual disorder	17%
Fever	59%	Leukopenia	16%
Asthenia	49%	Malaise	15%
Chills	46%	Palpitations	8%
Myalgia	44%	Dyspnea	8%
Sweating	23%	Injection site necrosis	2%

Source: The IFNB Multiple Sclerosis Study Group. Interferon beta-1b is effective in relapsing remitting multiple sclerosis: Clinical results of a multicenter randomized double blind, placebo controlled trial. Neurology 1993; 43:655–661; also ref. 93.

Fourteen of the 24 (58%) Betaseron patients developed neutralizing IgG antibody (NAb) activity against an NIH IFN-β standard. However, the occurrence of NAb was independent of the clinical effect on exacerbation frequency and was not associated with untoward reactions over the prolonged period of clinical observation. No direct relationship could be established between these antibody titers and exacerbation rates or the proportion of patients with side effects in the pilot study. The titers appeared to peak within the first 1.5–2.5 years of treatment and then subsequently declined. The clinical significance of these antibodies has remained uncertain.

d. Conclusions This pilot study was initiated to investigate the safety profile of Betaseron based on the desire to further test the potential therapeutic role for this form of interferon in the treatment of RR MS. Three major issues were of significant concern at the outset: (1) route of administration, (2) safety profile, and (3) side-effect profile. Was there a dose of Betaseron which would show efficacy when administered subcutaneously and yet have a sufficiently low side-effect profile to allow double-blinding to be maintained over a prolonged period of clinical study? A corollary issue of concern was the evaluation of the efficacy of Betaseron in reducing the number, duration, and severity of exacerbations in RR MS.

This pilot study demonstrated a dose-related trend in both the reduction of exacerbation frequency and the side-effect profile following the subcutaneous administration of Betaseron three times weekly (see Fig. 21). This suggested the s.c. route of administration for Betaseron was effective. The fewest exacerbations were observed a dose of 16 MU, but patients directly initiated at this dosage level most often experienced intolerable fatigue leading to dose reduction. The annualized exacerbation rates for the 8.0 and 0.8 MU groups also showed a decrease as compared with placebo and had fewer dose reductions than the highest dose. The 8-MU dose was selected for further study, because it had the maximum benefit relative to its side-effect profile when compared with placebo. In fact, to maximize the dose effectiveness, it was planned to use an alternate-day dosing schedule in the pivotal trial, so that a total of seven doses could be delivered every 2 weeks, in comparison with the six doses every 2 weeks that had been used in the pilot study.

In the laboratory, there was a dose-dependent reflection of Betaseron's biological effects. There was a dose-dependent association between serum neopterin levels and repeated Betaseron dosing (Table 15), providing a biochemical marker for the impact of Betaseron on these patients (20). Samples were collected prior to the first injection and then again within 14 days of the 6th week of treatment. The mean neopterin values at 6

Table 15 Serum Neopterin Levels After Repeated Subcutaneous Injections of Betaseron at Different Doses

| | Treatment group | | | | |
	Placebo	0.8 mU	4 mU	8 mU	16 mU
N	6	5	6	4	4
Baseline mean[a]	4.52	3.09	2.66	3.64	2.26
Std. dev.	2.46	1.32	0.24	1.67	0.93
D43 mean[b]	4.73	4.14	6.41	6.20	10.14
Std. dev.	1.45	0.57	2.09	2.15	4.02
Mean difference	0.22	1.05	3.75	2.55	7.89[d]
p value[c]	0.73	0.18	0.02	0.09	0.02

[a] Mean serum neopterin concentration, nmoles/ml.

[b] Blood samples were collected on study day 43 ± 14 days.

[c] Test that the mean paired difference is equal to zero, using one-way analysis of variance model to adjust for the effects of assay run.

[d] The mean increase in the 16-mU group was significantly different from the mean increase in the other four treatment groups ($p < 0.05$, taking multiple comparisons into consideration). Data were obtained in the Betaseron pilot trial undertaken in 1986, and demonstrate dose-dependent effects of Betaseron injection on serum neopterin levels. The greatest neopterin level, measured at approximately 6 weeks after the start of therapy, was associated with the highest dose of Betaseron.

Source: Knobler RL, Greenstein JI, Johnson KP, et al. Systemic recombinant human interferon-β treatment of relapsing-remitting multiple sclerosis: Pilot study analysis and six-year follow up. J IFN Res 1993; 13:333–340.

weeks were significantly higher than those at baseline, and the increase for the 16-MU dose group was significantly greater than for any of the other treatment groups ($p < .05$, taking multiple comparisons into consideration). Note that neopterin is largely induced by IFN-γ (84). This suggests that very high doses of IFN-β may have unexpected consequences and that even if IFN-γ were induced a therapeutic effect of Betaseron remained.

Betaseron was safely administered to patients with RR MS. Exacerbations were not induced in Betaseron recipients. In fact, the data showed that Betaseron use was associated with a reduced exacerbation frequency in RR MS (20). This observation was borne out in a multicenter trial comparing placebo with doses of 1.6 and 8.0 MU of Betaseron every other day in RR MS (16,21,52) (see below).

Betaseron was reasonably well tolerated. Injection site reactions and other side effects, although common (see Table 14), were relatively mild, usually dose related, and generally abated after several months of treatment. When patients dropped out of the study, it was primarily for personal reasons or for more steroid-treated exacerbations than permitted under the terms of the protocol rather than because of intolerable side effects. Though comparison of the side-effect profile at each dose, it was surmised that a gradual escalation of dose would lead to tachyphylaxis and greater acceptability of the Betaseron.

Neutralizing antibody titers were detected in some Betaseron recipients, and these could be quite high. These antibodies were of the IgG class, and they fluctuated independently of clinical changes in the side-effect profile. There was no evidence to suggest a detrimental effect from these antibodies. NAb titers fell spontaneously during prolonged treatment. A relationship to clinical outcome could not be appreciate and the eventual drop in NAb titers suggests that any interference with the clinical effect of IFN-β could be temporary. The pilot study helped to establish a long-term safety profile of Betaseron. However, the best dose regimen to achieve maximal therapeutic effect in the treatment of MS was not determined. Dosage optimization remains a future goal.

2. Betaseron Pivotal Trial

The multicenter pivotal trial of Betaseron was initiated at seven centers in the United States and four in Canada in the summer of 1988. Treatment was continued in a double-blinded fashion through early 1993. This provided almost 5 full years of data for analysis. The major conclusions of this trial were that Betaseron at a dose of 8 MU every other day led to at least a 30% reduction in the frequency of acute attacks of RR MS and a 50% reduction in moderate and severe attacks as compared with placebo, and that this effect was maintained throughout the duration of 5 years of study (21,52).

a. Design After signing an informed consent, three hundred and seventy-two patients of both sexes between the ages of 18 and 50 with clinically definite RR MS were randomized into three groups. Patients were enrolled between June, 1988, and July, 1989. Women of childbearing potential agreed to use contraceptive methods during the period of the study, and they were made aware of the unknown but potential risk of IFN therapy to the developing fetus. Patients all had active, clinically definite RR MS (86), with at least two exacerbations in the 2-year period prior to entry into the study. Patients met the same entry criteria as for the pilot study (20), which required ambulatory patients with a Kurtzke EDSS ranging up to 5.5 (ambulatory without assistance). Patients were evaluated in a similar fashion to the pilot study to preserve blinding.

Each group received either placebo or 1.6 or 8.0 MU of Betaseron delivered in a s.c. injection of 1 ml. The 1.6-MU dose was requested by the FDA to ensure that a low dose would be tested. Patients were taught self-injection or had a "significant other" available who was taught how to inject IFN. Dosing was carried out every other day to offer one extra dose in every 2-week period as compared with the pilot study protocol to take advantage of the dose-dependent response noted in that trial (20). The supplies of Betaseron and placebo were identical in appearance. The placebo was a solution of 15 mg human serum albumin plus 15 mg dextrose per 1 ml vial.

Kurtzke EDSS and Scripps NRS scores were again used to quantitate neurological status. Withdrawal criteria included the following: steady progression of disability (greater than one point on the EDSS), for a period of 6 months; treatment with more than three courses of ACTH or steroids in a 1-year period; failure to continue scheduled use of study medication for more than two consecutive weeks; and persistence or recurrence of moderate or severe drug toxicity after withdrawal and rechallenge with half-strength dosage.

MRI evaluation was incorporated into this study in three ways. First, as a screening tool to be certain that each patient had a pattern of lesions consistent with the diagnosis of MS. Second, for all centers, there was a required annual MRI examination, with strict repositioning so that follow-up studies could be compared with assess changes in the pattern of lesion burden and evaluate the effects of treatment. Third, a subset of patients at the University of British Columbia were subjected to a frequent MRI protocol at 6-week intervals.

Neutralizing antibodies to Betaseron were determined by the reduction of IFN activity in a bioassay using an endpoint of cytopathic effect. Neutralizing titers were expressed relative to an NIH standard, with the limit of detection at 20 neutralizing units per milliliter.

b. Outcome   The fewest exacerbations were seen in patients treated with the highest dose of Betaseron [Fig. 21 (left)]. This achieved statistical significance as compared with placebo (21), and this was maintained throughout the 5-year period of study (52). Adverse effects, including fever, fatigue, and injection site reactions were present in all treated groups allowing blinding to be maintained.

Over the study period, there was a longer time period to the first exacerbation for patients on 8 MU Betaseron as compared with those on placebo, and this difference was statistically significant (21). The proportion of exacerbation-free patients was also significantly greater in the Betaseron group than in the placebo group. The most dramatic difference between placebo- and Betaseron-treated patients was in the reduced severity of attacks in the 8 MU Betaseron group. There were 50% fewer moderate and severe attacks in this treatment group than in the placebo group [Fig.

	Placebo (n = 112)	IFNB	
		1.6 MIU (n = 111)	8 MIU (n = 115)
Patients with exacerbations	94	88	79
Number of exacerbations	266	242	173
Total patient-years on study	209.2	207.0	207.0
Annual rate			
Mild	0.54	0.62	0.45
Moderate and severe	0.45	0.32	0.23
Unknown	0.28	0.22	0.15
Totals	1.27	1.17	0.84

Placebo vs 8 MIU for moderate/severe, $p = 0.002$.
Overall for moderate/severe, $p = 0.007$.

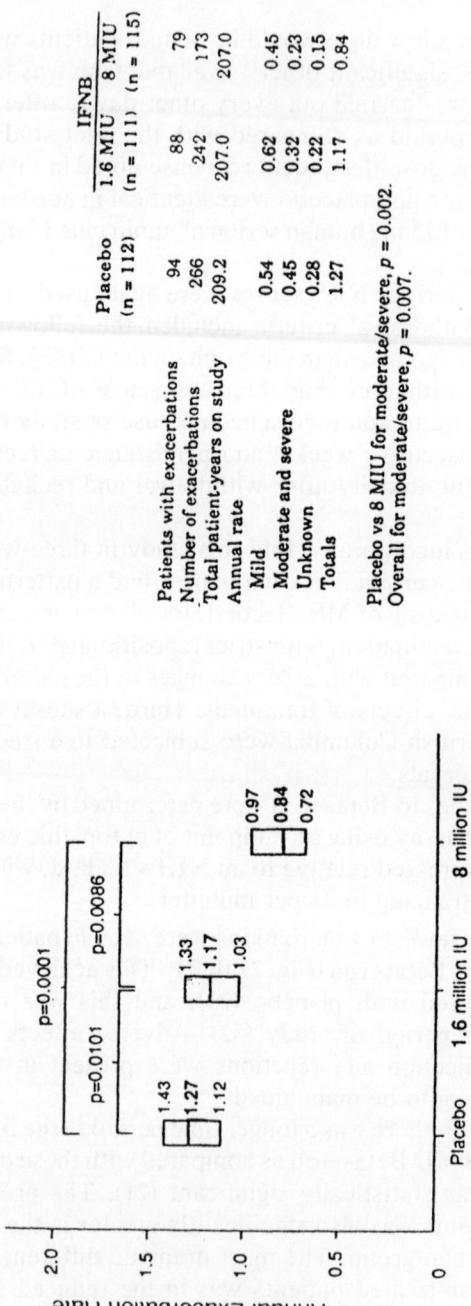

Figure 21 The pivotal trial of Betaseron, initiated in 1988, demonstrated a 30% reduction in exacerbation frequency, (left), and a 50% reduction in the occurence of moderate and severe exacerbations (right), for the first 2 years of the study. (From The IFNB Multiple Sclerosis Study Group. Interferon beta-1b is effective in relapsing-remitting multiple sclerosis. I. Clinical results of a multicenter, randomized, double-blind, placebo-controlled trial. Neurology 1993; 43:655–661.)

21 (right)]. The low-dose regimen (1.6 MU), caused an intermediate response between placebo and 8 MU.

The study was not adequately powered to demonstrate statistically significant changes from baseline for either the EDSS or SNRS scores as measures of disability (and criteria for statistical change were strict), although the trends in the 8 MU Betaseron–treated group were in the direction of clinical stabilization, whereas the trends for the placebo-treated group were in the direction of clinical worsening over the period of the study. This observation may be of some significance, since placebo groups of therapeutic clinical trial in MS as a rule do better than would be predicted for an age- and sex-matched population of MS patients. Placebo-treated patients are under closer scrutiny and hence the subject of better overall care than nonstudy patients.

From another perspective (nonclinical, and potentially less subject to examiner bias), disability status as measured by use of the visual evoked potential (VEP) was stabilized in high-dose patients. Careful analysis of the annually collected VEP data obtained for the first 2 years of the study demonstrated stabilization of the VEP in the 8 MU Betaseron–treated group, whereas there was worsening of VEP slowing in the placebo group (Fig. 22). These data are currently under further analysis and will be reported in more detail at a later date.

Because of its objectivity, the most convincing data regarding the impact of Betaseron on MS was obtained through the use of MRI (16,52). This showed a dramatic reduction in both new lesion activity and in accumulated lesion burden [Fig. 23 (left)] and was reinforced by the frequent MRI subset analysis of 52 patients at the University of British Columbia [Fig. 23 (right)] (see Chapter 15).

c. Side Effects The most frequently occurring adverse clinical events, as had been noted in the pilot study, were fatigue ("myasthenia"), headache, sense of weakness ("asthenia"), and skin reaction at the injection sites (see Table 13). These were most pronounced in the Betaseron groups, but they also were present to some degree in the placebo group, thus allowing preservation of blinding.[89a] However, depression and suicides were concentrated within the treatment groups. Although differences between groups were not statistically significant, the trend raised the possibility that depression was more than a coincidence (see Chapter 6).

The most notable laboratory abnormalities were lymphopenia (<1000/ mm^3 and elevation of liver enzymes, which were more common in the Betaseron-treated than in placebo patients. These side effects tended to abate after several months of treatment, independently of the dose with

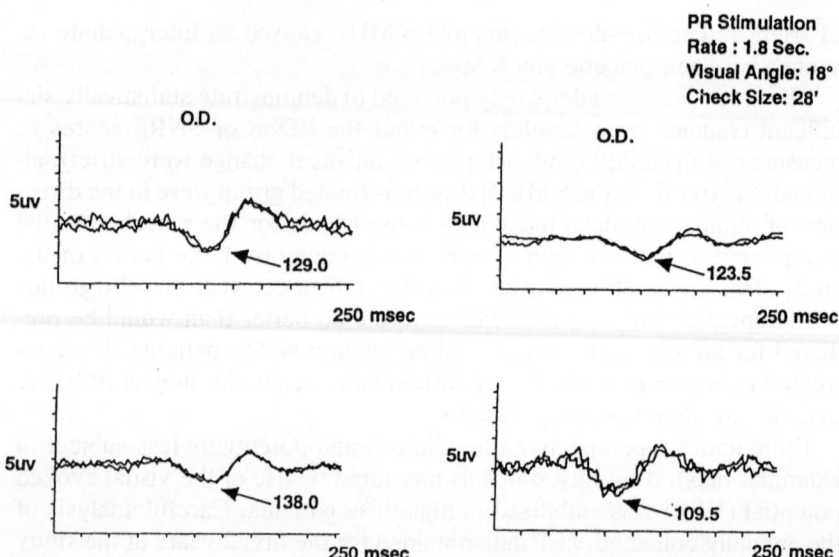

Figure 22 The VEP for study participants at Jefferson was analyzed over the first 2 years of treatment with Betaseron. There were 13 studies in the placebo group, and 13 studies in the 8 MIU Betaseron group. There was a mean worsening of 11.036 msec in the placebo group, with a p value of 0.0233, while there was a mean decline of 2.921 in the 8 MIU group, with a p value of 0.686, indicating that the latter group did not sustain a significant change. A sample of a placebo patient over a 2-year interval is shown on the left, and for an 8 MIU patient (From Wolfe WR, Wolfe RI, Streletz LJ, et al. Betaseron treatment prevents worsening of VEP in MS. Electroenceph Clin Neurophys 1995; 95:12P–13P.)

which they were associated in the study. However, skin irritation tended to persist for 1 year or longer in some patients.

Some Betaseron patients developed neutralizing IgG antibody activity against an NIH IFN-β standard. The titers could be quite high and were noted to fluctuate independently of exacerbation rates, the proportion of patients with side effects, or the side-effect profile. Antibody titers often fell spontaneously during prolonged treatment. Unfortunately, NAb titers were often quite variable, suggesting technical problems with the assay. The detection of antibodies in the neutralization assay indicates that the antibodies interfere with the antiviral activity of Betaseron. There is no information at present as to whether this antiviral activity of Betaseron provides the mechanism of action in reducing exacerbation frequency and severity in MS. Current thinking is centered on an immunological basis

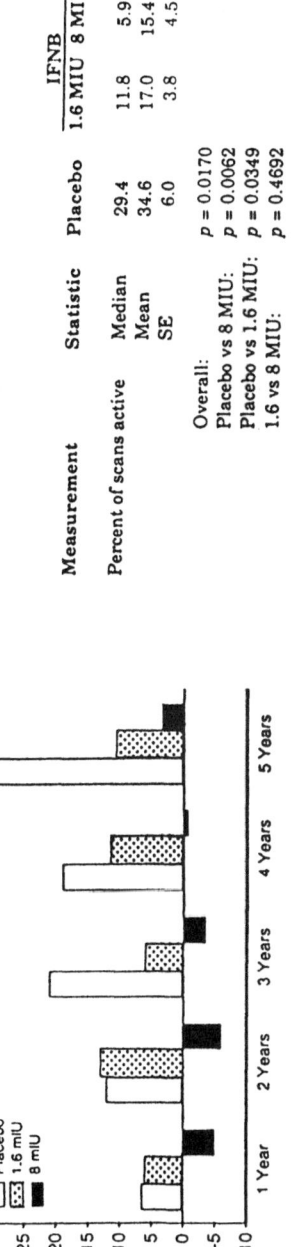

Measurement	Statistic	Placebo	IFNB 1.6 MIU	IFNB 8 MIU
Percent of scans active	Median	29.4	11.8	5.9
	Mean	34.6	17.0	15.4
	SE	6.0	3.8	4.5
Overall:		$p = 0.0170$		
Placebo vs 8 MIU:		$p = 0.0062$		
Placebo vs 1.6 MIU:		$p = 0.0349$		
1.6 vs 8 MIU:		$p = 0.4692$		

Figure 23 (Left) Cumulative MRI lesion burden median change from baseline in patients with annual scans. (Right) Results of a substudy with scans every 6 weeks ($n = 57$) corroborate these findings, showing the percentage of scans with lesion activity (new lesions or increase in size of older lesions). (From: The IFNB Multiple Sclerosis Study Group and the University of British Columbia MS/MRI Analysis Group. Interferon beta-1b in the treatment of multiple sclerosis: Final outcome of the randomized controlled trial. Neurology 1995; 45:1277–1285; Paty DW, Li DKB, UBC MS/MRI Study Group, et al. Interferon beta-1b is effective in relapsing-remitting multiple sclerosis. II. MRI analysis results of a multicenter, randomized, double-blind, placebo-controlled trial. Neurology 1993; 43:662–667.)

for MS, and antiviral NAb may not be the optimum assay against blockade of immune effects of IFN-β. However, further analyses are currently underway to develop a more reliable assay and to determine if there is a specific type of antibody which correlates with either more severe side effects or poor clinical outcome. Increased MRI lesion burden would be expected as an additional finding if these antibodies interefered with clinical effectiveness. At this point, the short- and long-term consequences of serum NAb to IFN-β are unknown.

The available data on the effectiveness of Betaseron in the reduction of exacerbation frequency and severity imply that these responses are dependent on a different portion of the molecule from that mediating antiviral activity. This issue is currently under further analysis and can only be resolved when the epitope specificity of the neutralizing antibodies is determined through mapping to specific fragments of the Betaseron molecule.

d. Conclusions Betaseron has been well tolerated in MS patients. Injection site reactions and other side effects, although common, were relatively mild, usually dose related, and had generally abated after several months of treatment. When patients left the study, it was primarily for personal reasons or for more steroid-treated exacerbations than permitted under the terms of the protocol rather than because of intolerable side effects. Although demonstrating effectiveness, this study did not ascertain the maximal potential therapeutic effect of Betaseron in the treatment of MS. The inclusion of a low-dose regimen, 1.6 MU, served to provide evidence of a dose response, indicating that further studies to evaluate dosage optimization are warranted.

The reduction in new lesion formation in Betaseron-treated patients on MRI (16,52) indicates that the mechanism of action of the agent is mediated through interruption of cell trafficking into the CNS of the MS patient. This provides a focal point for further studies exploring the mechanism of action of Betaseron in the treatment of MS. It also reinforces the usefulness of the MRI as a surrogate marker of MS disease activity, and provides an indicator of the effectiveness of treatment.

3. Betaseron Poststudy Experience

The pivotal study of Betaseron in the treatment of MS was concluded in the spring of 1993. The FDA preliminary hearing regarding approval of Betaseron for the treatment of RR MS was held on Friday, March 11, 1993. The clinical data was impressive and statistically significant, but the use of an additional objective measurement—comparison of the accumulated cerebral MRI lesion area in the placebo-treated versus the Betaseron-treated patients—proved to be the most convincing. The FDA approval of the use of Betaseron in the treatment of RR MS, by late August, 1993, was very rapid, and had at least three consequences.

First, in this, "the decade of the brain," FDA approval of a biotechnological industry therapy for MS would ensure the economic viability of this approach to other neurological diseases. Second, all future MS trials would certainly incorporate the use of the MRI as an adjunct to the clinical evaluation of the patient. Third, there was so much excitement about the prospect of a new treatment of MS that demand was great despite the admonition that Betaseron was not the "cure" for MS (90).

Expectations were out of proportion to what the drug could deliver, and nearly everybody with MS wanted Betaseron in September, 1993. The FDA, as it usually does, approved guidelines for prescribing Betaseron (these appeared in the package insert), which closely followed study entry criteria. These guidelines limited availability of Betaseron to only those individuals strictly meeting the criteria of ambulatory RR MS with a history of at least two documented exacerbations, a selection process which was closely scrutinized by third-party payers. Matters were further complicated by the limited supply of Betaseron available at that time, reflecting hesitation to gear up production of this drug until approval was certain, and by the cost of $10,000 per year ($55.56/dose for 180 doses per year) of treatment.

The Quality Standards Subcommittee of the American Academy of Neurology broadened the guidelines for use of Betaseron (91) to include patients older than age 50, patients with RP disease, as well as those with strictly RR MS, and nonambulatory patients (EDSS >6). This increased the demand and use of Betaseron at a time when experience with its use was limited. Furthermore, because the initial supplies of Betaseron were limited, Berlex opted to utilize a "lottery" for determining the distribution of Betaseron during the earliest phase of drug rollout. This meant that anyone with MS, regardless of whether ambulatory or even with RR MS, could have their name submitted by their physician (neurologists or non-neurologists alike) for entry into the lottery. If patients could afford the drug or have its use justified to their insurance carriers, and they had a lottery number which was selected, they could have treatment initiated.

This use of a lottery had consequences which have subsequently influenced drug utilization. For example, training on how to self-inject the drug and what to expect regarding its side effects and efficacy was highly variable. This resulted in many people feeling worse on drug than they had prior to its initiation because of poorly managed side effects. As a result, many people discontinued the use of Betaseron. In addition, failure of patients to notice clinical improvement led to disappointment and non-compliance, even though the report of describing the pivotal trial clearly stated that Betaseron reduced exacerbation rates and did not usually cause clinical improvement. This led to more people discontinuing the drug.

In hindsight, many of these issues could have been avoided by restricting the drug to the original 11 study centers in a phase IV safety program, gaining more knowledge in the process of how to fine tune the administration of the drug than presently stated in the package insert. This is an important lesson for future programs.

Postmarketing analysis has provided some observations on a base of 40,000 patients that did not emerge from the initial experience on the original 372 trial patients. Side effects such as increased spasticity, transient global weakness, "ulcerative" skin reactions, severe depression, and suicide have been recognized as potentially severe reactions to Betaseron. Pregnancies have occurred in women receiving Betaseron, and although there have not been problems observed, this remains an area in which caution is urged. With this base of experience, it has become apparent that there are steps that can be taken to make the initiation of dosing more tolerable for the patient.

4. Determination of Who Should Get Betaseron and When Should It Be Started?

It is sometimes a difficult decision to determine who should be treated with Betaseron and when therapy should begin. Betaseron should be given only to those in whom a diagnosis of clinically definite or laboratory supported MS has been established (86). Patients with a clinical course of either RR or relapsing/progressive (RP) MS which is clinically active are certainly potential candidates.

However, some individuals may be minimally affected clinically, yet show significant activity on the cerebral MRI. They are also viable candidates, since experience with frequent MRI analyses (8–10) indicates that their disease is active, and that they will eventually develop progressive symptoms and signs of MS. This population may experience more initial difficulty from side effects of Betaseron compared with their minimal symptoms of MS. This highlights the need for patient counseling and flexibility in dosage initiation to minimize such side effects. A possible exception to this group would be those individuals affected solely by sensory symptoms, since they, as a group, have the best overall prognosis.

Patients with a primary progressive course—spinal cord disease predominance with minimal, if any, cerebral involvement—may or may not be good candidates for Betaseron. The reasons for their different lesion distribution are not known, but the lack of demonstrated effectiveness of Betaseron on progressive lesions, at current dosing regimens, makes it difficult to justify treatment at this time. Perhaps this will change with additional experience, particularly with greater facility at following MS lesions with newer imaging techniques.

There is no clinical evidence, as yet, to support the use of Betaseron in secondary progressive MS (MS that was initially relapsing-remitting and became progressive). This issue is currently under study in a multicenter clinical trial in which disease progression is an important endpoint. Even greater doses than presently approved will be studied in this trial based on earlier small studies of dose-dependent responses. However, frequent relapses in a patient with secondary progressive MS at the present time warrant consideration for treatment with currently available doses of Betaseron.

Patients who demonstrate hypersensitivity to the material injected should not receive Betaseron. Betaseron hypersensitive individuals do not represent a large group; however, women of childbearing age represent a much bigger group. MS is almost twice as common in women, as well as being commonly of the relapsing-remitting course during their years of childbearing age. Patients who are pregnant are not candidates for treatment with Betaseron, specifically because of the potential threat to the unborn fetus. This reflects the known antiproliferative effects of Betaseron, which could disrupt growth the many rapidly dividing cell populations of the fetus.

One approach has been to take women contemplating pregnancy off Betaseron until 6 weeks after delivery. It is recognized that exacerbations are often less common during pregnancy, but more common after delivery (92). Breastfeeding can be carried out during the 6-week period after delivery, but not after the Betaseron has been restarted, because there is no information on the ability of Betaseron to cross into the newborn through breast milk.

Another group for whom there is concern regarding limiting access to Betaseron are patients who are severely depressed and considered at risk for suicide. These problems are more common in MS patients than in the general population (93). Treatment of these patients requires careful monitoring and an intact support system, with willingness to withdraw therapy, provide a drug holiday, or treat the patient on a reduced dose regimen until there is symptomatic improvement in the depression. Comanagement of these symptoms with a psychiatrist is an important consideration.

There are now recognized techniques which can be used to make the dose initiation phase go quite smoothly. These are illustrated in the next section.

5. Initiation of Betaseron Therapy

Although the recommended dose of Betaseron is 8 MU in 1 ml, and this is generally well tolerated by many for whom the drug is approved and targeted, there are some people who will react adversely when this full-strength dose is first given. Dose initiation may often have associated fever, chills, weakness, spasticity, and fatigue among other transient symptoms. Word of such side effects has spread rapidly throughout the MS community, and generates fear and trepidation that is unwarranted, and which serves to discourage patients from willingly trying Betaseron.

The cost of the drug is another factor that has discouraged patients from using Betaseron. This is compounded by the anxieties about the ability the to self-inject and being disturbed because of the possibility of feeling worse from receiving Betaseron injections than from the MS. With these prospects in mind, why initiate therapy, and in whom?

  a. What Side Effects Should Be Expected Side effects on dose initiation are directly due to the effects of Betaseron, such as lymphopenia or flu-like symptoms of fever and chills, or are due to secondary effects on the MS brain. The latter include increased spasticity or transient clinical symptoms such as global weakness or quadriparesis from elevations of core body temperature. Some symptoms may be due to either Betaseron or MS, such as fatigue and spasticity. Pain has been observed in some. This can be limb pain, which is most likely a reflection of increased spasticity, and close attention to its relation to injection time should be sought. Headache can also occur and may be quite unpleasant. Once again, the relationship of this symptom to the injection time should be sought, as well as ascertaining whether there had been a preexisting headache problem.

The patient should be closely observed, since these symptoms frequently disappear with continued treatment. Other causes of these symptoms should also aggressively be sought, specifically urinary tract infections, so that appropriate treatment can be initiated. Sometimes drugs that are used for the management of MS symptoms or seizures can lead to heightened elevation of liver enzymes. Drugs like acetominophen, baclofen, and carbamaeziepine, in particular, have this association. However, although elevated, these liver enzyme profiles remain stable at the heightened level rather than continually increasing. Therefore, repetitive testing to determine trends is warranted. When in doubt, a drug holiday will determine if there is a rapid return of enzyme values to their normal range with cessation of therapy.

All in all, patients should be advised of potential side effects and the possibility that they may feel worse for a period of time after the initiation of Betaseron therapy, and that this is not cause for alarm. Continued follow-up, suggested at 6 weeks after dose initiation initially and then at 3-month intervals, helps to provide a constant source of professional supervision throughout the course of therapy.

If a true exacerbation does occur, there is no contraindication to treatment with either a course of intravenous ACTH or methylprednisolone (see Table 4). In contrast to the potential impact on the unborn fetus, if an MS patient on Betaseron therapy must undergo a surgical procedure, there is no reason to withold the Betaseron.

b. The Betaseron Initiation Regimen Slow escalation of dose over a 4-week period; administration before bedtime; the use of analgesic/antipyretic medications, such as acetaminophen or nonsteroidal anti-inflammatory drugs (NSAIDs); and a brief course of either intravenous (3-day pulse at 1 g/day) or oral methylprednisolone (20 mg daily for 3–4 weeks), all serve to lessen the impact of initiating therapy. Autoinjectors are now available, as well, which ease the burden of self-injection. Even the most frightening of side effects, transient paralysis in those with a particularly large lesion burden, have not lasted longer than 10–12 hr. Severely affected patients appear to be the ones at greatest risk for this side effect, and appropriate caution in the form of adequate explanation of the transient nature of this side effect should be provided.

Acetaminophen will ameliorate side effects of fever, fatigue, and flu-like symptoms associated with initiation of Betaseron therapy. It is an important adjunct because of known worsening of MS symptoms with transient elevation of core body temperature. Regular use of acetominophen, starting with 1 g 1–2 hr before nighttime dosing, will facilitate sleeping through the flu-like symptoms, and then later continuing at 4-hr intervals for as long as needed, will help to reduce these symptoms. Flu-like symptoms usually stop after the second or third dose, but, may take up to several months to resolve in others. The reasons for these differences are not yet apparent.

It also has been learned that NSAIDs, such as aspirin, ibuprofen, or naprosyn, are well tolerated and aid in reducing of flu-like side effects, especially if coupled with an IFN dose–esclalation program. Curiously, NSAIDs sometimes increase the area of the redness at the injection site.

Another point of interest relates to the concomitant use of steroids during initial dosing. During the clinical trial, the first IFN β-1b was given at least 30 days after the last dose of steroids because of the trial design. However, after approval, it was anecdotaly observed that people started on Betaseron while on steroids had far fewer or no associated side effects. This may be because steroids suppress the ability of IFN-β to transiently stimulate IFN-γ (or other cytokine) production during the first month of therapy (84). Therefore, dosing patients with either a 3-day, 1 g per day,

methylprednisolone pulse, or a 4-week, 10–20 mg per day course, of prednisone, will empirically reduce the occurrence of side effects, making the
drug better tolerated.

c. Dose Initiation: Dose Escalation   Through trial and error and a
dose-escalation study, it has been learned that initiating therapy at one
0.25 dose (0.25 ml or 2 MU) and then gradually escalating by 0.25 ml at
weekly intervals facilitates tachyphylaxis to Betaseron side effects, so
that the full dose is then better tolerated. This second strategy to help
improve acceptance of the drug is commonly employed with other neurological therapies, such as gabapentin and carbamazepine, among others.
It is also likely that because people vary greatly in their body weight, and
a fixed dose has been recommended for use, lighter-weight patients will
need more time to equilibrate than heavier patients (52). Slow escalation
of dose provides greater equilibration time. The downside to this recommendation has been a financial concern regarding this regimen, because
the unused portion of the dose cannot be preserved for later use. However,
in my opinion, the trade-off of fewer side effects is worth the added effort
and expense. (Editor's note: One commercial provider of graded doses
of IFN β-1b has frozen the IFN without obvious adverse effects.)

d. Injection-Site Reactions   It is not unusual for injection site reactions to occur when substantial quantities of protein are injected subcutaneously. This has been the case with Betaseron therapy as well. Skin
reactions range in severity from local redness to ulcerated necrosis, with
the possibility of secondary infection. In some patients, there has been
worsening of psoriatic skin lesions (94), whereas others have experienced
itching and then frank ulceration (94). The mechanism of this reaction has
not yet been characterized, but it is tempting to speculate that this is the
consequence of immune complex deposition in the skin, hypothesizing
that there is local combination of antibodies to IFN-β with Betaseron.
Biopsy at the time of skin ulceration would not be expected to reveal the
presence of immune complexes within the skin lesions, since these are
known to disappear from lesions within 12 hr of their formation (95).
Further study of this phenomenon is currently underway. (See also Chapter 16.)

Some treatments will lessen the occurrence of the more superficial skin
reactions. These include the use of a cautious injection technique, cutting
the injection site to disperse the subcutaneous bolus of IFN, postinjection
application of ice to the injection site, application of steroid cream, or
application of diphenhydramine cream. Anecdotally, I have noted far
fewer such reactions after pretreatment with oral steroids and when the
injections of IFN are in the buttocks. In contrast to success with the

buttocks site, in some patients, injections of IFN over the arms and abdomen have been quite painful. The reasons for these differences are not immediately apparent.

ACKNOWLEDGMENTS

I would like to thank the continuing participation of the individuals affected by multiple sclerosis and their families, as well as my many colleagues who have played such an important role in both the studies that are the basis for this chapter and the development of the management strategies for day-to-day problems encountered in providing care to the patients affected by MS. Most importantly, I would like to thank my family for their continued understanding and encouragement of my interest in providing a cure for this disease.

REFERENCES

1. McFarlin DE, McFarland HF. Multiple sclerosis. N Engl J Med 1982; 307: 1183–1188, 1246–1251.
2. Yednock TA, Cannon C, Fritz LC, et al. Prevention of experimental autoimmune encephalomyelitis by antibodies against α-4-β-1 integrin. Nature 1992; 356:63–66.
3. Raine CS, Cross AH. Axonal dystrophy as a consequence of long-term demyelination. Lab Invest 1989; 60:714–725.
4. Waxman SG. Membranes, myelin, and the pathophysiology of multiple sclerosis. N Engl J Med 1982; 306:1529–1532.
5. Stone LA, Smith ME, Albert PS, et al. Blood-brain barrier disruption on contrast-enhanced MRI in patients with mild relapsing-remitting multiple sclerosis: Relationship to course, gender, and age. Neurology 1995; 45: 1122–1126.
6. Knobler RL, Marini JC, Goldowitz D, Lublin FD. Distribution of the blood-brain barrier in heterotopic brain transplants and its relationship to the lesions of EAE. J Neuropathol Exp Neurol 1992; 51:36–39.
7. Smith ME, Stone LA, Albert PS, et al. Clinical worsening in multiple sclerosis is associated with increased frequency and area of gadopentate dimeglumine-enhancing magnetic resonance imaging lesions. Ann Neurol 1993; 33: 480–489.
8. Frank JA, Stone LA, Smith ME, et al. Serial contrast-enhanced magnetic resonance imaging in patients with early relapsing-remitting multiple sclerosis: Implications for treatment trials. Ann Neurol 1994; 36(Suppl):S86–S90.
9. Thompson AJ, Miller D, Youl B, et al. Serial gadolinium-enhanced MRI in relapsing/remitting multiple sclerosis of varying disease duration. Neurology 1992; 42:60–63.

10. Paty DW. Magnetic resonance in multiple sclerosis. Curr Opin Neurol Neurosurg 1993; 6:202–208.

11. Rao SM, Leo GJ, Haughton VM, et al. Correlation of magnetic resonance imaging with neuropsychological testing in multiple sclerosis. Neurology 1989; 39:161–166.

12. Minden SL, Schiffer RB. Affective disorders in multiple sclerosis. Arch Neurol 1990; 47:98–104.

13. Swirsky-Sacchetti T, Mitchell DR, Seward J, et al. Neuropsychological and structural brain lesions in multiple sclerosis: A regional analysis. Neurology 1992; 42:1291–1295.

14. Kurtzke JF. Rating neurologic impairment in multiple sclerosis: An expanded disability status score (EDSS). Neurology 1983; 33:1444–1452.

15. Gonzalez C, Vinitski S, Lublin FD, et al. Tissue segmentation and volumetric measurements as a marker of disease activity in MS (abstract). Neurology 1995; 45(Suppl):4.

16. Paty DW, Li DKB, The IFNB Multiple Sclerosis Study Group. Interferon beta 1b is effective in relapsing-remitting multiple sclerosis: MRI results of a multicenter randomized double blind, placebo controlled trial. Neurology 1993; 43:662–667.

17. Whitaker JN, McFarland HF, Rudge P, et al. Outcomes assessment in multiple sclerosis clinical trials: A critical analysis. Mult Scler 1995; 1:37–47.

18. Sipe JC, Knobler RL, Braheny SL, et al. A neurologic rating scale (NRS) for use in multiple sclerosis. Neurology 1984; 34:1368–1372.

19. Knobler RL, Panitch HS, Braheny SL, et al. Systemic alpha-interferon therapy of multiple sclerosis. Neurology 1984; 34:1273–1279.

20. Knobler RL, Greenstein JI, Johnson KP, et al. Systemic recombinant human interferon-β treatment of relapsing-remitting multiple sclerosis: Pilot study analysis and six-year follow up. J IFN Res 1993; 13:333–340.

21. The IFNB Multiple Sclerosis Study Group. Interferon beta 1B is effective in relapsing remitting multiple sclerosis: Clinical results of a multicenter randomized double blind, placebo controlled trial. Neurology 1993; 43:655–661.

22. Sipe JC, Romine JS, Koziol JA, et al. Cladribine in treatment of chronic progressive multiple sclerosis. Lancet 1994; 344:9–13.

23. Eldridge R, Anaylotos CP, Schlesinger S, et al. Hereditary adult-onset leukodystrophy simulating chronic progressive multiple sclerosis. N Engl J Med 1984; 311:948–953.

24. Moser H. Leukoencephalopathies caused by metabolic disorders. In Koetsier JC, ed. Demyelinating Diseases. Vinken PJ, Bruyn GW, Klawans HL, series eds. Handbook of Clinical Neurology, Revised Series 3. Amsterdam: Elsevier, 1985; 47:583.

25. Johns DR, et al. Pitfalls in the molecular genetic diagnosis of Leber hereditary optic neuropathy (LHON). Am J Hum Genet 1993; 53:916–920.

26. Ebers GC, Bulman DE, Sadovnick AD, et al. A population-based twin study in multiple sclerosis. N Engl J Med 1986; 315:1638–1642.

27. McFarland HF. Twin studies and multiple sclerosis (editorial). Ann Neurol 1992; 32:722–723.
28. Compston A. The epidemiology of multiple sclerosis: Principles, achievements, and recommendations. Ann Neurol 1994; 36 (Suppl 2):S211–S217.
29. Zavala C, Morton NE, Rao DC, et al. Complex segregation analysis of diabetes mellitus. Hum Hered 1979; 29:325–333.
30. Kalman B, Lublin FD, Alder H. Mitochondrial DNA mutations in multiple sclerosis. Mult Scler 1995; 1:32–36.
31. Sibley WA, Bamford CR, Clark K. Clinical viral infections and multiple sclerosis. Lancet 1985; 1:1313–1315.
32. Kahn SH, Knobler RL, McGeady SJ, et al. The incidence and specificity of allergies in patients with multiple sclerosis. J Neuroimmunol 1991; (Suppl 1):184.
33. Boos J, Kim JH. Evidence for a viral etiology of multiple sclerosis latent viruses. In: Cook SD, ed. Handbook of Multiple Sclerosis, New York: Marcel Dekker, 1990:41–61.
34. Voskuhl RR, Robinson ED, Segal BM, et al. HLA restriction and TCR usage of T lymphocytes specific for a novel candidate autoantigen, X2 MBP, in multiple sclerosis. J Immunol 1994; 153:4834–4844.
35. Fujinami, RS. Virus-induced autoimmunity through molecular mimicry. In Raine CS, ed. Advances in Neuroimmunology. Ann NY Acad Sci 1988; 540: 210–217.
36. Martenson RE. Myelin: Biology and Chemistry. Boca Raton, FL: CRC Press, 1993.
37. Selmaj K, Brosnan CF, Raine CS. Expression of heat shock protein-65 by oligodendrocytes in vivo and in vitro: Implications for multiple sclerosis. Neurology 1992; 42:795–800.
38. Johnson HM, Russell JK, Pontzer CH. Superantigens in human disease. Sci Am 1992; 266(4):92–101.
39. Hickey WF. Migration of hematogenous cells through the blood-brain barrier and the initiation of CNS inflammation. Brain Pathol 1991; 1:97–105.
40. Wisniewski HM, Bloom BR. Primary demyelination as a nonspecific consequence of a cell-mediated immune reaction: Bystander demyelination. J Exp Med 1975; 141:346–359.
41. Hofman FM, Hinton DR, Johnson K, et al. Tumor necrosis factor identified in multiple sclerosis brain. J Exp Med 1989; 170:607–612.
42. Selmaj KW, Raine CS. Tumor necrosis factor mediates myelin and oligodendrocyte damage in vitro. Ann Neurol 1988; 23:339–346.
43. Soliven B, Szuchet S, Nelson DJ. Tumor necrosis factor inhibits K^+ current expression in cultured oligodendrocytes. J Membr Biol 1991; 124:127–137.
44. Lublin FD, Marini JC, Perreault M, et al. Autoimmune inflammation of astrocyte transplants. Ann Neurol 1992; 31:519–524.
45. Rose AS, Kuzma JW, Kurtzke JF, et al. Cooperative study in the evaluation of therapy in multiple sclerosis: ACTH vs. placebo. Final Report. Neurology 1970; 20(Suppl):1–59.

46. Myers LW. Treatment of multiple sclerosis with ACTH and corticosteroids. In: Rudick RA, Goodkin DE, eds. Treatment of Multiple Sclerosis: Trial Design, Results and Future Perspectives. Heidelberg, Germany: Springer-Verlag, 1992:135–156.

47. Beck RW, Cleary PA, Anderson MM Jr, et al. A randomized, controlled trial of corticosteroids in the treatment of acute optic neuritis. N Engl J Med 1992; 326:581–588.

48. Miller DH, Thompson AJ, Morrissey SP, et al. High dose steroids in acute relapses of multiple sclerosis: MRI evidence for a possible mechanism of therapeutic effect. J Neurol Neurosurg Psychiatry 1992; 55:450–453.

49. Beck RW, Cleary PA, Trobe JD, et al. The effect of corticosteroids for acute optic neuritis on the subsequent development of multiple sclerosis. N Engl J Med 1993; 329:1764–1769.

50. Sanders DB, Scopetta C. The treatment of patients with myasthenia gravis. Neurol Clin 1994; 12(2):343–368.

51. Goldberg E, Kelley CL, Trantas F, et al. Urinary tract infection frequency in MS exacerbations. J Neuroimmunol 1994; 54:173.

52. The IFNB Multiple Sclerosis Study Group and the University of British Columbia MS/MRI Analysis Group. Interferon beta-1b in the treatment of multiple sclerosis: Final outcome of the randomized controlled trial. Neurology 1995; 45(7):1277–1285.

53. Isaacs A, Lindenmann J. Virus interference. I. The interferons. Proc R Soc Lond B Biol Sci 1957; 147:258–273.

54. Friedman RM. Interferons: A Primer. New York: Academic Press, 1981.

55. Rueda BR, Naivar KA, George EM, et al. Recombinant interferon-tau regulates secretion of two bovine endometrial proteins. J IFN Res 1993; 13: 303–309.

56. Charlier M, L'Haridon R, Boisnard M, et al. Cloning and structural analysis of four genes encoding interferon-omega in rabbit. J IFN Res 1993; 13: 313–322.

57. Soos JM, Subramaniam PS, Hobeika AC, et al. The IFN pregnancy recognition hormone IFN-tau blocks both development and superantigen reactivation of experimental allergic encephalomyelitis without associated toxicity. J Immunol 1995; 155:2747–2753.

58. Fog T. Interferon treatment of multiple sclerosis patients: A pilot study. In: Boese A, ed. Search for the Cause of Multiple Sclerosis and Other Chronic Diseases of the Nervous System. Weinheim: Verlag Chemie, 1980:491–493.

59. Cantell K, Hirvonen S. Large-scale production of human leukocyte interferon containing 10^8 units per ml. J Gen Virol 1978; 39:541–543.

60. Volz MA, Kirkpatrick CH. Interferons 1992. How much of the promise has been realised? Drugs 1992; 43:285–294.

61. Durelli L. Effects of interferon alpha on cytokines and immune function in MS. In: Reder AT, ed. Interferon Therapy of Multiple Sclerosis. New York: Marcel Dekker, 1997, Chapter 12.

62. Neighbor PA, Bloom BR. Absence of virus-induced lymphocyte suppression and interferon production in multiple sclerosis. Proc Natl Acad Sci USA 1979; 76:476–480.

63. Arnason BGW, Reder AT. Interferons and multiple sclerosis. Clin Neuropharm 1994; 17(6):495–547.

64. Knobler RL. Systemic interferon therapy of multiple sclerosis: The pros. Neurology 1988; 38(Suppl 2):58–61.

65. Fox, C. Waiting for interferon. Harper's, 1982; 265(September):32–46.

66. Jacobs L, O'Malley J, Freeman A, Ekes R. Intrathecal interferon in multiple sclerosis. Science 1981; 214:1026–1028.

67. Rice GPA, Woelfel EL, Talbot PJ, et al. Immunological complications in multiple sclerosis patients receiving interferon. Ann Neurol 1985; 18: 439–442.

68. Kastrukoff L, Oger J. Natural interferon alpha in the treatment of MS. In: Reder AT, ed. Interferon Therapy in Multiple Sclerosis. New York: Marcel Dekker, 1997, Chapter 11.

69. Camenga DL, Johnson KP, Alter M, et al. Systemic recombinant alpha 2 interferon therapy in relapsing remitting multiple sclerosis. Arch Neurol 1986; 43:1239–1246.

70. Panitch HS, Hirsch RL, Haley AS, Johnson KP. Exacerbations of multiple sclerosis in patients treated with gamma interferon. Lancet 1987; 1:893–895.

71. Panitch HS, Hirsch RL, Schindler J, Johnson KP. Treatment of multiple sclerosis with gamma interferon: Exacerbations associated with activation of the immune system. Neurology 1987; 37:1097–1120.

72. Traugott U, Lebon B. Demonstration of alpha, beta and gamma interferon in active chronic multiple sclerosis lesions. In: Raine CS, ed. Advances in Neuroimmunology. Ann NY Acad Sci 1988; 540:309–311.

73. Lublin FD, Knobler RL, Kalman B, et al. Monoclonal anti-gamma interferon antibodies enhance experimental allergic encephalomyelitis. Autoimmunity 1993; 16:267–274.

74. Jacobs L, Salazar AM, Herndon R, et al. Multicentre double-blind study of effect of intrathecally administered natural human fibroblast interferon on exacerbations of multiple sclerosis. Lancet 1986;2:1411–1413.

75. Jacobs L, Salazar AM, Herndon R, et al. Intrathecally administered natural human fibroblast interferon reduces exacerbations of multiple sclerosis: Results of a multicenter, double-blinded study. Arch Neurol 1987; 44:589–595.

76. Joseph J, Knobler RL, D'Imperio C, Lublin FD. Down-regulation of interferon gamma induced class II expression on human glioma cells by recombinant interferon beta: Effects of dosage treatment schedule. J Neuroimmunol 1988; 20:39–44.

77. Noronha A, Toscas A, Jensen MA. Interferon β decreases T cell activation and interferon γ production in multiple sclerosis. J Neuroimmunol 1993; 46: 145–154.

78. Antel J, Arnason BGW, Medof ME. Suppressor cell function in multiple

sclerosis: Correlation with clinical disease activity. Ann Neurol 1979; 5: 338–342.

79. Noronha A, Toscas A, Arnason BGW, et al. Interferon beta augments suppressor cell function in multiple sclerosis. Ann Neurol 1990; 27:207–210.
80. Witt P. In: Reder AT, ed. Interferon Therapy in Multiple Sclerosis. New York: Marcel Dekker, 1997, Chapter 3.
81. Borden EC, Hawkins MJ, Sielaff KM, et al. Clinical and biological effects of recombinant interferon beta administered intravenously daily in phase I trial. J IFN Res 1988; 8:357–366.
82. Spear GT, Paulnock DM, Jordan RL, et al. Enhancement of monocyte class I and II histocompatibility antigen expression in man by in vivo beta interferon. Clin Exp Immunol 1987; 69:107–115.
83. Basham TY, Merigan TC. Recombinant interferon-gamma increases HLA-DR synthesis and expression. J Immunol 1983; 130:1492–1494.
84. Dayal AS, Jensen MA, Lledo A, Arnason BGW. Interferon-gamma-secreting cells in multiple sclerosis patients treated with interferon beta-1b. Neurology 1995; 45:2173–2177.
85. Knobler RL, Greenstein JI, Johnson KP, et al. A pilot trial of recombinant human beta interferon in the treatment of relapsing-remitting multiple sclerosis. In Gonsette RE, Delmotte P, eds. Recent Advances in Multiple Sclerosis Therapy. Amsterdam: Elsevier 989:121–124.
86. Poser CM, Paty DW, Scheinberg LC, et al. New diagnostic criteria for multiple sclerosis: Guidelines for research protocols. Ann Neurol 1983; 13: 227–231.
87. Antonelli G. Development of neutralizing and binding antibodies to interferon (IFN) in patients undergoing IFN therapy. Antiviral Res 1994; 24: 235–244.
88. Huber C, Batchelor JR, Fuchs D, et al. Immune response associated production of neopterin release from macrophages primarily under control of interferon gamma. J Exp Med 1984; 160:310–316.
89. Johnson KP, Knobler RL, Greenstein J, et al. Recombinant human interferon beta treatment of relapsing-remitting multiple sclerosis: Pilot study results. Neurology 1990; 40(Suppl 1):261.
89a. Sibley WA, Ebers GC, Panitch HS, Reder AT, van den Noort S. Interferon beta treatment of multiple sclerosis. Reply from the authors. Neurology 1994; 44:186–190.
90. Arnason BGW. Interferon beta in multiple sclerosis. Neurology 1993; 43: 641–643.
91. Report of the Quality Standards Subcommittee of the American Academy of Neurology. Practice advisory on selection of patients with multiple sclerosis for treatment with Betaseron. Neurology 1994; 44:1537–1540.
92. Birk K, Ford C, Smeltzer S, et al. The clinical course of multiple sclerosis during pregnancy and the puerperium. Arch Neurol 1990; 47:738–742.
93. Betaseron (Interferon beta-1b). Package insert. Berlex Laboratories, Richmond, CA, 1995.

94. Webster GF, Knobler RL, Lublin FD, et al. Cutaneous ulcerations and pustular psoriasis flare caused by recombinant interferon beta injections in patients with multiple sclerosis. J Am Acad Dermatol 1996; 34:365–367.

95. Braverman IM, Yen A. Demonstration of immune complexes in spontaneous and histamine-induced lesions and in normal skin of patients with leukocytoclastic angitis. J Invest Dermatol 1975; 64:105–112.

15

Effects of Interferon β-1b on Multiple Sclerosis Lesions Evaluated by Magnetic Resonance Imaging and Other Magnetic Resonance Techniques

Robert A. Koopmans, David K. B. Li, Guo Jun Zhao, Elana Brief, Alex MacKay, Irene Vavasour, Ken Whittall, and Donald W. Paty

The University of British Columbia, Vancouver, British Columbia, Canada

I. MULTIPLE SCLEROSIS

A. Clinical Course

The clinical course of multiple sclerosis (MS) is unpredictable and varies from death within weeks of onset to a completely asymptomatic course after initial symptoms. The diagnosis of MS rests on the ability to demonstrate white matter lesions in the central nervous system (CNS) disseminated both in time and space. Magnetic resonance imaging (MRI) is the imaging procedure of choice for the diagnosis of MS. MRI can also evaluate the progression of pathology and has become important in monitoring clinical trials. As of yet there is no cure for MS, although recently it has been shown with the aid of MRI that interferon β-1b (IFN β-1b) therapy reduces disease activity and may delay the progression of the disease (1).

B. Etiology and Pathogenesis

The cause and pathogenesis of MS are unknown, but there appears to be an autoimmune response targeted against myelin and/or oligodendrocytes. The pathological hallmark is the demyelinated plaque. Within the early plaque, axons are usually preserved. Prineas, in looking at the early lesion (2), has found that macrophages strip myelin off the axons. The active macrophages contain myelin debris, including neutral fat, in their cytoplasm. Initially, computed tomography (CT) (3) and more recently and with greater sensitivity MRI (4) have shown that the first event in the evolution of MS lesions that can be identified is breakdown of the blood-brain barrier (BBB) followed by dynamic size changes in what must be initially a purely inflammatory lesion. Serial follow-up MRI studies (5–9) show that these dynamic lesions can go through many cycles, waxing and waning in size, before they become confluent and permanent. The sequence of events in the evolution of a single MS lesion has been hypothesized to be as follows: (1) The BBB becomes leaky, (2) edema and/or inflammation develops around the leaky vessel, (3) demyelination occurs, (4) followed by gliosis, and (5) finally, axonal loss. The critical pathological feature that is irreversible and guaranteed to produce a permanent deficit is axonal loss. In contrast, BBB disruption, edema, and inflammation may resolve and recur several times before demyelination occurs. There is some evidence that remyelination may also occur (2). Moreover, autopsy studies (10), CT (3), and more recently MRI studies (11) have shown that many MS lesions are asymptomatic.

II. MAGNETIC RESONANCE

The physical principle of nuclear magnetic resonance (NMR) was first demonstrated in 1946 by the physicists Bloch and Purcell, who shared the Nobel Prize for this work. Since then, it has been possible to obtain in vitro NMR spectra from small samples in liquid or solid form. With the development of modern computer techniques (similar to those used in CT scanning) came the possibility of converting NMR signals into cross-sectional images. MRI produces multiplanar images and in essence maps the protons contained in tissue in the form of water and lipids. MRI contrast is largely determined by intrinsic tissue parameters—proton density, spin-lattice relaxation (T_1), and spin-spin relaxation (T_2). MRI is very sensitive in differentiating among various soft tissues and in detecting pathology. This sensitivity is largely due to differences in water T_1 and T_2 relaxation times that exist among various tissues.

In the early 1980s, shortly after its introduction to clinical medicine, MRI became the imaging procedure of choice for the diagnosis of MS (12). MRI of the brain is the most sensitive diagnostic test to demonstrate lesion dissemination in space; it is more sensitive than CT, evoked potential, or cerebrospinal fluid (CSF) studies (13). Multiple periventricular white matter lesions are characteristic of MS. They are typically ovoid and aligned perpendicular to the long axis of the ventricles, Dawson's fingers, and consist of lymphocytic infiltration along periventricular medullary veins (which radiate from the ventricular surface). The cerebellar and cerebral peduncles as well as the corpus collosum and spinal cord are also often affected. Lesions vary in size from tiny solitary foci to large confluent plaques.

Several serial MRI studies (5–9) of the natural history of MS have been carried out, both in relapsing-remitting (RR) and chronic progressive (CP) MS patients. These studies conclude that although clinically MS is often phasic in nature, the pathology is a much more continuous process. MRI evidence for disease activity is much more frequent (typically 5–10 times) than clinical evidence. When comparing the RR form of MS with CP disease, the rate of new lesions appearing on MRI is much greater in the CP group. The pattern of change of new and enlarging lesions, however, is the same in both forms of MS. Each lesion increases to maximum size in about 4 weeks and then gradually declines in size over a further 4–8 weeks. It is not unusual to see some lesions enlarging while others are simultaneously decreasing in size.

MRI, therefore, besides being diagnostically useful, provides a comprehensive method for monitoring progression of pathology. This capability has become especially relevant with the implementation of new therapies and monitoring of clinical trials. MR techniques have enhanced our understanding of the in vivo (biochemical) pathology of demyelination. A distinction between acute, potentially reversible lesions, from chronic, irreversible lesions is now possible and is of great importance when evaluating new therapies. MR can help detect the effects of therapy more accurately, more objectively, and after a shorter duration of follow-up than clinical monitoring alone.

Serial MRI measurements of burden of disease (BOD) and lesion activity (with or without gadolinium) are now the established MRI outcome measures for monitoring therapy in MS. BOD measurements provide a quantification of the pathological extent of the disease. In untreated MS, there is on average a 10% increase in BOD per year (1,14–16). However, the pattern of lesion activity varies widely among patients. Some patients have mostly new lesions. Others predominantly show enlargement of preexisting lesions. Some patients have discrete multifocal disease, whereas others have large confluent lesion loads. In the latter cases, important changes in activity of individual lesions may be obscured by the extensive background of disease, without a significant overall BOD change. The appearance of *new* lesions, which are usually small, probably is the fundamental process in MS. However, these new lesions may go unnoticed if BOD measures alone are used. Therefore, a separate analysis of individual lesions that show change on yearly (or more frequent) MRI scans may provide an additional sensitive and detailed measure of therapeutic effect.

MRI has been used in several clinical trials, including systemic lymphoblastoid IFN therapy (14) and cyclosporin A therapy of CP MS (15). In both studies, two separate analysis methods were used. Both methods enabled demonstration of progression of MS pathology over time. The first method was an analysis of MS lesion activity. The second method was a manually traced computer-assisted quantification of the BOD. Although there was a trend toward improvement for the lymphoblastoid IFN–treated group after 6 months, the MRI endpoint data showed that both lymphoblastoid IFN and cyclosporin were ineffective in the treatment of CP MS. On average, a 10% increase in BOD per year was seen for both placebo and treated patients. The MRI results supported the clinical findings in both studies. The BOD increase also correlated ($R = 0.186$, $P = .018$) with the increase in clinical impairment during the cyclosporine study.

III.   IFN β-1b TRIAL OF MS

A more recent MRI-monitored 5-year clinical trial of IFN β-1b showed exciting therapeutic results (1,16). MRI was used to monitor a randomized, double-blind placebo-controlled multicenter trial of two doses of IFN β-1b (1.6 and 8 million international units [MIU] injected subcutaneously on alternate days) in ambulatory patients with RR MS in Canada and the United States (1,16). Three hundred and seventy-two patients entered the study. Each patient had an annual cranial MRI scan (proton density and T_2-weighted images; gadolinium enhancement was not used). Two hundred and seventeen patients completed 4 or 5th year annual scans after baseline. A subgroup of 52 patients from one center (Vancouver) had additional frequent MRI scans every 6 weeks for the first 2 years of the study in order to measure lesion activity.

A.   MRI Outcome

The yearly MRI scans were evaluated using the BOD measurement, based on a manually traced computer-derived analysis of total lesion area. There were significant positive effects of IFN β-1b on BOD measurements, based on yearly MRI scans (1,16). There was a significant increase in MRI lesion burden in comparison with baseline in the placebo and 1.6-MIU group. In contrast, there was no significant increase in lesion burden, either yearly or for the entire duration of the study, in the 8-MIU treatment arm. The mean percentage increase in BOD in the placebo arm was approximately threefold higher than that seen in either the low- or high-dose IFN-treated arms (Table 1).

Table 1 Percentage Change in MRI Lesion Area from Baseline in 217 Patients Having at Least Four Annual Scans After Baseline

		Placebo	Low IFN-β	High IFN-β	P value
Baseline area (mm²)	N	73	66	78	
	Median	1503	1066	1525	0.1996
	Mean	1691	1727	2011	
	SE	180	241	189	
1 Year	N	72	62	77	
	Median	6.7	5.7	−4.9	0.0012
	Mean	110.6	11.0	5.4	
	SE	93.6	4.1	5.1	
2 Years	N	72	62	77	
	Median	11.9	12.4	−5.6	0.0015
	Mean	43.8	19.3	9.4	
	SE	14.0	5.7	8.5	
3 Years	N	70	59	73	
	Median	21.0	6.1	−3.8	0.0002
	Mean	161.5	34.4	14.2	
	SE	108.6	15.8	8.9	
4 Years	N	72	61	75	
	Median	18.7	11.7	−0.8	0.0055
	Mean	69.5	35.6	25.0	
	SE	26.4	14.9	13.7	
5 Years	N	14	16	19	
	Median	30.2	10.6	3.6	0.0363
	Mean	99.6	21.9	11.3	
	SE	55.0	12.4	9.2	

Source: From ref. 17.

The efficacy of IFN β-1b was confirmed by an independent analysis of MS lesion activity, based on yearly scans of 342 RR MS patients (Zhao et al, manuscript in preparation). In this study, an analysis of lesion activity on yearly MRI scans also demonstrated the therapeutic effect of IFN β-1b, and at the same time provided more detailed information on the effects of IFN β-1b. A total of 1396 MRI scans from 342 MS patients from 11 centers were analyzed (all scans that were analyzed were from patients who had at least a baseline and one other scan). Lesion activity was defined as either new lesions (never seen before) or enlargement of preexisting lesions. Table 2 shows the MS lesion activity events by treatment group over the duration of the study (5 years). With this analysis, it was

Table 2 MS Lesion Activity Events by Treatment Group

Type of lesion activity event (5 years)		Placebo (n = 115)	1.6 MIU (n = 116)	8 MIU (n = 111)
Total Events	Mean	6.44	3.92	3.08
	SE	0.88	0.47	0.42
Overall	P = .001			
Placebo vs 8.0 MIU	P = .001			
Placebo vs 1.6 MIU	P = .007			
1.6 MIU vs 8.0 MIU	P = .260			
New Lesions	Mean	3.57	2.01	1.80
	SE	0.44	0.28	0.26
Overall	P < .001			
Placebo vs 8.0 MIU	P = .001			
Placebo vs 1.6 MIU	P = .001			
1.6 MIU vs 8.0 MIU	P = .717			
Enlargements	Mean	2.65	1.83	1.23
	SE	0.52	0.26	0.20
Overall	P = .027			
Placebo vs 8.0 MIU	P = .022			
Placebo vs 1.6 MIU	P = .133			
1.6 MIU vs 8.0 MIU	P = .100			
Recurrences	Mean	0.22	0.09	0.05
	SE	0.10	0.03	0.03
Overall	P = .130			
Placebo vs 8.0 MIU	P = .103			
Placebo vs 1.6 MIU	P = .179			
1.6 MIU vs 8.0 MIU	P = .453			

Source: UBC MS/MRI Study Group, in preparation.

found that high-dose IFN β-1b (8 MIU) reduced the appearance of new and enlarging lesions by 50%. Interestingly, low-dose (1.6 MIU) IFN β-1b was almost equally as effective as high-dose IFN β-1b in the reduction of new lesions. However, the low-dose had no beneficial effects on lesion enlargements. In addition, there were significantly fewer patients with active disease (≥ 1 active lesion) in both IFN β-1b–treated groups when compared with placebo ($P \leq .05$) (Table 3).

In the subgroup of 52 patients who had frequent (every 6 weeks) MRI scans for 2 years, the treated patients showed a 70% decrease in active

Table 3 Patients with MRI Active Disease by Treatment Group

	Placebo (n = 115)	1.6 MIU (n = 116)	8 MIU (n = 111)
No. active (%)	96 (83.5%)	82 (70.7%)	72 (64.9%)
Overall $P = .005$			
Placebo vs 8.0 MIU $P = .001$			
Placebo vs 1.6 MIU $P = .011$			
1.6 MIU vs 8.0 MIU $P = .408$			

Source: UBC MS/MRI Study Group, in preparation.

lesions when compared with placebo. There was, however, no significant dose-response effect. Interestingly, after just 6 weeks of therapy, the mean percentage of patients with active scans, per scan week was reduced by approximately 50% in the patients treated with IFN β-1b (approximately 15% of IFN β-1b–treated patients vs 30% placebo-treated patients had active scans)—but again, no dose-response effect was seen. This treatment effect became statistically significant after 1 year and was maintained throughout the 2 years of study.

Stone et al. (17), from the US National Institutes of Health (NIH) examined the effect of IFN β-1b on contrast-enhanced MRI. Fourteen patients with RR MS were enrolled in this study. They had been followed previously by serial monthly gadolinium-enhanced MRI in a study designed to examine the natural history of MS using MRI. The contrast-enhanced lesion rate during a 7-month baseline period was compared with the enhanced lesion rate for the 6-month period following the initiation of treatment with 8 MIU of IFN β-1b. T_1-weighted, contrast-enhanced images were reviewed and the number of enhancing lesions were counted by consensus of a least two trained observers to determine the number of total and new enhancing lesions. Lesions were considered "new" if they showed no enhancement on the previous month's scan.

There was a significant reduction in the total lesion rate from 3.06 per month during the 7-month pretreatment baseline to 0.48 per month during treatment ($P = .002$). Since the patients had previously been entered in a study of the natural history of MS by monthly MRI, longer pretreatment baseline periods ranging from 6–58 months (mean = 26.4 months) were available for analysis in 12 of the 14 patients. During IFN β-1b treatment, the new lesion frequency decreased from 2.73 per month to a frequency of 0.23 per month, whereas the total lesion frequency for the entire baseline changed from 3.46 per month to 0.48 lesions per month. In 13 of the 14 patients, there was a reduction in enhancing lesion frequency during the 6-month treatment period. Five of these patients had no contrast-enhancing lesions during the treatment period. These findings suggest that IFN β-1b has a mechanism of action that at least temporarily inhibits the opening of the BBB in RR MS patients.

B. Clinical Outcome

The clinical outcome of the IFN β-1b trial (1,16) showed a significant reduction in clinical relapse rate of approximately 30% for each year of the study in the 8-MIU group. Over the 5-year period, the overall relapse rate was 1.12 relapses per patient per year in the placebo group; in the high-dose treatment group, the rate was 0.76 (Table 4). In parallel, confirmed disease progression (defined as a persistent increase of one or more expanded disability status score (EDSS) points confirmed on two consecu-

Table 4 Annual Exacerbation Rates by Year of Study

	Rx Group	N	Rate of Exacerbations (8 MIU vs Placebo)	Decrease (Placebo vs 8 MIU) (%)	Significance
Year 1	Placebo	123	1.44	33	$P < .001$
	1.6 MIU	125	1.22		
	8 MIU	124	0.96		
Year 2	Placebo	110	1.18	28	$P = .030$
	1.6 MIU	114	1.04		
	8 MIU	124	0.96		
Year 3	Placebo	96	0.92	28	$P = .084$
	1.6 MIU	95	0.80		
	8 MIU	95	0.66		
Year 4	Placebo	82	0.88	24	$P = .166$
	1.6 MIU	76	0.68		
	8 MIU	89	0.67		
Year 5	Placebo	56	0.81	30	$P = .393$
	1.6 MIU	52	0.66		
	8 MIU	58	0.57		

Source: From ref. 17.

tive evaluations 3 months apart) occurred in fewer patients in the high-dose treatment arm (35%) than in the placebo arm (46%) (P = .096).

C. Correlation Between MRI and Clinical Measures

There were significant correlations (P < .001) between MRI BOD measures and EDSS at baseline and endpoint; also between MRI BOD and the Scripps neurological rating scale (NRS) at baseline and endpoint; and between MRI BOD and exacerbation rate and change of EDSS and change in MRI BOD. Although these were highly significant statistically (P < .001), the R values were only modest (0.2–0.3). This suggests that factors other than T_2-weighted lesions were involved and could be measured with more pathologically specific or biochemically specific MRI techniques.

D. Conclusion

In this study, MRI has played a key role in the evaluation of drug therapy and was a major reason for US Food and Drug Administration (FDA) approval of IFN β-1b for the therapy of MS in 1993. The MRI data showed that in RR patients, treatment with IFN β-1b reduced the rate of formation of new lesions significantly and therefore had affected disease activity at a fundamental level. In addition, the MRI data strongly and objectively supported the clinical results.

IV. NEW MRI TECHNIQUES

Although conventional serial MRI is now generally accepted for treatment monitoring in MS trials, there are limitations with this technique. MRI is very sensitive in detecting the lesions of MS and is an excellent tool for studying dynamic gross morphological changes of MS pathology. However, except for gadolinium DTPA enhancement, which demonstrates BBB disruption, conventional MRI cannot characterize the MS lesions pathologically or biochemically. Ideally, imaging should differentiate among edema, inflammation, demyelination, axonal loss, and remyelination. All of these may have different implications for the clinical activity and eventual course of MS.

Magnetic resonance spectroscopy (MRS) offers the potential to address this issue, because it provides a means of observing the chemical pathology in demyelinating lesions. MRS can measure various biochemical abnormalities in vivo, including myelin breakdown products (18). In addition, relaxation MRI (19), which estimates myelin content, and magnetization transfer imaging (MTI) (20), may provide new methods to assess pathology in vivo and may provide a more comprehensive method for monitoring therapy of MS.

A. Magnetic Resonance Spectroscopy

MRS can provide in vivo biochemical information from a localized region within the brain. MRS can be conducted with clinical scanners (1.5 tesla [T]) and requires no contrast agents. Since it is a noninvasive and nondestructive technique, patients can be scanned repeatedly, and the progress of a disease can be monitored.

In MRS, spectra (i.e., plots of MR signal vs frequency) are acquired from a localized volume (a voxel) within the brain. The frequency of the MR signal is determined by the local chemical environment of the nucleus. Each signal frequency represents a specific molecular site on a brain metabolite. Signal intensity is proportional to molecular concentration. Therefore, MRS can be used to determine the concentrations of specific brain metabolites.

Proton (^{1}H) and phosphorus (^{31}P) are the two main nuclei employed in MRS of brain. A typical ^{1}H spectrum from a healthy human brain is shown in Fig. 1 (the x-axis is in parts per million [ppm], a standard unit

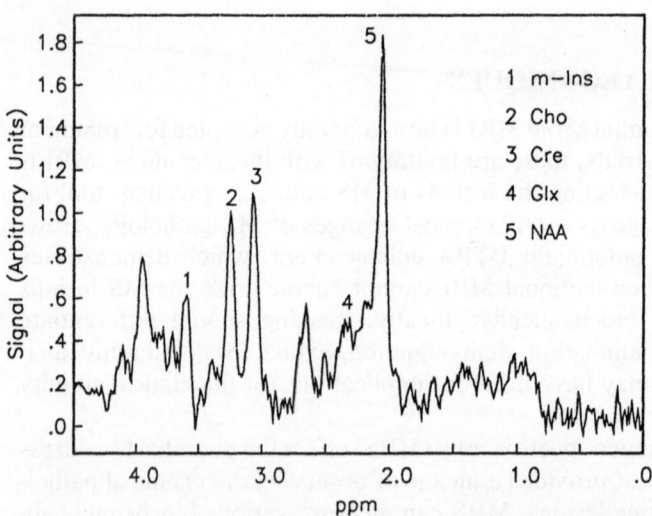

Figure 1 Normal proton MRS spectrum. MRS from white matter (8 cm³ voxel) in a normal volunteer (age 24 years). Five peaks are identified. The acquisition sequence was STEAM, TE 30 msec, TR 1500 msec, TM 13.7 msec.

which normalizes frequency). The peak at 2.0 ppm is from the methyl group (CH_3) on N-acetyl aspartate (NAA), the 3.2 ppm peak is from the CH_3 groups on the choline-containing compounds (Cho), and the CH_3 on creatine and phosphocreatine (Cr + PCr) give the 3.0 ppm peak. Lipids and lactate (1.3 ppm) are only seen in disease. Additional peaks for myo-inositol (m-Ins) and glutamine/glutamate (Glx) are shown in the Fig. 1. The ^{31}P MR spectrum contains signals from inorganic phosphates (P_i), phosphomonoesters (PME), phosphodiesters (PDEs), phosphocreatine (PCr), and the α, β, and γ phosphates of adenosine triphosphate.

For reliable clinical interpretation of MRS results, the spectrum must be analyzed. A common practice is to measure the signal areas from each metabolite and calculate ratios of peak areas. This method provides only relative concentrations. For determination of absolute brain metabolite concentrations, the spectrum must be corrected for relaxation effects and then calibrated to a known reference concentration. Internal and external references, such as in vivo creatine and in vitro doped water, have been used (21).

One limitation of MRS is its inherent low sensitivity. For better signal to noise ratios, spectra must be acquired from relatively large volumes (>1 ml). In single-voxel MRS (21), a spectrum is acquired from a single volume in the brain. In spectroscopic imaging (22,23), spectra are acquired from multiple voxels in one acquisition. Voxels should be placed in regions where this is optimal magnetic homogeneity and no contamination of the spectra from adjacent bone, fat, or air.

MRS research of MS, to date, has attempted to find answers for the following:

1. What are the metabolic changes in MS?
2. Is a chronic lesion distinguishable from an acute lesion?
3. Can one distinguish between demyelination and inflammation?
4. Is there a correlation between Gd-DTPA–enhancing lesions and metabolite levels?
5. Future research may use MRS to help determine more specific mechanisms of action of drug therapy.

MS lesions have consistently shown a decrease of the NAA/(Cr + PCr) levels. Since NAA is thought to be restricted to neurons (24), reductions in NAA may reflect secondary axonal injury or degeneration and or loss of function (25). An increase in Cho/Cr + PCr) and myo-inositol (mI/Cr + PCr) has also been reported (18,26–28). Choline-containing phospholipids are thought to increase with myelin breakdown (18). The change in mI is not understood (26). Another change seen has been an increase in lactate. Lactate has been considered a marker of relatively severe edema

(25). All investigators have assumed Cr + PCr remains constant, and use it as a standard in the ratios above. This assumption may not be valid (see Section IV.A.1).

Differences between acute and chronic lesions have been investigated in serial studies. NAA/(Cr + PCr) in chronic lesions continues to fall over time (18,25,28). In acute lesions, however, NAA/(Cr + PCr) rises somewhat after its initial decrease (always staying below its original level) (25,26,30). This possibly indicates a partial return of neuronal function. One report (25) distinguishes between acute and chronic lesions as follows: (1) an acute plaque is characterized by decreased NAA/(Cr + PCr), increased Cho/(Cr + PCr), and an occasional increase in lactate (Lac); and (2) a chronic plaque has decreased NAA/(Cr + PCr) and normal Cho/(Cr + PCr).

A short echo-time (TE) spectrum is shown in Fig. 2A from the voxel defined in Fig. 2B. Peaks can be seen at 0.9 and 1.33 ppm. These peaks have been attributed to lipid (31). Lipid is a myelin breakdown product. Several investigators have demonstrated lipid peaks within Gd-DTPA–enhancing lesions, whereas others have not (32–34). This suggests that en-

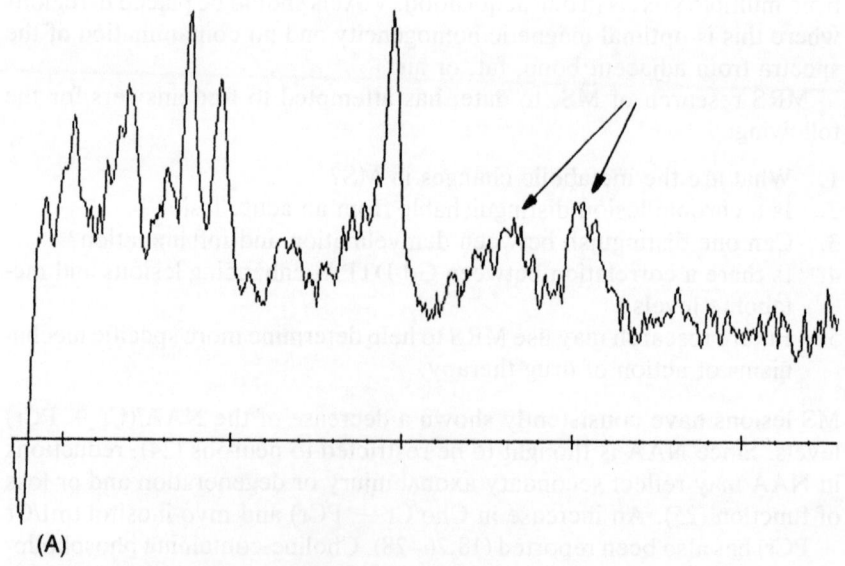

(A)

Figure 2 Proton MRS of MS. MRS spectrum (A) from 8 cm³ white matter voxel located in an MS lesion (B). Note decreased NAA and the increased intensities in the lipid region (arrows). Scan parameters same as for Figure 1.

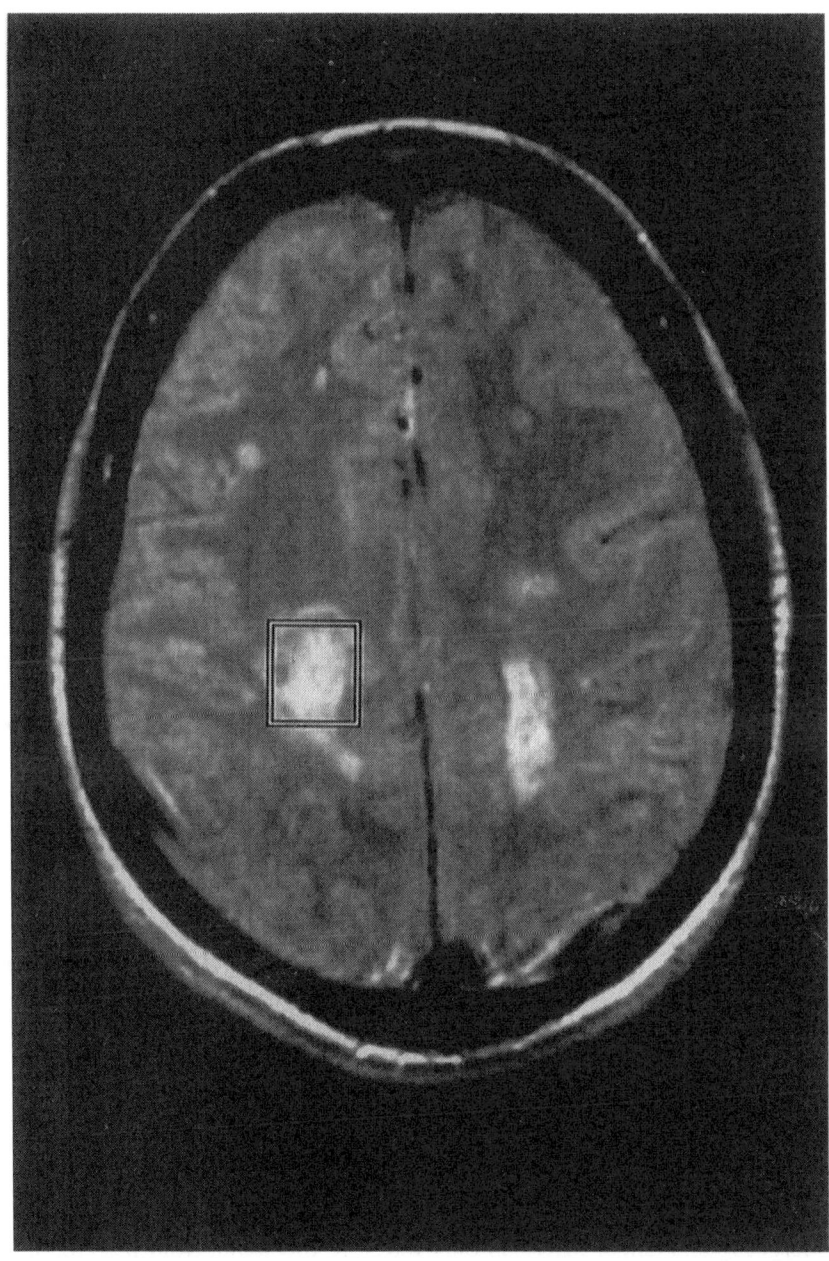

(B)

hancing lesions without lipid signals are edematous and not demyelinating (32). On average, lipid remains detectable for 5 months after the lesion has ceased to enhance (18,26,32,35). This finding indicates that MRS can provide important additional information about the natural history of MS lesions.

1. Pitfalls in MRS

Most groups interpret the decrease in NAA/(Cr + PCr) as being entirely due to NAA. The question arises as to how valid the assumption is that Cr + PCr is a constant. One study using ^{31}P MRS has demonstrated that PCr increases in a chronic lesion (36). This casts doubt on the accepted assumption. A rise in PCr (leading to a rise in the signal from Cr + PCr) would decrease the NAA/(Cr + PCr) ratio. Future studies should include full quantification of the signals so that absolute concentrations could be determined. Relying on relative changes in metabolite levels can lead to incorrect conclusions concerning the biochemistry of the brain.

2. Conclusions

MRS already provides insight into the progression of MS. NAA is consistently decreased in MS lesions, suggesting a loss of neuronal viability and function. However, the decline may be reversible in some instances. Furthermore, MRS detects (new) lipids and elevated inositol and choline levels in MS lesions. These changes may well reflect the breakdown of myelin membrane phospholipids. Some groups have also reported differences between acute and chronic lesions and between edema and demyelination. MRS appears to monitor changes in lesions not seen by standard MRI scans; MRS signals indicate that demyelination continues for months after Gd DTPA enhancement has stopped.

B. Magnetization Transfer

MTI is a relatively new MR imaging technique which produces a novel form of contrast (37).

The basic mechanism for MTI is an exchange of magnetization between two pools of protons in the brain (Fig. 3). One is a mobile pool which is composed of free water protons with a long T_2 (>1 msec). The other is a motionally restricted pool. These protons have a very short T_2, because they are attached to macromolecules such as lipids and proteins and their signal therefore decays in microseconds. Both proton pools are constantly undergoing exchange. MRI can only measure the signal from the mobile protons. If the motionally restricted pool is saturated, that is, the magnetization is set to zero, then the signal from the mobile pool is reduced owing to exchange (transfer of magnetization) between the two pools.

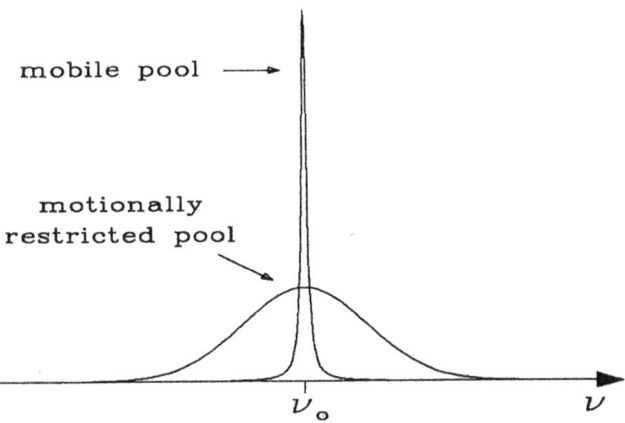

Figure 3 Magnetization transfer. The two proton pools found in the brain are shown. The wide pool (10 kHz) is associated with motionally restricted protons which are bound to macromolecules. The narrow line (10–100 Hz) is associated with the mobile protons of free water. Both lines are centered on the water resonance. Note that the drawing is not to scale. V = frequency; V_0 = resonance frequency.

This provides an indirect method of measuring the motionally restricted pool through its effect on the mobile pool.

In order to quantify the results, a magnetization transfer ratio is taken:

$$MTR = \frac{M_0 - M_s}{M_0}$$

M_0 is the intensity of the image without the saturation pulse and M_s is the intensity of the image with saturation.

Myelin is composed of lipids and proteins whose protons belong to the motionally restricted pool. The theory is that there is greater MT for regions in the brain with intact myelin. As demyelination occurs, the amount of magnetization transfer will decrease, thus decreasing the MTR. Therefore, MT is sensitive to the state of myelination of a lesion. A conventional proton density image and a MTR image of an MS patient is shown in Fig. 4A, B. In the MTR image, the intensity represents the MTR calculated for each pixel. Demyelinated lesions are of low signal on this image, since there is less magnetization transfer and therefore lower MTR.

Dousset et al. (20) showed that purely edematous lesions have a slightly decreased MTR, whereas demyelinated lesions have a greater decrease with a much smaller MTR. The small decrease for edema is probably

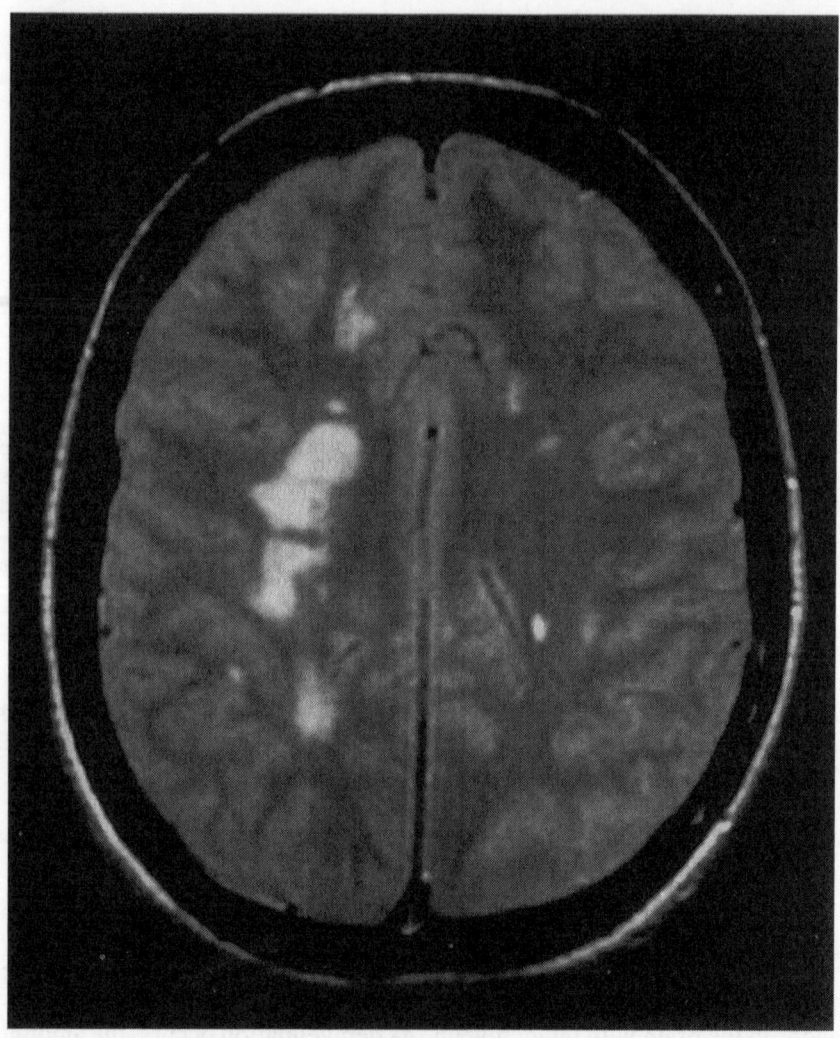

(A)

Figure 4 Magnetization transfer. (A) A proton density image (TE 30 msec, TR 2500 msec) from an MS patient. (B) The difference between an image of the slice in (A) with and without magnetization transfer. Scan parameters were spin echo, TE 16 msec, TR 1000 msec, slice thickness 5 mm, FOV 22 cm, and the saturation was provided by a sinc pulse 2 kHz off resonance. Several MS lesions appear as dark foci.

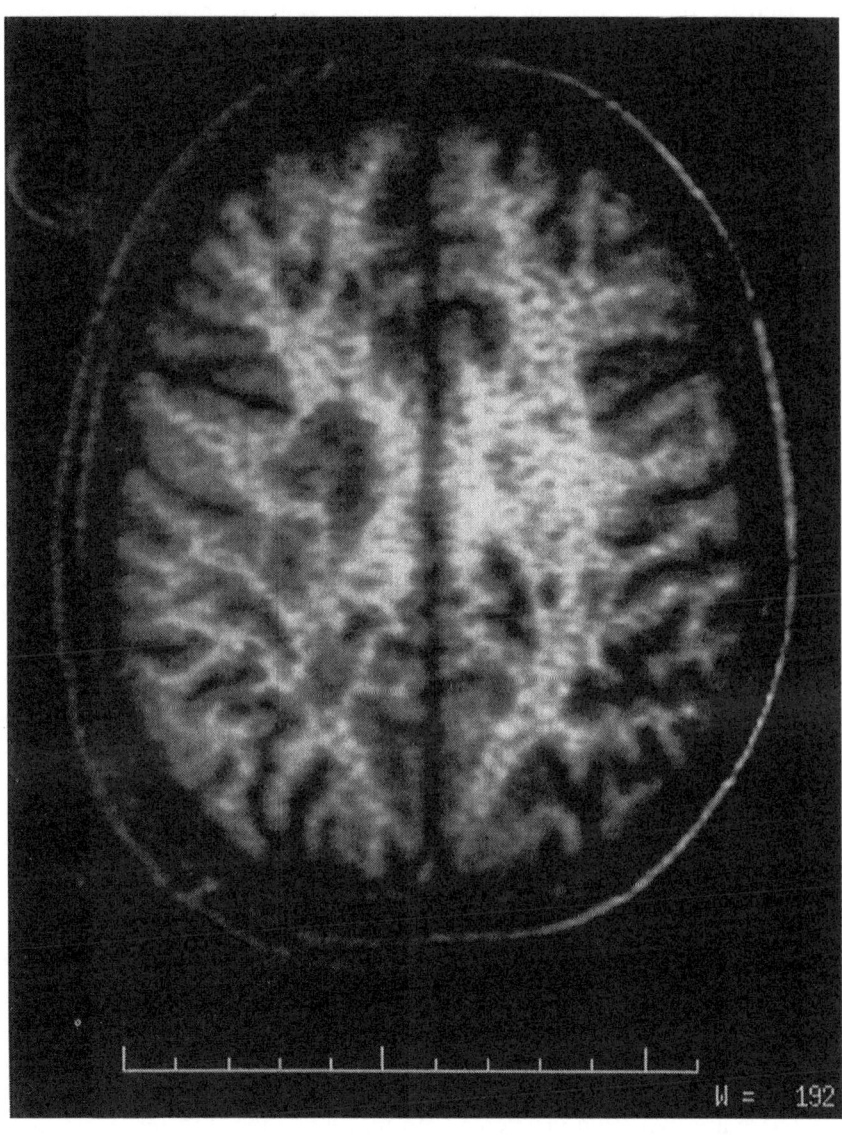

(B)

caused by the increase in the free water pool which dilutes the effect of the magnetization transfer from the motionally restricted pool. With demyelination, the motionally restricted pool is being decreased and therefore there is less interaction between the two pools. This would cause the larger decrease in the MTR.

Although Gd enhancement shows BBB breakdown, it cannot be used to determine the myelination state of a lesion (38). MT was combined with gadolinium enhancement to see whether there was a correlation between enhancing lesions and MTR. The MTR was decreased in MS lesions, yet MTR did not correlate with enhancement. Importantly, lesions which were hypointense on T_1-weighted images ("black holes" suggesting demyelination) had a smaller MTR than lesions which were isointense. Also, for ring-enhanced lesions, the central (more demyelinated) portion had a lower MTR than the enhancing ring. Thus, MTR may be better able to distinguish areas of demyelination from edema compared with conventional MRI.

MTI has also been used to study normal-appearing white matter (NAWM) in MS patients. Filippi et al. (38) found a lower mean MTR for NAWM in MS patients compared with controls. This suggests there are microscopic areas of demyelination even in NAWM in MS. In CP MS, the MTR of NAWM was lowest around lesions visible on MRI and increased progressively away from the lesion. This gradient might indicate that there are more disturbances in the white matter closer to lesions.

At present, it has been difficult to correlate the BOD, as detected with conventional MRI, with clinical disability. The 5-year data correlation was between 0.2–0.3 in the IFN β-1b trial (1). This is partly due to the fact that lesions cannot be categorized as to their stage of demyelination and axonal loss. With MT, however, there is a strong inverse correlation between lesion MTRs and EDSS (39). Interestingly, the MTR in patients with benign MS was higher than the MTR seen in patients with secondary progressive MS. MT has also been used to determine a correlation between the age of lesions and their MTR. Lesions less than a year old have a much lower MTR than lesions older than a year (40), possibly reflecting gliosis or remyelination in the older lesions. Therefore, it may be possible to differentiate between acute and chronic lesions using MT.

There are two main problems with magnetization transfer. First, misregistration due to motion during the acquisition of the images, with and without saturation, can cause errors in determining the MTRs. The second problem is the partial volume effect as a result of the slice having fixed dimensions. True quantification of MT is also difficult, since all the factors that affect MT are not known (myelination is only one of them). As MTRs depend greatly on which pulse sequence was used, different investigators will tend to have different results and the results cannot be easily compared. The main advantage is that MT can be acquired on the whole brain quickly and no new hardware is needed to implement it. The pulse sequences are also relatively easy to implement.

Comparison between MT and MRS has been done by Hiehle et al. (41). They compared MTRs for different lesions to MRS data such as the concentration of NAA and the concentration of a composite peak between 2.1 and 2.6 ppm, termed "marker peaks." These peaks are probably due to amino acid products such as γ-aminobutyric acid and glutamate which would be present after demyelination. The MTR did not correlate well with the NAA, Cho, or Cr/PCr concentrations but did correlate with the concentration of the marker peaks. These two methods characterize white matter differently, but the methods appear to be linked and complementary. MRS indicates biochemical changes and MT indicates structural changes such as degree of myelination.

It is still unclear whether MT will prove to be truly quantitative, as opposed to other methods such as T_2 relaxation (see further). Preliminary comparisons between the techniques seem to indicate that T_2 relaxation is a more rigorous method for measuring myelin content, whereas MT provides a quick qualitative assessment of myelin distribution (42).

In conclusion, MT imaging evaluates the integrity of tissue structure by probing the interactions of water with the surface of tissue components. Pathologically proven demyelinated plaques have a low MT transfer rate. Decreased MTR indicates a loss of tissue structure, and MTR images may prove useful in estimating the degree of demyelination in MS lesions and help determine drug efficacy. A long-term goal for the field would be true quantification of MT. At present, it is possible to differentiate between edema and demyelination. Determining whether there is remyelination of the axon cannot yet be done. MT combined with other techniques is a promising method for distinguishing between edema and demyelination, since it can be quickly acquired and can be used to look at the whole brain.

C. MR Relaxation Studies and MS

Since most of clinical MRI is dependent on image contrast provided by T_1 and T_2 relaxation, measurements of T_1 and T_2 times of tissue should provide increased specificity. Earlier relaxation studies (43) yielded little to support this expectation. However, with the recent implementation of more quantitative methodologies, there is reason to be more optimistic about the future of relaxation time measurements in MRI.

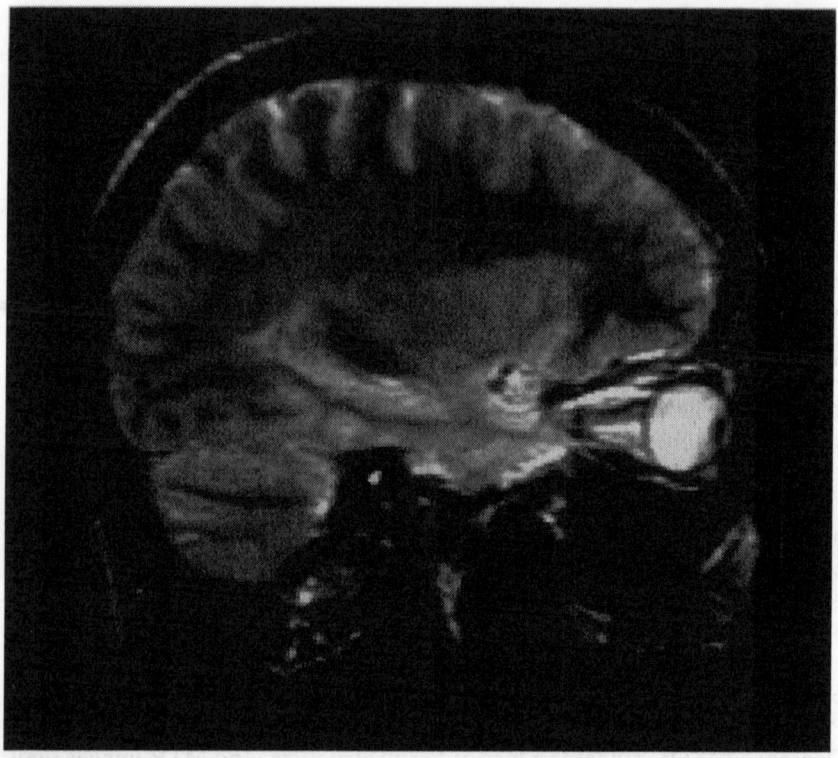

(A)

Figure 5 Conventional MR and T_2 relaxation images of a normal volunteer. (A) Sagittal image (TE 30 msec, TR 3000 msec) from a normal volunteer; (B) corresponding myelin water map. The myelin water content, which is proportional to the fraction of the signal possessing T_2 time between 15 and 50 msec, was estimated from the relaxation decay obtained from a single-slice 32 echo sequence with echo spacing 15 msec, TR 3000 msec, slice thickness 10 mm, and FOV 22 cm.

The mechanisms for T_1 and T_2 relaxation of water in normal and pathological brain are not understood quantitatively; however, it is well known that tissue water relaxation times are sensitive to their microscopic local environment. Edema and/or inflammation generally result in increased relaxation times, and hemorrhage results in decreased relaxation times. When the tissue water environment in the voxel is homogeneous, T_1 and T_2 measurements yield single exponential component relaxation decays.

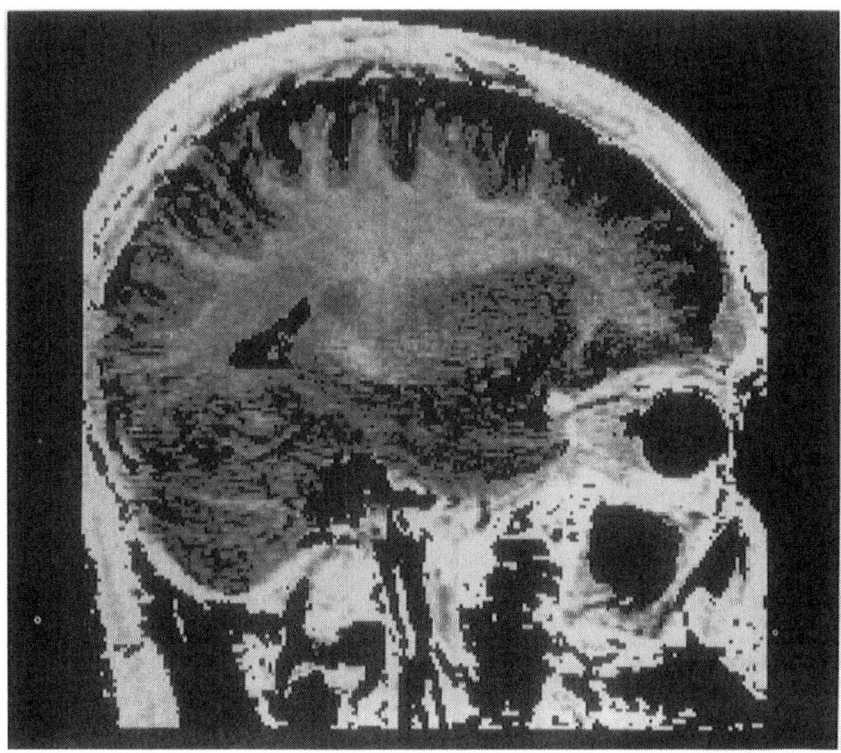

(B)

However, more than one water environment in the image voxel causes multiexponential relaxation decays. For example, if the voxel contains gray matter and CSF, the T_2 decay curve contains two exponential components: one with T_2 about 75 msec from the gray matter, and the other with T_2 several seconds long from the CSF. In vivo measurement of relaxation times in the presence of multiexponential decay curves is a challenging problem (44–46).

Multiple sclerosis plaques are visible on proton density, and on T_2 weighted MR images because of their increased water content and elevated T_2 times. Larsson et al. (47,48) reported that in MS plaques, T_1 times increased from 50 to 350% and T_2 times increased from 25 to 500% compared with the values for normal white matter. Armspach et al. (49) measured a similar range of T_2 times in MS lesions. Larsson et al. (50) found their measurements of T_1 and T_2 in MS patients had a reproducibility

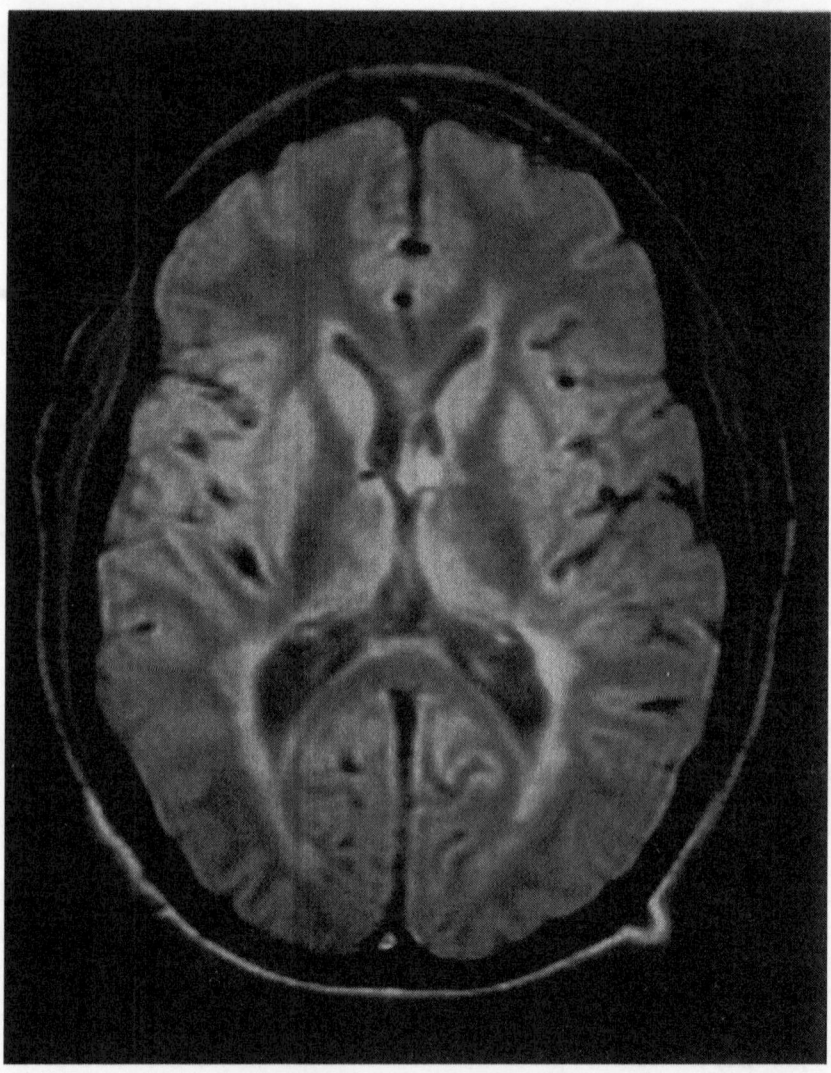

(A)

Figure 6 Conventional MR and T_2 relaxation image of a MS patient. (A) Axial image (TE 30 msec, TR 3000 msec) image from a MS patient; (B) corresponding myelin water map. The myelin water content, which was proportional to the fraction of the signal with T_2 time between 10 and 50 msec, was estimated from the

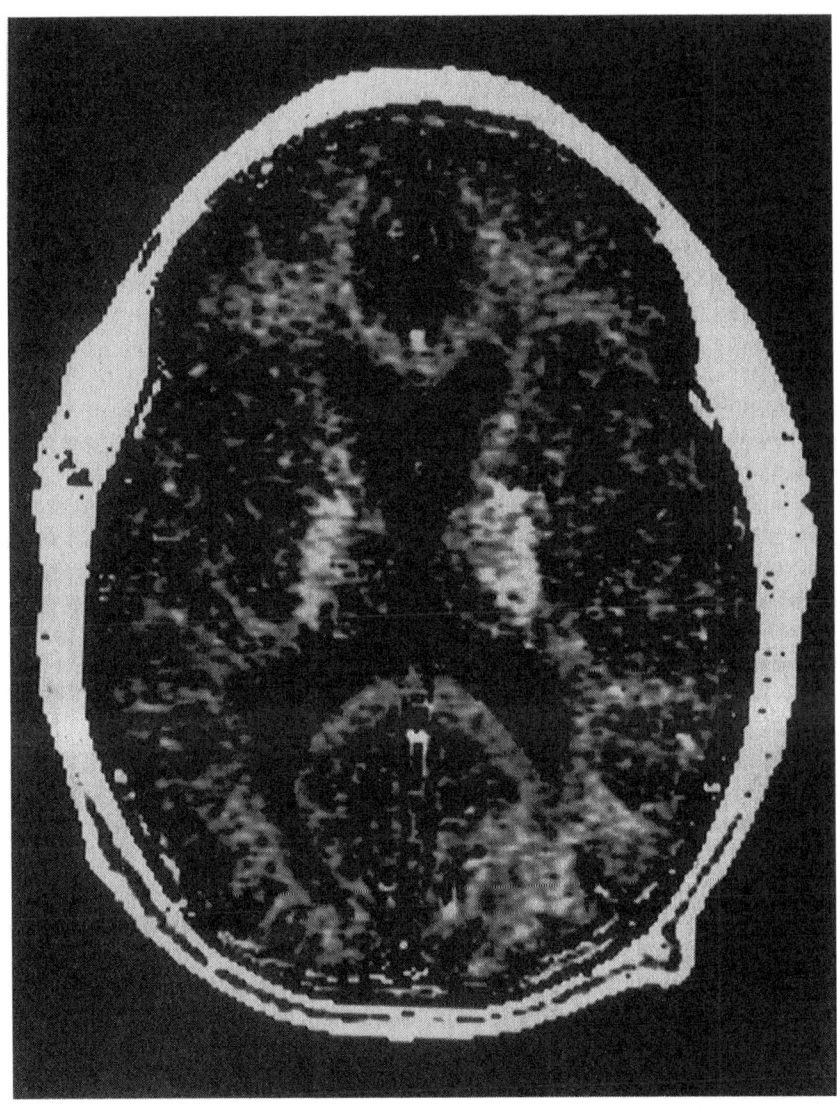

(B)

relaxation decay obtained from a single-slice 32 echo sequence with echo spacing 10 msec, TR 3000 msec, slice thickness 5 mm, and FOV 22 cm. Note that MS lesions in the myelin water map have reduced signal intensity, which is associated with demyelination.

within approximately 10%; hence changes of greater than 10% in measured times were considered to be statistically significant. The wide range in relaxation times reported in MS lesions is likely due to microscopic changes in the tissue. However, the current understanding of relaxation mechanisms in tissue is too primitive to enable us to use these results to obtain more detailed information about MS pathology.

Using a cat model, Barnes et al. (51) found that cerebral edema caused elevated T_1 and T_2 relaxation times and increased the proportion of the signal from the slower component of the biexponential relaxation decay curves (see above). This increase was related to the amount of edema. The same group (52) found that gliosis in a cat model resulted in slightly elevated T_1 and increased proton density but had little effect on T_2. These two studies should lead to a means of distinguishing between lesions which are primarily gliotic (elevated T_1 and proton density) and those containing significant amounts of edema (elevated T_1 and T_2).

Larsson et al. (48) found no difference in T_1 or T_2 relaxation times between acute and chronic MS lesions (both types of lesion had longer relaxation times compared with normal brain). However, they observed that acute plaques gave rise to single-component decay curves when measured within 20 days of onset, but usually exhibited biexponential decays at some later time. Multiexponential decays in tissue are indicative of inhomogeneity of the water environment. Potential sources of this inhomogeneity are myelinated axons, gliosis, inflammation, and edema. Armspach et al., in a related study (49), observed two-component T_2 relaxation decays in 87% of MS lesions. Barnes et al. (53) studied an MS patient group with long-standing lesions (at least 4 years old). They found elevated T_1 and T_2 times in lesions with a wide range of ages. About one-fifth of the lesions showed a blood-brain barrier defect visible with Gd-DTPA. This effect was dynamically different from that seen in acute inflammatory lesions, where maximum enhancement appears after 5 to 15 min; maximum enhancement in chronic lesions occurred from 15 to 60 min after Gd-DTPA injection. Filippi et al. (54) examined T_2 relaxation times in two groups of patients—one with benign MS (EDSS <3) and the other with secondary progressive MS (EDSS >5). They measured slightly longer T_2 relaxation times in chronic lesions from the benign group ($T_2 = 142$) than from the secondary progressive group ($T_2 = 123$ msec). Chronic lesions in the secondary progressive group were more likely to produce biexponential relaxation.

Larsson et al. (47) found that the T_2 time of normal-appearing white matter in MS was significantly longer than that in white matter of normal controls. Barbosa et al. (55) found in patients with RR MS that about 30% of the volume in normal-appearing white matter possessed elevated T_1

and T_2 times. This volume was made up of small regions, typically only one or two voxels in size, which were scattered throughout the white matter. The abnormal regions tended to occur on or near the boundary between gray and white matter. This study suggested that normal-appearing white matter may contain many microscopic lesions surrounded by otherwise normal brain tissue. Miller et al. (56) found small but measurable differences between T_1 and T_2 times from normal-appearing white matter in MS patients compared with those from white matter in normal controls and patients with systemic lupus erythematosus and cerebral sarcoidosis. Filippi et al. (54) found no significant difference between the T_2 times of normal-appearing white matter in benign MS patients and secondary progressive MS patients, suggesting that small areas of abnormality are present in both types of MS. Haughton et al. (57) found a weak correlation between abnormal values in the T_1 of normal-appearing white matter in MS patients and patient disability as measured by the Kurtzke EDSS. Therefore, evidence from MR relaxation suggests that in MS patients, disease not visualized in MRI as distinct foci of abnormal signal intensity may still contribute to disease burden and disability.

Using a technique designed to measure the complete T_2 relaxation decay curve, MacKay et al. (19) found three distinct T_2 components in the brain of normal volunteers. These three components, which had previously been measured in vitro (58,59), were (1) a minor component with T_2 about 20 msec assigned to water compartmentalized between myelin bilayers, (2) a major component with T_2 about 80 msec assigned to water in cytoplasmic and extracellular spaces, and (3) a component with T_2 longer than 1 sec assigned to cerebrospinal fluid. Previous in vivo studies were sensitive to only the latter two T_2 components. The former 20-msec component, which makes up 16% of the water in white matter on average, may provide an in vivo measure of myelin content. Initial tests on MS patients demonstrated that many MS lesions had reduced signal from the "myelin water" component. This technique may be able to characterize the myelination state of MS lesions and normal appearing white matter. A comparison between a conventional MRI scan and a myelin water image of normal and MS brain is shown in Figs. 5 and 6.

V. CONCLUSIONS

The MR findings proven or potentially able to give a pathological assessment of MS are summarized in Table 5.

Conventional serial MRI with or without Gd-DTPA is now generally accepted as an outcome measure for treatment monitoring in MS trials. In the future, additional techniques will provide a more comprehensive

Table 5 Magnetic Resonance in MS

Pathological feature	Anticipated MRI and MRS change in MS
BBB disruption	Gd-DTPA enhancement
Edema/inflammation	Expanding/contracting lesions on conventional serial MRI
Demyelination	Decreased MTR
	Selective loss of "short" T_2 signal
	Neutral lipid, choline increase, inositol increase on MRS
Gliosis	N-acetylaspartate decrease on MRS
Axonal loss	N-acetylaspartate decrease on MRS

method for monitoring therapy of MS. These include serial MRS measurements of myelin breakdown products and metabolic lesion activity, as well as advanced imaging techniques including T_2 relaxation assessment of overall myelin content, and MT measurements of demyelination. Any or all of these techniques may help assess in vivo whether therapy can modify lesion development and prevent demyelination, axonal loss, and end-stage sclerosis.

REFERENCES

1. The IFNB Multiple Sclerosis Study Group and the University of British Columbia MS/MRI Analysis Group. Interferon beta-1b in the treatment of multiple sclerosis: final outcome of the randomized controlled trial. Neurology 1995; 45:1277–1285.
2. Prineas JW. The neuropathology of multiple sclerosis. In: Vinken PJ, Bruyn GW, Klawans HL, Koetsier JC, ed. Handbook of Clinical Neurology. Vol. 3(47). Demyelinating Diseases Amsterdam: Elsevier, 1985:213–257.
3. Aita JF, Bennett DR, Anderson RE, et al. Cranial CT appearance of acute multiple sclerosis. Neurology 1978; 28:251–255.
4. Kermode AG, Tofts PS, Thompson AJ, et al. Heterogeneity of blood-brain barrier changes in multiple sclerosis: an MRI study with gadolinium-DTPA enhancement. Neurology 1990; 40:229–235.
5. Johnson MA, Li DKB, Bryant DJ, Payne JA. Magnetic resonance imaging: serial observations in multiple sclerosis. AJNR 1984; 5:495–499.

6. Isaac C, Li DKB, Genton M, et al. Multiple sclerosis: a serial study using MRI in relapsing patients. Neurology 1988; 38:1511–1515.
7. Willoughby EW, Grochowski E, Li DKB, Oger J, Kastrukoff LF, Paty DW. Serial magnetic resonance scanning in multiple sclerosis: a prospective study in relapsing patients. Ann Neurol 1989; 25:43–49.
8. Koopmans RA, Li DKB, Jardine C, et al. Chronic progressive multiple sclerosis: MRI assessment of disease activity over a six month period. Ann Neurol 1989;
9. Grossman RE, Braffman BH, Brorson JR, Goldberg HI, Silberberg DH, Gonzalez-Scarano F. Multiple Sclerosis: serial study of gadolinium-enhanced MR imaging. Radiology 1988; 169:117–122.
10. Engell T. A clinical patho-anatomical study of clinical silent multiple sclerosis. Acta Neurol Scand 1989; 79:428–430.
11. Koopmans RA, Li DKB, Grochowski E, Cutler PJ, Paty DW. Benign versus chronic progressive multiple sclerosis. magnetic resonance imaging features. Ann Neurol 1989; 25:74–81.
12. Young IR, Hall AS, Pallis CA, Legg NJ, Bydder GM, Steiner RE. Nuclear magnetic resonance imaging of the brain in multiple sclerosis. Lancet 1981; 2:1063–1066.
13. Paty DW, Asbury AD, Herndon RM, McFarland HF, McDonald WI, McIlroy WJ, Prineas JW, Scheinberg LC, Wolinsky JS. Use of magnetic resonance imaging in the diagnosis of multiple sclerosis: policy statement. Neurology 1986; 36:1575.
14. Koopmans RA, Li DKB, Redekop WK, Zhao GJ, Palmer MR, Kastrukoff LF and Paty DW. The use of magnetic resonance imaging in monitoring therapy of multiple sclerosis. J Neuroimag 1993; 3:163–168.
15. Koopmans RA, Li DKB, Zhao GJ, Redekop WK, Palmer MR and Paty DW. MRI assessment of cyclosporine therapy of MS in a multi-center trial. Neurology 1992; 42(suppl 3):210.
16. Paty DW and Li DKB. Interferon beta-1b is effective in relapsing-remitting multiple sclerosis. II. MRI analysis results of a multicenter, randomized, double-blind, placebo-controlled trial. UBC MS/MRI Study Group and the IFNB Multiple Sclerosis Study Group. Neurology 1993; 43:662–667.
17. Stone LA, Frank JA, Albert PS, et al. The effect of interferon β on blood brain barrier disruptions demonstrated by contrast-enhanced magnetic resonance imaging in relapsing/remitting multiple sclerosis. Ann Neurol 1995; 37:611–619.
18. Koopmans RA, Li DKB, Zhu G, Allen PS, Penn A, Paty DW. Magnetic resonance spectroscopy of multiple sclerosis: in vivo detection of myelin breakdown products. Lancet 1993; 341:631–632.
19. MacKay AL, Whittall KP, Adler J, Li DKB, Paty DW, Graeb D. In vivo visualization of myelin water in brain by magnetic resonance. Magn Reson Med 1994; 31:673–677.
20. Dousset V, Grossman RI, Ramer KN, Schnall MD, Young LHJ, Gonzalez-Scarano F, Lavi E, Cohen JA. Experimental allergic encephalomyelitis and

multiple sclerosis: lesion characterization with magnetization transfer imaging. Radiology 1992; 182:483–491.

21. Frahm J, Bruhn H, Gyngell ML, Merboldt KD, Hanicke W, Sauter R. Localized high-resolution proton nmr spectroscopy using stimulated echoes: Initial applications to human brain in vivo. Magn Reson Med 1989; 9:79–93.

22. Husted CA, Goodin DS, Hugg JW, Maudsley AA, Tsuruda JS, de Bie SH, Fein G, Matson GB, Weiner MW. Biochemical alterations in multiple sclerosis lesions and normal-appearing white matter detected by in vivo ^{31}P and ^{1}H spectroscopic imaging. Ann Neurol 1994; 36:157–164.

23. Arnold DL, Matthews PM, Francis GS, O'Connor J, Antel J. Proton magnetic resonance spectroscopic imaging for metabolic characterization of demyelinating plaques. Ann Neurol 1992; 31:235–241.

24. Birken DL, Oldendorf WH. N-acetyl-l-aspartic acid: A literature review of a compound prominent in the ^{1}H-NMR spectroscopic studies of brain. Neurosci Biobehav Rev 1989; 13:23–31.

25. Matthews PM, Francis GAntel J, Arnold DL. Proton magnetic resonance spectroscopy for metabolic characterization of plaques in multiple sclerosis. Neurology 1991; 41:1251–1256.

26. Davic CA, Hawkins CP, Barker GJ, Brennan A, Tofts PS, Miller DH, McDonald WI. Serial proton magnetic resonance spectroscopy in acute multiple sclerosis lesions. Brain 1994; 117:49–58.

27. Larsson HBW, Christiansen P, Jensen M, Fredericksen J, Heltberg A, Olesen J, Henricksen O. Localized in vivo proton spectroscopy in the brain of patients with multiple sclerosis. Magn Res Med 1991; 22:23–31.

28. Van Hecke P, Marchal G, Johannik K, Demaerel P, Wilms G, Carton H, Baert AL. Human brain proton localized NMR spectroscopy in multiple sclerosis. Magn Res Med 1991; 18:199–206.

29. Miller DH. Magnetic resonance in monitoring the treatment of multiple sclerosis. Ann Neurol 1994; 36:S91–S94.

30. Arnold DL, Riess GT, Matthews PM, Francis GS, Collins DL, Wolfson C, Antel JP. Use of proton magnetic resonance spectroscopy of monitoring disease progression in multiple sclerosis. Ann Neurol 1994; 36:76–82.

31. Davie CA, Hawkins CP, Barker GJ, Brennan A, Tofts PS, Miller DH, McDonald WI. Detection of myelin breakdown products by proton magnetic resonance spectroscopy. Lancet 1993; 341:630–631.

32. Grossman RI, Lenkinski RE, Ramer KN, Gonzalez-Scarano F, Cohen JA. MR proton spectroscopy in multiple sclerosis. Am J Neuroradiol 1992; 13: 1535–1543.

33. Wolinsky JS, Narayana PA. Proton magnetic resonance spectroscopy and multiple sclerosis. Lancet 1991; 337:362.

34. Wolinsky JS, Narayana PA, Fenstermacher MJ. Proton magnetic resonance spectroscopy in multiple sclerosis. Neurology 1990; 40:1764–1769.

35. Petroff OAC, Rothman DL, Behar KL. Metabolites and macromolecules changes within the MS plaque measured in vivo with serial ^{1}H NMR spectroscopy. Proc Soc Magn Reson 1994; 1:586.

36. Minderhoud JM, Mooyaart EL, Kamman RL, Teelken AW, Hoogstraten MC, Vencken LM, Gravenmade EJ, van den Brug W. In vivo phosphorous magnetic resonance spectroscopy in multiple sclerosis. Arch Neurol 1992; 49:161–165.
37. Wolff SD, Balaban RS. Magnetization transfer contrast (MTC) and tissue water proton relaxation in vivo. Magn Reson Med 1989; 10:135–144.
38. Filippi M, Campi A, Dousset V, Baratti C, Martinelli V, Canal N, Scotti G, Comi G. A magnetization transfer imaging study of normal appearing white matter in multiple sclerosis. Neurology 1995; 45:478–482.
39. Gass A, Barker GJ, Kidd D, Thorpe JW, MacManus D, Brennan A, Tofts PS, Thompson AJ, McDonald WI, Miller DH. Correlation of magnetization transfer ratio with clinical disability in multiple sclerosis. Ann Neurol 1994; 36:62–67.
40. Tomiak MM, Rosenblum JD, Prager JM, Metz CE. Magnetization transfer: a potential method to determine the age of multiple sclerosis lesions. AJNR 1994; 15:1569–1574.
41. Hiehle JF, Lenkinski RE, Grossman RI, Dousset V, Ramer KN, Schnall MS, Gohen JA, Gonzalez-Scarano F. Correlation of spectroscopy and magnetization transfer imaging in the evaluation of demyelinating lesions and normal appearing white matter in multiple sclerosis. Magn Reson Med 1994; 32:285–293.
42. Vavasour I, MacKay AL, Whittall KP. In preparation
43. Bottomley PA, Hardy CJ, Argersinger RE and Allen-Moore G. A review of ^1H nuclear magnetic resonance relaxation in pathology: Are T_1 and T_2 diagnostic? Med Phys 1987; 14:1–37.
44. Kroeker RM and Henkelman RM. Analysis of biological NMR relaxation data with continuous distributions of relaxation times. J Magn Reson 1986; 69:218–235.
45. Provencher SW. A constrained regularization method for inverting data represented by linear algebraaic or integral equations. Comput Phys Commun 1982; 27:213–227.
46. Whittall KP and MacKay AL. Quantitative interpretation of NMR relaxation data. J Magn Reson 1989; 84:134–152.
47. Larsson HBW, Rederiksen J, Kjaer L, Henriksen O, Olesen J. In vivo determination of T_1 and T_2 in the brain of patients with severe but stable multiple sclerosis. Magn Reson Med 1988; 7:43–55.
48. Larsson HBW, Frederikson J, Petersen J, Nordenbo A, Zeeberg I, Henriksen O and Olesen J. Assessment of demyelination, edema, and gliosis by in vivo determination of T_1 and T_2 in the brain of patients with acute attack of multiple sclerosis. Magn Reson Med 1989; 11:337–348.
49. Armspach JP, Gounot D, Rumbach L and Chambron J. In vivo determination of multiexponential T_2 relaxation in the brain of patients with multiple sclerosis. Magn Reson Imaging 1991; 9:107–113.
50. Larsson HBW, Christiansen P, Zeeberg I and Henriksen O. In vivo evaluation of the reproducibility of T_1 and T_2 measured in the brain of patients with multiple sclerosis. Magn Reson Imaging 1992; 10:579–584.

51. Barnes D, McDonald, Johnson G, Tofts PS and Landon DN. Quantitative nuclear magnetic resonance imaging: Characterization of experimental cerebral edema. J Neurol Neurosurg Psychiatry 1987; 50:125–133.

52. Barnes D, McDonald WI, Landon DN and Johnson G. The characterization of experimental gliosis by quantitative nuclear magnetic resonance imaging. Brain 1988; 111:83–94.

53. Barnes D, Munro PMG, Youl BD, Prineas JW, MacDonald WI. The long standing MS lesion. Brain 1991; 114:1271–1280.

54. Filippi M, Barker GJ, Hosfield MA, Sacares PR, MacManus DG, Thompson AJ, Tofts PS, McDonald WI, Miller DH. Benign and secondary progressive multiple sclerosis: A preliminary quantitative MRI study. J Neurol 1994; 241: 246–251.

55. Barbosa S, Blumhardy LD, Roberts N, Lock T and Edwards RHT. Magnetic resonance relaxation time mapping in multiple sclerosis: Normal appearing white matter and the invisible lesion load. Magn Reson Imaging 1994; 12: 33–42.

56. Miller DH, Johnson G, Tofts PS, MacManus D and McDonald WI. Precise relaxation time measurements of NAWM in inflammatory CNS disease. Magn Reson Med 1989; 11:331–336.

57. Haughton VM, Yetkin FZ, Rao SM, Rimm AA, Fischer ME, Papke RA, Breger RK and Khatri BO. Quantitative MR in the diagnosis of multiple sclerosis. Magn Reson Med 1992; 26:71–78.

58. Menon RS and Allen PS. Application of continuous relaxation distributions to the fitting of data from model systems and excised tissue. Magn Reson Med 1992; 20:214–227.

59. Stewart WA, MacKay AL, Whittall KP, Moore GRW, Paty DW. Spin-spin relaxation in experimental allergic encephalomyelitis. Analysis of CPMG data using a non-linear least squares method and linear inverse theory. Magn Reson Med 1993; 29:767–775.

16

Adverse Effects of Interferons

Richard Cirelli, Kathleen B. Herne, Monica L. McCrary, and Stephen K. Tyring

University of Texas Medical Branch, Galveston, Texas

I. CLASSIFICATION OF INTERFERONS

Interferons (IFNs) are classified into three major groups, α, β, and γ, on the basis of their antigenicity and the relatedness of their nucleotide sequences. IFNs were previously named according to the cell preparations from which they are derived. IFN-α was known as leukocyte, or lymphoblastoid, IFN, and IFN-β as fibroblast IFN. IFN-γ was known as immune IFN, because it had been derived from immunologically stimulated T lymphocytes. Type I IFNs comprise IFN-α and IFN-β, both of which bind to the same cell receptor, the type I IFN receptor. Type II IFN, IFN-γ, binds with type II receptor.

II. MAXIMUM TOLERATED DOSE, DOSE-LIMITING TOXICITIES, AND DOSE-DEPENDENT TOXICITIES

Determining maximum tolerated dose (MTD), dose-limiting toxicities (DLT), and dose-dependent toxicities (DDT) from the use of IFN is complicated by the fact that these determinations have been performed with patients suffering from a wide spectrum of diseases. The baseline condition of the patient no doubt influences how well the IFN will be tolerated. Also, not all phase I studies to determine optimal dosing took advantage of "acquired tolerance." Higher doses can often be achieved when the dose is gradually escalated because of acquired tolerance to adverse effects. Nonetheless, these studies provided a rough idea of what to expect with the use of IFNs.

A. Interferon-α

It has been suggested that intramuscular (i.m.) or subcutaneous (s.c.) administration is less well tolerated than intravenous (i.v.) administration of IFN-α (1). The contrary point of view has also been maintained (2). Intramuscular and s.c. injections do, however, increase the duration of adverse effects compared with bolus intravenous administration, probably because of more continuous and prolonged exposure (2–4). The dose relationship for i.m. or s.c. IFN-α, as determined by Quesada (1) is as follows:

1 to 5 million units (MU): tolerated for prolonged periods
6–10 MU: tolerated for a few weeks; usually a brief hiatus in treatment
   or decrease in dose will improve tolerance
>10 MU: often results in significant toxicity within days

Probably the best data for studying high-dose effects of IFN-α (MTD) comes from phase II/III studies of Kaposi's sarcoma. Although usually given i.m. or s.c. for Kaposi's sarcoma, some studies have used i.v. administration at high doses (5,6). Even at doses at 50 MU/m^2 daily, IFN-α was well tolerated and caused only flu-like symptoms and mild hematological and hepatic toxicity. Few patients discontinued treatment because of adverse effects.

One study with 52 advanced cancer patients, however, found that the MTD for i.m. IFN was 36 MU or greater (7). The DLTs in this study were fatigue/asthenia, weight loss, and elevation of transaminase levels. These DLTs required frequent interruption or reduction in dose or cessation of treatment. Myelosuppression was severe in some patients with multiple myeloma but rare in other patients. All toxicities were reversible on discontinuation of treatment.

One study using i.m. IFN-α_{2a} in patients with solid tumors attempted to determine dose-dependent toxicities (DDT) (8). One to 30 MU/injection i.m. daily was used for 14 days and then weekly for a further 10 weeks. DDTs were acute and chronic. Acute reactions took the form of an influenza-like syndrome consisting of chills, rigors, headache, tremor, nausea, vomiting, and myalgia. With these acute symptoms, tachyphylaxis developed with continued dosing. Symptoms that were not so dose dependent were more chronic in nature and tended to become more severe with prolonged treatment. These consisted of malaise, lethargy, fatigue, anorexia, and confusion. Objective toxicity consisted of myelosuppression and liver dysfunction. The investigators recommended 3–10 MU daily and 10 and 30 M twice were as tolerable i.m. doses for phase II/III studies.

A few studies have administered IFN-α by a circadian rhythm-based infusion rate (9,10). For example, maximum delivery would occur between 6 PM and 3 AM. Side effects are lessened with nighttime administration, possibly because the infusion takes place before and during the nocturnal rise in serum cortisol. This has been done with both i.v. and the s.c. routes (11). It appears that the circadian schedule allows delivery of higher doses of drug with less toxicity.

B. Interferon-β

Adverse effects with IFN-β are similar to those seen with IFN-α. Common IFN-β adverse effects are usually mild to moderate even at relatively high i.v. doses, and these include fever, chills, arthralgias, fatigue, and acral cyanosis (reported as frequent in one study) (4,12–14). Less frequent adverse effects are nausea, transient renal and hepatic dysfunction (elevated creatinine and transaminases), leukopenia, thrombocytopenia, myalgia, diarrhea, headache, and confusion (15–18). Hypotension and paresthesia have also been reported (15). Phase I studies indicate that IFN-β is less toxic than IFN-α. Kinney et al. state that although IFN-β uses the same membrane receptor as IFN-α, IFN-β_{ser}, (IFN β-1b is tolerated at a dose 5-fold to 10-fold higher than is IFN-α (14).

Intravenous infusion IFNβ_{ser} two or three times a week is tolerated at doses equal to or greater than 100 MU (12,14–21). (See note on IFN β-units in Chapter 3. These are old units. With the recalculation, differences between IFN and IFN-β are present but are less dramatic. Although most patients tolerate these high doses, particularly when the doses are gradually escalated, other patients do experience a lower MTD. MTDs for both natural IFN-β and IFN-β_{ser} have ranged from 9 to 50 MU for a single dose to greater than 500 MU after doses have been gradually increased (4,13–16,18,22–24). For example, Hu et al. found the MTD in patients with advanced cancer to be 100 MU IFN-β_{ser} i.v. on a three times a week schedule (18). MTD was defined in this study as the dose tolerated by >67% of patients.

Pertcheck et al. administered IFN-β_{ser} by rapid i.v. push to 15 patients with advanced refractory cancer in escalating doses up to 500 MU/m^2. (This would be equivalent to 930 MU for someone weighing 154 lb with a height of 5 ft 10 in.*) (24). Usually doses above 400 MU, however, cannot be tolerated unless tolerance is carefully developed (15,16). Grunberg et al. demonstrated such acquired tolerance in a study of 12 patients with advanced cancer given escalating doses of IFN-β_{ser} by i.v. infusion over 4 hr twice a week (15). Dose escalation within individual patients was allowed to a maximum dose of 400 MU/m^2. Fever, chills, fatigue, and acral cyanosis were commonly seen and increased in frequency at higher doses, but no conventional maximal tolerated dose could be defined, since several patients underwent escalation to the highest allowable dose and also developed tolerance to acute toxicities. Importantly, a maximal starting dose of 10 MU/m^2 was identified—those begun at this level or below tolerated semiweekly dose escalation, whereas those begun at 30 MU/m^2 could not tolerate continued therapy.

DLTs vary among i.v. studies. The most prevalent toxicities include fever, severe chills (associated with cardiac rhythm disturbance in one study), malaise, fatigue, anorexia, leukopenia, hypotension, and bradycardia (4,13–16,18,21–24). Most of the toxicities encountered increase in frequency at higher doses (15,16).

With i.m. administration, there is usually an absence of measurable titers in serum, yet the same adverse effects occur as those seen with i.v. administration (16). There have been few phase I (dose escalation studies of IFN-β administered by s.c. or i.m. routes. Chang et al. conducted a phase I study using IFN-β_{ser} s.c. in 14 patients with advanced cancer (25). Six patients received 10 MU and eight patients received 100 MU daily for 6 weeks. Those who did not show disease progression then received thrice weekly maintenance therapy at the same dose level. All toxicities were mild to moderate and reversible, and there were no DLTs. DDTs, however, were fever >38.5°C (12 of 14 patients), leukopenia (4 of 14), skin reaction (4 of 14), and hypertransaminasemia (4 of 14). A similar study using i.m. IFN-β_{ser} was performed with 20 cancer patients. Ten patients received 10 MU and 10 patients received 100 MU IFN-β_{ser} i.m. (26). DLTs toxicities were documented in three patients receiving the 100 MU: two patients because of fatigue and one patient because of SGOT elevation. Dose-dependent flu-like symptoms such as fever were experienced by all

---

* The equation for body surface area is

$$BSA \ (m^2) = \sqrt{\frac{Ht \ (cm) \times Wt \ (kg)}{3600}}$$

Hence, for someone weighing 154 lb (70.0 kg) with a height of 5 ft, 10 in (177.8 cm), the calculated body surface area is 1.86 m^2. At 500 MU/m^2, this person would be receiving 930 MU.

patients, and also myelo-suppression (leukopenia and thrombocytopenia) were experienced by three patients.

Phase II trials lasting for more extended periods also demonstrated the safety of IFN-β (27,28). Borden et al. administered 90 MU IFN β-1b i.v. daily for 10-day cycles separated by a period of 21 days (27), whereas Johnson et al. administered 4.5, 22.5, 45.0, or 90.0 MU (old units) s.c., twice a week for at least 6 months (28). Fever and fatigue were more frequent at higher doses in each trial, but were the major symptoms encountered.

The IFNB Multiple Sclerosis Study Group has provided the most complete information concerning the adverse effects of IFN-β_{ser} administered s.c. every other day (q.o.d.) over a prolonged period of time; that is, 3 years at publication (29). The only dose-related adverse effects significantly associated with 8 MU were fever, chills, myalgia, sweating, malaise, and injection site reactions. Laboratory abnormalities were mild, clinically insignificant, and sporadic neutropenia, anemia, and thrombocytopenia. All of the adverse effects were statistically dose related, and they were more common with 8 than with 16. With the exception of injection site reactions, all adverse side effects decreased after 3 months and approached the rate found in placebo-treated patients at 1 year.

Among the 16 patients at 2 years who withdrew from the study because of treatment side effects, 1 was in the placebo group, 5 were in 1.6-MU dose arm, and 10 were in the 8-MU dose arm. Reasons for withdrawal due to treatment effects were abnormal liver enzymes (three patients), injection site pain (three patients), fatigue (three patients), cardiac arrhythmias, allergic reactions, nausea, headache, flu-like syndrome, confusion, and "felt sick" (one patient each). In the third year, a suicide in 1.6-MU group was the only adverse-event withdrawal. (This patient had a history of depression and had stopped IFN treatment 100 days before the suicide.) At these doses of IFN β-1b, there was an absence of the severe systemic CNS side effects reported in many of the studies described in this chapter.

C. Interferon-γ

As with IFN-β, IFN-γ appears to be better tolerated than IFN-α (30). The most common toxicities with the use of IFN-γ, by either i.v., i.m., or s.c. administration, are constitutional symptoms such as fever, chills, myalgias, headache, and malaise; but sometimes they include the neurotoxic effect of fatigue/lethargy; the cardiovascular effect of hypotension (often an orthostatic hypotension [31,32]); and the hematological effect of leukopenia (usually a granulocytopenia but also a monocytopenia [33]) (3,30,34–37,37–44). Nausea and vomiting (31,32,37,45), anorexia (30,31,39,46,47), and increases in liver transaminases (and sometimes bilirubin) (32,40,45,48) are frequently encountered. Less frequently observed adverse effects include tachyarrhythmias (40), hypertriglyceridemia (39,49), and reversible first-degree atrioventricular block (37). Infrequent toxicities include hypocalcemia, diarrhea, constipation, and alopecia (45).

Longer i.v. infusion rates are usually associated with greater toxicity. For example, 12-hr infusion rates were more toxic than 6-hr infusion rates using the same dose of rIFN-γ (3,40), and 6-hr infusion rates were more toxic than 2-hr infusion rates (41,49). One study, however, found no difference in toxicity among infusion rates of 20 mins, 4 hr, and 24 hr (31).

MTDs with i.v. administration of rIFN-γ vary among different studies from 0.5 MU/m² (2,45) to 400 MU/m² (231), with most studies showing a MTD of 10–80 MU/m² (232,36,40,41,47–49). DLTs include the common constitutional symptoms of fever, chills, rigors, myalgias, headache, and malaise (40,45,48). Other DLTs include orthostatic hypotension, prolonged systolic hypotension, fatigue, anorexia, weight loss, leukopenia, hepatotoxicity, hypertriglyceridemia, lethargy and confusion (3,31,39,40,45,47,48). Toxicities are reversible, although dose-limiting occurs sporadically throughout all dosage levels (45). DDTs include the DLTs already mentioned along with nausea and vomiting and reversible first-degree atrioventricular block (37). Some studies however, find no relationship between fever, chills, and other flu-like symptoms and dose (3,37,38,42).

Far fewer studies have tried to determine the MTD with i.m. or s.c. administration of rIFN-γ. The MTD for i.m. administration is 1–5 MU/m²/day (32,43). DLTs include fatigue, malaise, and orthostatic hypotension (32,47). DDTs include the DLTs plus anorexia, weight loss, leukopenia, hepatotoxicity, and hypertriglyceridemia. One phase I study that investigated s.c. administration found 10 MU/m² was the MTD per injection (44). The DLTs from s.c. administration included headache, rigors, pyrexia, and leukopenia.

Toxicity varies considerably among patients. Some patients experience severe constitutional symptoms at low doses, whereas others treated at the MTD have few side effects. IFN in combination with chemotherapy agents, radiotherapy, or other cytokines may exhibit an additive toxic effect. The CNS and the bone marrow are particularly affected (1). Toxicities associated with IFN are usually fully reversible within days of stopping treatment.

III. SYSTEMIC ADVERSE EFFECTS

All the IFN families cause qualitatively the same systemic effects. These effects are induced at commonly used dosages and can be separated into two types: those of acute onset and those of delayed onset, which actually fall into the category of neurotoxicity (see Section IV). Both acute and delayed types have the potential to be dose limiting.

The acute effects are influenza-like in nature and characterized by a febrile reaction preceded by chills. This reaction is usually accompanied by myalgias, malaise, and headaches, or less frequently by arthralgias, mild nausea, tachycardia, and diaphoresis (1,2,50–57).

For IFN-α, the incidence of flu-like symptoms appears to be >90%, which makes fever the most common adverse effect (57). Table 1 lists the incidence of various adverse effects for IFN-α and IFN-β. For IFN-β, the most common adverse effects again are flu-like symptoms. The IFN-β Multiple Sclerosis Study Group found the incidence of flu-like symptoms was 76%; however, after 1 year, the incidence was equal to that of controls (29). Flu-like symptoms also predominate with IFN-γ.

IFN-α administered i.m. even at low doses (1–9 MU) induces fever (often 38–40°C) within 6 hr of administration (54). The temperature usually peaks at 4–8 hr following administration of IFN (58), and the fever usually lasts for 4–8 hr. IFN β-1a administered i.m. at 6 MU induces fever (usually <38°C) that may begin at 4 hr, peak at 8–10 hr, and lasts 12 hr postinjection (59). IFN-γ administered i.m. or i.v. at dosages >0.2 MU/m^2 induces fever (often >38°C) that usually peaks at 6–12 hr. IFN-γ–induced fever tends to last longer than the fever caused by IFN-α/β (31,52). The late peak after IFN-γ administration suggests that a second mediator is induced by IFN-γ. IFN-α and IFN-β induce fever probably by a combination of mechanisms. They stimulate the hypothalamus to secrete prostaglandin E$_2$, explaining why inhibitors of prostaglandin synthesis are able to prevent the adverse effect (58). They also cause the release of tumor necrosis factor (TNF) and interleukin-1 (IL-1, an endogenous pyrogen) (60).

IFN-γ also stimulates the production of IL-1 and TNF, but possibly not prostaglandin E$_2$, which may explain the difference in the pattern of fever it produces (52).

The mechanisms of tolerance and tachyphylaxis are poorly understood. Some of the adverse systemic, immune, and dermatological effects are discussed in ref. 61.

Quesada describes a dose effect for these acute-onset side effects, but there is significant person-to-person variability. IFN-α at low doses (1–9 MU) induces fever and chills which may be accompanied by myalgias, headaches, arthralgias, and other flu-like symptoms. At higher doses, patients administered IFN-α experience a high fever, with severe rigors, vasoconstriction, nausea, vomiting, intense myalgias, headaches, and exhaustion. At doses >50 MU, transient hypotension and syncope have been described (1).

Tolerance does develop against these symptoms. With IFN-α, using daily or alternate-day dosing, the febrile response and accompanying

Table 1 IFN-α and IFN-β Adverse Event Incidence (%)

Adverse events	IFN-α at varying doses in a mixed population[57]	IFN β-1b 8 MU in MS patients (n = 124)[29,57a]	Placebo in MS patients (n = 123)[29,57a]
Acute toxicity			
injection site reaction		85	37
injection site necrosis		1–5	0
flu-like symptoms:	>90[a]	76	56
fever	80–100	58	41
chills	60	47	19
myalgia	50	41	28
headache	40	70[c]	60
arthralgia	15		
diaphoresis	10	23	11
malaise		15	3
nausea and vomiting	20–50[b]		
hypotension	5–15[b]		
hypertension			
tachycardia			
Subacute or chronic toxicity			
asthenia/fatigue	30–90[b]	49	35
gastrointestinal disorders:	85[b]		
anorexia	30–60		
diarrhea	30		
dysgeusia	10–15		
weight loss	18		
menstrual disorder		17	8
dyspnea		8	2
palpitations		8	2
central nervous system disturbances:			
vertigo	20		
decreased mental status	12		
somnolence	11	6	
confusion	8		
depression	5		
paraesthesia	7		
abnormal taste	13		
cardiovascular effects:			
severe cardiotoxicity	<2		
myocardial infarction	<1		
dermatological effects:			
rash	4		

Table 1 (*continued*)

Adverse events	IFN-α at varying doses in a mixed population[57]	IFN β-1b 8 MU in MS patients (n = 124)[29,57a]	Placebo in MS patients (n = 123)[29,57a]
pruritus	4		
hair loss	5–30		
lab abnormalities			
leukopenia	25–70	16	5
thrombocytopenia	15–70		
anemia	30–60		
elevated transaminases	30–77	19	4
increased bilirubin	8–31		
increased alkaline phos.	22		
hypertriglyceridemia	32		
proteinuria	15–25		

A blank space in any of the columns signifies unknown.
[a] Controversial whether dose related.
[b] Dose-dependent adverse effects; that is, significantly increased with dosages >18 MU/ day IFN-α.
[c] Not a statistically significant increase over placebo.

symptoms usually decrease and disappear within the first few weeks. Longer dosing intervals appear to delay the onset of tolerance. With IFN-γ, fever is more persistent despite daily continuous administration (1).

Although there is not necessarily a direct relationship between dose (concentration) and toxicity, there appears to be a serum concentration threshold which if exceeded promotes a markedly more severe reaction (45,61). Dosage regimens have been proposed with these threshold and tolerance concepts in mind. Low doses are administered initially so as to limit acute adverse effects while at the same time inducing tolerance. Doses are then increased to achieve the target dose once tachyphylaxis to adverse events develops (2). For example, it has been recommended that multiple sclerosis patients start IFN β-1b at 4 MU per dose for the first 2 weeks and then change to 8 MU per dose thereafter (62).

Acetaminophen or inhibitors of prostaglandin synthesis ameliorate of these flu-like symptoms (63). Corticosteroids have also been successfully used without altering the clinical response (64). There is, however, the possibility that corticosteroids will block the antiviral activity of at least IFN-α (65).

IV. NEUROTOXICITY

An important adverse effect of IFNs, is neurotoxicity, particularly with IFN-α and apparently IFN-γ. The overall incidence of neurotoxicity in a review of 1403 patients who received IFN-α was 33% (55). At high doses of IFN-α, nearly all patients appear to develop clinical or subclinical neurotoxic effects (66). Most instances of neurotoxicity occur with high doses of IFN, doses much higher than those used to treat MS. (See also Chapter 3)

A. Central Nervous System

With continued administration of IFN-α, a persistent syndrome can occur (1,53). This syndrome is characterized by fatigue, asthenia, tiredness, lassitude, anorexia, weight loss, drowsiness, and possibly confusion. Fatigue is one of the most frequent DLTs, but the syndrome can be more serious than just fatigue. If persistent, it can reduce patients to a catabolic state with weight loss of 10% or more of body weight (55,62). It can be severe at doses above 20 MU IFN-α, particularly in elderly patients and in patients with a poor clinical condition (1). At doses above 50 MU/day of IFN-α, there may be marked somnolence, lethargy, and, very rarely, coma may occur (54,63). Very high doses ($\geq$100 MU IFN-α) can cause a syndrome of somnolence, lethargy, confusion, loss of taste and smell, mental and motor slowing with expressive dysphasia, obtundation, and, in extreme instances, coma (54,67–70). This syndrome promptly subsides on discontinuation of IFN-α. Rare cases of presenile dementia and mania have been described (54). Reversible generalized tonic-clonic convulsions and status epilepticus with unilateral seizures have occasionally been reported in patients receiving low doses of IFN-α (71–74). Low doses may produce other subclinical neurological disturbances detectable on EEG (68–70,75,76). Other rare neurological adverse effects include vertigo, cramp, ataxia, apraxia, tremor, dizziness, and extrapyramidal symptoms resembling Parkinson's disease and akathisia (57). Reversible upper motor neuron deficits of the legs have also been reported (68).

IFN-α sometimes produces psychiatric disturbances. These include behavior and emotional changes such as psychomotor slowing with lethargy, hypersomnia, loss of interest and verbal or motor spontaneity, lack of initiative, affective disorders, depression or mania, irritability, agitation, and aggressiveness. There have been cases of encephalopathy with visual hallucinations, dementia, and delirium, and of severe depression with suicidal potential (69,77). Cognitive disorders have also been reported. (See Chapter 3.)

EEG has documented diffuse or localized cerebral changes, predominantly in the anterior regions. The changes consist of slowing of dominant α rhythms, predominantly in the frontal lobes, with occasional appearance of diffuse or frontal δ or intermittent θ activity (69,70,78,79). Although electroencephalographic (EEG) changes are dose-related, no clear correlation between EEG disorders and neurological symptoms has been found (70).

IFN-γ produces similar neurophysiological changes (75). Adverse effects from recombinant IFN-γ have included fatigue, disorientation, headache, decreased alertness and confusion, dizziness, memory impairment, drowsiness, lethargy, and mild depression (38,40,45,80). Some of these effects seem to be dose related. As with IFN-α, resolution occurs on withdrawal of therapy. Seizures have occurred in IFN-γ–treated patients with brain metastasis (45). IFN-γ causes a more frequent exacerbation of relapsing-remitting multiple sclerosis (RR MS), and is considered to be contraindicated in these patients (81). A possible contributing factor is an increase of circulating monocytes bearing class II (HLA-DR) surface antigen, suggesting a deleterious IFN-γ–induced immune response.

IFN-β, by contrast, is believed to be less neurotoxic (82). Nonetheless, headache, fatigue, lethargy, depression, somnolence, weakness, agitation, malaise, and confusion or reduced ability to concentrate have been reported during IFN-β therapy, particularly with higher doses (23,27,59,83). Potentially neurotoxic effects of IFN β-1b reported in the IFN β-1b study (29) were confusion in two patients, which led to their withdrawal, and somnolence which was noted by 6% of the treated patients. Depression induced by IFN-β was a possible cause of four attempted suicides and one successful suicide (on the 1.6-MU dose) among 372 study patients receiving IFN-β over a 3-year period in the IFNβ Multiple Sclerosis Study Group trial (29). With IFN-α, the incidence of depression increases with duration of treatment, but there was no evidence of this in the IFN β-1b trial (77). Since MS patients have a higher incidence of suicide and depression, it is difficult to separate the effects of the disease from the drug.

Neurotoxic effects of high-dose i.v. IFN-β (90–540 MU three times weekly) caused early withdrawal of 10% of malignant glioma patients (23). All adverse effects were severe and included dementia, headache, fatigue, agitation, disorientation, and personality changes. Resolution of symptoms occurred on withdrawal of therapy. Mild-to-moderate CNS symptoms were observed in an additional 7% of patients, and these improved with dose reduction. In this study, malaise worsened with continued treatment, and it was the most common cause for dose reduction.

B. Peripheral Nervous System

Distal paraesthesias occurred in 7% of patients receiving high doses of IFN-α (53,68). An acute peripheral neuropathy was confirmed by electromyography in several patients receiving low doses (3–10 MU/day) of IFN-α. The patients suffered from a sensory neuropathy as well as motor polyneuropathy after at least 3 weeks of therapy. The neuropathy improved partially after dose reduction, but symptoms recurred after reintroducing IFN-α. Predisposing conditions were found in some cases.

C. Mechanisms of Neurological Disorders

IFN-α does not readily cross the blood-brain barrier. Even with doses higher than 50 MU/day, the blood concentration is only 0.1% of the plasma concentration (63,84). The other IFNs are likewise inhibited by this barrier. Because a direct effect of IFN is unlikely, indirect effects are postulated to account for the neurotoxicity. IFN-α binds to endothelial-glial cells, leading to the release of various mediators (63). IFNs may induce the release of substances such as endorphins, neurotransmitters, neuroendocrine hormones, or cytokines (IL-1, IL-2, TNF) that induce a similar toxicity profile (57). Based on clinical and EEG changes, the subcortical frontal region is proposed cause the neurasthenia and neuropsychological abnormalities, although this is contested (57).

V. HEMATOLOGICAL TOXICITIES

In a review of 1019 patients with a variety of cancers who received IFN-α_{2a}, the incidence of hematologic toxicity was leukopenia (69%), mild anemia (65%), neutropenia (58%), and thrombocytopenia (42%). Leukopenia was more common with a daily dosage schedule (56). Hemoglobin was decreased in 6.3% and hematocrit in 12.5% of patients. IFN-α often decreases peripheral white blood cell counts, particularly granulocytes, by 25–50%, and platelets by 5–50% within days of initiating treatment (1,55,85). A patient's baseline hematological health will influence the toxic effect of IFN. For example, thrombocytopenia occurs in 25–50% of patients with hematological malignancies but in only 5–10% of patients with solid malignancies (1).

Usually cytopenias are mild, self-limiting, dose dependent, predictable, and well tolerated. If severe, they respond to a dose adjustment or discontinuation of IFN (56,57). Although leukopenia and thrombocytopenia can occur at all doses, they usually become clinically significant and dose limiting only at high IFN doses (86). For all forms of IFN-α (i.e., natural and recombinant), cytopenias are seen at doses of 10–200 MU/day, depending on the route and schedule of administration (85).

Moderate normochromic, normocytic anemia may develop in patients receiving long-term therapy (54). More serious is elevated hematocrits and the development of severe and even fatal erythrocytosis in several patients during low-dose IFN-α therapy for hairy cell leukemia (87).

Protracted myelosuppression is rare even after long-term treatment. In a few patients with chronic myelogenous leukemia, however, life-threatening and sustained pancytopenias with bone marrow hypoplasia were observed during or after receiving IFN-α or IFN-γ (88,89).

Although IFN has strong antiproliferative/antidifferentiation properties in vitro, studies suggest that the decrease in leukocytes is a consequence of redistribution through a reversible inhibition of cell release from the bone marrow or the depletion and sequestration of peripheral mature cells rather than the inhibition of stem cells (57,62). It has also been suggested the IFNs suppress hematopoiesis by activating marrow suppressor T and/ or natural killer cells (88). The mechanism responsible for anemia may involve inhibition of erythropoiesis. This is suggested by the fact that anemia generally requires weeks to months to resolve, as compared to the brisk recovery from leukopenia (90).

Other hematological abnormalities are occasionally caused by IFN-α. These include mild or severe autoimmune hemolytic anemia, a positive direct Coombs' test without clinical hemolysis, a non–immune-mediated hemolytic anemia, an immune-mediated peripheral platelet destruction following IFN-α and IFN-β administration with widespread purpura, and reversible coagulation abnormalities (57).

IFN-β appears to have a higher maximum tolerated dose and induce less hematological toxicity than IFN-α (91,92). As with IFN-α and IFN-β, IFN-γ can cause a dose-dependent and reversible leukopenia, usually with granulocytopenia, and also like IFN-α/β, infrequent thrombocytopenia and anemia (38,93,94).

VI. HEPATOTOXICITY

Mild asymptomatic rises in aminotransferases have been observed in 25–30% of patients with low or moderate doses and in as many as 80% of those receiving high doses of IFN-α (50–80 MU twice weekly) (54,57). Increases in alkaline phosphatase, lactic dehydrogenase, and bilirubin have also been noted (53,54). Some patients without viral markers and consequently misdiagnosed with hepatitis C were later found to have autoimmune hepatitis. Some experienced an exacerbation of their disease on receiving IFN-α (95,96). (see also Section XII). Liver biopsies of patients with elevated hepatic enzyme levels show fatty metamorphosis of the liver (54).

Severe IFN-associated hepatotoxicity is rare. Fatal hepatic decompensation with ascites, jaundice, or encephalophy occurred within 2 months of receiving IFN-α in 9 of 2490 patients treated for chronic hepatitis B or C (97). Possibly this hepatic decompensation was the result of their viral disease, and indeed five patients had showed signs of decompensation before treatment. Nonetheless, patients with very active chronic hepatitis B may be predisposed to severe exacerbation and require closer monitoring of liver function during treatment.

As with IFN-α, IFN-β therapy can cause elevation in serum transaminases (27,59). Such elevations are reversible and there have been no reports of severe long-term hepatic dysfunction.

IFN-γ therapy elevates liver enzymes and serum bilirubin with relative frequency (38,40,45,80). As many as 76% of malignant melanoma patients had elevated liver enzymes after a twice weekly 2-hr i.v. infusion of IFN-γ (80). The elevations are reversible on cessation of therapy.

VII.   GASTROINTESTINAL DISORDERS

Nausea and vomiting occur in 10–30% of patients following dosages <18 MU/day of IFN-α and in 40–60% of patients during high-dose regimens of >18 MU/day (53,55). Tachyphylaxis to gastrointestinal effects usually develops. Mild watery diarrhea and abdominal pain have been reported in as many as 25% of patients and were more severe at higher doses. Anorexia is also relatively common.

Nausea and vomiting occurred in 52% of renal carcinoma patients during a 10-day i.v. course of IFN-β (27). Anorexia and occasional diarrhea have also been reported with IFN-β. IFN-γ, likewise, has produced nausea, vomiting, anorexia, and also a stomatitis (38,40,45,80,93).

VIII.   RENAL AND ELECTROLYTE DISTURBANCES
AND CATABOLISM OF IFNs

IFN-α is both catabolized and eliminated by the kidney; hepatic metabolism and biliary excretion serve as only minor elimination pathways (2,98–100). Although the kidney is the main elimination site for IFN-α, the mean total body clearance of IFN-α_{2a} is 1.8 times the glomerular filtration rate, indicating that extrarenal mechanisms (and renal tubular secretion and renal catabolism) contribute to elimination (2). Some IFN-α is rapidly inactivated in body fluids and tissue. Because of the body's conservation of amino acids inherent to the catabolism of proteins, negligible amounts of intact IFN-α are excreted in urine or bile (101). This is true also for IFN-β (102) and IFN-γ (103).

The liver appears to be an important catabolic site for IFN-β, possibly because it is glycosylated (104). It is important to note that IFN β-1b and some forms of IFN-α are not glycosylated, and their metabolism may differ from the metabolism of glycosylated forms of IFN-β. Both the liver and kidney are important catabolic sites for recombinant IFN-γ (unglycosylated) and natural (glycosylated) IFN-γ (103). (Unlike IFN-α or nonglycosylated IFN-γ, IFN-β and natural glycosylated IFN-γ are poorly absorbed from muscle or skin, and serum levels are often not detectable (106)).

Proteinuria is the most common renal disorder associated with the use of IFN and affects 15–25% of IFN-α recipients (54–56). The proteinuria is mild, clinically insignificant, and reversible. Benign and asymptomatic proteinuria has also been associated with IFN-β and IFN-γ (20,93).

Kurchel et al. performed a prospective study of IFN-α_{2b} nephrotoxicity in 58 patients with myeloproliferative syndromes. There was glomerular damage with moderate proteinuria in 10–20% and subclinical tubular injury in all patients (106). Serum creatinine was temporarily elevated in 10% of patients. Of 1019 patients with solid or hematological malignancies receiving IFN-α, 14% developed increased leukocytes in the urine, 4.5% increased erythrocytes in the urine, 10% an increased BUN, 10% an increased serum creatinine, and 15% an increased uric acid (53).

Oliguric and nonoliguric acute renal failure have developed with both IFN-α and IFN-γ. With IFN-α, examples include a recurrent nephrotic syndrome with a biopsy showing acute interstitial nephritis and minimal change nephropathy, (107) and an acute renal failure with a biopsy showing severe glomerular changes (108). With IFN-γ, a focal segmental glomerulosclerosis with acute tubular necrosis and interstitial edema has been reported (109). Using a combination of IFN-α and IFN-γ, one patient developed a nephrotic syndrome and acute renal failure (110).

Although renal disorders usually occur within the first weeks of therapy, renal insufficiency has been reported after a low-dose IFN-α maintenance regimen (between 2.5 and 6.5 years) (108). Renal function usually returns to normal after stopping IFN; however, irreversible or incomplete resolution of renal function has been rarely noted with IFN-α and IFN-γ (108,110–112). The mechanism of the proteinuria is not known but is probably not a direct effect of IFN. Acute renal failure and nephrotic syndrome are seemingly independent of the dose given (107). No significant renal disorder were seen in the pivotal IFN β-16 trial (29).

The syndrome of inappropriate antidiuretic hormone secretion (SIADH) resulting in hyponatremia has been described with IFN-α in cancer patients (54). Farkkila et al. described SIADH in six patients with amyotrophic lateral sclerosis receiving IFN-α-n3 (human leukocyte IFN) at 100–200 MU daily i.v. (113). Other electrolyte disturbances have also been reported with including significant decreases in serum calcium, and urinary excretion of magnesium high doses of IFN-α (114). On ceasing treatment, these effects were reversed.

The mechanism of nephrotoxicity is not clearly established. Possibly there is a direct nephrotoxic effect (109) and/or immune related damage. Theories for the mechanism of immune damage include enhancement of cellular immunity (107) and attack by activated lymphocytes after IFN-α–induced expression of human leukocyte (HLA)–DR antigens on the renal cells (106).

IX. CARDIOVASCULAR EFFECTS

The IFN-induced febrile reaction can affect the cardiovascular system by causing tachycardia, vasomotor reactions with distal cyanosis, diaphoresis, or occasionally hypotension. These reactions may jeopardize a patient with a limited heart reserve by precipitating congestive heart failure (1). Also, increased oxygen demand caused by fever, chills, and tachycardia may render an already compromised patient susceptible to infarction or arrhythmia (115). In one review study of 44 cancer patients with IFN-induced cardiotoxicity of a serious nature, none of 12 patients who had preexisting heart disease developed cardiomyopathy, but instead they developed arrhythmia or myocardial infarction (116). The cardiotoxicity was caused by either recombinant IFN-α (most patients) or IFN-γ; none of the patients had received IFN-β. The cardiotoxic effect was not related to total amount of IFN received or to duration of treatment. Hence, it was not necessarily related to the febrile reaction. The most common cardiotoxicity was arrhythmia. Twenty-five patients experienced supraventricular and ventricular arrhythmias. Supraventricular arrhythmias were reversed by antiarrhythmic drugs or dose reduction, and IFN treatment could be continued or reintroduced. However, 10 patients suffered a myocardial infarction or sudden death, and 5 developed a cardiomyopathy.

A prospective study looking at severe cardiovascular toxicity followed 138 IFN-α$_{2a}$ recipients (117). There were cardiac complications in six patients (4.3%), including septal hypokinesia compatible with myocardial infarction, angina pectoris, asymptomatic deterioration of cardiac function on echocardiography, complete atrioventricular block, and recurrent atrial fibrillation. Although symptoms resolved after cessation of treatment, full recovery was observed in only half of the patients.

Despite these reports, serious IFN-related cardiotoxicity, including arrythmia, is very uncommon. In a review of 15 phase I trials involving a total of 432 patients, most of whom where given recombinant IFN-α or IFN-γ and a few IFN-β, no significant cardiotoxic adverse effects of IFN were reported (118). Benign cardiovascular toxicity such as moderate hypotension and sometimes hypertension, uncomplicated tachycardia, and distal cyanosis occurs in 5–15% of IFN recipients within the first days of treatment (54,55,119). Unlike the more serious toxicities, these benign effects appear more dose related, are more severe in aged patients, and occur transiently during the initial febrile reaction.

Reviews of adverse effects of IFN-α encompassing more than 2000 patients from various clinical trials found cardiovascular effects in 5–15% of patients. The most frequent cardiovascular adverse effects were hypotension occurring in 5–6% of patients, chest pain in 3%, and myocardial infarction in 1% (53,56). A causal relation between IFN-α and the cardiovascular event could not be fully assessed.

The febrile reaction is a mechanism for some of the cardiovascular effects of IFN. Coronary spasm, peripheral vascular effects, altered adenosine triphosphate (ATP) levels (120), overstimulation of norepinephrine release (121), and autoimmune or inflammatory reactions have also been proposed. The inflammatory and immune-related causes have not been borne out in histological studies of the myocardium (122).

Since patients with previous heart disease have shown aggravation of ischemic symptoms during therapy, IFN should not be given in the presence of unstable angina. In patients with effort angina or previous ischemic events, careful cardiac observation should follow the first dose of IFN until cessation of the flu-like reaction. Sonnenblick et al. recommend commencing treatment with small doses and increasing them gradually in patients with a cardiac history (116).

X. DERMATOLOGICAL TOXICITY

Cutaneous reactions such as dryness, itching, transient skin rashes, diffuse erythema or urticaria, and nonspecific skin lesions occur with a frequency of about 5–12% (54,55).

Severe necrotizing cutaneous lesions complicating treatment with IFN β-1b have been reported. Sheremata et al. (123) reported marked acanthosis associated with superficial and deep perivascular and interstitial lymphocytic and histiocytic infiltrates mixed with neutrophils. Focal thrombosis of vessels was seen in deeper sections. Oeda and Shinohara (124) described a case of cutaneous necrosis caused by the injection of IFN-α. They stated that the pathogenesis of the cutaneous necrosis was unknown but may be related to a local inflammatory process (125). Trautinger and Knobler (126), however, propose that the explanation may be unintentional periarterial or intra-arterial injection with subsequent cutaneous infarction. Sheremata et al. (127) subsequently reported, however, that no arterial or arteriolar thrombosis was seen in a patient treated with IFN-α_{2b} who developed skin necrosis. The investigators did see capillary and venous thrombosis, leading them to suggest that preexisting factors contribute to a hypercoagulable state and increased the risk of ulceration.

New onset psoriasis and exacerbation of existing psoriasis have been reported with IFN-α (128). Psoriatic lesions have also been reported at the injection site of s.c. IFN-β (129) and IFN-γ (130); the latter in 10 of 42 patients treated for psoriatic arthritis. In the IFN-γ study of psoriatic arthritis patients, placebo and insulin injections did not produce psoriatic lesions.

Mild alopecia is rare at low dosage but is the most frequent cutaneous adverse effect in patients receiving higher doses of IFN-α (1). It is thought to be secondary to telogen effluvium and occurs in 23–30% of patients after several weeks of IFN-α therapy (131).

The mechanisms responsible for the various cutaneous effects of IFNs are not known, although a depot effect with less diffusion of IFN-β than of IFN-α (131a), increased production of epidermal IL-1 (132), and immunostimulating effects are likely to be involved (57). (See also Chapter 13.)

XI. ENDOCRINE AND METABOLIC DISORDERS

Cortisol and corticotropin secretion increase significantly after single dose of IFN-α (115,133,134) and IFN-γ (135). The effect is dose dependent, since a dose of 10 MU increased corticotropin plasma concentration, but a dose of 3 MU did not (136). These effects disappear after 3–4 weeks' treatment with IFN-α, suggesting desensitization (115). There is no elevation in serum cortisol with long-term IFN β-1b therapy (138).

Plasma norepinephrine increased following injection of IFN-α_{2a} 3 MU in healthy volunteers. In contrast, epinephrine plasma levels decreased in patients in the standing position (134).

IFN-α and IFN-β cause a sustained but reversible increase in plasma cholesterol by 15–40% within the first few days of treatment (137–141). Both low-density and high-density lipoproteins are affected.

Infectious diseases are associated with hypertriglyceridemia. Serum triglycerides increase after long-term treatment with IFN-α for viral hepatitis (142), and with IFN-α treatment of acquired immune deficiency syndrome (AIDS) patients. The serum concentration of IFN-α in these patients correlates with the triglyceride level (143). IFNs also induce triglycerides in the absence of infection. IFN β-1b at 8 MU s.c. every other day also elevates triglycerides (144), and IFN-γ is associated with a reversible and dose-dependent hypertriglyceridemia in cancer patients (145).

Prolonged prothrombin and partial thromboplastin times in leukemic patients have been described. This is associated with a decrease in activity of vitamin K–dependent factor and factor XIII (1).

XII. AUTOIMMUNITY AND IMMUNE DISORDERS

About 20–60% of patients may present with isolated autoantibodies after IFN treatment (57). Following IFN therapy, autoantibodies have developed against microsomal, thyroid, thyroglobulin, nuclear, and parietal cell antigens. At least one type of autoantibody, which failed to produce clinical symptoms, was found in 87% of 31 previously autoantibody-negative patients receiving IFN-α 10 MU/m^2 two to three times weekly (146). Lower dosages of IFN-α produce fewer autoantibodies. IFN-α at 4.5–5.0 MU three times weekly produced only asymptomatic antinuclear antibodies in 18% of 28 previously autoantibody-negative patients; assays for 11 other autoantibodies were negative (147).

The development of autoantibodies rarely causes autoimmune disease. Nonetheless, autoimmune diseases have been associated with the use of IFN and include autoimmune thyroiditis, hemolytic anemia and thrombocytopenia, systemic lupus erythematosus (SLE), rheumatoid arthritis, and exacerbation of psoriasis (148).

A. Thyroid Dysfunction

A number of investigators have reported thyroid dysfunction after IFN-α therapy (149–160). Hypothyroidism is more common than hyperthyroidism by at least twofold. Both may also appear together in the same patient in a condition similar to Hashimoto's thyroiditis, which begins with a transient hyperthyroidism followed by hypothyroidism (149,157,161). The experience with IFN-β and IFN-γ is limited in regard to thyroid autoimmunity. Presently, it appears they induce few antithyroid antibodies, although with more studies, particularly with IFN-γ, a greater association will probably be found. In studies specifically looking for signs of thyroid autoimmunity, none was detected in 20 patients treated with IFN-β (162) nor in 29 patients given recombinant IFN-γ (163,164). Patients with a history of autoimmune thyroid disorders are more likely to be affected with IFN-associated thyroid dysfunction than patients with no such history (156,157).

B. Systemic Lupus Erythematosus and Rheumatoid Symptoms

Both IFN-α and IFN-γ have been implicated in the occurrence of a SLE-like syndrome and a multiorgan flare of preexisting mild SLE (165–171). Patients usually present with arthralgia, proteinuria, anemia, and exanthema. Antinuclear antibody and anti–double-stranded DNA titers are increased. Complete clinical remission is usually achieved by withdrawing IFN or by using immunosuppressive drugs. However, there are cases of life-threatening or fatal IFN-associated SLE (167,172).

A number of inflammatory arthropathies have been associated with IFN-α. These include symmetrical seropositive (or seronegative) polyarthritis (173–176). Monoarthritis (177,178), and symmetrical seronegative polyarthritis with cutaneous psoriasis (179). IFN-γ was implicated in the development or reactivation of seronegative arthritis in three of nine patients treated for cutaneous psoriasis (180). Symptoms began 10–12 weeks after initiation of therapy and resolved with the cessation of IFN-γ, but one patient developed a recurrence following subsequent administration of IFN. IFN-γ induces MHC class II antigens on synovial cells, which may account for induction or exacerbation of immune-mediated arthritis (181).

The incidence of SLE-like disease and rheumatoid symptoms was assessed in 125 patients with chronic myelogenous leukemia (CML) and in 12 patients with essential thrombocythemia who received either IFN-α alone or a combination of IFN-α and low-dose IFN-γ (165). Twenty-seven of the 137 patients (20%) developed rheumatoid symptoms, three of which fulfilled the criteria for SLE. Elevated ANA titers were found in 5 of 19 (26%) of CML patients at the time of diagnosis and in 3 of 18 (17%) of patients treated with hydroxyurea or busulfan. After a median of 6 months of IFN treatment, however, 18 of 25 tested patients (72%) had elevated ANA titers. Some also had elevated levels of IgG, IgM, serum complement, rheumatoid factor, and other autoantibodies. In 15 of the ANA-positive patients, clinical signs of autoimmune disease appeared. These occurred after a median of 20 months of treatment and consisted mostly of myalgia, arthralgia or arthritis, and Raynaud's phenomenon. All these patients were in remission of disease and most were females by a 2:1 ratio. Severity of side effects led to the discontinuation of IFN treatment in three patients.

C. Other Autoimmune Diseases

IFN-α has been implicated in the development of insulin-dependent diabetes mellitus in one patient treated for hepatitis C after a 6-month course of treatment (182). Although the patient seroconverted to positive for islet cell antibodies, the patient had low titers of insulin autoantibodies and thyroid microsomal antibodies before treatment, suggesting genetic susceptibility.

IFN-γ resulted in the exacerbation of multiple sclerosis in 7 of 18 patients. There was a concomitant increase in circulating monocytes bearing class II (HLA-DR) surface antigen, suggesting the attacks were immunologically mediated.

D. Predisposing Factors and Mechanisms of Autoimmune Disorders

Most patients who develop clinical symptoms of autoimmunity with IFN therapy have preexisting autoantibodies (149,153,157). For example, in patients with malignant carcinoid who developed autoimmune thyroid disease during IFN-α therapy, 61% had preexisting antithyroid antibodies (149). There is a much lower incidence of thyroid disease in untreated autoantibody-positive healthy controls. It appears that the likelihood of developing an autoimmune disorder is increased with IFN-α/IFN-γ combinations (165) and in irradiation/IFN-α combination (158) therapy. High dose and/or long duration IFN-α therapy also appears to be a contributing factor (149,153,183).

Exactly how IFNs cause autoantibody development and autoimmune disease is unclear. Possibly the immunological actions of IFN cause a dysregulation between self-tolerance and activation of cells recognizing autologous antigens. This could occur through an increase in pathogenic autoantibodies; enhanced cytotoxic T-cell activity; inhibition of T suppressor cell function; the activation of cytokine-secreting immune cell induction of HLA class I antigen expression; and through aberrant or enhanced expression of MHC class II antigens on previously HLA-DR–negative cells with subsequent enhancement of self-antigen presentation (57,62,148). (See also Chapter 7.)

XIII. SAFETY IN PREGNANCY

IFN-α has produced no mutagenic or teratogenic effects in experimental models (57). Nor does IFN-α inhibit DNA synthesis. A study that used ex vivo placental perfusion suggests IFN-α does not cross the placenta (184).

Seven patients treated for chronic myelogenous leukemia or essential thrombocythemia with IFN-α during different stages of pregnancy, including the first trimester in five cases and the whole pregnancy in three, resulted in uncomplicated and successful pregnancies (185–188). Six went full-term and one premature at 34 weeks. After 2 and 3 years, those babies followed normal growth and development (175–187). Because of IFN's antiproliferative effects and the lack of experience using IFN-α during pregnancy, it is recommended that IFN-α treatment be delayed till after pregnancy, unless it is necessary to treat a life-threatening disease (57).

IFN-γ, on the other hand, has caused a dramatic decrease in fetal weight, increase in abortion rate, and several other fetal abnormalities in murine studies. This suggests its contraindication in pregnant women (189).

XIV. CONCLUSIONS

IFNs have a broad spectrum of action in that they induce a number of very active proteins and play a critical role in the body's immune system. Consequently, it is not surprising that IFNs induce a broad variety of adverse effects. These toxicities, however, should not detract from the important therapeutic uses of these agents.

Often low doses are as effective as high doses. If high doses are needed, gradually building up to them while developing tolerance to some of the more debilitating adverse effects is a good strategy. More will be learned about adverse effects of IFNs, but it is already clear that IFNs have a high therapeutic index in the treatment of a number of infections and neoplastic diseases, as well as in diseases of unknown etiology such as multiple sclerosis.

ACKNOWLEDGMENT

Data were managed and analyzed using the General Clinical Research Center Computerized Data Management and Analysis System (CDMAS), supported by grant M0)1 RR-00073 from the National Center for Research Resources, National Institutes of Health, USPHS.

REFERENCES

1.　Quesada JR. Toxicity and side effects of interferons. In: Baron S, Coppenhaver DH, Dianzani F, et al, eds. Interferon: Principles and Medical Applications. Galveston: The University of Texas Medical Branch at Galveston, Department of Microbiology, 1992:427–432.

2.　Wills RJ. Clinical pharmacokinetics of interferons. Clin Pharmacokinet 1990; 19:390–399.

3.　Kurzrock R, Quesada JR, Rosenblum MG, Sherwin SA, Gutterman JU. Phase I study of IV administered recombinant gamma interferon in cancer patients. Cancer Treat Rep 1986; 70:1357–1364.

4. Borden EC, Hawkins MJ, Sielaff KM, Storer BM, Schiesel JD, Smalley RV. Clinical and biological effects of recombinant interferon-beta administered intravenously daily in phase I trial published erratum appears in J Interferon Res 1988 8(5):704. J Interferon Res 1988; 8:357–366.

5. Volberding PA, Mitsuyasu RT, Golando JP, Spiegel RJ. Treatment of Kaposi's sarcoma with interferon alfa-2b (Intron A). Cancer 1987; 59: 620–625.

6. Groopman JE, Gottlieb MS, Goodman J, et al. Recombinant alpha-2 interferon therapy for Kaposi's sarcoma associated with the acquired immunodeficiency syndrome. Ann Intern Med 1984; 100:671–676.

7. Quesada JR, Hawkins M, Horning S, et al. Collaborative phase I–II study of recombinant DNA-produced leukocyte interferon (clone A) in metastatic breast cancer, malignant lymphoma, and multiple myeloma. Am J Med 1984; 77:427–432.

8. Wagstaff J, Chadwick G, Howell A, Thatcher N, Scarffe JH, Crowther D. A phase I toxicity study of human rDNA interferon in patients with solid tumours. Cancer Chemother Pharmacol 1984; 13:100–105.

9. Iacobelli S, Garufi C, Irtelli L, et al. A phase I study of recombinant interferon-α administered as a seven-day continuous venous infusion at circadian-rhythm modulated rate in patients with cancer. Am J Clin Oncol 1995; 18:27–31.

10. Depres-Brummer P, Levi F, Di Palma M, et al. A phase I trial of 21-day continuous venous infusion of alpha-interferon at circadian rhythm modulated rate in cancer patients. J Immunol 1991; 10:440–447.

11. Ludwig CU, Ludwig-Hagemann R, Obrist R, Obrecht JP, Holdener EE, Sutter-Melde C. Improved tolerance of interferon alpha-2a by continuous subcutaneous infusion. Onkologie 1990; 13:117–122.

12. Bukowski RM, Sergi JS, Sharfman WJ, et al. Phase I trial of natural human interferon beta in metastatic malignancy. Cancer Res 1991; 51:836–840.

13. Allen J, Packer R, Bleyer A, Zeltzer P, Prados M, Nirenberg A. Recombinant interferon beta: a phase I–II trial in children with recurrent brain tumors. J Clin Oncol 1991; 9:783–788.

14. Kinney P, Triozzi P, Young D, et al. Phase II trial of interferon-beta-serine in metastatic renal cell carcinoma. J Clin Oncol 1990; 8:881–885.

15. Grunberg SM, Kempf RA, Venturi CL, Mitchell MS. Phase I study of recombinant beta-interferon given by four-hour infusion. Cancer Res 1987; 47:1174–1178.

16. Hawkins M, Horning S, Konrad M, et al. Phase I evaluation of a synthetic mutant of beta-interferon. Cancer Res 1985; 45:5914–5920.

17. Liberati AM, Cinieri S, Senatore MG, et al. Phase I–II trial on natural beta interferon in chemoresistant and relapsing multiple myeloma. Haematologica 1990; 75:436–442.

18. Hu E, Horning SJ. Phase I study of recombinant human interferon beta in patients with advanced cancer. J Biol Resp Mod 1987; 6:121–129.

19. Rinehart JJ, Young D, Laforge J, Colborn D, Neidhart JA. Phase I/II trial

of interferon-beta-serine in patients with renal cell carcinoma: immunological and biological effects. Cancer Res 1987; 47:2481–2485.

20. Sarna G, Pertcheck M, Figlin R, Ardalan B. Phase I study of recombinant beta ser 17 interferon in the treatment of cancer. Cancer Treat Rep 1986; 70:1365–1372.

21. Borden EC, Kim K, Ryan L, et al. Phase II trials of interferons-alpha and -beta in advanced sarcomas. J Interferon Res 1992; 12:455–458.

22. Liberati AM, Biscottini B, Fizzotti M, et al. A phase I study of human natural interferon-beta in cancer patients. J Interferon Res 1989; 9:339–348.

23. Yung WK, Prados M, Levin VA, et al. Intravenous recombinant interferon beta in patients with recurrent malignant gliomas: a phase I/II study (see comments). J Clin Oncol 1991; 9:1945–1949.

24. Pertcheck M, Figlin R, Sarna G. Phase I study of beta ser 17 interferon by rapid intravenous push. Proc Am Soc Clin Oncol 1985; 4:226.

25. Chang AYC, Pandya KJ, Asbury RF, et al. Phase I study of recombinant beta interferon ser (rIFN-βser) in cancer patients by subcutaneous (sc) injection. Proc Am Soc Clin Oncol 1985; 4:226.

26. Chang AYC, Asbury RF, McCune C, et al. Phase I study of human recombinant beta interferon (IFN-βser) in cancer patients by intramuscular injection. Proc Am Soc Clin Oncol 1986; 5:233.

27. Borden EC, Rinehart JJ, Storer BE, Trump DL, Paulnock DM, Teitelbaum AP. Biological and clinical effects of interferon-beta ser at two doses. J Interferon Res 1990; 10:559–570.

28. Johnson KP, Knobler RL, Greenstein JI, et al. Recombinant human beta interferon treatment of relapsing-remitting multiple sclerosis: pilot study results (abstr). Neurology 1990; 40(suppl 1):261.

29. IFNB Multiple Sclerosis Study Group. Interferon beta-1b is effective in relapsing-remitting multiple sclerosis. I. Clinical results of a multicenter, randomized, double-blind, placebo-controlled trial. Neurology 1993; 43: 655–661.

30. Foon KA, Sherwin SA, Abrams PG, et al. A phase I trial of recombinant gamma interferon in patients with cancer. Cancer Immunol Immunother 1985; 20:193–197.

31. Laszlo J, Goldstein D, Gockerman J, et al. Phase I studies of recombinant interferon-gamma. J Biol Resp Mod 1990; 9:185–193.

32. Perez R, Lipton A, Harvey HA, et al. A phase I trial of recombinant human gamma interferon (IFN-gamma 4A) in patients with advanced malignancy. J Biol Resp Mod 1988; 7:309–317.

33. Aulitzky WE, Tilg H, Vogel W, et al. Acute hematologic effects of interferon alpha, interferon gamma, tumor necrosis factor alpha and interleukin 2. Ann Hematol 1991; 62:25–31.

34. Creagan ET, Schaid DJ, Ahmann DL, Frytak S. Disseminated malignant melanoma and recombinant interferon: analysis of seven consecutive phase II investigations. J Invest Dermatol 1990; 95:188S–192S.

35. German Lymphokine Study Group. Double blind controlled phase III multi-

center clinical trial with interferon gamma in rheumatoid arthritis. Rheumatol Int 1992; 12:175–185.

36. Rinehart JJ, Young D, Laforge J, Colburn D, Neidhart J. Phase I/II trial of recombinant gamma-interferon in patients with renal cell carcinoma: immunologic and biologic effects. J Biol Resp Mod 1987; 6:302–312.

37. Boue F, Pastran Z, Spielmann M, et al. A phase I trial with recombinant interferon gamma (Roussel UCLAF) in advanced cancer patients. Cancer Immunol Immunother 1990; 32:67–70.

38. Boman BM, Gagen MM, Bonnem E, et al. Phase I study of recombinant gamma-interferon (rIFN-gamma). J Biol Resp Mod 1988; 7:438–446.

39. Quesada JR, Kurzrock R, Sherwin SA, Gutterman JU. Phase II studies of recombinant human interferon gamma in metastatic renal cell carcinoma. J Biol Respir Mod 1987; 6:20–27.

40. Ernstoff MS, Trautman T, Davis CA, et al. A randomized phase I/II study of continuous versus intermittent intravenous interferon gamma in patients with metastatic melanoma. J Clin Oncol 1987; 5:1804–1810.

41. Vadhan-Raj S, Al-Katib A, Bhalla R, et al. Phase I trial of recombinant interferon gamma in cancer patients. J Clin Oncol 1986; 4:137–146.

42. van der Burg M, Edelstein M, Gerlis L, Liang CM, Hirschi M, Dawson A. Recombinant interferon-gamma (immuneron): results of a phase I trial in patients with cancer. J Biol Resp Mod 1985; 4:264–272.

43. Kurzrock R, Quesada JR, Talpaz M, Hersh EM, Reuben JM, Sherwin SA. Phase I study of multiple dose intramuscularly administered recombinant gamma interferon. J Clin Oncol 1986; 4:1101–1109.

44. Wagstaff J, Smith D, Nelmes P, Loynds P, Crowther D. A phase I study of recombinant interferon gamma administered by s.c. injection three times per week in patients with solid tumours. Cancer Immunol Immunother 1987; 25:54–58.

45. Brown TD, Koeller J, Beougher K, Golando J, Bonnem EM, Spiegel RJ. A phase I clinical trial of recombinant DNA gamma interferon. J Clin Oncol 1987; 5:790–798.

46. Rinehart JJ, Malspeis L, Young D, Neidhart JA. Phase I/II trial of human recombinant interferon gamma in renal cell carcinoma J Biol Resp Mod 1986; 5:300–308.

47. Sherwin SA, Foon KA, Abrams PG, et al. A preliminary Phase I trial of partially purified interferon-gamma in patients with cancer. J Biol Resp Mod 1984; 3:599–607.

48. Garnick MB, Reich SD, Maxwell B, Coval-Goldsmith S, Richie JP. Phase I/II study of recombinant interferon gamma in advanced renal cell carcinoma. J Urol 1988; 139:251–255.

49. Vadhan-Raj S, Nathan CF, Sherwin SA, Oettgen HF, Krown SE. Phase I trial of recombinant interferon gamma by 1-hour i.v. infusion. Cancer Treat Rep 1986; 70:609–614.

50. Quesada JR, Gutterman JU, Hersh EM. Clinical and immunological study of beta interferon by intramuscular route in patients with metastatic breast cancer. J Interferon Res 1982; 2:593–599.

51. McPherson TA, Tan YH. Phase I pharmacotoxicology study of human fibroblast interferon in human cancers. J Natl Cancer Inst 1980; 65:75–79.
52. Kurzrock R, Rosenblum MG, Sherwin SA, et al. Pharmacokinetics, single-dose tolerance, and biological activity of recombinant gamma-interferon in cancer patients. Cancer Res 1985; 45:2866–2872.
53. Jones GJ, Itri LM. Safety and tolerance of recombinant interferon alfa-2a (Roferon-A) in cancer patients. Cancer 1986; 57:1709–1715.
54. Quesada JR, Talpaz M, Rios A, Kurzrock R, Gutterman JU. Clinical toxicity of interferons in cancer patients: a review. J Clin Oncol 1986; 4:234–243.
55. Spiegel RJ. The alpha interferons: clinical overview. Semin Oncol 1987; 14:1–12.
56. Gauci L. Management of cancer patients receiving interferon alfa-2a. Int J Cancer Suppl 1987; 1:21–30.
57. Vial T, Descotes J. Clinical toxicity of the interferons. Drug Saf 1994; 10:115–150.
57a. Goodkin DE. Interferon beta-1b. Lancet 1994; 344:1057–1060.
58. Dinarello CA, Bernheim HA, Duff GW, et al. Mechanisms of fever induced by recombinant human interferon. J Clin Invest 1984; 74:906–913.
59. Liberati AM, Horisberger MA, Palmisano L, et al. Double-blind randomized phase I study on the clinical tolerance and biological effects of natural and recombinant interferon β. J Interferon Res 1992; 12:329–336.
60. Dianzani F. Interferon treatments: how to use an endogenous system as a therapeutic agent. J Interferon Res 1992; Spec No:109–118.
61. Wills RJ, Dennis S, Spiegel HE, Gibson DM, Nadler PI. Interferon kinetics and adverse reactions after intravenous, intramuscular, and subcutaneous injection. Clin Pharmacol Ther 1984; 35:722–727.
62. Arnason BG, Reder AT. Interferons and multiple sclerosis. Clin Neuropharmacol 1994; 17:495–547.
63. Bocci V. Central nervous system toxicity of interferons and other cytokines. J Biol Regul Homeost Agents 1988; 2:107–118.
64. Visco G, Boumis E, Noto P, Comandini UV. Prevention of side-effects of interferon (letter). Lancet 1991; 337:741.
65. Witter FR, Woods AS, Griffin MD, Smith CR, Nadler P, Lietman PS. Effects of prednisone, aspirin, and acetaminophen on an in vivo biologic response to interferon in humans. Clin Pharmacol Ther 1988; 44:239–243.
66. Niiranen A, Laaksonen R, Iivanainen M, Mattson K, Farkkila M, Cantell K. Behavioral assessment of patients treated with alpha-interferon. Acta Psychiatr Scand 1988; 78:622–626.
67. Adams F, Quesada JR, Gutterman JU. Neuropsychiatric manifestations of human leukocyte interferon therapy in patients with cancer. JAMA 1984; 252:938–941.
68. Smedley H, Katrak M, Sikora K, Wheeler T. Neurological effects of recombinant human interferon. Br Med J (Clin Res Ed) 1983; 286:262–264.
69. Renault PF, Hoofnagle JH, Park Y, et al. Psychiatric complications of long-term interferon alfa therapy. Arch Intern Med 1987; 147:1577–1580.

70. Suter CC, Westmoreland BF, Sharbrough FW, Hermann RC, Jr. Electroencephalographic abnormalities in interferon encephalopathy: a preliminary report. Mayo Clin Proc 1984; 59:847–850.

71. Crockett DM, McCabe BF, Lusk RP, Mixon JH. Side effects and toxicity of interferon in the treatment of recurrent respiratory papillomatosis. Ann Otol Rhinol Laryngol 1987; 96:601–607.

72. Dierckx RA, Michotte A, Schmedding E, Ebinger G, Degeeter T, van CampB. Unilateral seizures in a patient with hairy cell leukemia treated with interferon. Clin Neurol Neurosurg 1985; 87:209–212.

73. Janssen HL, Berk L, Vermeulen M, Schalm SW. Seizures associated with low-dose alpha-interferon (letter). Lancet 1990; 336:1580.

74. Hibi H, Itoh K, Kamiya T, Yamada Y, Shimoji T. [Grand mal like attack by interferon injection in case of renal cell carcinoma] (Japanese). Hinyokika Kiyo 1991; 37:69–72.

75. Born J, Spath-Schwalbe E, Pietrowsky R, Porzsolt F, Fehm HL. Neurophysiological effects of recombinant interferon-gamma and -alpha in man. Clin Physiol Biochem 1989; 7:119–127.

76. McDonald EM, Mann AH, Thomas HC. Interferons as mediators of psychiatric morbidity. An investigation in a trial of recombinant alpha-interferon in hepatitis-B carriers. Lancet 1987; 2:1175–1178.

77. Prasad S, Waters B, Hill PB, Portera FA, Riely CA. Psychiatric side effects in interferon alpha-2b in patients treated for hepatitis C (abstr). Clin Res 1992; 40:340A.

78. Mattson K, Niiranen A, Iivanainen M, et al. Neurotoxicity of interferon (letter). Cancer Treat Rep 1983; 67:958–961.

79. Rohatiner AZ, Prior PF, Burton AC, Smith AT, Balkwill FR, Lister TA. Central nervous system toxicity of interferon. Br J Cancer 1983; 47:419–422.

80. Creagan ET, Loprinzi CL, Ahmann DL, Schaid DJ. A phase I-II trial of the combination of recombinant leukocyte A interferon and recombinant human interferon-gamma in patients with metastatic malignant melanoma. Cancer 1988; 62:2472–2474.

81. Panitch HS, Hirsch RL, Haley AS, Johnson KP. Exacerbations of multiple sclerosis in patients treated with gamma interferon. Lancet 1987; 1:893–895.

82. Liberati AM, Biagini S, Perticoni G, Ricci S, D'Alessandro P, Cinieri S. Electrophysiological and neuropsychological functions in patients treated with interferon-beta. J Interferon Res 1990; 10:613–619.

83. Caselmann WH, Eisenburg J, Hofschneider PH, Koshy R. Beta- and gamma-interferon in chronic active hepatitis B. A pilot trial of short-term combination therapy. Gastroenterology 1989; 96:449–455.

84. Smith RA, Norris F, Palmer D, Bernhardt L, Wills RJ. Distribution of alpha interferon in serum and cerebrospinal fluid after systemic administration. Clin Pharmacol Ther 1985; 37:85–88.

85. Ernstoff MS, Kirkwood JM. Changes in the bone marrow of cancer patients treated with recombinant interferon alpha-2. Am J Med 1984; 76:593–596.

86. Balmer CM. The new alpha interferons. Drug Intell Clin Pharm 1985; 19: 887–893.

87.   Steis RG, VanderMolen LA, Lawrence J, et al. Erythrocytosis in hairy cell leukaemia following therapy with interferon alpha. Br J Haematol 1990; 75: 133–135.

88.   Mangan KF, Zidar B, Shadduck RK, Zeigler Z, Winkelstein A. Interferon-induced aplasia: evidence for T-cell-mediated suppression of hematopoiesis and recovery after treatment with horse antihuman thymocyte globulin. Am J Hematol 1985; 19:401–413.

89.   Talpaz M, Kantarjian H, Kurzrock R, Gutterman JU. Bone marrow hypoplasia and aplasia complicating interferon therapy for chronic myelogenous leukemia. Cancer 1992; 69:410–412.

90.   Ingimarsson S, Bergstrom K, Brostrom LA, Cantell K, Strander H. Effect of long-term treatment with human leukocyte interferon on various laboratory parameters. Acta Med Scand 1980; 208:155–159.

91.   Miles SA, Wang HJ, Cortes E, Carden J, Marcus S, Mitsuyasu RT. Beta-interferon therapy in patients with poor-prognosis Kaposi sarcoma related to the acquired immunodeficiency syndrome (AIDS). A phase II trial with preliminary evidence of antiviral activity and low incidence of opportunistic infections. Ann Intern Med 1990; 112:582–589.

92.   Rinehart J, Malspeis L, Young D, Neidhart J. Phase I/II trial of human recombinant beta-interferon serine in patients with renal cell carcinoma. Cancer Res 1986; 46:5364–5367.

93.   Sriskandan K, Garner P, Watkinson J, Pettingale KW, Brinkley D, Tee DE. A toxicity study of recombinant interferon-gamma given by intravenous infusion to patients with advanced cancer. Cancer Chemother Pharmacol 1986; 18:63–68.

94.   Di Bisceglie AM, Rustgi VK, Kassianides C, Lisker-Melman M, Park Y, Hoofnagle JH. Therapy of chronic hepatitis B with recombinant human alpha and gamma interferon. Hepatology 1990; 11:266–270.

95.   Papo T, Marcellin P, Bernuau J, Durand F, Poynard T, Benhamou JP. Autoimmune chronic hepatitis exacerbated by alpha-interferon (see comments). Ann Intern Med 1992; 116:51–53.

96.   Vento S, Di Perri G, Garofano T, Cosco L, Concia E, Ferraro T. Hazards of interferon therapy for HBV-seronegative chronic hepatitis (letter). Lancet 1989; 2:926.

97.   Janssen HL, Brouwer JT, Nevens F, Sanchez-Tapias JM, Craxi A. Fatal hepatic decompensation associated with interferon alfa. European concerted action on viral hepatitis (Eurohep). Br Med J 1993; 306:107–108.

98.   Bino T, Edery H, Gertler A, Rosenberg H. Involvement of the kidney in catabolism of human leukocyte interferon. J Gen Virol 1982; 59:39–45.

99.   Bino T, Madar Z, Gertler A, Rosenberg H. The kidney is the main site of interferon degradation. J Interferon Res 1982; 2:301–308.

100. Bocci V, Di Francesco P, Pacini A, Pessina GP, Rossi GB, Sorrentino V. Renal metabolism of homologous serum interferon. Antiviral Res 1983; 3: 53–58.

101. Bocci V. Distribution, catabolism and pharmacokinetics of interferons. In:

Finter NB, et al., eds. In Vivo and Clinical Fluids. New York: Elsevier, 1985:47–72.

102. Abdi EA, Kamitomo VJ, McPherson TA, Konrad MW, Inoue M, Tan YH. Extended phase I study of human beta-interferon in human cancer. Clin Invest Med 1986; 9:33–40.

103. Bocci V, Pacini A, Pessina GP, Paulesu L, Muscettola M, Lunghetti G. Catabolic sites of human interferon-gamma. J Gen Virol 1985; 66:887–891.

104. Bocci V, Pacini A, Bandinelli L, Pessina GP, Muscettola M, Paulesu L. The role of liver in the catabolism of human alpha- and beta-interferon. J Gen Virol 1982; 60:397–400.

105. Billiau A, De Somers P, Edy VG, De Clercq E, Heremans H. Human fibroblast interferon for clinical trials: pharmacokinetics and tolerability in experimental animals and humans. Antimicrob Agents Chemother 1979; 16: 56–63.

106. Kurschel E, Metz-Kurschel U, Niederle N, Aulbert E. Investigations on the subclinical and clinical nephrotoxicity of interferon alpha-2B in patients with myeloproliferative syndromes. Ren Fail 1991; 13:87–93.

107. Averbuch SD, Austin HA, Sherwin SA, Antonovych T, Bunn PA, Jr., Longo DL. Acute interstitial nephritis with the nephrotic syndrome following recombinant leukocyte a interferon therapy for mycosis fungoides. N Engl J Med 1984; 310:32–35.

108. Lederer E, Truong L. Unusual glomerular lesion in a patient receiving long-term interferon alpha. Am J Kidney Dis 1992; 20:516–518.

109. Ault BH, Stapleton FB, Gaber L, Martin A, Roy S, Murphy SB. Acute renal failure during therapy with recombinant human gamma interferon. N Engl J Med 1988; 319:1397–1400.

110. Nair S, Ernstoff MS, Bahnson RR, et al. Interferon-induced reversible acute renal failure with nephrotic syndrome. Urology 1992; 39:169–172.

111. Sawamura M, Matsushima T, Tamura J, Murakami H, Tsuchiya J. Renal toxicity in long-term alpha-interferon treatment in a patient with myeloma (letter). Am J Hematol 1992; 41:146.

112. Noel C, Vrtovsnik F, Facon T, et al. Acute and definitive renal failure in progressive multiple myeloma treated with recombinant interferon alpha-2a: report of two patients (letter). Am J Hematol 1992; 41:298–299.

113. Farkkila M, Iivanainen M, Roine R, et al. Neurotoxic and other side effects of high-dose interferon in amyotrophic lateral sclerosis. Acta Neurol Scand 1984; 70:42–46.

114. Farkkila AM, Iivanainen MV, Farkkila MA. Disturbance of the water and electrolyte balance during high-dose interferon treatment. J Interferon Res 1990; 10:221–227.

115. Gisslinger H, Svoboda T, Clodi M, Gilly B, Ludwig H, Havelec L. Interferon-alpha stimulates the hypothalamic-pituitary-adrenal axis in vivo and in vitro. Neuroendocrinology 1993; 57:489–495.

116. Sonnenblick M, Rosin A. Cardiotoxicity of interferon. A review of 44 cases (review). Chest 1991; 99:557–561.

117. Mansat-Krzyzanowska E, Dreno B, Chiffoleau A, Litoux P. Cardiovascular manifestations associated with interferon alfa-2A. Ann Med Interne (Paris) 1991; 142:576–581.

118. Takai Y, Herrmann SH, Greenstein JL, Spitalny GL, Burakoff SJ. Requirement for three distinct lymphokines for the induction of cytotoxic T lymphocytes from thymocytes. J Immunol 1986; 137:3494–3500.

119. Mattson K, Niiranen A, Pyrhonen S, Farkkila M, Cantell K. Recombinant interferon gamma treatment in non-small cell lung cancer. Antitumour effect and cardiotoxicity. Acta Oncol 1991; 30:607–610.

120. Lampidis TJ, Brouty-Boye D. Interferon inhibits cardiac cell function in vitro. Proc Soc Exp Biol Med 1981; 166:181–185.

121. Bialock JE, Stanton JD. Common pathways of interferon and hormonal action. Nature 1980; 283:406–408.

122. Deyton LR, Walker RE, Kovacs JA, et al. Reversible cardiac dysfunction associated with interferon alfa therapy in AIDS patients with Kaposi's sarcoma (see comments). N Engl J Med 1989; 321:1246–1249.

123. Sheremata WA, Taylor JR, Elgart GW. Severe necrotizing cutaneous lesions complicating treatment with interferon beta-1b. N Engl J Med 1995; 332:1584.

124. Oeda E, Shinohara K. Cutaneous necrosis caused by injection of α-interferon in a patient with chronic myelogenous leukemia. Am J Hematol 1993; 44:213–214.

125. Shinohara K. More on interferon-induced cutaneous necrosis. N Engl J Med 1995; 333:1222.

126. Trautinger F, Knobler RM. Chronic pancreatitis. N Engl J Med 1995; 333: 1222–1223.

127. Sheremata WA, Taylor JR, Elgart GW. Chronic pancreatitis. N Engl J Med 1995; 333:1223–1224.

128. Quesada JR, Gutterman JU. Psoriasis and alpha-interferon. Lancet 1986; 1:1466–1468.

129. Kowalzick L, Weyer U. Psoriasis induced at the injection site of recombinant interferons [letter; comment]. Arch Dermatol 1990; 126:1515–1516.

130. Fierlbeck G, Rassner G, Muller C. Psoriasis induced at the injection site of recombinant interferon gamma. Results of immunohistologic investigations (see comments). Arch Dermatol 1990; 126:351–355.

131. Tosti A, Misciali C, Bardazzi F, Fanti PA, Varotti C. Telogen effluvium due to recombinant interferon alpha-2b. Dermatology 1992; 184:124–125.

131a. Billiau A, de Somer P, Edy VG, de Clercq E, Heremans H. Human fibroblast interferon for clinical trials: pharmacokinetics and tolerability in experimental animals and humans. Antimicrob Agents Chemother 1979; 16: 56–63.

132. Dreno B, Huart A, Billaud E, Litoux P, Godefroy WY. Alpha-interferon therapy and cutaneous vascular lesions (letter). Ann Intern Med 1989; 111: 95–96.

133. Muller H, Hiemke C, Hammes E, Hess G. Sub-acute effects of interferon-alpha 2 on adrenocorticotrophic hormone, cortisol, growth hormone and prolactin in humans. Psychoneuroendocrinology 1992; 17:459–465.

134. Pende A, Musso NR, Vergassola C, et al. Neuroendocrine effects of interferon alpha 2-a in healthy human subjects. J Biol Regul Homeost Agents 1990; 4:67–72.

135. Krishnan R, Ellinwood EH, Laszlo J, Hood L, Ritchie J. Effect of gamma interferon on the hypothalamic-pituitary-adrenal system. Biol Psychiatry 1987; 22:1163–1166.

136. Barreca T, Picciotto A, Franceschini R, Varagona G, Corsini G, et al. Effects of acute administration of recombinant interferon alpha 2b on pituitary hormone secretion in patients with chronic active hepatitis. Curr Ther Res 1992; 52:695–701.

137. Dixon RM, Borden EC, Keim NL, Anderson S, Spennetta TL, Tormey DC. Decreases in serum high-density-lipoprotein cholesterol and total cholesterol resulting from naturally produced and recombinant DNA-derived leukocyte interferons. Metabolism 1984; 33:Clinical &-Clinical &4.

138. Reder AT, Lowy MT. Interferon-β treatment does not elevate cortisol in multiple sclerosis. J Interferon Res 1992; 12:195–198.

139. Massaro ER, Borden EC, Hawkins MJ, Wiebe DA, Shrago E. Effects of recombinant interferon-alpha 2 treatment upon lipid concentrations and lipoprotein composition. J Interferon Res 1986; 6:655–662.

140. Rosenzweig IB, Wiebe DA, Borden EC, Storer B, Shrago ES. Plasma lipoprotein changes in humans induced by beta-interferon. Atherosclerosis 1987; 67:261–267.

141. Schectman G, Kaul S, Mueller RA, Borden EC, Kissebah AH. The effect of interferon on the metabolism of LDLs. Arterioscler Thromb 1992; 12:1053–1062.

142. Ruiz-Moreno M, Carreno V, Rua MJ, Cotonat T, Serrano B, Santos M. Increase in triglycerides during alpha-interferon treatment of chronic viral hepatitis (letter). J Hepatol 1992; 16:384.

143. Grunfeld C, Kotler DP, Shigenaga JK, et al. Circulating interferon-alpha levels and hypertriglyceridemia in the acquired immunodeficiency syndrome. Am J Med 1991; 90:154–162.

144. Byskosh PV, Reder AT. IFN β-1b effects on cytokine mRNA in peripheral mononuclear cells in multiple sclerosis. Multiple Sclerosis 1996; 1:262–269.

145. Kurzrock R, Rohde MF, Quesada JR, et al. Recombinant gamma interferon induces hypertriglyceridemia and inhibits post-heparin lipase activity in cancer patients. J Exp Med 1986; 164:1093–1101.

146. Schattner A. Interferons and autoimmunity (review). Am J Med Sci 1988; 295:532–544.

147. Mayet WJ, Hess G, Gerken G, et al. Treatment of chronic type B hepatitis with recombinant alpha-interferon induces autoantibodies not specific for autoimmune chronic hepatitis. Hepatology 1989; 10:24–28.

148. Fattovich G, Betterle C, Brollo L, Giustina G, Pedini B, Alberti A. Induction of autoantibodies during alpha interferon treatment in chronic hepatitis B. Arch Virol 1992; 4(suppl):291–293.

149. Rönnblom LE, Alm GV, Öberg KE. Autoimmunity after alpha-interferon therapy for malignant carcinoid tumors. Ann Intern Med 1991; 115:178–183.

150. Saracco G, Touscoz A, Durazzo M, et al. Autoantibodies and response to alpha-interferon in patients with chronic viral hepatitis. J Hepatol 1990; 11: 339–343.

151. Lisker Melman M, Di Bisceglie AM, Usala SJ, Weintraub B, Murray LM, Hoofnagle JH. Development of thyroid disease during therapy of chronic viral hepatitis with interferon alfa. Gastroenterology 1992; 102:2155–2160.

152. Burman P, Totterman TH, Oberg K, Karlsson FA. Thyroid autoimmunity in patients on long term therapy with leukocyte-derived interferon. J Clin Endocrinol Metab 1986; 63:1086–1090.

153. Gisslinger H, Gilly B, Woloszczuk W, Mayr WR, Havelec L, Linkesch W. Thyroid autoimmunity and hypothyroidism during long-term treatment with recombinant interferon-alpha. Clin Exp Immunol 1992; 90:363–367.

154. Schultz M, Muller R, von zur Muhlen A, Brabant G. Induction of hyperthyroidism by interferon-alpha-2b (letter). Lancet 1989; 1:1452.

155. Picciotto A, Varagona G, Cianciosi P, Franceschini R, Garibaldi A. Thyroid function and interferon treatment in chronic hepatitis C (letter; comment). Gut 1993; 34:574.

156. Marcellin P, Pouteau M, Renard P, et al. Sustained hypothyroidism induced by recombinant alpha interferon in patients with chronic hepatitis C (see comments). Gut 1992; 33:855–856.

157. Conlon KC, Urba WJ, Smith JW, Steis RG, Longo DL, Clark JW. Exacerbation of symptoms of autoimmune disease in patients receiving alpha-interferon therapy. Cancer 1990; 65:2237–2242.

158. Giles FJ, Worman CP, Jewell AP, Goldstone AH. Recombinant alpha-interferons, thyroid irradiation and thyroid disease. Acta Haematol 1991; 85: 160–163.

159. Kamikubo K, Takami R, Suwa T, et al. Case report: silent thyroiditis developed during alpha-interferon therapy. Am J Med Sci 1993; 306:174–176.

160. Koizumi S, Mashio Y, Mizuo H, et al. Graves' hyperthyroidism following transient thyrotoxicosis during interferon therapy for chronic hepatitis type C. Intern Med 1995; 34:58–60.

161. Sauter NP, Atkins MB, Mier JW, Lechan RM. Transient thyrotoxicosis and persistent hypothyroidism due to acute autoimmune thyroiditis after interleukin-2 and interferon-alpha therapy for metastatic carcinoma: a case report. Am J Med 1992; 92:441–444.

162. Pagliacci MC, Pelicci G, Schippa M, Liberati AM, Nicoletti I. Does interferon-beta therapy induce thyroid autoimmune phenomena? Horm Metab Res 1991; 23:196–197.

163. Kung AW, Jones BM, Lai CL. Effects of interferon-gamma therapy on thyroid function, T-lymphocyte subpopulations and induction of autoantibodies. J Clin Endocrinol Metab 1990; 71:1230–1234.

164. Bhakri H, Sriskandan K, Davis T, Pettingale K, Tee D. Recombinant gamma interferon and autoimmune thyroid disease (letter). Lancet 1985; 2: 457.

165. Wandl UB, Nagel Hiemke M, May D, et al. Lupus-like autoimmune disease induced by interferon therapy for myeloproliferative disorders. Clin Immunol Immunopathol 1992; 65:70–74.

166. Machold KP, Smolen JS. Interferon-gamma induced exacerbation of systemic lupus erythematosus. J Rheumatol 1990; 17:831–832.

167. Graninger WB, Hassfeld W, Pesau BB, Machold KP, Zielinski CC, Smolen JS. Induction of systemic lupus erythematosus by interferon-gamma in a patient with rheumatoid arthritis. J Rheumatol 1991; 18:1621–1622.

168. Schilling PJ, Kurzrock R, Kantarjian H, Gutterman JU, Talpaz M. Development of systemic lupus erythematosus after interferon therapy for chronic myelogenous leukemia. Cancer 1991; 68:1536–1537.

169. Ronnblom LE, Alm GV, Oberg KE. Possible induction of systemic lupus erythematosus by interferon-alpha treatment in a patient with a malignant carcinoid tumour. J Intern Med 1990; 227:207–210.

170. Tolaymat A, Leventhal B, Sakarcan A, Kashima H, Monteiro C. Systemic lupus erythematosus in a child receiving long-term interferon therapy. J Pediatr 1992; 120:429–432.

171. Mehta ND, Hooberman AL, Vokes EE, Neeley S, Cotler S. 35-year-old patient with chronic myelogenous leukemia developing systemic lupus erythematosus after alpha-interferon therapy [letter]. Am J Hematol 1992; 41:141.

172. Machold KP, Neumann K, Smolen JS. Recombinant human interferon gamma in the treatment of rheumatoid arthritis: double blind placebo controlled study. Ann Rheum Dis 1992; 51:1039–1043.

173. Chazerain P, Meyer O, Kahn MF. Rheumatoid arthritis-like disease after alpha-interferon therapy (letter; comment) (see comments). Ann Intern Med 1992; 116:427.

174. Ueno Y, Sohma T. Alpha-interferon-induced nodular rheumatoid arthritis in renal cell carcinoma (letter; comment). Ann Intern Med 1992; 117:266–267.

175. Taylor HG, Davis MJ, Hothersall TE. Hairy cell leukaemia and rheumatoid arthritis (letter; comment). Br J Rheumatol 1991; 30:391–392.

176. Maccari S, Bassi C, Giovannini AG, Plancher AC. A case of arthropathy and hypothyroidism during recombinant alpha-interferon therapy. Clin Rheumatol 1991; 10:452–454.

177. Chan GC, Lee SS, Yeoh EK. Mono-arthritis in a chronic hepatitis B patient after alpha-interferon treatment. J Gastroenterol Hepatol 1992; 7:432–433.

178. Kiely PD, Bruckner FE. Acute arthritis following interferon-alpha therapy (letter). Br J Rheumatol 1994; 33:502–503.

179. Jucgla A, Marcoval J, Curco N, Servitje O. Psoriasis with articular involvement induced by interferon alfa (letter). Arch Dermatol 1991; 127:910–911.

180. O'Connell PG, Gerber LH, Digiovanna JJ, Peck GL. Arthritis in patients with psoriasis treated with gamma-interferon. J Rheumatol 1992; 19:80–82.

181. Amento EP, Bhan AK, McCullagh KG, Krane SM. Influences of gamma interferon on synovial fibroblast-like cells. Ia induction and inhibition of collagen synthesis. J Clin Invest 1985; 76:837–848.

182. Fabris P, Betterle C, Floreani A, et al. Development of type 1 diabetes mellitus during interferon alfa therapy for chronic HCV hepatitis (letter) (see comments). Lancet 1992; 340:548.

183. Fonseca V, Thomas M, Dusheiko G. Thyrotropin receptor antibodies fol-

lowing treatment with recombinant alpha-interferon in patients with hepatitis. Acta Endocrinol 1991; 125:491–493.

184. Waysbort A, Giroux M, Mansat V, Teixeira M, Dumas JC, Puel J. Experimental study of transplacental passage of alpha interferon by two assay techniques. Antimicrob Agents Chemother 1993; 37:1232–1237.

185. Baer MR, Ozer H, Foon KA. Interferon-alpha therapy during pregnancy in chronic myelogenous leukaemia and hairy cell leukaemia. Br J Haematol 1992; 81:167–169.

186. Reichel RP, Linkesch W, Schetitska D. Therapy with recombinant interferon alpha-2c during unexpected pregnancy in a patient with chronic myeloid leukaemia. Br J Haematol 1992; 82:472–473.

187. Crump M, Wang XH, Sermer M, Keating A. Successful pregnancy and delivery during alpha-interferon therapy for chronic myeloid leukemia (letter). Am J Hematol 1992; 40:238–239.

188. Petit JJ, Callis M, Fernandez de Sevilla A. Normal pregnancy in a patient with essential thrombocythemia treated with interferon-alpha 2b (letter) (see comments). Am J Hematol 1992; 40:80.

189. Vassiliadis S, Tsoukatos D, Athanassakis I. Interferon-induced class II expression at the spongiotrophoblastic zone of the murine placenta is linked to fetal rejection and developmental abnormalities. Acta Physiol Scand 1994; 151:485–495.

17

Interferon-τ: A Potential Treatment for Inflammatory Central Nervous System Disease

Jeanne M. Soos

Brigham and Women's Hospital, Boston, Massachusetts

Joel Schiffenbauer and Howard M. Johnson

University of Florida, Gainesville, Florida

Carol H. Pontzer

University of Maryland, College Park, Maryland

I. INTRODUCTION

Interferon-τ (IFN-τ) is a recently discovered IFN that possesses activities similar to those observed for the other type I IFNs, α and β; however, IFN-τ functions in the absence of normally associated toxicity (1–5). In light of the recent success of IFN β-1b treatment for multiple sclerosis (MS), IFN-τ has been examined for its ability to prevent the development of experimental allergic encephalomyelitis (EAE), an animal model of antigen-induced autoimmunity that has been widely studied to gain insight into MS (6). IFN-τ has been shown to prevent the development and superantigen-induced exacerbations of EAE in the absence of toxicity (7). Sections of this chapter cover the background of IFN-τ, an overview of IFN-τ structure-function studies, including its lack of toxicity as well as the development of IFN-τ for use as an immunotherapy for EAE.

II. IDENTIFICATION AND CHARACTERIZATION OF IFN-τ

A. Discovery of IFN-τ

Ovine IFN-τ (OvIFN-τ) was the first IFN-τ to be identified. In 1979, several isoforms of an 18-kDa protein were identified in conceptus homogenates (8). The conceptus is the embryo and the surrounding membranes.

Subsequently, a low molecular weight protein released into conceptus culture medium was purified and shown to be both heat labile and susceptible to proteases (9). It was originally called ovine trophoblast protein-one (oTP-1), because it was the primary secretory protein initially produced by trophectoderm of the sheep conceptus. The question immediately arose as to the function of this protein. It was produced in surprisingly high amounts, approximately 250 μg/day (10). Further, the timing of its secretion (from days 13–21 of pregnancy) coincided with the time frame for maternal recognition of pregnancy (9). This signal from the embryo to the mother is necessary for successful continuation of the pregnancy.

Functionally, IFN-τ infusion into the uterine horn of nonpregnant ewes prolonged the estrous cycle and the life span of the corpus luteum (11,12). In the cycling ewe, uterine oxytocin receptors increase prior to luteolysis (13). Oxytocin produced by the anterior pituitary or the corpus luteum acts on uterine oxytocin receptors to induce the pulsatile secretion of prostaglandin $F_{2\alpha}$ ($PGF_{2\alpha}$) by the uterus. These $PGF_{2\alpha}$ pulses travel in a retrograde fashion to the ovary and act on the corpus luteum to produce regression. Regression of the corpus luteum is associated with the lack of progesterone secretion; hence, no pregnancy. In contrast, in the pregnant ewe, oxytocin receptor numbers are downregulated by IFN-τ (1,14). Consequently, $PGF_{2\alpha}$ pulses are not triggered by oxytocin. The corpus luteum is maintained, the requisite progesterone is produced, and establishment of pregnancy occurs.

Types of IFN-τ with similar characteristics and activities have been isolated from other ruminant species, including cows and goats (15,16). Antisera to all these types of IFN-τ cross react. This is not unexpected, since the species-specific forms of IFN-τ are more closely homologous to each other than to an IFN-α from the identical species (17). Antiviral activity, identified by immunoneutralization as resulting from a type I IFN, has also been detected in conceptus cultures of nonruminant species such as mice, pigs, horses, and rabbits, although it is on the order of 1000 U rather than 10^6 U (17). The human gene which encodes for an equivalent protein is discussed in detail below.

Thus, IFN-τ acts to signal maternal recognition of pregnancy in ruminants, just as chorionic gonadotropin does in humans. Its function, though, is more appropriately described as antiluteolytic rather than luteotrophic, since it acts on the uterus rather than directly on the corpus luteum.

B. Identification of IFN-τ as a Member of the IFN Family of Molecules

IFN-τ was purified from conceptus cultures by ion exchange chromatography and gel filtration. It shared size (19 kDa) and charge (pl = 5.5–5.7) with IFN-α (18). The cDNA was obtained by probing a sheep blastocyst library with a synthetic oligonucleotide representing the N-terminal amino acid sequence (18). The predicted amino acid sequence was 45–55% homologous with IFN-α from human, mouse, rat, and pig and 70% homologous with bovine IFN-α_2, now referred to as IFN-ω. Currently, several cDNA sequences have been reported which represent different isoforms (19–21). All are approximately 1 kb with a 585-base open reading frame that codes for a 23–amino acid leader sequence and a 172–amino acid mature protein. The predicted structure of IFN-τ as a four-helical bundle with the amino- and carboxy-termini in apposition further speaks to its being classified as a type I IFN (22).

In addition to its novel reproductive function, IFN-τ displays all of the activities classically associated with the type I IFNs (Table 1). Its antiviral activity is as potent as any known IFN (23). Upregulation of 2',5'-oligoadenylate synthetase, a mechanism for IFN-induced antiviral protection, has also been demonstrated for IFN-τ (24). IFN-τ also displays antiretroviral activity, inhibiting reverse transcriptase of both the feline and human immunodeficiency viruses (3,25). It exhibits antiproliferative activity against a variety of cell lines, including Madin-Darby bovine kidney (MDBK), murine L929, and human WISH cells, retarding their entry into S phase of the cell cycle (4). Since cell lines from different species are responsive to OvIFN-τ, it has cross-species activity. Further, IFN-τ inhibits the mixed lymphocyte reaction as well as both mitogen- and superantigen-induced lymphocyte proliferation (5,26). All the activities described above can be observed at IFN-τ concentrations similar to those of IFN-α. An advantage to the use of IFN-τ is the ability to use high concentrations of IFN-τ without cellular toxicity (1–5).

Despite the classification of IFN-τ as a type I IFN, considerable differences exist between it and other type I IFNs. All type I IFNs, except

Table 1 Overview of the IFNs

Types	Type I			Type II
	α & ω	β	τ	γ
Produced by	Leukocyte	Fibroblast	Trophoblast	Lymphocyte
Effects				
antiviral	+	+	+	+
antiproliferative	+	+	+	+
antitumor	+	+	?	+
MHC regulation	+	+	?	+
Pregnancy signaling	–	–	+	–

IFN-τ, are induced readily by viruses and double-stranded RNA (17). Induced IFN-α and IFN-β expression is transient, lasting approximately a few hours. In contrast, IFN-τ synthesis is maintained over a period of days (9). On a per cell basis, 300-fold more IFN-τ is produced than other type I IFNs (27). Interestingly, IFN-τ expression is restricted to a particular stage (primarily days 13–21) of conceptus development in ruminants (9). However, preliminary studies suggest that the human form of IFN-τ is constitutively expressed throughout pregnancy (28). Ruminant forms of IFN-τ show cell-specific expression in that only cells of trophoblast origin transcribe IFN-τ (27). For example, transfection of the human trophoblast cell line JAR with the gene for bovine IFN-τ resulted in antiviral activity, whereas transfection with the bovine IFN-ω gene did not. This implies unique transacting factors involved in IFN-τ gene expression. Consistent with this is the observation that whereas the proximal promoter region (from − 126 to the transcriptional start site) of IFNτ is highly homologous to that of IFNα and IFNβ, the region from − 126 to − 450 is not homologous and enhances only IFN-τ expression (27). Thus, different regulatory factors appear to be involved in IFN-τ expression as compared with the other type I IFNs.

In binding studies using endometrial membranes and spleen cells, only IFN-τ has been cross linked to both the 100-kDa binding chain of the type I IFN receptor and a 70-kDa–associated protein (29). Cross linking to this 70-kDa protein may be indicative of altered orientation at the receptor, or it may represent an accessory protein unique to the elicitation of IFN-τ reproductive or cell-tolerant activities. An important IFN-τ distinction is that it displays a function which until now would have been unheard of for an IFN; that is signaling pregnancy in ruminants. IFN-α is far less efficient in this function, since it has been shown that to induce pseudopregnancy in nonpregnant ewes much higher concentrations of IFN-α are required (30). Finally, the most advantageous characteristic of IFN-τ may prove to be its lack of toxicity at high doses (1–5).

C.   Structure-Function Studies of OvIFN-τ

Studies have been undertaken to identify sites important for function and receptor binding on the OvIFN-τ molecule. To accomplish this, the synthetic peptide approach was employed in which overlapping synthetic peptides corresponding to the entire primary sequence of OvIFN-τ were synthesized using FMOC chemistry. The effects of the peptides and antipeptide antisera on the interaction of OvIFN-τ with the type I IFN receptor as well as the antiviral and antiproliferative activities of OvIFN-τ were assessed. Using a radioligand binding assay, the regions 1–37, 62–92,

139–172, and to a lesser extent 119–150 of OvIFN-τ were shown to be involved in interaction with the type I receptor, as antipeptide antisera raised against peptides encompassing these regions inhibited IFN-τ binding to receptor (31). Likewise, these same regions of OvIFN-τ were also shown to be important for antiviral activity (31). In contrast, antiproliferative activity exerted by OvIFN-τ appears to be linked more closely the C-terminus of the molecule. Regions 119–150, 90–122, and 139–172 of OvIFN-τ were able to block the antiproliferative effects of OvIFN-τ in cell culture. Inhibition by C-terminal peptides was also observed in the cell cycle distribution of OvIFN-τ–treated MDBK cells over a 24-hr period. Taken together, these data suggest that multiple functional domains are present in the IFN-τ molecule through which different functions may be elicited. A summary of OvIFN-τ regions involved in binding and function is presented in Table 2.

In order to gain more insight into the functional regions of IFN-τ and their orientation in the molecule, a model of the three-dimensional structure was generated (22). To achieve this goal, the secondary structure of the IFN-τ molecule and IFN-τ peptides was first assessed using circular dichroism (CD) analysis. The IFN-τ molecule exhibited approximately 70% α-helix, whereas four of six IFN-τ peptides also showed the presence of α-helical structure. Identification of α-helical structure in the IFN-τ peptides supported the CD analysis of the intact protein and provided the basis for location of α-helical segments within the intact molecule.

To generate a predicted three-dimensional structure for IFN-τ, the CD analysis of IFN-τ and the IFN-τ peptides and a comparison of IFN-τ with IFN-β were used. The x-ray crystal structure of IFN-β is known (32) and

Table 2 Summary of OvIFN-τ Regions Important for Type 1 IFN Receptor Binding and Function

OvIFN-τ peptides	Receptor binding	Antiviral activity	Antiproliferative activity
1–37	+ + +	+ + +	−
34–64	−	−	−
62–92	+ + +	+ +	−
90–122	−	−	+ +
119–150	+	+ +	+ + +
139–172	+ + +	+ + +	+

Plus and minus signs indicate level of inhibition: (+ + +), excellent; (+ +), good; (+), significant; (−), none.
Source: From ref. 31.

was employed as a template for predicting the overall topology of IFN-τ. A comparison of amino acid residues based on conservative substitutions revealed a similarity of 50% between IFN-τ and IFN-β. However, when a comparison of the location of hydrophobic residues residing in the IFN-τ and IFN-β molecules was made, a similarity of 75% was observed. This is of importance, since hydrophobicity is considered to be a critical factor in driving protein folding, making the IFN-β molecule a valuable tool for predicting IFN-τ structure. The predicted structure of OvIFN-τ with the functional domains highlighted is presented in Fig. 1. From the predicted three-dimensional IFN-τ structure, it appears that five α-helical segments comprise the main portion of the molecule. The regions of IFN-τ, 1–37, 62–92, and 139–172, which are involved in receptor interaction, are in close proximity in the three-dimensional structure. This may explain how sequentially noncontiguous residues of IFN-τ are involved in binding to

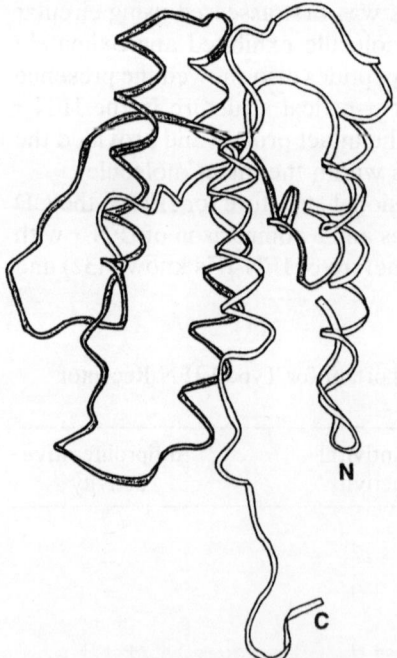

Figure 1 Predicted structure and proposed location of functional domains of OvIFN-τ. The functionally important peptide sequences of OvIFN-τ are shaded and a side view of the molecule is presented. The N- and C-termini are labeled as N and C, respectively.

receptor. Clearly the insight gained from the knowledge of the predicted three-dimensional structure of the IFN-τ molecule will facilitate our understanding of its functional activities and receptor interactions.

D. IFN-τ Lacks Toxicity

One of the most unique aspects of the activity of IFN-τ is its remarkable lack of toxicity. Toxicity induced by other IFNs, including the type I IFNs, IFN-α and IFN-β, as well as type II IFN-γ, has been well documented (33,34). Detrimental toxic effects exerted by these IFNs have been observed during clinical trials and patient treatment. Symptoms relating to IFN-induced toxicity include flu-like symptoms such as fever, chills, nausea, weight loss, leukopenia, and neutropenia. Toxicity has also been shown by testing in animals models and in tissue culture. Thus far, IFN-τ has shown no toxicity either in vivo as tested in animal models or in tissue culture (Table 3) (1–5,7).

The first observation of a lack of toxicity for IFN-τ was made in studying its antiproliferative effects. MDBK cells exhibited reduced viability

Table 3 Parameters Demonstrating the Toxicity of IFN-α and β, but the Lack of Toxicity by IFN-τ

	Toxicity		
	IFN-τ	IFN-α	IFN-β
In vitro (cell viability)			
Mouse L929 (50,000–200,000 U/ml of IFN)	−	+	+
Bovine MDBK (at 50,000 U/ml of IFN)	−	+	ND
Human WISH (at 50,000 U/ml of IFN)	−	+	ND
Human peripheral lymphocytes (at 50,000 U/ml of IFN)	−	+	+
HIV-infected human peripheral lymphocytes (50,000–500,000 U/ml of IFN)	−	+	ND
In vivo (NZW mice)			
White blood cell count	−	+	+
Lymphocyte depression	−	+	+
Weight measurement	−	+	±

ND, not determined.
Plus and minus signs indicate toxicity or lack there of induced by treatment with the various type I IFNs. For in vivo studies, 10^5 U was administered per injection and cell counts and weights were evaluated at either 12 or 24 hr after injection.
Source: From refs. 1–4 and 7.

when cultured in the presence of IFN-α at a concentration of 50,000 U/ml, whereas IFN-τ was not toxic (4). This observation has also held true for the human WISH and murine L929 cell lines. A direct comparison of IFN-τ and IFN-β on L929 cells showed IFN-τ to lack toxicity at a concentration as high as 200,000 U/ml, whereas IFN-β reduced viability at concentrations much lower than 200,000 U/ml (7). A panel of tumorigenic cell lines was also tested and IFN-τ was found to lack toxicity on these as well, but did inhibit cell replication (C.H. Pontzer, personal observation). In addition to transformed cell lines, comparisons of IFN-τ with other IFNs have been made on human peripheral mononuclear cells (HPMCs) and human immunodeficiency virus (HIV)–infected HPMCs. IFN-τ did not exhibit toxic effects on cultured HPMCs, whereas both IFN-α and IFN-β reduced cell viability at 50,000 U/ml (5). Human lymphocytes infected with HIV-1 and feline lymphocytes infected with feline immunodeficiency virus (FIV) also did not exhibit reduced viability in the presence of IFN-τ (3). These findings suggest that a lack of toxicity by IFN-τ observed using long-term cell lines also applies to human peripheral blood.

The lack of toxicity by IFN-τ has also been compared with IFN-β and IFN-α in certain animal models. As part of the studies in which IFN-τ was shown to prevent development of EAE, white blood cell counts, lymphocyte percentages, and total body weights of NZW mice injected with the various IFNs were followed over time (7). Twelve hours after injection with 10^5 U of murine IFN-α (MuIFN-α), mice exhibited decreased white blood cell counts and lymphopenia. Injection of 10^5 U of MuIFN-β also resulted in lymphopenia, whereas injection of an equal amount of OvIFN-τ had no effect on either white blood cell counts or percentages of lymphocytes (7). In the case of weight measurements, mice injected with 10^5 U of MuIFN-α showed substantial weight loss, whereas injection of MuIFN-β caused minimal weight loss to be observed. IFN-α has been previously demonstrated to induce a higher degree of toxicity than that observed for IFN-β. In the case of OvIFN-τ, no detectable weight loss was observed. Thus, OvIFN-τ did not induce toxicity at the dosage required for prevention of EAE.

The question arises as to the nature of the mechanism underlying IFN-τ's lack of toxicity. Such a mechanism may occur at one or multiple levels, including, interaction with the type I receptor, induction of transcription factors, and ultimately gene activation. At the receptor level, a differential binding with type I IFN receptor subunits unique to IFN-τ may partially explain differences in toxicity. Additionally, differences in affinity between IFN-τ and other type I IFNs for binding to receptor may influence signaling events intracellularly. At the level of intracellular signaling, IFN-τ may activate different or as yet to be identified kinases and transcription factors. Signaling for IFN-α has been shown to involve the actions of the Janus kinases, JAK 1 and TYK 2, as well as the transcription factors, STAT1α/β and STAT2 (35–38). IFN-τ does induce activation of TYK 2-like IFN-α; therefore, this does not contribute to the lack of toxicity observed for IFN-τ (38a). However, the combination of STAT protein interactions may vary for IFN-τ, as the biological effects of IFN-τ and IFN-α vary. Levels of transcription factor activation as evidenced by phosphorylation of the relevant STAT proteins may also play a role. As a direct consequence of differences at the transcription factor level, differential gene activation may occur between IFN-τ and other type I IFNs. Either of these differences could potentially contribute to the lack of toxicity exhibited by IFN-τ. Currently, there are a number of lines of inquiry under investigation regarding the mechanism by which IFN-τ lacks toxicity.

III. EFFECTIVENESS OF IFN-τ IN THE EAE MODEL FOR MS

A. OvIFN-τ Can Prevent Development of EAE

OvIFN-τ, which possesses immunomodulatory activity in the absence of toxicity, is an attractive candidate for testing as an immunotherapy for autoimmune disease. OvIFN-τ has been examined for its ability to prevent the development of EAE in mice (7), an animal model of antigen-induced autoimmunity that is widely studied to gain insight into human MS. When treatment consisted of a single dose of 10^5 U of OvIFN-τ injected intraperitoneally (i.p.) on the day of immunization with MBP, development of clinical signs of disease was delayed by 7 days when compared with an untreated control group (7). Like OvIFN-τ, a single dose of 10^5 U of MuIFN-β also caused a 7-day delay in the development of disease.

In seeking full protection from the development of EAE, treatment with OvIFN-τ was increased to three doses of 10^5 U given 48 hr prior to immunization with MBP, on the day of immunization with MBP, and 48 hr after immunization with MBP. This schedule of OvIFN-τ treatment blocked all clinical signs of EAE. In addition, OvIFN-τ was as effective as MuIFN-β in blocking EAE at this dosage. A time course of the mean severity from the experiments described above is presented in Figure 2. Data shown in this figure are for treatment groups which received either a single dose of OvIFN-τ, three doses of OvIFN-τ, or no OvIFN-τ. It would appear that OvIFN-τ is an effective immunotherapy for the prevention of EAE and is as effective a treatment as MuIFN-β in this model for autoimmune disease.

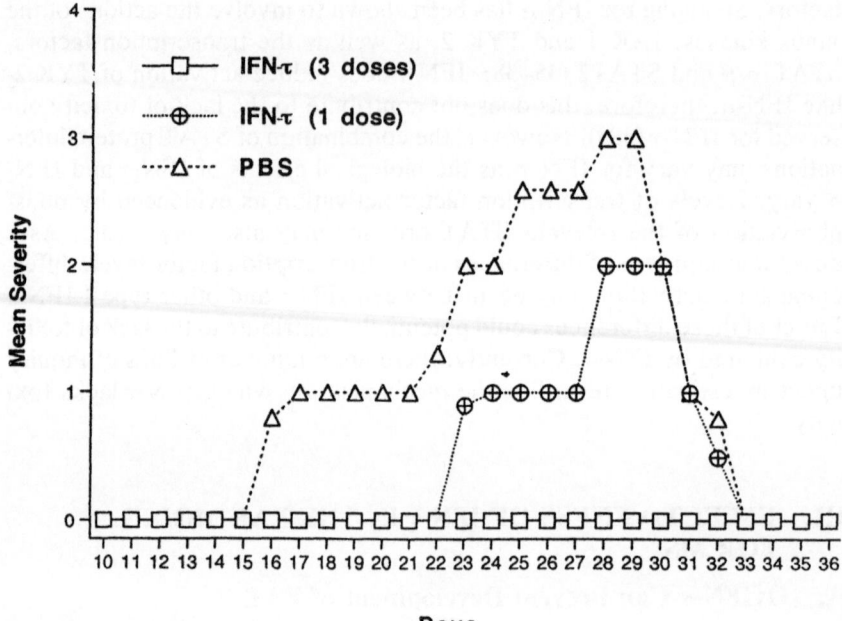

Figure 2   A time course of the mean severity of NZW mice immunized with MBP for induction of EAE and treated with either a single dose of OvIFN-τ (crossed circles), three doses of OvIFN-τ (squares), or no OvIFN-τ (triangles).

B.   OvIFN-τ Can Prevent Superantigen Reactivation of EAE

The symptomatology of MS can often be observed to occur in a relapsing-remitting manner. This form of MS consists of the onset of clinical symptoms of MS followed by periods of remission. How relapses and exacerbations occur and what causes the reactivation of autoimmune disease has been a topic of much speculation. It has been suggested that environmental influences may contribute to or even be responsible for exacerbations of autoimmune disease. Such influences from one's environment potentially include exposure to infectious agents as well as factors possessing immunostimulatory activity. One class of proteins which is ubiquitous in our environment are the microbial superantigens.

Microbial superantigens are toxins produced by a variety of bacteria, viruses, and other organisms such as *Mycoplasma* that possess extremely potent immunostimulatory activity (39–41). They are responsible for a number of maladies, including food poisoning and toxic shock syndrome

(42,43). Such powerful immunostimulation by superantigens is based on their ability to engage major histocompatibility complex (MHC) class II molecules and then together as a binary complex bind to the T-cell receptor in a β chain variable region (Vβ)–specific manner (44–48). Such binding triggers T-cell activation leading to proliferation of as much as 20% of a T-cell repertoire (44). Superantigen-induced T-cell proliferation is accompanied by massive amounts of cytokine production, including interleukin-2 (IL-2), IFN-γ, and tumor necrosis factor-α (TNF-α). Of the cytokines whose production is induced by superantigen stimulation, IFN-γ and TNF-α have been implicated as mediators of autoimmune pathogenesis. IFN-γ has been shown to cause exacerbations of MS in clinical trials (49,50). Production of TNF-α is a requirement for the encephalitogenicity of certain T-cell lines used adoptively to transfer EAE (51) as well as causing myelin-producing oligodendrocyte death in vitro (52).

Exacerbation evidenced as a clinical relapse of EAE was first demonstrated by the administration of a microbial superantigen. In the PL/J mice strain, acute episodes of EAE usually resolve and clinical relapses do not occur (53). After resolution of all clinical signs of EAE induced by immunization with MBP, administration of either of the staphylococcal enterotoxin (SE) superantigens, SEB or SEA, was shown to cause reactivation of disease (54). An outline of experiments and their results demonstrating the ability of bacterial superantigens to reactivate EAE is presented in Figure 3. Multiple episodes of disease exacerbation over a 4-month period were also shown in which EAE could be reactivated and resolved based on multiple injections of SEB (54). Reactivation of EAE by SEB has also been shown to occur in other susceptible strains, including NZW (J. Schiffenbauer, personal observation). SEB can also reactivate disease when an acetylated amino-terminal peptide of MBP is employed as the immunogen (55).

In addition to reactivation of EAE, SEB can also prevent EAE when administered prior to immunization with MBP (56,57). Anergy and or deletion of the Vβ8$^+$ T-cell subset which is responsible for the initial induction of EAE appears to be the mechanism for this protection. Targeting of a Vβ-specific T-cell population does not, however, provide absolute protection from the development of EAE. When mice protected from development of EAE by SEB pretreatment are exposed to SEA (which has a different Vβ T-cell specificity from SEB), induction of EAE does occur (58). This SEA-induced EAE is characterized by severe paralysis and accelerated onset of clinical symptoms. Thus, the effects of microbial superantigens introduce a profound complexity to autoimmune disease models such as EAE akin to the complexity of the pathogenesis observed in MS.

A

Induction of EAE

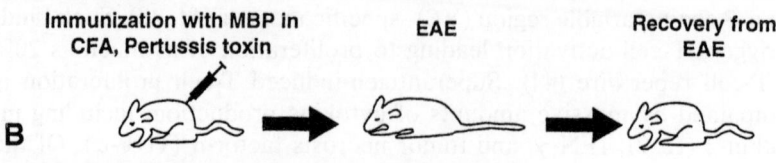

Immunization with MBP in   EAE   Recovery from
CFA, Pertussis toxin   EAE

B

Reactivation of EAE by superantigen in recovered mice

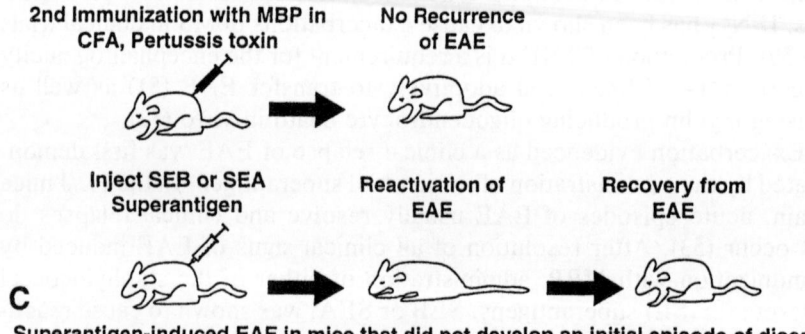

2nd Immunization with MBP in   No Recurrence
CFA, Pertussis toxin   of EAE

Inject SEB or SEA   Reactivation of   Recovery from
Superantigen   EAE   EAE

C

Superantigen-induced EAE in mice that did not develop an initial episode of disease

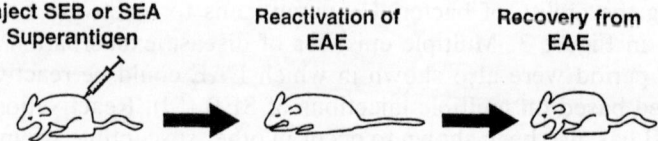

Inject SEB or SEA   Reactivation of   Recovery from
Superantigen   EAE   EAE

Figure 3 Reactivation of EAE by the staphylococcal enterotoxin superantigens, SEB and SEA. (A) PL/J mice employed for reactivation studies were initially immunized with MBP in complete Freund's adjuvant (CFA) and injected with pertussis toxin on the day of immunization and 48 hr later. Mice developed EAE on or about days 10–14 and were allowed to recover from clinical symptoms for at least 2 weeks to 1 month. (B) After resolution of clinical symptoms of EAE, injections with the superantigens, SEB or SEA, were given. A significant number of mice developed a clinical reactivation of EAE on or about 7 days after exposure to superantigen. Previous experiments have shown that a second immunization of MBP can not reactivate EAE. (C) Injection of superantigens can also induce an initial episode of clinical disease in PL/J mice that had been immunized with MBP but did not develop EAE.

We have examined the effect of OvIFN-τ treatment on exacerbations of EAE induced by superantigen and have shown that OvIFN-τ can also prevent superantigen reactivation of EAE (7). Treatment with OvIFN-τ when administered in three doses of 10^5 U (48 hr prior to SEB injection, on the day of SEB injection, and 48 hr after SEB injection) blocked EAE reactivation by superantigen. In comparison, untreated control groups exhibited superantigen reactivation of EAE consistent with previous studies (54). The observation that OvIFN-τ can block superantigen-induced exacerbations of EAE may be a corollary to the reduction in disease exacerbations in MS patients undergoing treatment with IFN β-1b (59). A summary of the studies showing that OvIFN-τ can prevent development and superantigen reactivation of EAE is presented in Figure 4.

OvIFN-τ's lack of toxicity and ability to ameliorate EAE form a persuasive argument for the clinical testing of IFN-τ as an immunotherapy for MS. If lack of toxicity by IFN-τ holds true in humans, the dosage of IFN-

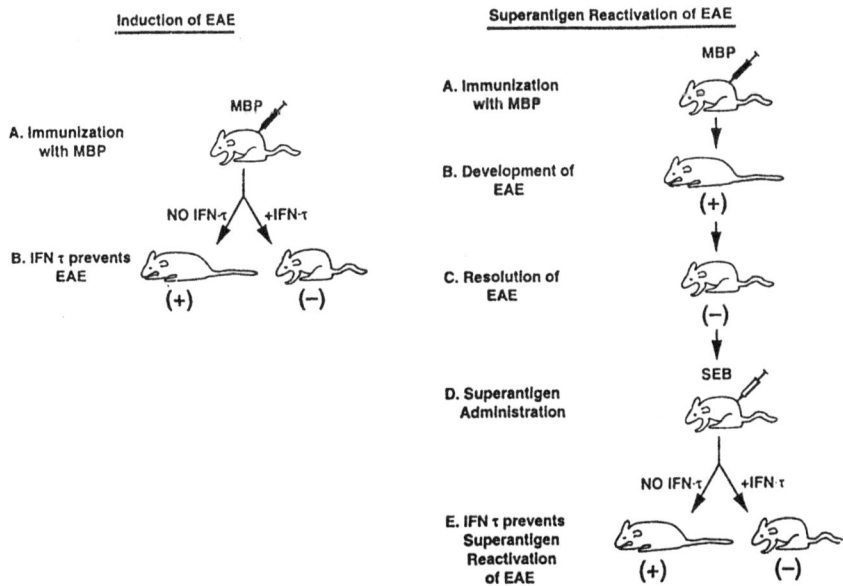

Figure 4 IFN-τ blocks development and superantigen reactivation of EAE. In the case of initial induction of EAE, treatment with IFN-τ can prevent the development of disease. IFN-τ can also block superantigen-induced exacerbations of EAE akin to the reduced exacerbations of disease observed in IFN β-1b–treated MS patients. Plus signs indicate induction of disease. Minus signs indicate absence of clinical disease.

τ treatment may not be limited as is the dosage of IFN β-1b owing to toxic side effects. Therapeutic effects exerted by IFN β-1b have been shown to be dose dependent with higher dosages providing greater beneficial effects. If dosage limits are not of concern in the use of IFN-τ, MS patients who did not show improvement at IFN β-1b's indicated dosage or could not tolerate IFN β-1b owing to toxicity may benefit from treatment with IFN-τ. In addition, the development of neutralizing antibodies has been demonstrated in IFN β-1b–treated patients (60). If such neutralizing antibodies prove to impede the effectiveness of IFN β-1b, IFN-τ may be an important alternative therapy as antibody cross reactivity is unlikely to occur. Finally, IFN-τ is an effective therapeutic for both the acute and relapsing-remitting forms of EAE when orally fed. This suggests that oral IFN-τ therapy may be the desired route of administration for treatment of disease (JM Soos, M Mustafa, HM Johnson, manuscript submitted).

C. Potential Mechanisms for IFN-τ Amelioration of EAE

It is quite probable that a number of immunomodulatory activities exerted by IFN-τ contribute to the mechanisms by which its amelioration of EAE occurs. Among these potential mechanisms are:

Reduced T-cell responses to specific peptide antigen
Reduced T-cell responses to microbial superantigens
Reduced production of exacerbatory cytokines (such as IFN-γ and TNF-α)
Induced production of beneficial cytokines (such as IL-4 or TGF-β)
Increased suppressor T-cell function
Altered cell migration into the central nervous system (CNS)
Downregulation of the expression of certain adhesion molecules
Downregulation of the expression of MHC class I and class II molecules
Altered production of anti-MBP antibodies

OvIFN-τ has been shown to inhibit MBP-specific as well as superantigen-induced T-cell proliferation (5,7). OvIFN-τ can also inhibit superantigen-induced Vβ-specific T-cell expansion and IL-2 and TNF-α production (5,7). OvIFN-τ-induced suppressor cell function can also reduce MBP-specific T-cell proliferation as well as delay onset of EAE via synergism of the Th2 type cytokines, IL-10 and TGF-β (M Mustafa, JM Soos, HM Johnson, manuscript submitted). Likewise, splenic cells from OvIFN-τ-treated MBP T-cell receptor transgenic mice produce IL-10 when stimulated in vitro with MBP (JM Soos, HM Johnson, SS Zamvil, unpublished data). Clearly, several areas of research remain to be explored to fully elucidate the mechanisms by which OvIFN-τ ameliorates EAE.

IV. HUMAN IFN-τ: DEVELOPMENT FOR USE AS AN IMMUNOTHERAPY

Unlike the role of IFN-τ in ruminants, the human form of IFN-τ does not act to signal maternal recognition of pregnancy. In humans, chorionic gonadotropin serves this important function. In spite of this difference, mRNA transcripts of several human IFN-τ genes have been shown to be expressed constitutively throughout pregnancy (28). Through in situ hybridization experiments, human IFN-τ mRNA could be localized to extravillous trophoblast cells of the placenta. In addition, IFN-τ mRNA transcripts could also be detected in both adult lymphocytes and amniocytes.

At least seven putative human IFN-τ genes have been identified (C.P. Liu, Pepgen Corp., Berkeley, CA, personal observation). The protein of one of the human IFN-τ genes has been expressed and appears to possess potent antiviral activity (unpublished data). This human IFN-τ protein is currently being examined in toxicity studies similar to those described in this chapter. In addition, this human IFN-τ is also being characterized with respect to its immunoregulatory, antiproliferative, antitumor, and other properties in addition to its antiviral activity. One may wonder then about the role human IFN-τ potentially plays in the reduced number of relapses observed in pregnant MS patients (61–63).

V. CONCLUSIONS

IFN-τ, a type I IFN, was originally identified because of its role in the reproductive cycle of ruminants such as sheep and cows. However, it also possesses all of the functions ascribed to the other type I IFNs, including antiviral, antiproliferative, and immunomodulatory activities, but it differs in that it is relatively nontoxic to cells at high concentrations. Several genes encoding for human forms of IFN-τ have recently been identified. IFN-τ was examined for its effect on the development of MBP-induced EAE in mice, an animal model for MS in humans. IFN-τ prevents development of EAE as effectively as IFN-β. IFN-β has recently been approved by the U.S. Food and Drug Administration for the treatment of MS. Unlike IFN-β, IFN-τ–treated mice did not develop leukopenia. We have recently shown that superantigens can induce relapses in EAE, similar to those that occur "spontaneously" in MS patients. IFN-τ blocked superantigen reactivation of EAE. The inhibitory effect of IFN-τ on the induction of EAE and reactivation by superantigen involves suppression of MBP and superantigen activation of T cells as well as suppressed induction of destructive cytokines such as TNF. IFN-τ thus has considerable potential for treatment of autoimmune disease, including MS.

ACKNOWLEDGMENTS

The authors gratefully acknowledge Amy C. Hobeika and Dr. Brian E. Szente for critical review of the manuscript and Roger Hoover for artwork. This research was supported by Grants CA 69959 and AI 25904 from the National Institutes of Health. Dr. Howard M. Johnson is a consultant to the Pepgen Corp., Berkeley, CA. Dr. Jeanne M. Soos is a Fellow of the National Multiple Sclerosis Society. This manuscript is University of Florida Agricultural Experiment Station No. R-05298.

REFERENCES

1. Bazer FW, Johnson HM. Type I conceptus interferons: maternal recognition of pregnancy signals and potential therapeutic agents. Am J Reprod Immunol 1991; 26:19–22.
2. Johnson HM, Bazer FW, Szente BE, Jarpe MA. How interferons fight disease. Sci Am 1994; 270(5):40–47.
3. Bazer FW, Johnson HM, Yamamoto JK. Effect of ovine trophoblast protein-1 (oTP-1) on replication of feline (FIV) and human (HIV) immunodeficiency viruses (abstr). Biol Reprod 1989; 40(suppl):63.
4. Pontzer CH, Bazer FW, Johnson HM. Antiproliferative activity of a pregnancy recognition hormone, ovine trophoblast protein-1. Cancer Res 1991; 51:5304–5307.
5. Soos JM, Johnson HM. Type I interferon inhibition of superantigen-induced stimulation: implications for the treatment of superantigen-associated disease. J IFN Cytokine Res 1995; 15:39–45.
6. Zamvil SS, Steinman L. The T lymphocyte in experimental allergic encephalomyelitis. Annu Rev Immunol 1990; 8:579–621.
7. Soos JM, Subramaniam PS, Hobeika AC, Schiffenbauer J, Johnson HM. The interferon pregnancy recognition hormone, interferon tau, blocks both development and superantigen reactivation of experimental allergic encephalomyelitis without associated toxicity. J Immunol 1995; 155:2747–2753.
8. Martal J, Lacroix MC, Loudes C, Saunier M, Wintenberger-Torres C. Trophoblastin, an anti-luteolytic protein present in early pregnancy in sheep. J Reprod Fertil 1979; 56:63–73.
9. Godkin JD, Bazer FW, Moffatt J, Sessions F, Roberts RM. Purification and properties of a major, low molecular weight protein released by the trophoblast of sheep blastocysts at day 13–21. J Reprod Fertil 1982; 65: 141–150.
10. Vallet JL, Bazer FW, Ashworth CJ, Johnson HM, Pontzer CH. Development

of a radioimmunoassay for ovine trophoblast protein-1, the antiluteolytic protein from the sheep conceptus. J Endocrinol 1988; 117:R5–R8.

11. Godkin JD, Bazer FW, Thatcher WW, Roberts RM. Proteins released by cultured day 15–16 conceptuses prolong luteal maintenance when introduced into the uterine lumen of cyclic ewes. J Reprod Fertil 1984; 71:57–64.

12. Vallet JL, Bazer FW, Fliss MFV, Thatcher WW. Effect of ovine conceptus secretory proteins and purified ovine trophoblast protein-1 on interoestrous interval and plasma concentrations of prostaglandin F2alpha and E and of 13,14-dihydro-15-keto prostaglandin F2alpha in cyclic ewes. J Reprod Fertil 1988; 84:493–504.

13. Flint APF, Sheldrick EL, McCann TJ, Jones DSC. Luteal oxytocin: characteristics and control of synchronous episodes of oxytocin and PGF2alpha secretion at luteolysis in ruminants. Domest Anim Endocrinol 1990; 7: 111–124.

14. Mirando MA, Ott TL, Harney JP, Bazer FW. Ovine trophoblast protein-one inhibits development of endometrial responsiveness to oxytocin in ewes. Biol Reprod 1990; 43:1070–1078.

15. Bartol FF, Roberts RM, Bazer FW, Lewis GS, Godkin JD, Thatcher WW. Characterization of proteins produced in vitro by peri-attachment bovine conceptuses. Biol Reprod 1985; 32:681–693.

16. Gnatek GG, Smith LD, Duby RT, Godkin JD. Maternal recognition of pregnancy in the goat: effects of conceptus removal on interestrus intervals and characterization of conceptus protein production during early pregnancy. Biol Reprod 1989; 41:655–664.

17. Roberts RM, Cross JC, Leaman DW. Interferons as hormones of pregnancy. Endocr Rev 1992; 13:432–452.

18. Imakawa K, Anthony RV, Kazemi M, Marotti KR, Polites HG, Roberts RM. Interferon-like sequence of ovine trophoblast protein secreted by embryonic trophectoderm. Nature 1987; 330:377–379.

19. Stewart HJ, McCann SHE, Northrop AJ, Lamming GE, Flint APF. Sheep antiluteolytic interferon: cDNA sequence and analysis of mRNA levels. J Mol Endocrinol 1989; 2:65.

20. Klemann SW, Imakawa K, Roberts RM. Sequence variability among ovine trophoblast interferon mRNA. Nucleic Acids Res 1990; 18:6724.

21. Charlier M, Hue D, Boisnard M, Martal J, Gaye P. Cloning and structural analysis of two distinct families of ovine interferon-alpha genes encoding functional class II and trophoblast (oTP-1) alpha-interferons. Mol Cell Endocrinol 1991; 76:161–171.

22. Jarpe MA, Johnson HM, Bazer FW, Ott TL, Curto EV, Rama Krishna N, Pontzer CH. Predicted structural motif of IFN tau. Protein Eng 1994; 7: 863–867.

23. Pontzer CH, Torres BA, Vallet JL, Bazer FW, Johnson HM. Antiviral activity of the pregnancy recognition hormone ovine trophoblast protein-1. Biochem Biophys Res Commun 1988; 152:801–807.

24. Mirando MA, Short EC, Geisert RD, Vallet JL, Bazer FW. Stimulation of

2,5-oligoadenylate synthetase activity in sheep endometrium during pregnancy, by intrauterine infusion of oTP-1, and by intramuscular administration of recombinant bovine interferon-alpha1. J Reprod Fertil 1991; 93:599.

25. Pontzer CH, Yamamoto JK, Bazer FW, Johnson HM. Potent anti-FIV and anti-HIV effect of interferon tau. J Immunol. In press.

26. Skopets B, Li J, Thatcher WW, Roberts RM, Hansen PJ. Inhibition of lymphocyte proliferation by bovine trophoblast protein-1 (type I trophoblast interferon) and bovine interferon-alpha1. Vet Immunol Immunopathol 1992; 34:81–96.

27. Cross JC, Roberts RM. Constitutive and trophoblast-specific expression of a class of bovine interferon genes. Proc Natl Acad Sci USA 1991; 88: 3817–3821.

28. Whaley AE, Reddy Meka CS, Hunt JS, Imakawa K. Identification and cellular localization of unique interferon mRNA from human placenta. J Biol Chem 1994; 269:10864–10868.

29. Hansen TR, Kazemi M, Keisler DH, Malathy PV, Imakawa K, Roberts RM. Complex binding of the embryonic interferon, ovine trophoblast protein-1, to endometrial receptors. J Interferon Res 1989; 9:215–225.

30. Stewart HJ, McCann SHE, Lamming GE, Flint APF. Evidence for a role for interferon in the maternal recognition of pregnancy. J Reprod Fertil 1989; 37(suppl):127–138.

31. Pontzer CH, Ott TL, Bazer FW, Johnson HM. Structure/function studies with interferon tau: evidence for multiple active sites. J Interferon Res. 1994; 14:133–141.

32. Senda T, Shimazu T, Matsuda S, Kawano G, Shimizu H, Nakamura KT, Mitsui Y. Three dimensional crystal structure of recombinant murine interferon beta. EMBO J 1992; 11:3193–3201.

33. Degré M. Influence of exogenous interferon on the peripheral white blood cell count in mice. Int J Cancer 1974; 14:699–703.

34. Fent K, Zbinden G. Toxicity of interferon and interleukin. Trends Pharm Sci 1987; 8:100–105.

35. David M, Larner AC. Activation of transcription factors by interferon-alpha in a cell free system. Science 1992; 257:813–815.

36. Schindler C, Shuai K, Prezioso VR, Darnell JE Jr. Interferon-dependent tyrosine phosphorylation of a latent cytoplasmic transcription factor. Science 1992; 257:809–813.

37. Valazquez L, Fellous M, Stark GR, Pellegrini S. A protein tyrosine kinase in the interferon α/β signaling pathway. Cell 1992; 70:313–322.

38. Ihle JN, Witthuhn BA, Quelle FW, Yamamoto K, Thierfelder WE, Kreider B, Silvennoinen O. Signaling by the cytokine receptor family: JAKs and STATs. Trends Biol Sci 1994; 19:222–227.

38a. Subramaniam PS, Khan SA, Pontzer CH, Johnson HM. Differential recognition of the type I interferon receptor by interferons tau and alpha is responsible for their disparate cytotoxicities. Proc Natl Acad Sci USA 1995; 92: 12270–12274.

39. Langford MP, Stanton GJ, Johnson HM. Biological effects of staphylococcal

enterotoxin A on human peripheral lymphocytes. Infect Immun 1978; 22: 62–68.

40. Carlsson R, Sjogren HO. Kinetics of IL-2 and interferon production, expression of IL-2 receptors, and cell proliferation in human mononuclear cells exposed to staphylococcal enterotoxin. A. Cell Immunol 1985; 96:175–183.

41. Johnson HM, Magazine HI. Potent mitogenic activity of staphylococcal enterotoxin A requires induction of IL-2. Int Arch Allergy Appl Immunol 1988; 87:87–90.

42. Bergdoll MS. The staphylococcal enterotoxins: an update. In: Jelijaszewicz J, ed. The Staphylococci. New York: Gustav Fischer Verlag, 1985:247–254.

43. Bergdoll MS, Crass BA, Reiser RF, Robbins RN, Davis JP. A new staphylococcal enterotoxin, enterotoxin F, associated with toxic shock syndrome Staphylococcus aureus isolates. Lancet 1981; 1:1071–1072.

44. Johnson HM, Russell JK, Pontzer CH. Staphylococcal enterotoxin superantigens FASEB J 1991; 5:2706–2712.

45. Janeway CA, Yagi J, Conrad PJ, Katz ME, Jones B, Vroegop S, Buxser S. T-cell responses to MIs and bacterial proteins that mimic its behavior. Immunol Rev 1989; 107:61–88.

46. White J, Herman A, Pullen AM, Kubo R, Kappler JW, Marrack P. The Vβ specific superantigen staphylococcal enterotoxin B: stimulation of mature T cells and clonal deletion in neonatal mice. Cell 1989; 56:27–35.

47. Carlsson R, Fischer H, Sjogren HO. Binding of staphylococcal enterotoxin A to accessory cells is a requirement for its ability to activate human T cells. J Immunol 1988; 140:2484–2488.

48. Fleischer B, Schrezenmeier H. T cell stimulation by staphylococcal enterotoxins. Clonally variable response and requirement for major histocompatibility complex class II molecules on accessory or target cells. J Exp Med 1988; 176:1697–1707.

49. Panitch HS, Hirsch RL, Haley AS, Johnson KP. Exacerbations of multiple sclerosis in patients treated with gamma interferon. Lancet 1987; 1:893–895.

50. Panitch HS, Hirsch RL, Schindler J, Johnson KP. Treatment of multiple sclerosis with gamma interferon: exacerbations associated with activation of the immune system. Neurology 1987; 37:1097–1102.

51. Powell MB, Mitchell D, Lederman J, Buckmeier J, Zamvil SS, Graham M, Ruddle N, Steinman L. Lymphotoxin and tumor necrosis factor alpha production by myelin basic protein specific T cell clones correlates with encephalolitogenicity. Int Immunol 1990; 2:539–544.

52. Selmaj KW, Raine CS. Tumor necrosis factor mediates myelin and oligodendrocyte damage in vitro. Ann Neurol 1988; 23:339–346.

53. Fritz RB, Chou CH, McFarlin DE. Relapsing murine experimental allergic encephalomyelitis induced by myelin basic protein. J Immunol 1983; 130(3): 1024–1026.

54. Schiffenbauer J, Johnson HM, Butfiloski E, Wegrzyn L, Soos JM. Staphylococcal enterotoxins reactivate experimental allergic encephalomyelitis. Proc Natl Acad Sci USA 1993; 90:8543–8546.

55. Brocke S, Gaur A, Piercy C, Gautam A, Gijbels K, Fathamn CG, Steinman

S. Induction of relapsing paralysis in experimental allergic encephalomyelitis by bacterial superantigen. Nature 1993; 365:642–644.

56. Soos JM, Schiffenbauer J, Johnson HM. Treatment of PL/J mice with the superantigen, straphylococcal enterotoxin B, prevents development of experimental allergic encephalomyelitis. J Neuroimmunol 1993; 43:39–44.

57. Kalman B, Lublin FD, Lattime E, Joseph J, Knobler RL. Effects of staphylococcal enterotoxin B on T cell receptor Vβ utilization and clinical manifestations of experimental allergic encephalomyelitis. J Neuroimmunol 1993; 45: 83–88.

58. Soos JM, Hobeika AC, Butfiloski EJ, Schiffenbauer J, Johnson HM. Accelerated induction of experimental allergic encephalomyelitis in PL/J mice by a non-Vβ8 specific superantigen. Proc Natl Acad Sci USA 1995; 92:6082–6086.

59. IFNβ Multiple Sclerosis Study Group. Interferon IFNβ-1b is effective in relapsing-remitting multiple sclerosis. I. Clinical results of a multicenter, randomized, double-blind, placebo controlled trial. Neurology 1993; 43:655.

60. Weinstock-Guttman B, Ransohoff RM, Kinkel RP, Rudnick RA. The interferons: biological effects, mechanisms of action, and use in multiple sclerosis. Ann Neurol 1995; 37:7–15.

61. Abramsky O, Lubetzki-Korn I, Evron S, Brenner T. Suppressive effect of pregnancy on MS and EAE. Prog Clin Biol Res 1984; 146:399–406.

62. Birk K, Ford C, Smeltzer S, Ryan D, Miller R, Rudnick RA. The clinical course of multiple sclerosis during pregnancy and the puerperium. Arch Neurol 1990; 47:738–742.

63. Runmarker B, Andersen O. Pregnancy is associated with a lower risk of onset and a better prognosis in multiple sclerosis. Brain 1995; 118:253–261.

18

Clinical Trials of Multiple Sclerosis

Jeremy C. Hobart and Alan J. Thompson

Institute of Neurology, London, England

I. INTRODUCTION

The recent emergence of interventions that effect some aspects of the disease process in multiple sclerosis (MS) has resulted in a resurgence of interest in the evaluation of these new agents in a way that produces clear, definitive results to guide patients, prescribers, and purchasers. This chapter addresses some of the complexities involved in undertaking studies to determine treatment effectiveness in MS. They are considered under three main headings: the disease process, identifying and measuring outcomes, and trial design. These headings are ordered in a logical fashion: it is impossible to identify outcome measurement without in-depth knowledge of the disease process and equally impossible to design a trial without a clear idea of the questions being asked and the outcomes that address those questions.

II. THE DISEASE PROCESS OF MS

MS is a condition of low incidence but high prevalence. It is a chronic inflammatory demyelinating disorder whose cause is unknown and whose pathogenesis is poorly understood. The clinical manifestations are diverse as most parts of the neuraxis may be involved. MS has little effect on longevity and it is not unusual for the condition to continue for 50 years following diagnosis.

MS is classified according to disease course. The majority of patients (90%) begin with a relapsing-remitting course. Initially, recovery (remission) from each episode of neurological deterioration (relapse) tends to be complete. However, with time, recovery may be incomplete and irreversible disability develops. This is further complicated in 60% of cases by the onset of progressive deterioration in the patient's condition, which is distinct from relapses and remissions, but may be associated with them. A minority of patients (10%) have different disease courses with either progressive deterioration from onset (primary progressive MS) or a single relapse either preceding or following the progressive phase.

It is essential to ensure that only patients with clinically definite, or laboratory-supported definite MS are included in clinical trials (1). However, even within this group it may be prudent to restrict studies to certain subgroups, particularly if there are clear-cut differences in clinical and MR activity as in primary versus secondary progressive MS (2). This desired goal has previously been hampered by the use of a wide range of poorly defined terms. Lublin and Reingold have recently addressed this issue and propose a clearly defined and well-understood classification of clinical course: relapsing-remitting MS; primary progressive MS; secondary progressive MS; benign MS; and progressive relapsing MS for patients who show progression from onset but with one or more acute relapses (3).

The key features of MS that mitigate against simple clinical trials include the unpredictability of its course, the diversity of its clinical manifestations, and its slow change over time (4). These features influence the numbers and selection of patients, the duration of the study, and the need for a placebo group. Definitive studies are likely to require large numbers of patients [there are 720 patients in the current European trial of Interferon (IFN) β-1b in secondary progressive MS (5)], preferably from one disease subgroup. This necessitates multi-center participation often involving a number of countries or states. The limited number of patients with this condition constitute a precious resource, an important consideration if, as is now the case, a number of new drugs require evaluation. The unpredictability of MS and the tendency to spontaneous recovery following relapse necessitates the presence of a placebo arm in any study of effectiveness. The chronicity of the disorder means that even studies carried out over 2–3 years are only a snapshot of the entire disease course, during which clinical change may be small.

III. OUTCOME MEASUREMENT

Determining the effectiveness of an intervention measuring the clinical outcomes is a particularly difficult area in MS (6). Which outcomes should be measured and how this process should be undertaken are fundamental questions that remain largely unresolved (7).

A. Which Outcomes Should Be Measured?

Considerable information exists showing that the perspectives of patients and their physicians differ (8,9). The impact on disease process does not necessarily equate with the impact on health status (10), and even an apparently good outcome may not meet with patient approval. It is also likely that increased longevity in the face of no meaningful function is a poor patient outcome. These discrepancies in perspective must be considered when evaluating the outcomes of therapeutic interventions on MS. Clinical outcomes should be considered at four levels:

1. Physiological parameters of disease (e.g., magnetic resonance imaging, MRI)
2. Crude clinical end-points (e.g., relapse rate)
3. Relevant aspects of health status (e.g., disability)
4. Health-related quality of life

Measurement at the first two levels constitutes the "physician-oriented outcomes." These provide cogent information on the presence, natural history, severity, and activity of MS, but very limited information about the diverse clinical consequences and fail to incorporate the patient's perspective. These shortcomings can be addressed by measuring "patient-oriented outcomes" (levels 3 and 4). Health-related quality of life is a uniquely personal perception denoting the way the individual patients perceive and react to their health status thereby allowing individual patients to incorporate their distinctive values and preferences into the assessment process (11,12).

Although these four levels are interrelated, their relationships are complex and poorly understood. For example, there is a lack of linear relationship between relapse rate and development of disability (13). Consequently each level provides different information concerning the impact of MS on patients and it is therefore unrealistic to expect a single instrument to cover all levels. Depending on the questions posed by individual studies, different levels will be required.

B. How Should Desired Outcomes Be Measured?

Physiological parameters of disease and crude clinical end-points present few inherent measurement difficulties, as subjective judgment plays a minor role and issues of reproducibility and validity are usually amenable to technological solutions (14). However, even frequency of relapse rate creates problems as there is no scientific way of defining a true relapse or of quantifying its severity and the degree of resolution. In addition, relapse frequency is unpredictable and may be influenced by age and duration of illness (15).

In contrast, aspects of health status and health-related quality of life are elusive, abstract, and complex concepts. To ensure that they are measured meticulously, instruments must be developed in accordance with rigorous predetermined guidelines; in short, they must be clinically useful (brief, user-friendly, appropriate to the population under study) and scientifically sound (reliable, valid, and responsive) (16).

Measures of health status and health-related quality of life can be either generic or disease-specific. While the former allow comparison of different disorders, they are likely to omit areas salient to specific diseases. On the other hand, disease-specific instruments are likely to be more responsive as their content is more relevant to patients and clinicians (17,18). The use of both types of instruments is recommended.

1. Physiological Parameters of Disease—MRI

There has been considerable enthusiasm over the use of MRI to monitor disease activity in MS and its role as a potential surrogate marker. While it demonstrates activity objectively and sensitively, its ability to predict outcome is less clear-cut. Although MR abnormalities correlate well with relapse activity and predict the development of MS in patients with clinically isolated syndromes (19), the role of MRI in predicting disability in patients with established disease is less clear-cut (20). For example, in the pivotal study of IFN β-1b a powerful effect on MR activity was not associated with a significant effect on disability (10). This may be related in part to the outcome measure used to evaluate disability, i.e., the lack of responsiveness of the EDSS (21), but also relates to the lack of pathological specificity of current MR techniques (22). Much of the emphasis in recent years has been on: (1) the development of more pathologically specific techniques including magnetization transfer imaging, MR spectroscopy, the evaluation of hypointense lesions on T1-weighted scans and atrophy of the spinal cord and brain (see Chapter 15) and (2) the improvement of measures of quantification of abnormalities in T_2-weighted scans (23). These developments have been summarized in a recent paper from an MS Task Force (24). At present, MRI is seen as very useful in screening potential therapies (monthly gadolinium-enhanced MRI for 6 months), but is not yet being used as a primary outcome measure in phase III studies.

2. Health Status Measurement in MS

Relevant aspects of health status that warrant measurement in MS patients include impairment, disability, handicap, psychosocial adjustment to illness, sexual function, fatigue, and mood. To date the main emphasis has focused on disability measurement, and the instrument seen as the gold (if somewhat tarnished) standard is the Kurtzke Expanded Disability Status Scale (EDSS) (21). This scale is based on findings of a large cohort of patients with MS, but has limited scientific data and has been much criticized (25,26). It is an ordinal scale that is multidimensional, mixing impairment and disability and virtually ignoring cognitive dysfunction. Limited inter- and intrarater reliability has been documented, which is particularly significant in the context of multicenter studies (27–29). Validity and responsiveness have yet to be comprehensively determined. The latter is clinically felt to be poor, thereby risking false negative results (type II error). Multiple alternative measures of disability exist (30–33) but few fulfill recommended criteria (34,35), and as yet there is no MS-specific disability measure that is clinically useful, scientifically sound, and widely accepted.

3. Health-Related Quality of Life

Clinician-reported measures (e.g., EDSS) fail to address the impact of MS on subjectively assessed function and psychosocial well-being, the so-called concept of health-related quality of life (HR-QOL). Consequently, the inclusion of patient-reported measures has been advocated as central to the evaluation of therapeutic interventions (36). One clinically useful and scientifically sound generic measure of HR-QOL is the Short Form -36 Health Survey (SF-36) (37,38). However, it appears to have significant limitations when used in MS patients, notably pronounced floor effect and lack of responsiveness (39), which may limit its role in the evaluation of therapeutic efficiency. Preliminary data are available concerning a new instrument, MSQOL-54 (40), based on the SF-36. However, it has yet to be evaluated in accordance with recommended guidelines (16,35) and in particular its responsiveness has yet to be addressed.

IV. TRIAL DESIGN IN MS

A. Blinding, Size, Controls, and Outcomes

Any study design is affected to some degree by two types of bias: first, those factors influencing the accuracy of results in the specific setting of the study (internal validity of the study); and second, those affecting extrapolation of the results to wider settings where the techniques, patients, indications, and other factors may be different (external validity of the study). The distinction between the efficacy (in research settings) and effectiveness (in routine practice) of an intervention reflects the concern that the level and quality of care might be different in research settings than in actual practice (41).

Double-blind, randomized, placebo-controlled studies are considered the gold-standard methodology for evaluating therapeutic effectiveness in MS (42,43). In theory the strength of this study design is its freedom from bias arising from: (1) patient selection (the purpose of randomization); (2) physician and patient awareness (the purpose of blinding); and (3) the placebo effect. However, blinded, randomized, placebo-controlled studies have their own inherent weaknesses (44). In particular, their external validity is sensitive to population bias, as the recruitment process and inclusion criteria often result in a narrowly defined set of patient indications (10), i.e., concerns that efficacy and efficiency differ.

To produce definitive results, the sample sizes of clinical trials in MS must be carefully computed using power calculations. Using the EDSS as the primary outcome measure, this is usually several hundred patients in each treatment arm. However, should a more responsive measurement instrument be used, such as MRI, the sample size may be reduced as the power calculation is dependent (in part) on the smallest change in the primary outcome considered significant (45). Power calculations can only be determined if the reliability and responsiveness of the outcome measures employed in a study have been defined previously. Consequently, only comprehensively evaluated instruments should be used in MS effectiveness studies.

The precise definition of the primary clinical outcome warrants careful consideration. Particularly important is confirmation of when that change is reached, given the fluctuating nature of MS. In relation to the EDSS, there is some evidence that using the concept of "time to confirmed treatment failure," rather than comparing differences in initial and final scores, may be more powerful (46). Although MRI is more straightforward, it is not yet accepted as a surrogate marker.

Phase III MS clinical trials invariably need to be multicentered, thus introducing administrative complexity and considerable expense. In addition, they demand standardization of outcome measurement among participating units, which may limit the potential pool of instruments to those with proven high interrater and intrainstitutional reliability. Even the relatively objective technique of MRI ideally requires analysis by a single evaluator (24).

Whilst the inclusion of a control group is essential, it is well established that patients in this arm do better than expected, in part from the placebo effect and also from regression to the mean (15). The behavior of the control group can substantially affect the power and outcome of a clinical trial if not anticipated. This issue has been comprehensively addressed in a recent publication (46).

Blinding patient and physician as to which arm of a study they have been randomized to, though preferable in theory (47), is difficult to achieve in practice as many of the drugs currently being evaluated in multiple sclerosis have well-documented side effects. The resultant patient and physician awareness as to who is receiving drug or placebo risks false positive findings suggesting efficacy (type 1 error) (4). Studies of long duration increase the likelihood of dropout from both treatment and placebo groups, reducing statistical power.

B. Ethical Considerations

Placebo controlling raises ethical issues (47,48). It prevents patients already receiving the drug being enlisted into studies and will stop those enrolled in trials from taking any drug that might be of benefit. In addition, it will not allow direct comparison between the drug being evaluated and any currently available medication. At present, placebo controlling remains both necessary and justifiable, as no therapeutic intervention has an overwhelmingly beneficial effect in MS (49).

A second ethical consideration relates to conflict of interest. Ideally the manufacturer of the drug should have no involvement in its evaluation and investigators should have no financial involvement in the sponsoring pharmaceutical company. Similarly, data safety and advisory committees should not include physicians actively involved in the drug under study, or in any other trial involving the sponsoring company. However, with an increasing number of pharmaceutical companies and therapeutic interventions, and the relatively small number of investigators with a particular interest in MS, it is almost impossible to adhere strictly to these guidelines. Furthermore, there has been a recent trend for investigators to establish their own companies and patent the intervention or technology under study. Early recognition and explicit confrontation of conflicts of interest is necessary if studies are to gain widespread ethical approval (50).

V. FUTURE PROSPECTS

It is clear from this brief overview that clinical trials in MS are complex. However, in looking toward the future there are at least two realistic goals: first, the development of an MR-based technique that gives a high, graded, and consistent correlation with disability, which can be used as a primary outcome measure in hospital-based studies involving relatively small numbers of patients; second, the development of instruments to measure relevant aspects of health status and health-related quality of life in a reproducible manner. The development of these instruments will necessitate patient involvement (the absence of which is striking in currently available tools) and will enable community-based studies involving large numbers of patient over a protracted period of time. Trial design in MS remains a challenging area, but recent developments are encouraging.

REFERENCES

1. Poser CM, Paty DW, McDonald WI, et al. New diagnostic criteria for multiple sclerosis: guidelines for research protocols. Ann Neurol 1983; 13: 227–231.
2. Thompson AJ, Kermode AG, Wicks D, et al. Major differences in the dynamics of primary and secondary progressive multiple sclerosis. Ann Neurol 1991; 29:53–62.
3. Lublin FD, Reingold SC. Defining the clinical course of multiple sclerosis: results of an international survey. Neurology 1996; 46:907–910.
4. Noseworthy JH. Immunosuppressive therapy in multiple sclerosis: pros and cons. Int MS J 1994; 1:79–89.
5. Polman CH, Dahlke K, Thompson AJ, et al. Interferon beta-1b in secondary progressive multiple sclerosis—outline of the clinical trial. Mult Scler 1995; 1:S51–S54.
6. Whitaker JN, McFarland HF, Rudge P, Reingold SC. Outcomes assessment in multiple sclerosis trials: a critical analysis. Mult Scler 1995; 1:37–47.
7. Rudick R, Antel J, Confavreux C, et al. Clinical outcomes assessment in multiple sclerosis. Ann Neurol (in press).
8. Gothan A, Brown R, Marsden C. Depression in Parkinson's disease: a quantitative and qualitative analysis. J Neurol Neurosurg Psychiatry 1986; 49: 381–389.
9. Brown R, MacCarthy B, Jahanshahi M, Marsden C. Accuracy of self-reported disability in patients with parkinsonism. Arch Neurol 1989; 46: 955–959.
10. The IFNB Multiple Sclerosis Study Group. Interferon beta-1b is effective in relapsing-remitting multiple sclerosis. I. Clinical results of a multi-center, randomised, double-blind, placebo-controlled trial. Neurology 1993; 43: 655–661.
11. Devinsky O. Outcomes research in neurology: incorporating health-related quality of life. Ann Neurol 1995; 37(2):141–142.
12. Gill TM. Quality of life assessment. J Roy Soc Med 1995; 88:680–682.
13. Runmarker B, Andersen O. Prognostic factors in a multiple sclerosis cohort with 25 years follow up. Brain 1993; 116:117–134.
14. Streiner DL, Norman GR. Health Measurement Scales: A Practical Guide to Their Development and Use, 2nd ed. Oxford: Oxford University Press, 1995.
15. Weinshenker BG. Natural history of multiple sclerosis. Ann Neurol 1994; 36:S6–S11.

16. Hobart JC, Lamping DL, Thompson AJ. Evaluating neurological outcome measures: the bare essentials. J Neurol Neurosurg Psychiatry 1996; 60: 127–130.
17. Guyatt G, Freeny D, Patrick D. Measuring health-related quality of life. Ann Intern Med 1993; 118:622–629.
18. Patrick D, Deyo R. Generic and disease specific measures in assessing health status and quality of life. Med Care 1989; 27(Suppl):217–232.
19. Morrisey SP, Miller DH, Kendall BE, et al. The significance of brain magnetic resonance imaging abnormalities at presentation with clinically isolated syndromes suggestive of multiple sclerosis. Brain 1993; 116:135–146.
20. Losseff NA, Kingsley DPE, Miller DH, McDonald WI, Thompson AJ. Clinical and magnetic resonance imaging in primary and secondary progressive multiple sclerosis. Mult Scler 1996; 1:218–222.
21. Kurtzke JF. Rating neurological impairment in multiple sclerosis: an expanded disability status scale (EDSS). Neurology 1983; 33:1444–1452.
22. McDonald WI, Miller DH, Thompson AJ. Are magnetic resonance findings predictive of clinical outcome in therapeutic trials in multiple sclerosis? The dilemma of interferon-β. Ann Neurol 1994; 36(1):14–18.
23. Fillipi M, Horsfield MA, Tofts PS, Barkof F, Thompson AJ, Miller DH. Quantitative assessment of MRI lesion load in monitoring the evolution of multiple sclerosis. Brain 1995; 118:1601–1612.
24. Miller DH, Albert PS, Barkhof F, et al. Guidelines for the use of magnetic resonance techniques in monitoring the treatment of multiple sclerosis. Ann Neurol 1996; 39:6–16.
25. Willoughby EW, Paty DW. Scales for rating impairment in multiple sclerosis: a critique. Neurology 1988; 38:1793–1798.
26. Noseworthy JH. Clinical scoring methods for multiple sclerosis. Ann Neurol 1994; 36:S80–S85.
27. Noseworthy JH, Vander voort MK, Wong CJ, Ebers GC. Interrater variability with the Expanded Disability Status Scale (EDSS) and Functional Systems (FS) in a multiple sclerosis clinical trial. Neurology 1990; 40:971–975.
28. Goodkin DE, Cookfair D, Wende K, et al. Inter- and intra-rater scoring agreement using grades 1.0 to 3.5 of the Kurtzke Expanded Disability Status Scale (EDSS). Neurology 1992; 42:859–863.
29. Francis DA, Bain P, Swan AV, Hughes RAC. An assessment of disability rating scales used in multiple sclerosis. Arch Neurol 1991; 48:299–301.
30. McDowell I, Newell C. Measuring Health: A Guide to Rating Scales and Questionnaires. Oxford: Oxford University Press, 1987.
31. Wilkin D, Hallam L, Doggett M-A. Measures of Need and Outcome for Primary Health Care. Oxford: Oxford University Press, 1994.
32. Bowling A. Measuring Disease: A Review of Disease Specific Quality of Life Measurement Scales. Buckingham, Philadelphia: Open University Press, 1995.
33. Sharrack B, Hughes RAC. Clinical scales for multiple sclerosis. J Neurol Sci 1996; 135:1–9.
34. American Education Research Association, American Psychological Associ-

ation and National Council on Measurement in Education. Standards for Education and Psychological Testing. Washington, DC: American Psychological Association, 1985.

35. Medical Outcomes Trust. Instrument review criteria. Med Outcomes Trust Bull 1995; 3(4):i–iv.

36. Fitzpatrick R. Applications of health status measures. In: Jenkinsin C, ed. Measuring Health and Medical Outcomes. London: UCL Press, 1994.

37. Ware JE, Sherbourne DC. The MOS 36-item short form health survey (SF-36). I. Conceptual framework and item selection. Med Care 1992; 30(6): 473–483.

38. McHorney CA, Ware JE, Raczek AE. The MOS 36-item Short-Form Health Survey (SF-36). II. Psychometric and clinical tests of validity in measuring physical and mental health constructs. Med Care 1993; 31(3):247–263.

39. Freeman JA, Langdon DW, Thompson AJ. The health-related quality of life of people with advanced multiple sclerosis. Arch Phys Med Rehabil (in press).

40. Vickrey BG, Hays RD, Harooni R, Myers LW, Ellison GW. A health-related quality of life measure for multiple sclerosis. Qual Life Res 1995; 4:187–206.

41. Eddy DM. Should we change the rules for evaluating medical technologies? In: Gelijns AC, ed. Modern Methods of Clinical Investigation. Washington, DC: National Academic Press, 1990:

42. Brown JR, et al. The design of clinical studies to assess therapeutic efficacy in multiple sclerosis. Neurology 1979; 21:2–23.

43. Herndon RM, Murray TJ. Proceedings of the international conference on therapeutic trials in multiple sclerosis. Arch Neurol 1983; 40:663–710.

44. Black N. Why we need observational studies to evaluate the effectiveness of health care. Br Med J 1996; 312(7040):1215–1218.

45. Nauta JJP, Thompson AJ, Barkhof F, Miller DH. Magnetic resonance imaging in monitoring the treatment of multiple sclerosis patients: statistical power of parallel-groups and crossover designs. J Neurol Sci 1994; 122:6–14.

46. Weinshenker B, Issa M, Baskerville J. Meta-analysis of the placebo treated groups in clinical trials of progressive MS. Neurology (in press).

47. Polman CH, Hartung HP. The treatment of multiple sclerosis: current and future. Curr Opin Neurol 1995; 8:200–209.

48. Ellison GW, Myers LW, Leake BD, et al. Design strategies for multiple sclerosis clinical trials. Ann Neurol 1994; 36:S108–S112.

49. Thompson AJ, Noseworthy JH. New treatment for multiple sclerosis: a clinical perspective. Curr Opin Neurol 1996; 9:187–198.

50. Foa R. Ethical considerations raised by clinical trials. In: Goodkin DE, Rudick RA, eds. Multiple Sclerosis: Advances in Clinical Trial Design, Treatment and Future Perspectives. London: Springer-Verlag, 1996.

19

The Incidence and Clinical Significance of Antibodies to Interferon-α

Kjell Öberg

University Hospital, Uppsala, Sweden

Rachel M. McKenna

Health Sciences Centre, University of Manitoba, Winnipeg, Manitoba, Canada

I. INTRODUCTION

Interferons (IFNs) are a family of biologically active proteins that are active against viruses and tumors. They comprise three main types, α, β, and γ, that are distinguished by the cell of origin, amino acid structure, production, and response to a given stimulus. Both the IFN-β and IFN-γ are coded by one gene each. IFN-α, in contrast, has at least 23 different genes on chromosome 9 coding for 15 different functional proteins (1).

Within a given subtype or locus of IFN-α, different allelic forms of the gene may exist. The IFN protein consists of 165–187 amino acids with molecular weights of 17–25 kD. Some of the natural IFNs are glycosylated. The natural IFNs contain about 13 different subtypes of IFN-α, as does the IFN which is derived from a malignant transformed cell line Namalwa (IFN α-N1, Wellferon). By recombinant DNA techniques, nonglycosylated single species of IFN-α are produced such as IFN α-2a (Roferon) and IFN α-2b (Intron-A) or IFN α-2c (2).

The mature IFN α-2a protein product (Roferon) is characterized by a lysine at position 23 and a histidine at position 34. In contrast, IFN α-2b encodes an arginine at position 23, and IFN α-2c has arginine residues at both positions 23 and 34. Recent studies which have examined the frequency of the different IFN α-2 variants in both white and Japanese individuals have concluded that the sequences corresponding to IFN α-2a and IFN α-2c are either minor variants of the IFN α-2b gene or that they only occur in immortalized cell lines grown in culture (2,4). In one study of human genomic DNA from 28,000 North American individuals, IFN α-2b was the predominant IFN-α species detected in a very small percentage of the population processing the IFN α-2c gene, and in none was the α-2a gene detected (5).

The antiviral and antitumor effects have been most widely studied by recombinant IFN α-2, but recent data indicate that other subtypes of IFN-α might also be potent (3). Very recently, IFN α-N1 has demonstrated significantly better effect in the treatment of patients with hepatitis C compared with those treated with Intron-A (3).

IFN-α has been approved and is under investigation for the treatment of a number of malignant diseases in the United States, Canada, Europe, Australia, and Japan. Clinical trials have shown significant antitumor effect in diseases such as hairy cell leukemia, human immunodeficiency virus (HIV)–related Kaposi's sarcoma, basal cell carcinoma, chronic myeloid leukemia (CML), cutaneous T-cell lymphoma, and multiple myeloma but also in solid tumors such as malignant carcinoid tumors, melanoma, ovarian cancer, and renal cell carcinoma (RCC) (6–9). IFN-α has demonstrated significant effects in viral diseases such as chronic hepatitis B, C, and more recently D (10). It has also shown beneficial effects in condyloma acuminatum and laryngeal papilomas when given intralesionally.

Therapy with recombinant and natural IFNs has been associated with the development of anti-IFN antibodies in variable proportions of the patients (11–13). Induction of IFN antibodies and the ability to detect them may depend on several factors such as type and stage of the underlying disease, previous and concomitant treatment, patient age, type of IFN, route of IFN administration, dose regimens and duration of treatment, cumulative IFN dose, and finally mode of serum sampling and type of assay used for the antibody detection. Last but not least, even when the same assay is used in different laboratories, great variation in the levels of anti-IFN antibodies can be encountered between the laboratories.

II.   ASSAYS TO DETECT ANTIBODIES TO IFN-α

The level of antibodies to IFN-α will vary with the assay used, and some assays are more sensitive than others, thus presenting problems of interpreting antibody data from various studies. Today, four different types of assays have been used to detect antibodies to IFN-α. The principle of each assay and their limitations are described below.

A. Neutralization Assays

In contrast to the other assay, the neutralization assay tests the ability of antibodies to interfere with one function of IFN; that is, the antiviral effect. Serum samples are incubated with a known amount of IFN-α, which can be a recombinant IFN or a natural leukocyte product. The ability of the serum-treated IFN to inhibit viral replication in a virus-sensitive cell line is then compared with the activity of the same amount of IFN which has not been treated with the serum. For quantitative neutralization bioassays, the preferred expression of the neutralizing potency of an antiserum is a titer, that is, the dilution of serum that reduces 10 laboratory units (LUs) per milliliter of the IFN to 1 LU/ml, the endpoint of most bioassays (14). This 10–1 LU/ml expression, which has been recommended by the World Health Organization for reporting the results of IFN neutralization by the constant IFN method, with varying dilutions of serum but can as well be used with a constant antibody method (with varying concentrations of IFN).

This assay is so far the only one which tests the ability of the antibodies to inhibit IFN function and is regarded as the "gold standard" assay for detecting antibodies to IFN. However, this assay does not directly measure immunoglobulin to IFN and can therefore be influenced by nonantibody serum factors which may inhibit the antiviral activity of IFN. In addition, being a bioassay, the sensitivity can vary from assay to assay and operator to operator. Other variables in the neutralizing assay can be the source of virus-sensitive cell lines used. To detect neutralizing antibodies to IFN-α, a variety of cell lines have been used, including human lung fibroblasts, human amniotic cells, and bovine kidney cells. Some cell lines are more sensitive to the action of one IFN-α subtype more than others. Thus, one bioassay may be more sensitive at detecting IFN activity and therefore may be more sensitive at detecting anti-IFN activity than others. Another limitation of this assay is that the antibody activity will only be detected if it interferes with one function of IFN; that is, viral replication. It does not measure other functions of IFN such as its ability to inhibit cell proliferation.

B. Radioimmunoassay

The radioimmunoassay is sometimes called an immunoradiometric assay (IRMA). It is an indirect assay which tests the ability of serum samples to compete with a radiolabeled monoclonal IFN-α antibody to bind to recombinant or natural IFN-α. Serum samples are incubated with a known amount of IFN-α followed by incubation with an I^{125}-labeled monoclonal antibody raised to a specific IFN. After further incubation, a bead coated with a polyclonal sheep antibody to IFN-α is added to the reaction mixture, creating a sandwich with IFN-α as the filling. A comparison of the amount of radioactivity detected in the absence and presence of the serum sample is made, and a significant reduction in the amount of radioactivity detected is taken as evidence for the presence of anti-IFN antibodies. This assay, like the neutralization assay, is an indirect assay for anti-IFN antibodies. It therefore is subjected to some of the same limitations as the neutralizing assay in that other serum factors which inhibit the ability to bind to radioactive antibodies cannot be distinguished. The method does not measure biological activity of IFNs.

C. ELISA

The enzyme-linked immunosorbent assay (ELISA) (16) is based on the direct detection of human immunoglobulin bound to an IFN-α–coated plate and has been used to detect antibodies to various IFN-α. Plastic wells of microtiter plates are coated with recombinant types of and serum samples are added to the wells and allowed to incubate with the IFN. The plates are washed and a goat antibody to human immunoglobulin conjugated to peroxidases is added to the wells. Unbound antibody is washed off and a colored substrate is added to the wells. The absorbency is then measured and used as an indication of the amount of antibody present. This assay has the advantage that it is relatively easy to perform and standardize and only detects immunoglobulin. However, this also means it will detect all antibodies to IFN, including those that do not interfere with its function. For this reason, it is usually used as a screening assay to detect antibodies in patient sera to IFN-α. If the serum is found to be positive by ELISA, it is further tested in a biological assay for neutralization activity.

D. Enzyme Immunoassay

The enzyme immunoassay (EIA) is a sandwich assay, that, the presence of antibodies to IFN-α, is measured by testing the ability of the serum to act as a bridge between two IFN molecules; one molecule is coupled to a solid phase and the other is conjugated to peroxidase. The serum is first incubated with a polystyrene bead coated with IFN-α. After washing away unbound material, IFN-α coupled to peroxidase is added to the reaction mixture, followed by substrate, and then the absorbency is determined. The color produced by the reaction is the function of the antibody concentration in the patient serum. The advantages of this assay are that it is relatively easy to perform and to be standardized. However, like the immunoassay, the EIA does not directly detect the presence of immunoglobulin but rather serum factors which can bind to IFN-α. Also, it does not test the ability of antibodies detected to inhibit the function of the IFN. For this reason, it has been used as a screening assay to detect antibodies to IFN-α. If the antibody is detected by this method, it is further tested for functional activity in a neutralization assay.

Recently, two new assays have been developed: an antiproliferation assay (O. Prümmer, personal communication) for IFN-α and a so-called MxA assay for both IFN-α and IFN-β (see Chapter 20).

III. DEVELOPMENT OF ANTIBODIES TO DIFFERENT IFN PREPARATIONS

It is clear that patients being treated with IFN-α can develop antibodies to the various IFN preparations. Some of the variables which have been proposed to influence the development of antibodies are the route of administration of IFN, the cumulative dose of drug received, the underlying disease, and the IFN preparation used. The role of each of these in the development of antibodies to IFN-α is discussed below (12,13).

A. Route of Administration

IFN-α can be administered intralesionally (e.g. in the treatment of condyloma acuminata) or systematically (e.g., intramuscularly, subcutaneously, or intravenously). The effect of the route of administration and the development of antibodies to IFN is difficult to assess, because the route of administration of the IFN is usually determined by the disease being treated and the preparation used. In the beginning, when recombinant IFN-α was introduced into clinical trials, many patients were treated with intramuscular injections, whereas during the last decade, most patients have been treated subcutaneously.

Differences in the rate of antibody development to IFN α-2a were reported in two studies in which patients with hairy cell leukemia (HCL) were administered IFN by two different routes. In one study, the patients received the IFN subcutaneously and 9% of them developed neutralizing antibodies (19). In a second study, the patients received the IFN intramuscularly and 19% of them developed antibodies (20). However, these results have to be interpreted cautiously. The patients who received IFN-α intramuscularly and developed the high rate of antibody response also received a higher cumulative dose of IFN.

The only way to evaluate the role of the route of administration of a preparation is to give the same preparation and the same dose to patients with the same disease using different routes of administration. This has only been reported for a group of patients receiving recombinant IFN-β. The incidence of ELISA-detectable antibody formation to IFN β-1b was much higher in the patients who received the drug intramuscularly as opposed to intravenously (21). It has been known for some time that the route of administration affects the immune response. The administration of an antigen intravenously tends to favor the development of tolerance to the antigen, whereas the subcutaneous or intramuscular route favors an immune response. Indeed, most vaccines are delivered by the latter two routes for this reason.

B. Cumulative Dose and Dosing Regimens

Larger doses of an antigen and more frequent administration of an antigen are more likely to lead to an immune response. Therefore, it is certainly theoretically possible that patients who receive high cumulative dose and/or more frequent administration of IFN-α are more likely to develop antibodies. However, in a study of patients with renal cell carcinoma (RCC) where the patients were entered into either a high-dose protocol (35–54 MU daily for 28 days) or low-dose protocol (3 MU daily for 48 weeks) with IFN α-2a, the frequency of the development of neutralizing antibodies to IFN in the group receiving the high dose was 50% compared with 74% of patients receiving the lower dose (22). In another study of high- and low-dose IFN α-2a administration to patients with RCC, the incidence of neutralizing antibodies were similar in patients receiving the high and low doses of IFN: 37% for high versus 33% for low doses in spite of the 10-fold difference in the dose (23). These findings suggest that in this disease, at least the dose of IFN α-2a does not influence the development of antibodies to IFN.

C. Role of Disease

The ability to develop an antibody response will be influenced by a given patient's immune system, which can certainly be influenced by disease status, especially cancer. This variable may, therefore, influence development of antibodies to IFN-α. In a study of 537 patients who received systemic therapy with IFN α-2b, the incidence of neutralizing antibody development varied from a low of 0% of patients treated with HCL up to 14.2% of patients treated for small cell lung cancer (12). In a similar study which looked at development of neutralizing antibodies to IFN-α in 559 patients treated with IFN α-2a, the incidence of antibodies also varied with disease with 4.6% for leukemias to 46% for patients with RCC (24). However, it should be mentioned that patients with different diseases may received different doses, regimens of doses, and duration of treatment, all of which may also contribute to the development of antibodies. For example, patients with RCC received much high doses of IFN than patients with HCL or hepatitis. Finally, the immune response in MS patients may differ from responses in cancer patients.

D. Role of Different IFN Preparations in Generating Antibody Responses

There have been suggestions that different IFN preparations differ with respect to their ability to induce an antibody response; that is, some preparations are more "antigenic" than others. Some reports have suggested that IFN α-2a is more likely to induce neutralizing antibodies than IFN α-2b. Counterarguments to this are that the route of administration, the cumulative dose of IFN, and the assay used to detect IFN antibodies influence the reported incidence of antibodies to IFN-α more than the preparation. Therefore, the best studies to examine differences in antigenecity between IFN-α preparations are the ones in which different IFN-α preparations were given to patients with the same underlying disease and using the same route of administration, dosing schedule, and antibody detection system.

A series of such studies have now been reported in a number of different diseases shown in Table 1. In each of these diseases, the frequency of antibody development was always greater in patients who received IFN α-2a compared with IFN α-2b. This varied from an almost twofold differ-

Table 1 Development of Neutralizing Antibodies to IFN-α

Study	Disease	IFN	% Incidence of Antibodies
Grander et al. (25)	Carcinoids	IFN α-2a	50 (6/12)
		IFN α-2b	0 (0/10)
Öberg et al. (26)	Carcinoids	IFN α-2a	37 (12/32)
		IFN α-2b	10 (21/208)
		HuLe IFN-α	1 (1/103)
		IFN α-N1	6 (1/16)
von Wussow et al. (27)	CML	IFN α-2a	28 (14/50)
		IFN α-2b	6 (2/33)
		IFN α-2a	20 (15/74)
Antonelli et al. (29)	Hepatitis	IFN α-2b	7 (10/144)
		Natural IFN-α	1 (1/78)

CML, chronic myeloid leukemia.

ence in patients with metastatic carcinoids (25,26) to a fourfold difference in patients with CML (27). This difference in incidence of antibody development was statistically significant when the data were analyzed using a stratified Mantle-Haenszel test ($P < .0001$) with an odds ratio of 4.98 for the development of antibodies in patients receiving IFN α-2a when compared to IFN α-2b (28). Interestingly, in patients who received nonrecombinant preparation of IFN-α, the incidence of antibody development was even lower than in patients who received either of the recombinant IFN α-2 products (26,29). A possible explanation for this is that recombinant proteins are not glycosylated, whereas the natural IFN proteins are. Furthermore, IFN α-2a and IFN α-2b differ only in one amino-acid at position 23. Recent unpublished studies have shown that the IFN α-2a preparation forms large aggregates in the vials, such as dimers and trimers (Nolte K.U., personal communication), which might be more antigenic than the IFN α-2b. Another explanation for the difference in antigenicity between IFN α-2a and IFN α-2b might be that the IFN α-2b subtype seems to be the most common allelic variant of IFN α-2. Therefore, the majority of patients will not form antibodies to a normal cell protein but may well form antibodies to a variant of the same protein.

IV. CLINICAL SIGNIFICANCE OF THE DEVELOPMENT OF ANTIBODIES TO IFN

Since the initial discovery that antibodies to IFNs could develop in patients treated with IFN, there has been much debate about the clinical significance of such antibodies. Some studies suggest that there are no adverse effects associated with the development of such antibodies to IFNs, and indeed that the development of antibodies in patients is associated with a good prognosis (11,13,22). Other studies have reported that the development of antibodies is associated with a poor outcome (30). As noted in the previous section, antibodies to IFN can be detected by a number of different techniques, which are basically divided into those that detect neutralizing and those which detect binding or nonneutralizing antibodies. As expected, only a proportion of the antibodies which are positive in the binding assay are also positive in the neutralization assay. In studies that have shown adverse effects to be associated with the development of IFN-α antibodies, this seems to be associated with only neutralizing antibodies (19,30,32).

A list of studies that have compared the response of treatment in patients who did and did not develop neutralizing antibodies is shown in

Table 2 Clinical Significance of Neutralizing Antibodies to IFN-α

Study	Disease	IFN	Resistance or Relapse		Significance $P^{a,b}$
			Antibody Positive (%)	Antibody Negative (%)	
Steis et al. (16)	HCL	IFN α-2a	6/16 (38)	0/35 (0)	.001
Quesada et al. (33)	HCL	IFN α-2a	518 (63)	0/32 (0)	.001
von Wussow et al. (19)	HCL	IFN α-2a	6/6 (100)	0/61 (0)	.001
Berman et al. (20)	HCL	IFN α-2a	6/6 (100)	9/26 (35)	.004
von Wussow et al. (31)	CML	IFN α-2b	5/5 (100)	0/20 (0)	.001
Freund et al. (34)	CML	IFN α-2b	7/8 (88)	7/19 (37)	.016
Öberg et al. (35)	Carcinoids	IFN α-2b	2/3 (66)	1/17 (7)	.007
Grander et al. (25)	Carcinoids	IFN α-2b	3[c]	4/10 (40)	
		IFN α-2a	5/6 (83)	4/6 (66)	.5
Quesada et al. (23)	RCC	IFN α-2a	7/7 (100)	0/5 (0)	.001
Prummer et al. (36)	RCC	IFN α-2a	8/25 (32)	13/61 (20)	.295

HCL, hair cell leukemia; CML, chronic myeloid leukemia; RCC, renal cell carcinoma.
[a] Chi-squared test for significance of association between the presence of neutralizing antibodies and the development of resistance to treatment relapse.
[b] An overall significance level is not reported as the odds ratios of the different studies were not homogenous as determined by a Breslow Day test for homogeneity.
[c] No patients developed antibodies.

Table 2. In four studies of patients with HCL, either resistance to treatment or relapse was more common in patients who developed neutralizing antibodies to IFN α-2a (19,20,30,33). This ranged from 38 to 100% of patients in the antibody-positive group to only 0–35% in the antibody negative group. This association of antibodies to IFN-α with resistance or relapse was statistically significant in all four studies. Similar results were seen in antibody-positive and antibody-negative patients with CML, where the incidence of resistance or relapse was 100 and 88% in the antibody-positive group and 0 and 37%, respectively, in the antibody-negative groups (31,34).

In patients with carcinoids who developed neutralizing antibodies to IFN α-2b, the relapse and resistance rate was higher in the antibody-positive group (two of three) compared with the antibody-negative group (one of seven). Interestingly, in patients with carcinoids who were treated with IFN α-2a, the relapse and resistance rates were similar in both antibody-positive (five of six) and antibody negative groups (four of six) (25).

Finally, in two studies, patients with RCC were monitored for the development of neutralizing antibodies to IFN α-2a. The relapse/resistance rate was higher in the antibody-positive groups (21,36).

Although the numbers in some of these studies are very small, it would appear that in at least four different malignancies, the development of neutralizing antibodies to IFN-α has been associated with adverse clinical effects. Sixty-three percent of patients who developed neutralizing antibodies had impaired effects versus only 13% of those who did not have a relapse or became resistant to treatment. Interestingly, the reactivity patterns of the neutralizing antibodies against recombinant IFN α-2a, usually also cross reacted with IFN α-2b, so that the substitution of one recombinant product for another was not possible (23,26,31). However, in a number of instances, these antibodies did not neutralize natural IFN-α, so antibody-positive patients could be successfully treated with nonrecombinant IFN-α products (23,30,35,37). Another important issue is the titer of neutralizing antibodies. In our studies of patients with carcinoids (26), as well as in the study of von Wussow et al. (27) in CML patients, a titer above 400 NU/ml is related to abrogation of therapeutic response.

V. SUMMARY AND CONCLUSION

Antibodies to IFN-α can develop in patients who have been treated with both natural and recombinant IFN-α products. However, high-titer neutralizing IFN antibodies are significantly more common in patients treated with recombinant IFN α-2a. The development of neutralizing antibodies to IFN-α is associated with a higher frequency of relapse or resistance to further IFN-α therapy. In patients receiving IFN-α who develop resistance to treatment or who relapse, it may therefore be useful to measure neutralizing antibodies to IFN-α so that alternative treatment modalities can be considered for antibody-positive patients. The significance of non-neutralizing antibodies to IFN-α is not clear, but they do not seem to be associated with the loss of therapeutic efficacy.

REFERENCES

1. Weissman C, Weber H. The interferon genes. Prog Nucleic Acid Res 1986; 33:251.
2. Gewert D, Salom C, Barber K, et al. Analysis of interferon-α2 sequences in human genomic DNA. J Interferon Res 1993; 13:227.
3. Tillman HL. Different HCV-genotypes and their response to interferon: IX European Interferon Workshop. Hannover, Germany, 1996, p. 40.
4. Hosoi H, Imai M, Yamanaka M. The interferon-α2β gene in Japanese patients with chronic viral hepatitis who developed antibodies after treatment with recombinant interferon-α2a. J. Gastroenterol Hepatol 1992; 7:411.
5. Liao MJ, Lee N, Hussain M, et al. Distribution of IFN-α2 genes in humans (abstr). VIII European Interferon Workshop. Hannover, Germany, 1994.
6. Spiegel RJ. Alpha interferons: a clinical overview. Urology 1989; 34:75.
7. Strander H. Interferon treatment of human neoplasia. In: Klein G, Weinhouse S, eds. Advances in Cancer Research, Vol 46. London: Academic Press, 1986:1–20.
8. Baron S, Tyring SK, Fleischmann WR, et al. The interferons. Mechanisms of actions and clinical applications. JAMA 1991; 266:1375.
9. Stuart-Harris RC, Lauchlan R, Day R. The clinical application of the interferons: a review. Med J Austral 1992; 156:869.
10. Dorr RT. Interferon-alpha in malignant and viral diseases. A review. Drugs 1993; 45:177.
11. Itri LM, Campion M, Dennin RA, et al. Incidence and clinical significance of neutralizing antibodies in patients receiving recombinant alpha-2a by intramuscular injection. Cancer 1987; 59:668.
12. Spiegel RJ, Spicehandler JR, Jacobs SL, et al. Low Incidence of serum neutralizing factors in patients receiving recombinant alpha-2b Interferon (Intron A). Am J Med 1986; 80:223.
13. Figlin RA, Itri LM. Anti-interferon antibodies: a perspective. Semin Hematol 1988; 25:9.
14. Kawade Y. Quantitation of neutralizing of interferon by antibody; Methods Enzymol 1986; 119:558.
15. Protzman WP, Jacobs SL, Minnicozzi M, et al. A radioimmunologic technique to screen for antibodies to α-2 interferon. J Immunol Methods 1984; 75:317.
16. Jacobs SJ, Sullivan LM, Salfi M, et al. Minimal antigenecity of Intron A in human recipients demonstrated by three analytical methods. J Biol Response Modifiers 1988; 7:447.
17. Grossberg SE. Human antibodies to interferons: report of National Institutes of Health Workshop, J Interferon Res 1988; 8:v.
18. Hennes U, Jucker W, Fischer EA, Krummenacher TH, Palleroni AV, Trown PW, et al. The detection of antibodies to recombinant interferon alfa-2a in human serum. J Biol Stand 1987; 15:231.
19. von Wussow P, Pralle H, Jakshies D, et al. Effective treatment of recombi-

nant interferon alpha-2 (IFN-α) antibody–positive hairy cell leukemia (HCL) patients with natural interferon alpha (nIFN) (abstr). Am Soc Hematol 1989.

20. Berman E, Heiler G, Kemoin S, et al. Incidence of response and long-term follow-up in a patient with hairy cell leukemia treated with recombinant interferon alfa-2a. Blood 1990; 75:839.

21. Konrad M, Childs A, Merigan T, et al. Assessment of the antigenic response in humans to a recombinant mutant interferon beta. J Clin Immunol 1987; 7:365–375.

22. Krown SE, Real FX, Einzig AI, et al. Treatment of Kaposi's sarcoma and renal cell carcinoma with recombinant leukocyte A interferon. In: Kirchner H, Schellekens H, eds. Biol Interferon Systems. Elsevier, 1985:523.

23. Quesada JR, Rios A, Swanson D, et al. Anti tumor activity of recombinant-derived interferon alpha in metastatic renal cell carcinoma. J Clin Oncol 1985; 3:1522.

24. Jones GJ, Itri LM. Safety and tolerance of recombinant interferon alfa-2a in cancer patients. Cancer 1986; 57:1709.

25. Grander D, Öberg K, Lundqvist ML, et al. Interferon-enhancement of 2'-5'-oligodenylate synthetase in mid-gut carcinoid tumours. Lancet 1990; 336: 337.

26. Öberg K. Autoimmunity and antibodies to interferons in patients with carcinoid tumors—clinical consequences (abstr). VIII European Interferon Workshop. Hannover, Germany, 1994.

27. von Wussow P, Hehlmann R, Nolte Ku, et al. IFN-α2A (Roferon) is more immunogenic than IFN-α-2B (Intron A) in patients with CML (abstr). VIII European Interferon Workshop. Hannover, Germany, 1994.

28. Breslow NE, Day NE. Classical methods of analysis of grouped data. In: Breslow NE, Day NE, eds. Statistical Methods in Cancer Research. Vol. 1. The Analysis of Case-Control Studies. Lyon: International Agency for Research on Cancer, 1980:122.

29. Antonelli G, Currenti M, Turriziani O, et al. Neutralizing antibodies to interferon-α: relative frequency in patients treated with different interferon preparations. J Infect Dis 1991; 163:882.

30. Steis RG, Smith JW, Urba WJ, et al. Resistance to recombinant interferon alfa-2a hairy cell leukemia associated with neutralizing anti-interferon antibodies. N Engl J Med 1988; 318:1409.

31. von Wussow P, Freund M, Block B, et al. Clinical significance of anti–IFN-α antibody titres during Interferon therapy. Lancet 1987; 2:635.

32. Gutterman JU, et al. The role of interferons in the treatment of hematologic malignancies. Semin Hematol 1988; 25:3.

33. Quesada JR, Itri L, Gutterman JU. Alpha Interferons in hairy cell leukemia (HCL). A five year follow up in 100 patients. J Interferon Res 1987; 7:678.

34. Freund M, von Wussow P, Diedrich H, et al. Recombinant human interferon (IFN) alpha-2b in chronic myelogenous leukemia. Dose dependency of response and frequency of neutralizing anti-interferon antibodies. Br J Hematol 1989; 72:350.

35. Öberg K, Alm G, Magnusson A, et al. Treatment of malignant carcinoid tumors with recombinant interferon alfa-2b: development of neutralizing interferon antibodies and possible loss of anti tumor activity. J Natl Cancer Inst 1989; 81:531.
36. Prümmer O. Interferon-alpha antibodies in patients with renal cell carcinoma treated with recombinant interferon-alpha-2A in an adjuvant multicenter trial. Cancer 1993; 71:1828.
37. Rönnblom LE, Janson ET, Perers A, et al. Characterization of anti-interferon antibodies appearing during recombinant interferon-α2a treatment. Clin Exp Immunol 1992; 89:330.

20

Quantitation and Characterization of Multiple Sclerosis Patient Antibodies to Interferon-β

Eirik Nestaas, James G. Files, Jeffrey W. Nelson, and Erno Pungor, Jr.

Berlex Biosciences, Richmond, California

I. INTRODUCTION

Chapter 19 (1) addressed antibodies to interferon-α (IFN-α) developed in patients treated with either natural or recombinant IFN-α products. This chapter presents data on antibodies generated in multiple sclerosis (MS) patients on IFN-β therapy.

Natural IFN-β is a glycosylated protein comprising 166 amino acids. Although IFN-β and types of IFN-α are structurally quite different, they are generally believed to target the same cellular receptors and to elicit similar cellular responses. They are on this basis commonly referred to as type 1 IFNs.

Two different recombinant forms of IFN-β are presently approved for chronic therapy in MS. These are Betaseron, a nonglycosylated form (IFN β-1b) expressed in *Escherichia coli,* and Avonex, a glycosylated form (IFN β-1a), expressed in Chinese hamster ovary (CHO) cells. Betaseron lacks the N-terminal methionine of the natural IFN-β and has an amino acid substitution in position 17 (cysteine to serine). These minor amino acid changes are not believed significantly to affect the biological activity of the molecule. Most of the clinical experience to date have been for MS patients on Betaseron therapy.

Just as with various types of IFN-α, chronic therapy with IFN-β will generate anti-IFN antibodies in many patients. This chapter describes novel methodologies to characterize such antibodies. Although these methods were specifically developed to monitor MS patients on Betaseron therapy, they should in principle apply equally well to long-term treatment with other type 1 IFN therapeutics.

II.   ASSAY METHODOLOGIES

Antibodies to IFN-β can be measured using the general methods described for IFN-α in Chapter 19. However, these commonly employed assays exhibit certain limitations affecting our ability to confidently interpret antibody data and their therapeutic relevance. For such reasons, we decided to develop new assay methodologies to improve the quantitation and characterization of antibodies generated in MS patients on Betaseron therapy. These new assays are summarized below.

A.   IFN Activity Assay

The commonly employed antiviral assays are not absolutely specific for type 1 IFNs; they will also respond to a number of other compounds present in human serum, such as platelet-derived growth factor (PDGF). In addition, antiviral assays are relatively imprecise, they are not always sufficiently sensitive (e.g., to measure circulating levels of IFN-β in blood; sensitivity is typically 20 IU/ml), and they can be cumbersome and exhibit poor reproducibility.

To minimize such limitations, we developed and validated a new activity assay based on the type 1 IFN–specific induction of the *MxA* gene in human cells (2–5). Gene induction is here measured by immunoassay of accumulated MxA protein in A549 cells (4,6). The immunoassay response (measured as chemiluminescence) can be quantitatively related to IFN activity. In this manner, the biological activity of IFNs can be determined reliably without virus infection of the indicator cell line. This assay is adaptable to measuring type I IFN activity in human sera. For such measurements the assay has a lower limit of quantitation of 1 IU Betaseron per mL serum and a precision of $\pm 18\%$ (6).

B.   Neutralizing Antibody Assay

The MxA induction assay is employed to measure neutralizing titers in patient sera based on the World Health Organization (WHO) recommended procedure outlined in Chapter 19. Its precision in titer determination is $\pm 0.2 \log_{10}$ units, and it can detect neutralizing titers of 10 or greater.

However, since not all neutralizing activity may be antibody mediated, a scrubbing procedure employing protein A–conjugated Sepharose was developed to selectively remove IgG from patient sera. The difference between neutralizing activity before and after the scrubbing thus represents antibody-mediated neutralization (i.e., IgG-mediated neutralization) (7).

C. Total Antibody Assay

An enzyme-linked immunosorbent assay (ELISA) to measure total Betaseron-binding antibodies (as IgG) in MS patient sera was developed and validated. Serial dilutions of sera are added to Betaseron-coated 96-well microtiter plates. The amount of captured antibody is detected employing goat antihuman IgG.

III. TESTING OF MS PATIENT SERA

Sera (309 samples) from 35 MS patients on Betaseron therapy were tested employing the new antibody assays. The neutralizing activities were compared with those obtained previously for these samples using an antiviral activity (CPE) assay. The patients included in this study were selected to

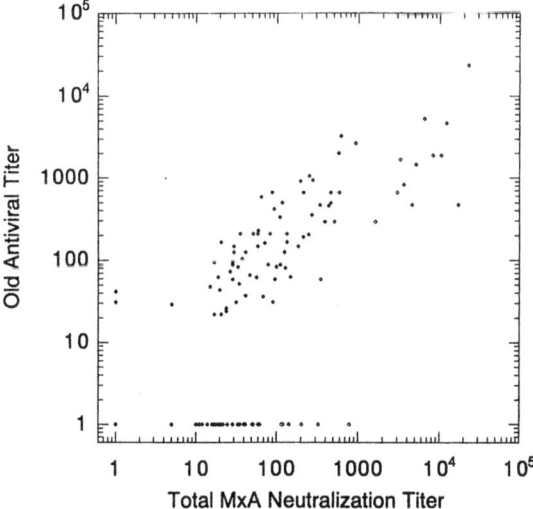

Figure 1 Neutralizing titers obtained previously ("old antiviral titer") versus neutralizing titers obtained recently with the new MxA induction bioassay. The chart represents 309 serum samples from 35 MS patients (30 on Betaseron therapy, 5 on placebo). Nonneutralizing samples are plotted as "1" to allow logarithmic charting.

cover a wide range of neutralizing antibody titers, from undetectable to several thousand. It should also be noted that some of these patients in previous tests (i.e., using the antiviral assay) showed persistent antibody responses while other only showed transient antibody responses. On the average, nine serum samples were analyzed per patient and spanning 3–5 years of Betaseron therapy. All samples were blinded prior to analyses.

Figure 1 demonstrates the overall good correlation between the old antiviral titers and the MxA neutralizing titers. This figure also illustrates that the MxA induction assay is more sensitive in identifying positive sera. False-positive rates (based on placebo serum samples) were low and similar for both assays. (Note that nonneutralizing samples are plotted as "1" to allow logarithmic charting.)

Figure 2 shows that virtually all measured neutralization was antibody-mediated (and IgG mediated). Only seven samples with moderate and low titers exhibited significant (but reproducible) neutralization owing to components other than antibodies. However, it should be emphasized that these serum samples had been stored for several years at −20°C and

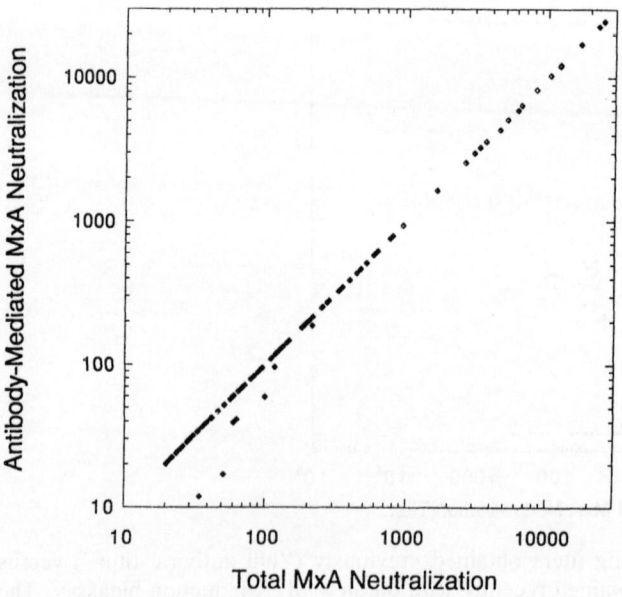

Figure 2 Total neutralizing titers (MxA induction bioassay) versus Neutralizing antibody titers (i.e., total neutralizing titers minus nonantibody-mediated titers determined after removal of all IgG). (See Fig. 1 for description of samples.)

that non-IgG antibodies and other neutralizing compounds may be more significant in fresher sera.

Figure 3a demonstrates the poor correlation between neutralizing antibodies and total antibodies to Betaseron: it is not possible to predict the

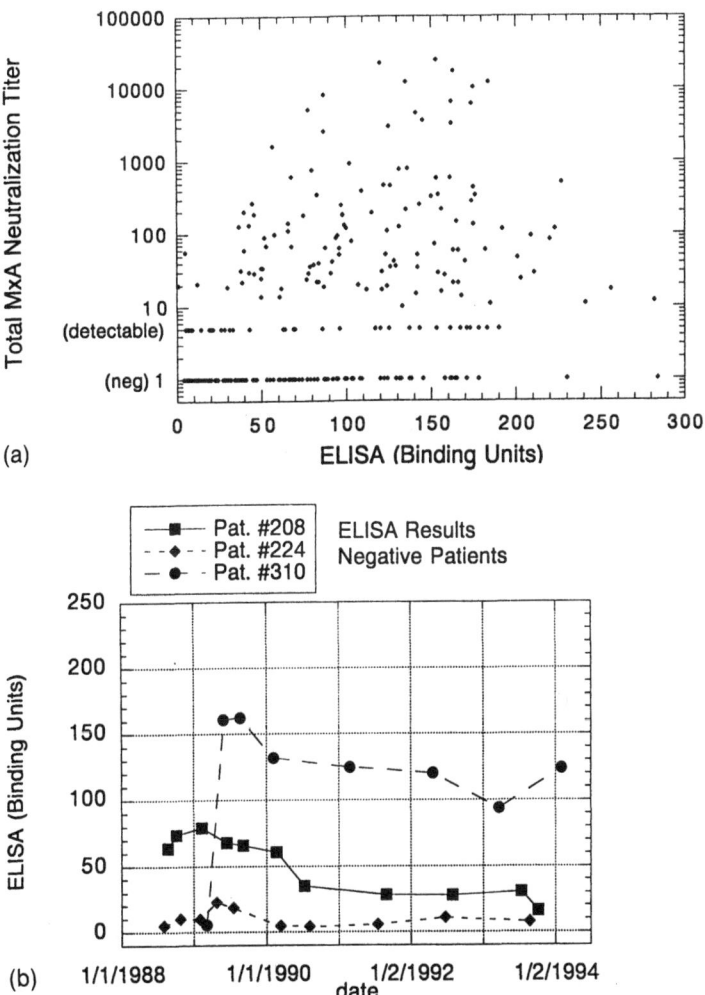

(a)

(b)

Figure 3 (a) Total neutralizing titers (MxA induction bioassay) versus total Betaseron binding antibodies (i.e., total IgG as "binding units"). (See Fig. 1 for description of samples.) (b) Changes in serum levels of Betaseron binding antibodies (IgG) during Betaseron therapy. None of the three patients represented here developed measurable neutralizing antibody titers at any time during therapy.

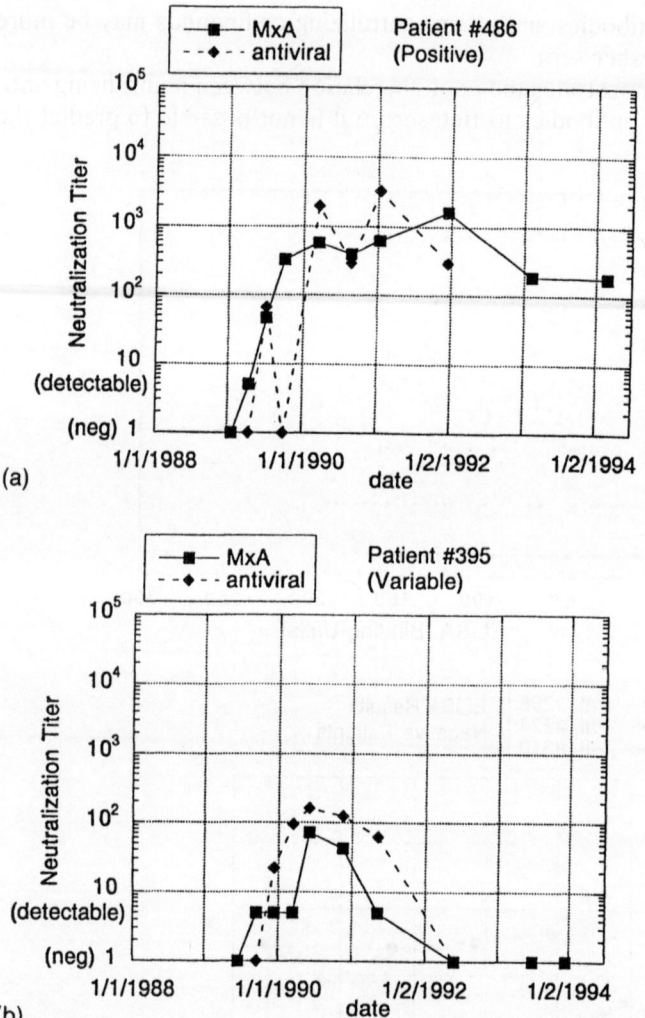

Figure 4 (a) Changes in neutralizing titers over time for one persistent neutraliz-ing antibody responder. Neutralizing titers obtained previously (antiviral titer) versus neutralizing titers obtained recently with the new MxA induction bioassay. (b) Changes in neutralizing titers over time for one transient neutralizing antibody responder. Neutralizing titers obtained previously (antiviral titer) versus neutraliz-ing titers obtained recently with the new MxA induction bioassay. Note that the neutralizing titers in this patient were confirmed to appear only transiently.

presence of neutralizing antibodies from total antibody data. This lack of predictability is exemplified by Figure 3b: MS patients who at no time during Betaseron therapy developed neutralizing antibody titers nevertheless could show consistently either high, moderate, or very low total antibody responses.

Although the MxA and antiviral assays measured similar neutralizing titers for each patient, the MxA induction assay data were generally more consistent and less variable. This is exemplified by Figure 4a (a persistent neutralizing antibody responder). It is also interesting that the MxA assay confirmed previous findings that neutralizing antibodies (Nabs) may appear and then ultimately disappear (Fig. 4b; a transient neutralizing antibody responder).

IV. CONCLUSIONS

Serum antibodies that neutralize IFN-β activity can be measured precisely and sensitively with a new assay methodology based on *MxA* gene induction in cultured human cells. Antibody-mediated (IgG-mediated) neutralization can be distinguished from other neutralizing activities. The MxA assay was validated against an antiviral assay and is currently being employed to establish the potential clinical relevance of neutralizing antibodies against IFN-β (Betaseron).

Data provided by this assay have confirmed earlier findings that in some MS patients on Betaseron therapy, neutralizing antibodies may develop only transiently. It was also shown that many patients developed Betaseron binding antibodies without ever developing neutralizing antibodies. The total antibody assays (ELISA) can therefore not substitute for activity assays (MxA or antiviral) for the determination or prediction of neutralizing antibodies.

REFERENCES

1. Öberg K, McKenna RM. The incidence and clinical significance of antibodies to interferon alpha. In: Interferon Therapy in Multiple Sclerosis; 1996: 509–521.
2. Ronni T, Melen K, Maygin A, Julkunen I. Control of IFN-inducible MxA gene expression in human cells. J Immunol 1993;150:1715–1726.
3. Simon A, Fah J, Haller O, Staehli P. Interferon regulated Mx-genes are not responsive to interleukin-1, tumor necrosis factor, and other cytokines. J Virol 1990; 65:968–971.
4. Towbin H, Schmitz A, Jakschies D, von Wussow P, Horisberger MA. A whole blood immunoassay for the interferon-inducible human Mx protein. J Interferon Res 1992; 12:67–74.

5. Von Wussow P, Jakschies D, Hochkeppel H-K, Fibich C, Penner L, Deicher H. The human intracellular Mx-homologous protein is specifically induced by type 1 interferons. Eur J Immunol 1990; 20:2015–2019.
6. Files JG, et al. A novel sensitive and selective bioassay for human type 1 interferons. 1996. Submitted.
7. Pungor E et al. Quantitation and characterization of therapy induced neutralizing antibodies against Betaseron®, a recombinant interferon beta. 1996. Submitted.

Index

About the Editor

ANTHONY T. REDER is an Associate Professor in the Department of Neurology, University of Chicago, Illinois. He is the author or coauthor of over 150 book chapters, original papers, and abstracts, and a member of the American Academy of Neurology, the American Association of Immunology, the American Neurological Association, the Society for Experimental Neuropathology, the International Society for Neuroimmunomodulation, and the International Society for Interferon Research, among others. Certified by the American Board of Psychiatry and Neurology, Dr. Reder received the B.S. degree (1974) in psychology and zoology, and the M.D. degree (1978) from the University of Michigan, Ann Arbor.